SIDE EFFECTS OF DRUGS ANNUAL 8 – 1984

Complementary to this volume:

SIDE EFFECTS OF DRUGS ANNUALS 1–7 (1977–1983)
Edited by M.N.G. Dukes

MEYLER'S SIDE EFFECTS OF DRUGS, 9TH EDITION – 1980
MEYLER'S SIDE EFFECTS OF DRUGS, 10TH EDITION – 1984
Edited by M.N.G. Dukes

SIDE EFFECTS OF DRUGS ANNUAL 8

A worldwide yearly survey of new data and trends

EDITOR:

M.N.G. DUKES M.D., M.A., LL.B.

Regional Officer for Pharmaceuticals and Drug Utilization,
The World Health Organization, Copenhagen, Denmark

ASSISTANT EDITOR:

J. ELIS M.D., D.Sc.

State Institute for Drug Control, Prague, Czechoslovakia

1984

ELSEVIER, Amsterdam – New York – Oxford

ISBN 0 444 90339 9
Library of Congress ISSN 78-644057

The representation of facts in this volume, as well as the conclusions and recommendations which are given, represent the medical and scientific judgment of the authors and editors, individually or in consultation. They do not imply the expression of any opinion on the part of the World Health Organization or other institutions with which the authors or editors may be associated. Neither these institutions nor the publisher shall be held responsible for statements made in this volume or any consequences ensuing from such statements.

Published by:
Elsevier Science Publishers B.V.
P.O. Box 1126
1000 BC Amsterdam

Sole distributors for the USA and Canada
Elsevier Science Publishing Co., Inc.
52 Vanderbilt Avenue
New York, NY 10017

Typeset by H Charlesworth & Co., Alphen a/d Rijn
Printed in the Netherlands by Casparie – Amsterdam

How to use this book

THE SCOPE OF THE 'ANNUAL'

Side Effects of Drugs Annual has been published in January of each year since 1977. It is designed to provide a critical and up-to-date account of new information relating to adverse drug reactions and interactions from the clinician's point of view. The Annual can be used independently or as a supplement to the standard encyclopedic work in this field, *Meyler's Side Effects of Drugs*, the ninth edition of which was published in March 1980, and the tenth edition of which will be published in June 1984.

SPECIAL REVIEWS

As new data appear, older findings may be discredited and existing concepts may require revision. Some fifty 'special reviews' deal critically with such topics, interpreting conflicting evidence and providing the reader with clear guidance. Special reviews are identified by the traditional prescription symbol and are printed in italic type. Older papers cited in these reviews are either listed by name or via cross references to previous Annuals or past editions of Meyler's Side Effects of Drugs, which can be found in most medical libraries.

SELECTION OF MATERIAL

In compiling the SED Annual particular attention is devoted to those publications which provide essentially new information or throw a new light on problems already recognized. In addition, some authoritative new reviews are listed. Publications which do not meet these criteria are omitted. Readers anxious to trace all references on a particular topic, including those which duplicate earlier work, are advised to consult *Adverse Reactions Titles*, a monthly bibliography of titles from approximately 3400 biomedical journals published throughout the world, compiled by the international Excerpta Medica abstracting service.

PERIOD COVERED

The present Annual reviews all reports presenting significant new information on adverse reactions to drugs from July 1st 1982 to June 30th 1983. Where possible more recent papers have been included. Subsequent Annuals will similarly cover the world literature appearing yearly between July 1st of one year and June 30th of the next.

CLASSIFICATION

Drugs are classified according to their main field of application or the properties for which they are most generally recognized. In borderline cases, however, some supplementary discussion has been included in other chapters relating to secondary fields of application. Fixed combinations of drugs are dealt with according to their most characteristic component.

DRUG NAMES

Drug products are in general dealt with in the text under their most usual non-proprietary names; where these are not available, chemical names have been used; fixed combinations usually have no non-proprietary connotation and here trade names have been used as necessary.

SYSTEM OF REFERENCES

References in the text are coded as follows:

R: In the original paper, the point is *reviewed* in some detail with reference to other literature.

r: The original paper *refers* only briefly to the point, on the basis of evidence adduced by other writers.

C: The original paper presents detailed *original clinical evidence* on this point.

c: The original paper provides *clinical evidence,* but only briefly.

The code has not been applied to animal pharmacological papers.

The various Editions of *Meyler's Side Effects of Drugs* are cited in the text as SED-8, SED-9, etc.; *SED Annuals 1–7* are cited as SEDA-1, SEDA-2, etc.

INDEXES

Index of Drugs: This index provides a complete listing of all references to a drug.

Index of Side Effects: This index is necessarily selective, since a particular side effect may be caused by very large numbers of compounds; the index is therefore mainly directed to those side effects which are acute or life-threatening or are discussed in special detail. Before assuming that a given drug does not have a particular side effect one should consult the relevant chapters.

The indexes have been compiled by Dr H. Kettner, Middelburg, The Netherlands.

Contributors

S.A. AGOSTON, M.D.
Institute of Clinical Pharmacology
Institute of Clinical Experimental Anesthesiology
State University
Bloemsingel 1
9713 BZ Groningen
The Netherlands

G. ANSELL, M.D., F.R.C.P., F.R.C.R.
Department of Radiology
Whiston Hospital, Prescot
Merseyside L35 5DR
United Kingdom

J.K. ARONSON, D.Phil., M.B., M.R.C.P.
MRC Clinical Pharmacology Unit
University Department of Clinical Pharmacology
Radcliffe Infirmary
Woodstock Road
Oxford OX2 6HE
United Kingdom

A.V. ASTAHOVA, M.D.
All-Union Center on Studying Side Effects of Drugs
Ministry of Health
Per. Rachmanovskij 3
Moscow 1–51
U.S.S.R.

E.A. BABAYAN, M.D.
Chairman, Narcotics Commission
Ministry of Health
Per. Rachmanovskij 3
Moscow 1–51
U.S.S.R.

T.H. BEWLEY, M.D.
Drug Dependence Units
St. Thomas' and Tooting Bec Hospitals
Tooting Bec Road
London SW17 8BL
United Kingdom

B. BLACKWELL, M.D.
University of Wisconsin Medical School
Department of Psychiatry
Mount Sinai Medical Center
950 North 12th Street
Milwaukee, Wisconsin 53201
U.S.A.

R. BOUILLON, M.D.
Laboratory for Experimental Medicine
Catholic University of Leuven
Rega Institute
Minderbroedersstraat 10
3000 Leuven
Belgium

E.J. BUURKE, M.D.
Westeinde Hospital
Lijnbaan 32
2512 VA The Hague
The Netherlands

H. BUURMA, M.Pharm.
Faculty of Pharmacology
State University
Anton Deusinglaan 2
9713 AW Groningen
The Netherlands

A. DANYSZ, Ph.D.
Department of Pharmacology
Institute for Drug Research and Control
Ul. Chelmska 30/34
00–725 Warsaw
Poland

G.A.B. DAVIES-JONES, M.D.
Department of Neurology
Hallamshire Hospital
Glossop Road
Sheffield S10 2JF
United Kingdom

A.C. DE GROOT, M.D.
Department of Dermatology
Willem Alexander Hospital
Deutersestraat 2
5200 MD 's-Hertogenbosch
The Netherlands

A. DEL FAVERO, M.D.
University of Perugia
Institute of Clinical Medicine
06100 Perugia
Italy

J. DESCOTES, M.D.
Laboratory of Pharmacology
Alexis Carrel Faculty of Medicine
Rue Guillaume Paradin
69008 Lyon
France

M.N.G. DUKES, M.D., M.A., LL.B.
Regional Officer for Pharmaceuticals and Drug Utilization
The World Health Organization
Scherfigsvej 8
DK-2100 Copenhagen Ø
Denmark

J. ELIS, M.D., D.Sc.
State Institute for Drug Control
Srobárova 48
100 41 Prague 10
Czechoslovakia

J.Cl. EVREUX, M.D.
Laboratory of Pharmacology
Alexis Carrel Faculty of Medicine
Rue Guillaume Paradin
69008 Lyon
France

Z. FASTNER, M.D.
Municipal Health Department
Korte Vleerstraat 140
2513 VK The Hague
The Netherlands

P.I. FOLB, M.D., F.R.C.P.
Groote Schuur Hospital
University of Cape Town
Medical School
Observatory 7925
South Africa

A.H. GHODSE
Drug Dependence Units
St. George's
St. Thomas' and Tooting Bec Hospitals
Tooting Bec Road
London SW17 8BL
United Kingdom

A.I. GREEN, M.D.
Senior Research Fellow in Psychiatry
Harvard Medical School
Boston, MA 02114
U.S.A.

W. HEYNS, M.D.
Department of Experimental Medicine
Catholic University of Leuven
Rega Institute
Minderbroedersstraat 10
3000 Leuven
Belgium

B. HOFMAN, M.D.
Rosariumlaan 24
3972 GJ Driebergen
formerly at
National Institute of Public Health
Antonie van Leeuwenhoeklaan 9
3721 MA Bilthoven
The Netherlands

J.E. IDÄNPÄÄN-HEIKKILÄ, M.D.
The National Board of Health
Siltasaarenkatu 18A
00530 Helsinki 53
Finland

T.C. JERRAM, B.A., M.B., B.Ch., M.R.C.P., M.R.C. Psych.
High Royds Hospital
Menston
Ilkley
West Yorkshire LS29 6AQ
United Kingdom

H.M.J. KRANS, M.D.
Department of Endocrinology and Metabolic Diseases
University Hospital
Rijnsburgerweg 10
2333 AA Leyden
The Netherlands

M.J.S. LANGMAN, M.D.
Department of Therapeutics
Floor C., South Block
University Hospital
Nottingham NG7 2UH
United Kingdom

H.P. LANSBERG, M.D.
Rembrandtlaan 47
3723 BG Bilthoven
formerly at
National Institute of Public Health
Antonie van Leeuwenhoeklaan 9
3721 MA Bilthoven
The Netherlands

J.R. LAWRENCE, M.D.
Department of Medicine
Dumfries and Galloway Royal Infirmary
Bankend Road
Dumfries DG1 4AP
United Kingdom

P.E. LEBECH, M.D.
Gynaekologisk-Obstetrisk Afdeling
Frederiksberg Hospital
DK-2000 Copenhagen F
Denmark

V.K. LEPÁKHIN, M.D.
Pharmacological Committee
Ministry of Health
Kropotkinskij Pereulok 25/9
Moscow
U.S.S.R.

E.A. LOELIGER, M.D.
Division of Hemostasis and Thrombosis Research
Hematology Section, Department of Medicine
University Hospital
Rijnsburgerweg 10
2333 AA Leyden
The Netherlands

A.S. LOPATIN, M.D.
All-Union Center on Studying Side Effects of Drugs
Ministry of Health
Per. Rachmanovskij 3
Moscow 1–51
U.S.S.R.

R.H.B. MEYBOOM, M.D.
Netherlands Center for Monitoring of Adverse Reactions to Drugs
Ministry of Welfare, Public Health and Culture
P.O. Box 439
2260 AK Leidschendam
The Netherlands

T. MIDTVEDT, M.D.
Institutionen för Medicinsk Mikrobiell Ekologi
Karolinska Institutet
Box 60 400
S-104 01 Stockholm
Sweden

J.P. NATER, M.D.
Department of Dermatology
University Hospital
Oostersingel 59
9713 EZ Groningen
The Netherlands

F.A. NELEMANS, M.D.
Center for Toxicology
Subfaculty for Pharmacy
State University
Vondellaan 14
3521 GE Utrecht
The Netherlands

I. NIR, M.D., Ph.D.
Department of Pharmacology and Experimental Therapeutics
The Hebrew University
Haddassah Medical School
Jerusalem
Israel

O.R. ØDEGAARD, M.D.
Department of Social Medicine
Aker Hospital
Trondheimsvn. 235
Oslo 5
Norway

B. OTTESEN, M.D.
Gynaekologisk-Obstetrisk Afdeling
Frederiksberg Hospital
DK-2000 Copenhagen F
Denmark

A. PIEKARCZYK, M.D.
National Research Institute of Mother and Child
Department of Pharmacology
Kasprzaka 17
01-211 Warsaw
Poland

B.C.P. POLAK, M.D.
Department of Ophthalmology
Erasmus University Eye Hospital
Schiedamse Vest 180
3011 BH Rotterdam
The Netherlands

C. REINICKE, M.D.
Laboratory of Clinical Pharmacology
Department of Internal Medicine
Friedrich Schiller University
Karl-Marx-Allee 101
6902 Jena-Lobeda-East
German Democratic Republic

H.D. REUTER, M.D.
Department of Medicine
University Hospital
Joseph Stelzmannstrasse 9
5 Cologne 41
Federal Republic of Germany

G. REYBROUCK, M.D.
Public Health Laboratory
School of Public Health
Catholic University
Vital Decosterstraat 102
3000 Leuven
Belgium

F.J. RICHARDSON, M.D.
Institute of Anesthesiology
State University
Bloemsingel 1
9713 BZ Groningen
The Netherlands

G.M. RUDENKO, M.D.
Scientific Secretary, Pharmacological Committee
Ministry of Health
Kropotkinskij Pereulok 25/9
Moscow
U.S.S.R.

C. SALZMAN, M.D.
Director of Psychopharmacology
Massachusetts Mental Health Center
74 Fenwood Road
Boston, Mass. 02115
U.S.A.

M. SCHOU, M.D.
The Psychopharmacology Research Unit
Institute of Psychiatry
Aarhus University
Psychiatric Hospital
DK-8240 Risskov
Denmark

J.A. STEINER, M.B., B.S., D.Phil., F.R.A.C.P.
The Royal Free Hospital
Pond Street, Hampstead
London NW3 2QG
United Kingdom

C.B.M. TESTER-DALDERUP, M.D.
Advisor, Netherlands Committee for the Evaluation of Medicines
Workers Compensation Board Alberta Canada
P.O. Box 11291
Edmonton T5J 3K5, Alberta
Canada

J. TUOMISTO, M.D.
Department of Pharmacology
University of Kuopio
Box 138
70101 Kuopio
Finland

F.A. VAN ASSCHE, M.D.
Department of Gynecology
University Hospital St. Rafael
Kapucijnenvoer 33
3000 Leuven
Belgium

C.P.H. VAN DIJKE, M.D.
Netherlands Center for Monitoring of Adverse Reactions to Drugs
Ministry of Welfare, Public Health and Culture
P.O. Box 439
2260 AK Leidschendam
The Netherlands

J. VANĚČEK, M.D., D.Sc.
President, Czechoslovak Society of Pharmacology
Charles University
Albertov 4
128 00 Prague 2
Czechoslovakia

M. VERSTRAETE, M.D.
Department of Medical Research
Catholic University of Leuven
Kapucijnenvoer 35
3000 Leuven
Belgium

A.G. VULTO, M.Pharm.
Rudolf Magnus Institute of Pharmacology
State University Utrecht
Vondellaan 6
3521 AW Utrecht
The Netherlands

B. WÁNKOWICZ, M.Sc.
National Research Institute of Mother and Child
Department of Pharmacology
Kasprzaka 17
01-211 Warsaw
Poland

K. WIERZBA, Ph.D.
National Research Institute for Mother and Child
Department of Pharmacology
Kasprzaka 17
01-211 Warsaw
Poland

J.R.B. WILLIAMS, M.D., F.R.C.Path.
Lister Hospital
Coreys Mill Lane
Stevenage, Herts SG1 4AB
United Kingdom

Contents

SIDE EFFECTS OF DRUGS ESSAY 1984

The seven pillars of foolishness

M.N.G. Dukes

The Editorial 'we', explicit or implied by anonymity, should by now have had its day. Editors, at least as vain as other mortals and probably more so, use and misuse it to impart to their pronouncements the majesty of plurality and the ponderousness of nameless authority. A medical editor may even find it a convenient way of suggesting to his colleagues and readers that he is speaking on their behalf. This, at all events, is not a pluralistic Essay; indeed, you may find it a very singular one. It is mine, and mine alone, and I shall not attempt to suggest that the views which I hold and the disgust which I feel at this moment are shared by anyone but myself. If you want facts about drugs, then set me aside and turn quickly over the next few pages so that you can feast upon the meat of the book without more ado. If, however you are interested in people, well or ill, please have a little patience.

Has it ever struck you that, for some of us who live in the world of drug therapy, a medicine so very easily becomes more important – certainly more central and more tangible – than the hundreds of thousands of people who take it? It has a name, protected by law and patent, whilst its users are but a grey, anonymous, heterogeneous mass. It is fathered by proud men in white coats, who conceived its origins upon laboratory blackboards. It is born in a retort. It is developed and nurtured like any infant to adulthood. It curtsies before the scientific world as might the most select of society *debutantes*, and then, somewhat incongruously, it is often promoted into fame in the medical marketplace in a manner of which a rock star might be envious. The mere patient has no say over the drug; he is ordered to take it by his physician, and if he does as he is bid the doctors pat him on the head and condescendingly call him compliant. If all goes well from the drug's point of view it has its long day of acclaim, bringing its industrial godfathers fame and fortune. If at any time its name and reputation are besmirched, grave advocates will be at hand to defend it. It may be a long time before the glory fades and other medicines take their place before the footlights. And even then, the old drug may be an unconscionable time a-dying.

I do not see any real alternative at present to this process; this is the way that technological society in the west chooses to advance and the way good business apparently must be done. If, in the interests of progress, mankind has to live with image-builders and the ever more subtle machinery of hidden persuasion, applied to a range of goods ranging from video-recorders and benzodiazepines to politicians, then there is not very much mankind can currently do about it. But somewhere limits must surely be set. One such limit must apply when one defines what can reasonably be regarded as progress, in the name of which this whole process is maintained. Not every new molecule which acquires a sales licence can claim to represent a step ahead; many a new drug is merely a step aside, some are quite distinctly a step backwards. How much sales talk can one tolerate for such fruits of pseudo-innovation? It has very often been argued that when a new drug appears in the medical marketplace it is still too early to decide whether or not it represents a useful advance in therapy, and that many a new drug should be given a chance to prove itself in this respect over a period of years before the world passes judgment. So it may be, but did you ever see a drug introduced to physicians like that? 'Dear Doctor', the introductory letter might run, 'we do not really know whether our new product is any better, or safer, or more convenient to use than those which you already have, but we surely hope so. We would also like to earn back some of the money which we have spent on developing it, so that we can go on trying. Will you kindly give it a chance?' Oddly, if medical society had not grown so used to hyperbole, such an honest approach might prove to have some appeal to the prescriber. But nothing of this: the physician is beaten about the ears with the name of the new nostrum, with its supposed advantages, and with pictures which imply what words must not promise; all this goes on until he is so conditioned (compliant, perhaps) that he begins to prescribe it. If the truth be exactly as its founder fathers may have believed at the start, namely that the drug has nothing new to offer, this will in due time become evident; but that will happen only very slowly, for it will be a matter, not merely of confirming or rejecting a calm hypothesis, but of gradually eroding the inflated image of the drug which Madison Avenue advertising has built around it. And if the truth of the matter be that the drug is in fact risky the slowness with which that truth emerges in the face of many triumphal fanfares can mean unnecessary suffering.

Lest anyone think that this is another diatribe against the drug industry and its promotional techniques, let me at once take some other people to task. Where a flicker of a risk seems to be emerging it is not merely the marketing managers who will at first be loathe to admit it. What about the regulators in their ministerial offices? They have only just licensed the drug. If it is indeed problematical, what will parliament be saying about their licensing policies and their technical competence? Then there is the doctor. He has prescribed it and his first few patients appear happy. Is he very anxious to hear that he has been reckless or uncritical? Are his patients willing to have the new remedy, with the hope which it might bring, taken away from them? All these things can delay the admission, even where convincing evidence comes forward, that a hypothesis of risk is anything more than a hypothesis. Once a drug has got onto the market, the dice are heavily loaded in favor of its remaining there, with the reputation originally accorded to it, for a long time.

It has been said often enough but I have to say it again: drug risks are inevitable. Much drug therapy as it exists today is still a lamentably crude means of influencing the workings of a machine as complex as the human body. It may one day be possible to make fine adjustments to physiological balances, and indeed there are a few instruments, such as the hormonal releasers, which render it possible to do so already; all too often however the only drugs available are pharmacotherapeutic blunderbusses which present a known or unknown degree of risk. That being so, one has to be extraordinarily careful about handling them socially and administratively in ways which may raise the measure of risk still further. Loading the dice in the way I have already described increases the risks; so for example does the use of fancy algorithms to test every shred of evidence of a drug's noxiousness before one is prepared to take it seriously. But the risks are raised to a wholly irresponsible degree if one puts the interests of the drug in the middle of the picture and those of the patient at the periphery. Yet that happens, and in some areas it is getting worse rather than better.

People still point to thalidomide as a monumental disaster, *the* monumental disaster, fortunately now a quarter of a century behind us; then they add blissfully that things like that do not happen nowadays. Unhappily they do. Not in exactly the same horrifying way, but in a multitude of others. During the last two years there has been a new epidemic of misery, and one cannot continue to pretend that all is well. The most unhappy aspect of it all has been that things have been made worse than they need have been; much of the misery could have been prevented entirely, much more cut short quickly, had society been awake, and honest, and interested.

Let me recall seven stories. They are seven aspects of the recent history of antirheumatic drug treatment, and since they have been well documented in these volumes and elsewhere I shall not repeat every detail; but I shall attempt to put all seven stories into some perspective. For they stand like seven pillars of foolishness, some taller than others, yet all monuments to human error, greed, vanity, self-interest, gullibility or shortsightedness. Thanks to such things, most of these stories are worse than they need have been.

Benoxaprofen

Benoxaprofen was (or is) an antirheumatic drug which was submitted to various drug regulatory agencies for licencing from about 1979 onwards. It was structurally related to many well-known antirheumatic drugs and most of its effects appeared very similar. There was, however, some qualitative shift as regards the relative importance of the two modes of action often described for these drugs; as compared with its predecessors, benoxaprofen seemed to have a little less effect on prostaglandin synthetase and a little more on leukocyte migration. The hypothesis was raised that this might result in a reduced incidence of those adverse effects – notably gastric bleeding – which seem to be linked to prostaglandin synthetase inhibition. The early clinical studies indeed suggested some practical benefit, but this is quite usual with most antirheumatic drugs of this type – the real gastric problems usually emerge later.

When the real problems emerged with benoxaprofen they were however more serious than with other drugs of its type. Not only was it causing the usual pattern of gastric irritation, but it was also apparently killing old people from hepatic disorders and it was inducing photosensitivity on a massive scale; it was also causing onycholysis in a frequency of anything up to fifteen percent. The brief and destructive career of benoxaprofen ended with its withdrawal in the summer of 1982 from the very few markets in which it had been accepted by regulatory agencies (1).

No party emerges very creditably from this story. The world's regulatory authorities found themselves from the start in disarray, handing down decisions on the original new drug application which ranged from complete rejection to open-armed acceptance. The company which marketed the drug, a highly respected and usually very sober organization, launched it with reckless, hysterical, preposterous advertising; whatever one may think of the words in which it was couched, visually it clearly conveyed the impression that one was dealing with a breakthrough of world-shattering importance. As a result, the drug was prescribed on a massive scale and when the troubles came they came in batallions. It seems probable that at least seventy elderly patients died and a great many more people suffered (2). Yet even then the foolishness was not over. Some regulatory agencies, conveniently forgetting the emphatic recommendation of the World Health Organization that drugs likely to be used in the elderly should be investigated in the elderly at an early stage, sought in retrospect to whitewash their acceptance of the drug despite the almost total lack of such geriatric trials. Company lawyers continued to deny cause and effect, no doubt in the hope of fending off liability proceedings. Even after the drug had been quietly abandoned, a vigorous defence of it was still being put up by gentlemen whose own adverse reaction monitoring systems had failed to detect the harm which was being done; in such cases, no doubt, one's own reputation weighs more heavily than anything else.

Benoxaprofen was a compound which seemed to bear promise of better things to come, and it is sad that it has gone; but the patients who were killed by benoxaprofen, many of them unnecessarily, are dead as well, no amount of whitewash and denial will bring them back to us.

Zomepirac

Like the benoxaprofen drama, that involving zomepirac was limited largely to one country – in this instance the United States. Zomepirac is basically a traditional antiinflammatory analgesic agent. It is extremely closely related to tolmetin which has been sold in some countries for many years as an antirheumatic drug. Tolmetin is a perfectly usable compound, though a little too prone to cause anaphylactoid reactions, and had zomepirac been presented as its twin sister it would no doubt have been used in the same way and treated with the same respect. But the image builders took over; zomepirac was selectively investigated as an analgesic; with its other properties relegated to the small print it took its bow in the advertising columns as heaven's own gift to pain sufferers. This time, the advertising men appear to have had not only the doctors but even the stock market and the regulators in their pockets; when zomepirac turned out to induce anaphylaxis on a scale commensurate with the scale of its promotion, astonishment and dismay were expressed on all sides. The drug was withdrawn in March 1983, and the accusations as to who was responsible for it all are still flying; but at least eight people are dead (2), and to judge from scattered news items rather more. Given a little more caution by everyone involved – need any of them have died at all?

Osmosin

Osmosin was laid to rest by its founder fathers in January 1984 (3); its victims had been laid to rest the previous year. Developed at a time when the patents on indometacin were running out, Osmosin provided it with an elegant but costly kinetic face-lift. Its osmotic tablets released the drug slowly through a semipermeable membrane as they travelled down the gastrointestinal tract, thereby prolonging the duration of activity and perhaps promising to reduce gastric irritation. Even at the time when it was developed, there were murmurings to the effect that in this way gastric problems might merely be shifted to a lower level. As things turned out, this is apparently what happened; the Osmosin tablets seem either to have adhered to the intestinal mucosa, became lodged in diverticula or peppered the gut with potassium which, astonishingly, was used as an excipient. When perforations resulted, the anti-inflammatory effect may well have masked the consequences until it was too late; certainly people who had tolerated plain indometacin well for a long time died when they were needlessly switched to Osmosin. In the drug's own obituary, the company claimed that extensive studies had failed to demonstrate any special risk (3); so they may have done, but that presumably only reflects the inadequacy of the studies. There is a splendid company there in Rahway which has done fine things for medicine and will do fine things again; it should not have its monuments in the churchyards.

Two butazones

The double story of phenylbutazone and oxyphenbutazone is quite a different one. These drugs have been with us for a generation. They arrived at a time when in the field of antirheumatic treatment there was little to choose from, and they found their place. They caused their problems, but the nature of these became known very early; the 1960 edition of Meyler's *Side Effects of Drugs* recorded a series of cases of agranulocytosis as well as a range of other complications and their incidence. Twenty years later, the 'butazones' as they were loosely called, were almost hidden among the throng of newer nonsteroidal antirheumatic agents which now jostled one another in the market place. Nevertheless they had retained something of their early reputation for the treatment of ankylosing spondylitis, though it is not clear whether they really deserved it. Things might have gone on as they were for another generation, with both products falling gently into obscurity, had not, in the summer of 1983, an internal memorandum from Messrs Ciba-Geigy dropped into the hands of Dr Sidney Wolfe of America's Public Citizen action group (4). The memorandum estimated that there had been 1182 deaths due to these drugs worldwide and it not unreasonably raised the question within the company whether it was not time to stop promoting them. Public Citizen called for an immediate ban on both drugs as an 'imminent hazard to public health'. Dr Ole Hansson of Sweden, who appears to be deeply convinced that Ciba-Geigy is incorrigibly wicked in its ways, took up the cry in the Scandinavian newspapers; on December 14th Norway banned both products and throughout the world regulatory agencies sat down to consider whether or not they should follow suit; some seemed very likely at least to make gestures of concern.

From what I have already said it will be clear that my main concern is with patients dying or suffering needless injury; but in the way in which society is now suddenly reacting to Dr Wolfe and Dr Hansson there is something very wrong as well (5). Most of the evidence of the harm which these drugs can do was available two decades ago, largely quantified. If it is true that, because of the arrival of somewhat safer products, one should reevaluate and perhaps discard these old stalwarts, then that could have happened any time from 1970 onwards, certainly by 1975, on the basis of a careful comparison of the benefit-to-risk ratio of all the compounds available. Alas, regulatory agencies do not usually do these things; they are too busy approving new drugs to take a hard look at old ones; when they do so, it all too often happens because people like Dr Wolfe and Dr Hansson have raised the hue and cry. I have a shrewd suspicion that aspirin has killed a multiple of those who are said to be victims of the butazones, and that several other drugs are rather worse than these two; but I have to suspend judgement because I do not have the comparative data available. Unhappily, neither does anyone else; the medical world too has been much too busy testing new antirheumatic drugs to learn much more about the comparative merits of those it already has. Is there not something amiss with our priorities?

Pyrithioxine

Pyrithioxine hydrochloride is what my friend Dr Leo Offerhaus calls a chameleon. It is a vitamin B6 derivative and reputed to be an anabolic for the brain, very good for contusion, behavioral disorders in children and senile dementia (6). Even for these purposes it is sold under thirty of the most musical names with which a drug was ever blessed, including Cerebrotrofina, Musa, Gladius, Scintidin, Tonomentis and Life. Small wonder that when it suddenly surfaced in France, chameleon-like, as an antirheumatic agent physicians had no idea what it was and compliantly prescribed it. When it began to cause rashes and stomatitis did one in a thousand physicians know of its structural link – the dithio group – to penicillamine, with which some of these rheumatic patients must have been treated earlier? Had they known, they might have prescribed it more critically. Some elderly rheumatic patients were indeed already receiving the same compound under another connotation for their ailing medical state. But do you know what the physician who asked about the chemical nature of this new antirheumatic drug was told? He was solemnly informed that it was 3,3′-dithiodimethylenebis(5-hydroxy-6-methyl-4-pyridylmethanol)dihydrochloride monohydrate. Mercy be with us – will doctors never insist on having generic names and some intelligible indication of what they are really dealing with before they write a prescription?

Oxametacin

Space is at a premium, and I must be brief. Oxametacin, by all accounts, is a miracle, for the clinical papers which I have seen conclude that it is the equivalent of indometacin without its side effects (7). I am nevertheless also assured that it has been discussed around certain regulatory tables and gave rise there to some amusement. Privately, all I can conclude is that the published material is not all of a standard which I would like to see, that the drug is metabolized in part as indometacin, and that the patients without side effects did not receive an effective dose. If better work proves the contrary, I shall be delighted to be corrected; so far, I am forced to believe that this is not the way to help rheumatic patients to avoid adverse reactions. This gem, should you require it, is to be found in the pharmacies of Italy; you will be hard put to it to find it in most other places.

Seven stories and many morals

The chain of stories could continue; the particular nastinesses or oddities associated with indoprofen, ibufenac, aclofenac, mefenamic acid, acemetacin, fenclofenac and glafenine are much in the same vein. For the present purpose, these seven tales must suffice. Not all of them had a tragic ending, but all of them illustrate some of the absurdities in the way in which the community has behaved and continues to behave when it deals with drug safety. Even from the purely scientific and epidemiological point of view it is difficult enough to come by reliable information on adverse reactions, and to spot it sufficiently early to prevent much injury being caused. Yet, even as the facts begin to emerge, any attempt to interpret and objectify them may be bedevilled by the machinations of people who have their own interests to defend and their own axes to grind. It is entirely proper that the truth about side effects and benefit-risk ratios should emerge from a weighing of a mass of conflicting evidence, but the process is immeasurably complicated and delayed where costly reputations and much money are at stake. Doctors, companies, regulatory agencies, politicians, consumers and nowadays even stockbrokers (yes, *stockbrokers*!) all throw up their own particular smokescreens when suspicions of major adverse reactions are discussed; all that one can do, and must do, is to set aside most of the commentary and interpretation that is cast around on such a vexed issue, go back to the patients who are at the centre of the problem and verify the facts. For let me say it once again; it is only the patient who matters. For him or her a serious side effect is of course not a side effect at all; it is a very central effect indeed, perhaps one of life and death.

These problems can arise in every field of drug therapy, but it is today tragically easy to identify them in the field of antirheumatic treatment. For two decades most nations have in good faith accepted the argument that every nonsteroidal antiinflammatory drug which shows promise must be given a chance, since it may contribute something to therapeutic progress. As a result, the financially profitable field of antirheumatic drug therapy has in many countries become a fairground, the noise in which is utterly confusing to pharmacologists, physicians and patients alike (8). No one particular segment of the community is really to blame; society has created a situation in which everyone is under pressure to behave in a particular way; if I had a good new antirheumatic drug to sell I too would be obliged to sell it with trumpets and bells, however distasteful I might find it, since otherwise no-one would notice. It is clear that too much injury is being caused by drugs in this field; the proportion of drugs which come, kill and go is too high, and amid all the clamour it is now impossible for the doctor to decide which risks are worth taking in his patient's interest.

Should one not, to begin with, look very carefully at the comparative merits of all the antirheumatic drugs currently known, sponsoring impartial research where necessary to find the data needed to prune the market and update the textbooks? If no-one else will do it, the drug regulatory agencies of the world, which are very slowly closing their ranks, might share out the task, if possible in collaboration with the pharmaceutical industry. It has to be done. As recently as January 1984 one could find statements in the medical literature to the effect that aspirin, after three generations, was still the drug of choice in rheumatoid arthritis (9). That may not always be true, but the fact that in 1984 it can still be said with some authority and backed by substantial evidence surely makes one wonder whether society has been using its resources optimally to find better and safer antirheumatic medicines. The fact alone that the number of nonsteroidal antiinflammatory drugs licensed for sale in various European countries varies sevenfold (10) reflects the uncertainty as to how the situation should now be handled.

Again, I think the medical profession should be taking a hard look at the way in which new antirheumatic drugs are currently sold to it, and the consequences which that has for everyone. More restrained promotion could be more informative and a great deal less wasteful. If only a fraction of the money currently being spent, at the community's expense, on breathless four-colour advertisements and double teams of detailmen were to be diverted into basic research in the better industrial laboratories society might be on the way to developing the truly new and truly safer antirheumatic drugs which patients need. Whether one believes that industry can regulate itself into a more balanced situation, or whether one expects governments to impose a solution will depend on one's own private philosophies, but I know it must happen if there are not going to be a series of other pillars of foolishness lining our way through the 'eighties'. Accidents will still happen, patients will still be injured and killed by the unforeseen and unforeseeable, but people will hopefully no longer die merely because society has been as hesitant to admit the risks as is currently the case.

There is an unhappy turn of phrase currently going around medical meetings which refers to patients as 'the people out there...' Perhaps that is merely symptomatic of the wrongheadedness which besets the world of drug experts. The patients are indeed out there, and the drugs are in here with us, being coddled in the warmth. It may be the destiny of the clinical pharmacologists to bring drug policies and policy makers back where they belong, at the bedside and in the consulting room, with the patient – every patient – at the heart of things, whilst the chemists, the stockbrokers, the image makers and the detailmen wait, cap in hand, at the door for judgement to be pronounced.

Copenhagen, January 1984

SELECTED REFERENCES

1. Anon (1982) Lilly suspends benoxaprofen worldwide. *Scrip, 717,* 1.
2. Offerhaus L (1983) Non-steroidal anti-inflammatory drugs in the treatment of rheumatic disorders: pitfalls and problems with the present plethora. *Neth. J. Med., 26,* 173.
3. Anon (1983) Osmosin not to return to market. *Scrip, 864,* 17.
4. Wolfe SM (1983) *Letter from Health Research Group* to Margaret Heckler, Department of Health and Human Services. Washington, December 28th.
5. Borchgrevink CF (1984) Tanker ved avregistrering av to medikamenter. *Tidskr. Norsk. Laegeforen., 104,* 255.
6. *Martindale: The Extra Pharmacopoeia, 28th Ed.,* London 1982, 1750.
7. Polderman J and Colin M (1979) Oxamethacin: a pilot field survey. *J. Int. Med. Res., 7,* 83.
8. Hvidberg E (1981) Hvad skal vi dog gøre ved de mange nye antireumatika? *Ugeskr. Laeg., 143,* 1040.
9. Hadler NM (1984) The argument for aspirin as the NSAID of choice in the management of rheumatoid arthritis. *Drug Intell. Clin. Pharm., 18,* 34.
10. Dukes MNG and Lunde I (1981) The regulatory control of non-steroidal anti-inflammatory agents. *Eur. J. Clin. Pharmacol., 19,* 3.

E.A. Babayan, A.V. Astahova, V.K. Lepakhin and A.S. Lopatin

1 Central nervous system stimulants and anorectic agents

CNS STIMULANTS

GENERAL

One of the principal and most serious side effects of certain CNS stimulants is their influence on mental status, mood and behavior, opening a door to abuse of these drugs and to narcomania. This represents a complex medical, social and legal challenge. For this reason, several CNS stimulants have been scheduled under the Convention on Psychotropic Substances and their use has in consequence been banned or restricted in a number of countries.

From the international legal point of view, the stimulants thus fall into two groups; the first comprises those which are subject to special national and international controls and the second those which are not subject to such special controls. In view, however, of the nature and mode of action of stimulants and their effects on the CNS, even the latter group must be regarded with caution since any of them may become the object of addiction and misuse in particular situations. Restrictive legislation has promoted the more cautious use of stimulant drugs in medical practice, but the continuing availability of various non-prescription stimulants in some countries for a variety of indications still provides a potential for abuse and for drug-induced morbidity and mortality.

Side Effects of Drugs Annual 8
M.N.G. Dukes, editor

ISBN 0 444 90339 9
$0.80 per article per page (transactional system)
$0.20 per article per page (licensing system)

USE, ABUSE AND MISUSE OF NON-PRESCRIPTION STIMULANTS

In recent years there has in some countries been a trend to an increase in the use and misuse of various non-prescription stimulants. The US National Clearing House for Poison Control Centers recently reported that the incidence of improper exposure to phenylpropanolamine products increased from 0.1% of all drug mentions in 1975 to 0.9% in 1980 (1^{C}).

Sawyer et al (2^{CR}) draw attention to the fact that many different non-prescription tablets and capsules are still widely distributed as safe and powerful stimulants, also being available through mail-order houses and in shops selling 'drug paraphernalia' throughout the United States; these same formulations are also being passed on the street as 'speed'. All contain (singly or in combination) the same basic active ingredients: phenylpropanolamine 25–30 mg, caffeine 100–200 mg, and ephedrine 25 mg.

These authors have reviewed the symptomatology and management of toxicity caused by non-prescription stimulants. They note that generally, toxic reactions involve excessive CNS stimulation (e.g. increased motor activity, anxiety, and agitation) and mildly elevated pulse rate and blood pressure that resolve in 6 to 8 hours without specific treatment. However, reactions following the ingestion of these stimulants have included severe hypertension, possible renal failure, cerebral hemorrhage, and cardiac arrhythmias.

Sawyer et al summarized 11 reports in the literature of toxicity following the ingestion of either phenylpropanolamine, ephedrine, or a combination of phenylpropanolamine and caffeine. The following

3 case reports illustrate important aspects in the symptomatology and management of such severe reactions associated with misuse of legally available stimulants.

A teenage girl developed fatal intracerebral bleeding following the ingestion of an unknown quantity of capsules containing phenylpropanolamine 50 mg, caffeine 100 mg, and ephedrine 25 mg. Cause-effect relationships were not proven; contents of ingested capsules were not analyzed.

A young man had symptomatic bradycardia following a suicide attempt with 10–15 capsules. Each capsule contained phenylpropanolamine 50 mg and caffeine 200 mg. His heart rate increased to more than 50 beats per min following the i.v. administration of atropine sulfate 0.4 mg. As his heart rate increased, his blood pressure increased to 190/120 mm Hg. Phentolamine 5 mg i.v. was administered, and there was a sustained decrease in blood pressure.

A 32-year-old man developed orthostatic hypotension accompanied by a blood pressure increase to 190/120 mm Hg (supine) approximately 1 hour after ingestion of 2 capsules containing phenylpropanolamine 50 mg and caffeine 200 mg. His symptoms resolved over 4 hours with no treatment.

Although patients generally have self-limiting symptoms following the ingestion of non-prescription stimulants, hypertensive crises with resultant end-organ damage may develop in susceptible individuals. Following phenylpropanolamine ingestion bradycardia has been observed, as opposed to tachyarrhythmias, which are also commonly seen.

Treatment

The authors' recommendations for treatment of patients who have taken an overdose are as follows:

General management

1. Establish respiration.
   Create artificial airway if necessary.
   Check adequacy of tidal volume.
2. Emesis should be initiated unless the patient is comatose, convulsing, or has lost the gag reflex. If any of these contraindications are present, endotracheal intubation should precede gastric lavage with a large-bore tube.
3. Administer activated charcoal (adults 60–100 g; children 30–60 g).
4. Administer cathartic. Magnesium sulfate (adults 30 g; children 250 mg/kg).
5. Monitor ECG and blood pressure.
6. Urinary output should be monitored and fluid replaced as appropriate.

Suggested management of specific complications:

1. Agitation, disorientation, increased motor activity, hallucinations, and tachypnea – supportive.
2. Seizures – treat seizures with i.v. diazepam (adults: up to 10 mg slowly, repeated if necessary; children: 0.1–0.3 mg/kg slowly).
3. *Arrhythmias*
   a. Bradycardia: atropine sulfate (adults: 0.4 mg i.v., repeat every 5 min, maximum 2 mg; children: 0.01 mg/kg i.v., not to exceed 0.4 mg).
   b. Frequent premature ventricular contractions or ventricular tachycardia: lidocaine (1 mg/kg i.v. bolus, repeat 0.5 mg/kg bolus if necessary and follow with 20–40 mg/kg/min infusion). If no response from lidocaine administration administer propranolol (adults: 0.025–0.10 mg/kg i.v. slowly over 2–3 min; children: do not exceed 2 mg with initial dose).
4. *Hypertension*
   a. Mild to moderate elevation in blood pressure – observation.
   b. Hypertensive crisis: nitroprusside (initiate 1 mg/kg/min i.v. infusion and adjust to control blood pressure, dose average 3 mg/kg/min) or phentolamine (adults: 2.5–5.0 mg i.v., repeat every 5 min until hypertension controlled, then 2–4 hr p.r.n.; children: 0.05–0.1 mg/kg dose, repeat every 5 min until hypertension controlled, then 1–4 hr p.r.n.).

In conclusion the authors emphasize that the easy availability of different non-prescription stimulants creates a potential for drug-induced morbidity and mortality. They believe that more intensive efforts to restrain the manufacture of these products and to remove the latter from the US market should be strongly encouraged.

Serious concern as to the increasing abuse of over-the-counter preparations containing combinations of phenylpropanolamine, ephedrine, and caffeine has been expressed by Weesner et al (3^C). The authors describe their experience with an adolescent who presented with complex cardiac arrhythmias, including ventricular tachycardia, following ingestion of such a combination.

The patient, a 14-year-old white female, ingested 15 to 18 capsules called RJ 8 (ephedrine 25 mg, caffeine 200 mg, phenylpropanolamine 50 mg) in a suicide gesture. Approximately 1.5 hr after the ingestion she complained of blurred vision, nervousness, tremor, and inability to walk. She was taken to a local hospital where she was given ipecac and activated charcoal. On admission her blood pressure was 104/62 mm Hg, with a heart rate of 180 beats/min and frequent aberrant beats and premature atrial contractions as well as short periods of ventricular tachycardia. The remainder of the physical examination was unremarkable. Because of the serious nature of the arrhythmias, lidocaine therapy (50 mg/kg i.v. bolus, followed by a constant infusion of 20 mg/kg/min) was instituted. This treatment did not alter the appearance of the arrhythmias. The patient was subsequently hospitalized for further treatment.

Upon arrival the patient remained alert and responsive but complained of palpitations, nervousness, and blurred vision. Examination revealed a pulse of 140 beats/min which was irregular, a blood pressure of 135/68 mm Hg, pupils that were 3 mm equal and reacted slowly to light, and generalized hyperreflexia. The lidocaine infusion was continued for 15 min after admission. Continuous ECG monitoring was remarkable for numerous ventricular premature contractions. Due to the lack of response to lidocaine, the patient received 1 mg propranolol as an intravenous infusion over 3 min, during which the heart rate converted to a normal sinus rhythm at a rate of 86 beats per min. The lidocaine infusion was discontinued, and the patient's recovery was uneventful with oral administration of propranolol without further arrhythmias.

Three cases of toxic reactions following relatively small doses of phenylpropanolamine are presented by Bernstein et al (4[CR]).

One patient had a hypertensive crisis and seizures after taking two Comtrex tablets for 'congestion'; the others had intracerebral hemorhages culminating in death after ingestion of two 'pick me up' capsules containing phenylpropanolamine 50 mg, caffeine 200 mg, and ephedrine 25 mg.

The second and third cases are dramatic examples of the effects of phenylpronanolamine in combination with caffeine and ephedrine. Severe hypertensive reactions have been reported when phenylpropanolamine was used concomitantly with monoamine oxidase inhibitors, foods containing tyramine, anti-hypertensive drugs such as methyldopa and oxprenolal, and indomethacin. But never before has death been reported resulting from intracerebral bleeding associated with the combination with ephedrine and caffeine. The combination and synergistic effect these drugs represent is a new problem arising from the attempt to find a substitute stimulant for the discredited amphetamine preparations. These 'look-alike' drugs contain as much as 50 mg phenylpropanolamine and 25 mg ephedrine, and because they usually do not give the user a high equivalent to amphetamine, the user seems more likely to take several pills at a time. Because phenylpropanolamine and ephedrine have a much more pronounced peripheral effect than do the amphetamines, the hypertensive reactions from these stimulants are, in the view of Bernstein et al, much greater.

Finally one must move to Australia, which has been a prominent source of reports on adverse reactions to phenylpropanolamine, particularly relating to the occurrence of cardiovascular complications following its (entirely legal) use as an 'over-the-counter' appetite suppressant drug. McEwen, Secretary of the Australian Drug Reactions Advisory Committee, has very recently presented reports on 8 apparently normotensive Australian women who developed hypertension after taking appetite-suppressant preparations which contained high doses of phenylpropanolamine (80[CR]). In Australia some such preparations at one time contained up to 85 mg phenylpropanolamine; later this was reduced to 50 mg. The dose actually taken by the 8 women in question ranged from 60 to 170 mg. Headache and nausea were the most usual symptoms; all 8 patients recovered.

It is notable that in the same issue of the Medical Journal of Australia, an editorial by Frewin (81[R]) reminds the reader that reports of hypertension with this drug have often been disputed; it raises at the same time the intriguing question as to the perhaps better availability of the phenylpropranolamine products marketed in Australia, which could explain the relatively large number of reports of complications emanating from that country. By and large, however, it does appear that there is an increasing weight of medical opinion that such high doses of phenylpropanolamine should not be available over the counter, either as decongestants or as anorectics.

MISUSE OF NASAL INHALERS

The history, epidemiology, and medical complications of nasal inhaler abuse have been reviewed by Anderson et al (5[R]). The first report on the oral use of the volatile amphetamine base from a nasal inhaler by entertainers appeared in 1946. In 1947 Monroe and Drell (6[C]) reported that 25% of an inmate population in a United States disciplinary barracks at Fort Benjamin Harrison, Indiana, used inhaler material for intoxicating purposes. Fourteen percent of this inmate population had abused the inhaler material prior to incarceration. In the mid-fifties, localized epidemics of intravenous injections of amphetamine inhaler contents were reported to the FDA.

The FDA took a decisive step in 1959 by invoking Section 503(b) of the Durham-Humphrey Amendment (of 1951) to the

Food, Drug and Cosmetic Act to cover the amphetamine inhaler because 'recurring reports of abuse and misuse indicate the potentiality for harmful effect' ([7C]). The amendment states: 'Because of toxicity or *other potentiality for harmful effect* or the method of its use, or the collateral measures necessary to its use', a drug may be considered safe for use only under the supervision of a physician. So ended the legal, over-the-counter sale of amphetamines in nasal inhalers. It was assumed that the misapplication of nasal inhalers was over.

To replace amphetamine inhalers a nasal inhaler was developed based on propylhexedrine which appeared to have minimal effects on the CNS. In 1972, however, Marsden and Sheldon ([8C]) reported an adult case of propylhexedrine poisoning complicated by myocardial infarction, shock, adult respiratory distress syndrome, thrombocytopenia, and gastrointestinal bleeding. Once again, the product had been misused and taken orally. By the early seventies, reports began to appear which described propylhexedrine-induced psychosis, similar to the schizophreniform psychosis induced by amphetamine. Some of the patients involved had previously been habituated to methamphetamine and during heavy use had been admitted to psychiatric hospitals for paranoid schizophrenia. Their habitual intake ranged from 2 to 11 inhalers, chewed or swallowed daily.

Between 1973 and 1979, 15 propylhexedrine-related deaths were reported from Dallas County (Texas) ([9C], [10C], [11C], [12C]). Twelve resulted directly from acute propylhexedrine intoxication, superimposed on chronic abuse. Two deaths represent homicides and one a suicide which occurred as part of an acute drug-induced psychosis. The method of administration was intravenous in each situation, but at least one victim also 'skin popped'. These deaths were sudden, often precipitated by a 'flight or fight' provocation. Unlike sudden death with intravenous heroin or cocaine, the victims often died many hours after injection. The postmortem findings of these victims revealed pulmonary granulomas in 9, intimal and medial proliferation of pulmonary arterioles in 8 and right ventricular hypertrophy in 9 of the victims. In all 12 victims dying of propylhexedrine intoxication, pulmonary edema was evident postmortem. The range of blood concentrations for propylhexedrine was 0.3 to 2.27 mg/l (mean 0.16 mg/dl) but this is somewhat skewed with lower values from victims surviving 8 to 12 hr before toxicology studies were obtained.

The mechanisms responsible for sudden death in these victims were not clear. Whatever the etiology, it was evident from the clinical picture of victims surviving to reach medical care that intravenous abuse of propylhexedrine could result in collapse, refractory shock, cardiac arrhythmias, and sudden death.

The authors urge that the possibility of propylhexedrine abuse be borne in mind in sudden death syndromes with evidence of intravenous drug abuse, and toxicological investigations should include screening for propylhexedrine when tests for other etiologic agents are negative. Propylhexedrine can be detected and quantitated in blood and tissue by gas chromatography after extraction by n-butyl chloride, using the procedure described by Foerster et al ([13C]).

The continuous search by the polydrug abuser for previously unrecognized sources of gratification may have led to the misapplication of the propylhexedrine nasal inhaler like its predecessor, amphetamine. The legal accessibility and the inexpensive nature of the instrument make the growth potential for abuse great. Propylhexedrine abuse is now endemic, but, as with an infectious disease, it may become epidemic unless preventive measures are taken.

Liggett ([14C]) describes a man who presented with agitation, tremor, sweating, hypertension, and tachycardia due to the deliberate ingestion of propylhexedrine as a substitute for amphetamine abuse.

A 29-year-old man had soaked the fibrous interior of a propylhexedrine nasal inhaler (Benzedrex, containing 250 mg of propylhexedrine) in a cup of hot tap water for 10 min and had drunk the mixture, which he described as greasy and bad tasting. About 30 min after ingestion, he became nauseated and restless, and after an hour he had hand tremors and extreme agitation. The euphoria he usually experienced from amphetamines was absent and instead he felt anxious and 'uneasy'. Physical examination 2 hours after ingestion revealed a talkative, restless man with coarse hand tremors and sweating of the face and hands. Oral temperature was 100.4°F (38°C), respiration 20/min and regular, pulse 100/min, and blood pressure 170/190 mm Hg. The pupils were not dilated and reacted normally to light. The hand tremors were rapid, coarse, irregular and of the postural type. Cardiac auscultation revealed a regular rate and rhythm. The deep tendon reflexes were 3 bilaterally; no pathologic reflexes elicitated. He showed no signs of psychosis or paranoia.

The patient was placed in a quiet, darkened examining room. His blood pressure 30 min later was 140/80 mm Hg and gradually decreased to 125/70, with a pulse of 70/min. The hand tremors subsided after 2 hours and he stated that he felt much better and was without nausea.

Some abusers, as already pointed out, use propylhexedrine intravenously; the nasal inhaler is disassembled, and the enclosed cotton plug, which contains 250 mg of drug, is soaked in water. Croft et al (15[C]) describe 4 chronic abusers of intravenous propylhexedrine who had severe left ventricular dysfunction most consistent with a congestive cardiomyopathy.

Between September 1978 and February 1982, 4 men who were chronic abusers of intravenous propylhexedrine were hospitalized with symptoms, signs, and radiographic evidence of severe left ventricular failure. The patients ranged in age from 26 to 36 years. Three patients showed echocardiographic evidence of right ventricular dilatation, and all 4 had left ventricular dilatation. At catheterization, the average forward cardiac index was 1.8 $l/min \cdot m^2$ body surface area, and all patients had markedly increased left ventricular end-diastolic and end-systolic volume indices, greatly depressed left ventricular ejection fractions, and severe global hypokinesis. Three patients had mild mitral regurgitation (presumably secondary to left ventricular dilatation), and one had mild aortic regurgitation. Two patients had moderate pulmonary hypertension, and in 3 patients there was a substantial difference between the pulmonary arterial diastolic pressure and the pulmonary capillary wedge pressure. Selective coronary arteriography showed normal coronary arteries in 2 patients; arteriography was not done in the other 2. In all patients serologic testing failed to show evidence of a recent viral infection. One patient was evaluated 14 months after the initial study, at which time he claimed to have curtailed his intravenous drug abuse. His symptoms had improved, and his left ventricular ejection fraction was 0.35 (increased from 0.12 at the initial study). The other 3 patients were lost to follow-up.

The authors suggest that cardiomyopathy could result from the sympathomimetic properties of propylhexedrine.

DYSTONIA DUE TO DECONGESTANTS

Dystonic reactions may rarely result from unrecognized long-term use of decongestants. Powers (16[C]) describes a 34-year-old man who had blepharospasm and orofacial dystonia of 3 months' duration. Despite his age, the patient was thought to have an idiopathic oral-facial dyskinesia consistent with Meige's disease. Habitual use of a decongestant spray several times daily for 10 years because of chronic nasal congestion was eventually acknowledged, and the dyskinesia decreased substantially when use was discontinued. The decongestant was a combination of 0.2% pheniramine maleate, 0.5% phenylephrine hydrochloride, and benzalkonium chloride. Long-term use of decongestants may affect central dopaminergic and cholinergic receptors. The full consequences of these effects are not known, but include a risk for development of chronic dyskinesia. The author proposes that persons with blepharospasm or orofacial dystonia be questioned specially about use of decongestants.

AMPHETAMINE ABUSE

Cerebrovascular complications of amphetamine abuse were described earlier in the Annuals (SEDA-6, 12).

Eriksson and Wibell (17[C]) have now reported a fatal case of *hemorrhagic cerebral infarction* associated with amphetamine abuse. This case illustrates a possible important pathophysiological mechanism for cerebrovascular damage. The authors conclude that a cerebrovascular event following amphetamine abuse, whether comprising an infarction or a hemorrhage is unlikely to have been caused directly by the drug; damage to the vessels or vascular spasm is likely to have been present.

The first report of *cerebral vasculitis* associated with oral dextroamphetamine overdose and followed by multiple CNS complications has been presented by Matick et al (18[CR]).

A 25-year-old man, a known abuser of amphetamines, was admitted in a semi-comatose state. He had ingested 50 dextroamphetamine sulfate tablets with the previous 24 hours. His blood pressure was 240/100 mm Hg. He rapidly became tachycardic and had a generalized seizure. Therapy was started with phenytoin sodium, phenobarbital sodium, and dexamethasone phosphate for cerebral edema.

The next day a 4-vessel cerebral angiogram revealed a 2 mm fusiform aneurysm of the left anterior temporal branch of the middle cerebral artery. There were multiple areas of luminal irregularity throughout the supratentorial circulation suggestive of a vasculopathy. A lumbar puncture yielded hemorrhagic non-clotting CSF, with 1,200 RBCs, a protein level of 70 mg/dl, no WBCs and a glucose level of 60 mg/dl. He remained obtunded.

A second computed tomographic scan was performed 4 days later. It showed a diffuse increase in density about the tentorium, suggesting a recent subarachnoid hemorrhage.

These authors suggested that, because of amphetamine abuse, a vasculitis was produced over time, which led in turn to aneurysm formation and then to subarachnoid bleeding. In the setting of amphetamine abuse and cerebrovascular deficits, CNS vasculitis should be sought for and diagnosed after infectious vasculitis or other causes have been ruled out.

The vascular changes associated with amphetamine abuse may produce deficits that may be chronic. Treatment consists of withdrawing the offending agent, treating concomitant infections and administering steroids.

Cerebral abscess as a fairly rare complication of amphetamine abuse is reported by Shibahashi et al (19[C]).

A 37-year-old man, who had been an amphetamine addict for 4 years was hospitalized under suspicion of a brain tumor. Neurological examination revealed somnolence, left homonymous hemianopsia, bilateral choked disks, mydriasis and sluggish response to light on the right, and left hemiparesis. CT scan showed a low density area with a markedly enhanced ring-blush in the right occipital lobe. Angiography showed an avascular area with a halo formation in the venous phase. A brain abscess was diagnosed and an emergent operation was performed. 50 ml of yellowish pus was aspirated through a right occipital craniotomy and the abscess totally extirpated. *Staphylococcus aureus* grew from the pus.

The possibility of brain abscess should be kept in mind when an addict shows focal neurological signs, or the signs of increased intracranial pressure. CT with contrast enhancement is the most useful diagnostic tool in such cases.

Call et al (20[C]) described a case of a woman who developed *acute cardiomyopathy* with myocardial dysfunction and pulmonary edema immediately after intravenous amphetamine abuse. Serious heart and lung complications from i.v. drug abuse have been well documented earlier, but most notably have involved either bacterial endocarditis or noncardiac pulmonary edema, the latter especially after i.v. use of heroin. However, i.v. drug abuse causing acute cardiomyopathy with left ventricular dysfunction has not been clearly demonstrated before.

Scandling and Spital (21[CR]) have added to the literature the case of a man who had a crush injury and myoglobinuric renal failure after oral ingestion of 50 amphetamine sulfate tablets in a suicidal gesture. There has been no previously documented case of *rhabdomyolysis due to a crush syndrome* after oral amphetamine ingestion in the absence of other serious complicating features. The authors suggest that patients abusing amphetamine should be observed for signs of muscle injury even in the absence of other myotoxic factors. Furthermore, myoglobinuric renal failure may result.

Paranoid psychosis may result from intoxication with or withdrawal from amphetamines. Deveaugh-Geiss and Pandurangi (22[C]) described 2 patients who were withdrawn from sympathomimetic amines, resulting in their having a confusional paranoid psychosis. In view of the widespread use of sympathomimetic drugs, one has to be aware not only of the depressive symptoms associated with withdrawal but also of the possibility of precipitating psychosis.

Djenderedjian and Tashjian (23[C]) reported for the first time in the literature a syndrome of *agoraphobia* precipitated by amphetamine abuse and withdrawal.

A 32-year-old woman was admitted to the hospital complaining of fears of leaving her house alone for the last 2 years. She had given up her job and was not able to go shopping or visiting. Her condition followed the sudden cessation of amphetamine abuse when she went through a psychotic withdrawal period at home, with visual hallucinations and paranoid ideations persisting for one week. One week following this experience, she became anergic and depressed. She developed anxiety symptoms with hyperventilation and hypochondria and remained housebound.

At the mental health center a trial course of imipramine 200 mg/day was given for 5 weeks with no improvement in her condition. After a drug-free period of 2 weeks, phenelzine 15 mg t.i.d. was instituted with diet instruction. After 2 weeks, she was able to leave her house alone and she reported improvement in her depressive, anxiety and phobic symptoms. One year follow-up revealed further improvement in the patient's condition with complete recovery from agoraphobia and depressive features. During this treatment period she had a relapse of her agoraphobia due to a temporary discontinuation of the phenelzine for dental work. One week following its resumption she was symptom-free once again and has been productive socially since.

MISUSE OF INDIVIDUAL DRUGS

Pseudoephedrine

Rosen (24[C]) reported a case of *angina* in an otherwise healthy woman associated with the ingestion of the oral pseudoephedrine-containing product Actifed.

Intracranial hemorrhage in association with pseudoephedrine overdose has been described by Loizou et al (25[C]).

A 17-year-old girl who had made an attempt at self-poisoning 12 months previously, but was not a drug abuser, was admitted 4 hours after ingesting 20 tablets containing pseudoephedrine hydrochloride 60 mg. She was slightly disoriented with a blood pressure of 120/70 mm Hg, and a pulse of 84/min, with sinus rhythm. Over the next 24 hours she developed headache, drowsiness, and a right hemiparesis with sensory deficit; blood pressure remained normal. Examination of the CSF on the 4th day of admission showed blood stained xanthochromic fluid under raised pressure. CT scan showed a hematoma in the left frontal area, and a small lucency in the head of the right caudate nucleus. Bilateral carotic angiograms on the 7th day of the illness confirmed the presence of an avascular space-occupying lesion in the left frontal region and, in addition, revealed widespread segmental narrowing of the major and smaller branches of the intracranial carotid arteries. She was managed conservatively and recovered rapidly. Six months later she was normal, and repeat CT scan showed resolution of the hematoma with a small residual cavity.

Pseudoephedrine has only rarely produced neurological complications, because it is a very weak sympathomimetic amine which has not achieved status as a drug of abuse or addiction. The present case, however, serves to illustrate its potential dangers.

Methylphenidate (Ritalin, Centedrin)

Drug abuse Haglund and Howerton (26[CR]) studied the use of methylphenidate among clients of drug abuse treatment programs. A consecutive series of admissions (N = 192) was examined for possible use of Ritalin during outpatient treatment for opiate dependency. It was found that the majority of patients were also addicted to Ritalin. Common adverse reactions in subjects using both Ritalin and opiates were as shown in Table 1.

Chillar et al (27[C]) reported two more cases of *hemiplegia* after accidental intracarotid injection of methylphenidate in addicts attempting to inject methylphenidate into the neck veins.

These authors have observed that the superficial veins seem rapidly to become sclerotic with methylphenidate abuse, increasing the risk of intracarotid drug injection.

Table 1. *Major symptoms*

	No.	%
Paranoid, other disturbances	12	(17)
Sweating, chills	13	(18)
Elevated heartbeat, breathing	15	(21)
Stomach irritation	5	(7)
Weak/run down	4	(6)
Abscess/rash	8	(11)
Sleep disturbance	7	(9)
Other symptoms	8	(11)

COMPLICATIONS OF STIMULANT THERAPY FOR ADD

Cowart (28[R]) has reviewed problems due to stimulant therapy for attention-deficit disorders (ADD) in children. Methylphenidate and dextroamphetamine are the two drugs most often prescribed for ADD and appear to favorably influence both attention and physical activity. Children on stimulants for these purposes do not become euphoric or 'high', nor does taking stimulant drugs for ADD appear to make a person more likely to become a drug abuser in later life.

Adverse reactions reported with the use of stimulant drugs in children include *suppression of height and weight development*, and appearance of *tics*. Since growth improvement occurs on an irregular basis careful monitoring of the growth pattern of a particular child receiving stimulants is sufficient. If a tic develops, stimulants should be withdrawn.

Lowe et al (29[CR]) have described 15 cases of *Gilles de la Tourette's syndrome* following treatment with stimulant medications for symptoms of attention deficit disorder in children. They stress that early signs of Tourette's syndrome may be difficult to distinguish from hyperactive and attention disordered symptoms, leading the clinician to consider treatment with stimulants. In these Tourette's-susceptible patients, stimulants may exacerbate severe motor and phonic tics, requiring discontinuation of administration of stimulants and institution of haloperidol therapy for tic control.

Although *toxic psychosis* is not generally considered among the major side effects of methylphenidate, it is essential that clinicians be aware of the psychotogenic potential of this medication (occasionally within the normal dosage range) and the variable forms the syndrome may take. These factors are illustrated by 2 case reports presented by Young (30[C]).

Methylphenidate was first prescribed to a child for hyperactivity when he was 6 years old. Soon after the start of his 5th-grade year, he began to complain of itching in his nose, ears and hair and frequently scratched and shook his head. These symptoms occurred most frequently during the school day but had also bothered him during the previous summer when he was in a camp. At that time he complained about mosquitoes, spiders and other bugs, which he thought were getting into his ears, eyes and nose. His methylphenidate dose during this period ranged from 20 to 30 mg/day. A month after the start of the school year, the methylphenidate was discontinued and the 'bug problem' ceased. However, a short time later he again became restless, inattentive, and began 'showing off to make the kids laugh'. When methylphenidate was reinstituted, he grew calmer but reported that 'the bugs came back. I felt the itching and saw the bugs'. When the medication was again discontinued these symptoms ceased. The hallucinations never included an olfactory or gustatory component, and there were no psychotic-like symptoms during drug-free periods.

A second child was first treated at the age of eight with methylphenidate in a dosage of 2.5 mg/day for 2 days, which was then increased gradually. When the dosage reached 7.5 mg/day, the child began to complain that he saw horseflies and became very passive. His parents thought that his complaint was related to a tingling or itching that also preoccupied him. As the dosage was further increased to 20 mg/day, he became fearful, his agitation increased, and he clung to his mother. He no longer wanted to go outside the house and continued to talk about the horseflies. The medication was then discontinued. His symptoms abated and the fearful behavior disappeared.

The appearance of these effects might suggest a careful reduction of dosage rather than the assumption of an idiosyncratic reaction, with consequent discontinuation of the stimulant. The delicate balance between activation of the presynaptic autoreceptor and stimulation of the postsynaptic receptor, as well as the sensitive interactions among monoamine neuronal systems, underscores the need for careful management of dosage and attention to individual metabolic differences in response.

Satterfield et al (31[C]) studied possible adverse effects of methylphenidate on normal growth and development, and on different physiological systems in hyperactive boys. They found no adverse effects on any of the physiologic systems monitored as evidenced by serial clinical laboratory studies or by cardiovascular or growth measures.

ADVERSE EFFECTS OF INDIVIDUAL STIMULANTS

Pemoline

The first known case of chorea associated with the use of magnesium pemoline in the usual dosage has been described by Singh et al (32[C]).

In 1975, at the age of 6, the boy was initially treated with chlorpromazine and diazepam because of uncontrolled hyperactivity and psychomotor retardation. At this time he was already suffering from a seizure disorder controlled by primidone, 50 mg twice daily.

In 1976 the patient became progressively hyperactive in spite of continuing therapy with chlorpromazine 75 mg twice daily. Primidone was discontinued and the patient was given phenytoin 50 mg twice daily, and diazepam 5 mg three times daily. Thioridazine 15 mg three times daily was given from March 1977 to March 1978 without improvement. From March 1978 to October 1979 methylphenidate at a dosage of 10 mg daily was tried without success.

In November 1979 magnesium pemoline 37.5 mg per day was started and increased to 75 mg daily after 5 weeks, resulting in an improvement in behavior. In July 1980 the patient was noted to have violent choreiform involuntary movements of all the extremities and dyskinetic movements of the face and tongue. Other findings were unchanged. Pemoline was discontinued, and the abnormal movements slowly diminished and completely disappeared over the next 48 hours. At present, the patient is taking phenytoin alone and is slowly becoming hyperactive again.

Epinephrine

During the last years it has been recognized that the efficacy and tolerance of drugs can depend very much on their mode of formulation. A report by Feldschuh and Gambino (33[C]) illustrated once more what the dramatic consequences of such variations may be.

A patient was found to have a femoral arterial pH of 6.53 during cardiac arrest. An investigation undertaken to determine the cause of this unusually low pH led to the finding that standard 1 mg single-dose 10 ml Abbott epinephrine which had been employed in this case contained a large unsuspected acid load as compared to a presumably identical Bristol product and an equivalent epinephrine solution prepared from Parke-Davis 1:1,000 epinephrine diluted with normal saline solution.

Oxiracetam

Itil et al (34[cr]) have reported results of a double-blind controlled trial of the clinical effects of oxiracetam, a new 'nootropic' compound, in a group of 60 elderly patients with organic mental disorders; comparison was with piracetam, each preparation being given to 30 patients. Most of the important target symptoms improved significantly over time, both subjectively (i.e. rating scales) and objectively (i.e. psychological tests) after administration of either drug. Twenty-four of the oxiracetam subjects reported symptoms at some time compared with 20 of the piracetam group. None of the symptoms were consistent across either of the drug groups, and only a few patients reported any one symptom.

In conclusion both drugs seemed to produce sleep disturbance, nausea, and head pressure. The symptoms seen predominantly with oxiracetam included headache, hearing impairment, hypertension, constipation, diarrhea. The symptoms seen with piracetam were dizziness, increased urinary frequency, blurred vision, tremor of the hands and dry mouth.

METHYLXANTHINES

Caffeine

Cardiovascular effects The cardiovascular effects induced by caffeine continue to attract investigational attention. Conrad et al (35[CR]) studied the effects of caffeine upon cardiovascular function in healthy elderly volunteers.

Ten volunteers were given 4 mg/kg of caffeine by infusion on 3 separate occasions. This resulted in mean peak plasma concentrations of caffeine of 7.4 ± 0.7 μg/ml. Immediately after each of the 3 caffeine infusions, the mean systolic blood pressures increased by 14.7 and 16 mm Hg, and the mean diastolic blood pressures increased by 7.4 and 7 mm Hg, respectively. Both the systolic and the disatolic blood pressures returned to preinfusion values within 4 hours. The QS_2 index and the left ventricular ejection time (LVET) index increased after caffeine, probably as a result of the caffeine-induced increase in arterial blood pressure. The pre-ejection period (PEP), the PEP/LVET ratio, and the diastolic time remained unchanged. Caffeine, in doses equal to those contained in 2 to 3 cups of coffee, produces an increase in blood pressure but has no demonstrable positive inotropic effect in healthy men.

In order to determine the arrhythmogenic effects of caffeine, electrophysiologic studies were performed by Dobmeyer et al (36[C]) on 9 patients before and after the administration of either 200 mg of caffeine in the form of coffee or intravenous caffeine citrate. Four of the patients gave a history of palpitation or syncope associated with the ingestion of caffeinated substances. Effective refractory periods decreased after caffeine for the high right atrium, low right atrium and right ventricle. Left atrial effective refractory periods increased after caffeine. All patients demonstrated increases in right ventricular repetitive responses after caffeine as determined by programmed ventricular stimulation. In addition, 4 patients developed sustained atrial flutter and 1 developed sustained supraventricular tachycardia after caffeine. Of the remaining 4 patients, 3 showed increases in nonsustained atrial flutter response to atrial programmed stimulation. A previous history of caffeine-induced symptoms correlated highly with the development of supraventricular tachyarrhythmias.

Caffeine poisoning The sympathomimetic effects of caffeine are well known and believed to result from inhibition of phosphodiesterase, an enzyme that degrades the beta-adrenergic messenger, cyclic adenisine monophosphate. Recently, it was shown that caffeine in doses that might be consumed in beverages increases plasma catecholamine concentrations. Benowitz et al

(37[C]) have observed a patient who took a suicidal overdose of caffeine and had a hyperadrenergic syndrome associated with markedly elevated circulating catecholamine concentrations. Their patient ingested 24 g of caffeine, far above the stated lethal dose of 10 g. The maximal caffeine concentration of 200 mg/l is the highest in a surviving patient. Assuming a volume distribution of total body load water, it is estimated that this patient had a total body load of 6 g. Recurrent emesis, a characteristic feature of caffeine poisoning, may have eliminated a substantial part of the ingested dose. Many of the metabolic abnormalities observed in this patient, including metabolic acidosis, hyperglycemia and ketosis, as well as sinus tachycardia, can be explained by the high circulating concentrations of catecholamines. Sustained adrenergic stimulation and/or caffeine-induced hyperventilation presumably explain the development of hypokalemia. The authors draw attention to the fact that caffeine poisoning should be considered along with diabetes and salicylate poisoning in the differential diagnosis of hyperventilation, metabolic acidosis, and hyperglycemia, particularly when associated with behavioral abnormalities.

Teratogenic effects of caffeine A retrospective survey to examine the relationship between caffeine consumption and the outcome of human pregnancy was carried out by Worthington-Roberts et al (38[R]). Caffeine easily crosses the placental barrier and enters the fetal circulation; to date, however, most studies that demonstrate caffeine's teratogenic potential have been conducted in animal models. Although no definite relationship in humans has been confirmed, these authors suggest that a pregnant woman should limit or discontinue the intake of caffeine.

Not all authors are so cautious. Martin (39[R]) reviewed the effects on the offspring of smoking and caffeine using pregnant women and animal models, concluding that the evidence for caffeine damage is neither compelling nor consistent, and unless a woman ingests extremely large quantities daily the fetus is probably not at risk. Obviously more controlled studies need to be performed.

Theophylline

General In a review by Smith (40) the known side effects of theophylline are described, and it is pointed out that clinical manifestations of toxicity correlate well with serum concentrations and vary with age and ability to metabolize the drug. Hendeles and Weinberger (41) have analyzed the literature on theophylline and conclude that serum concentration measurements are the only reliable means of predicting life-threatening toxicity from this drug. They believe that all serious toxicity associated with theophylline is both predictable and preventable.

Malignant hyperthermia: special risks? An interesting study was performed by Flewellen and Nelson (42[CR]), who sought to determine whether methylxanthines are contraindicated in malignant hyperthermia-susceptible patients. In the light of animal data, aminophylline (theophylline ethylenediamine) and caffeine have earlier been said to be contraindicated in such patients. The authors diagnosed 4 malignant hyperthermia-susceptible patients using the caffeine-halothane contracture response. Skeletal muscle fascicles from these patients were exposed in vitro to theophylline alone or in the presence of 1% halothane.

It was shown that the theophylline concentrations achieved clinically are far lower than those required in vitro to produce contracture. A similar conclusion was reached for the moderate consumption of caffeinated beverages by hyperthermia-susceptible patients. Theophylline is equipotent with caffeine when inducing in vitro contracture. Halothane increases the in vitro contracture sensitivity of skeletal muscle to either agent but the effect on caffeine is greater.

Miscellaneous adverse effects Clark and Devenport (79[C]) have described a case in which exacerbation of spasticity in a case of hemiplegia (following an ischemic cerebrovascular accident) was clearly a consequence of theophylline use. The effect, which was confirmed by rechallenge, may reflect the direct vasoconstrictor effect of theophylline on the cerebral circulation or an increase in neurotransmitter at the neuromuscular junction.

Use in children Some special studies of the efficacy and tolerance of theophylline preparations in children have been reported. Newth et al (43[cr]), in a double blind study, compared oral theophylline and nebulized sodium cromoglycate for controlling symptoms of chronic asthma in 26 pre-school children. Sodium cromoglycate was at least as effective as theophylline. Gastrointestinal and central nervous system symptoms were noted quite frequently during the early days of theophylline treatment phases. Ten patients suffered from episodes of vomiting without fever or diarrhea during the theophylline phase, 7 during the combined treatment period, but only 2 during the cromoglycate regimen. Other symptoms reported during theophylline phases were excessive restless activity and difficulty with concentration (6 patients) and insomnia (5 patients). In most patients the adverse effects gradually receded.

Evaluation of long-term oral administration of a sustained release theophylline preparation in children with chronic asthma was performed by Cantani et al (44[CR]). The children received initially 14 mg/kg/day in 2 divided doses. If the serum theophylline level was not in the therapeutic range, the dose was increased up to 21 mg/kg/day and sometimes given in 3 divided doses. Only 2 children experienced side effects such as nausea and mild abdominal pains. Two patients had a serum theophylline level higher than 20 μg/ml (23 and 25 μg/ml respectively), but without any signs of side effects.

Haddad and Sakai (45[c]) reported the case of a 4-month-old infant who accidentally ingested her mother's oxtriphylline tablets and survived a stormy hospital course and a peak theophylline level of 224.6 μg/ml. This case represents the highest theophylline level reported in an infant to survive massive intoxication.

Intoxication *Seizures* are a potentially fatal complication of theophylline therapy. This complication represents a distinct clinical entity with several unique features. Nevertheless, the clinical diagnosis and management of theophylline-induced seizures are not as well appreciated as in other forms of drug toxicity. Nakada et al (46[CR]) have concluded from their own work and the literature that theophylline-induced seizures tend to occur in neurologically intact patients and have only minor neurological sequelae or none if controlled early. They begin with focal motor seizures with or without secondary generalization and are followed by stupor or coma. They are responsive only to adjustment of theophylline dosage. Should the motor phenomena persist, they may develop into an epilepsia partialis continua. The electroencephalogram typically shows periodic lateralized epileptiform discharges, which may provide a diagnostic clue.

The *use of hemoperfusion* in the treatment of theophylline intoxication with or without seizures is disputed. Dean and Brown (47[C]) have described a case of massive theophylline overdose surviving without hemoperfusion, despite the highest blood theophylline level yet recorded, in an adult..

A 58-year-old woman was admitted to hospital because of an oxtriphylline overdose. The patient, with a history of chronic obstructive lung disease and alcohol abuse, had arrived at another hospital after having attempted suicide by ingesting approximately one hundred 200 mg tablets of oxtriphylline, which is equivalent to 12.8 g of anhydrous theophylline. Ipecac, 45 ml, had been given, and it produced emesis containing pill fragments.

On arrival at the hospital the patient's BP was 80 mm Hg systolic and the pulse rate 145 beats per min. Ventricular ectopy was noted, and lidocaine therapy, 3 mg/min, was begun. Lavage returned pill fragments, and activated charcoal was given. The blood theophylline level on admission was 203 μg/ml.

Shortly after arrival at the intensive care unit, progressive hypotension was noted, which failed to respond to fluid challenge. Dopamine hydrochloride infusion at 5 mg/kg was begun. Ventricular ectopy continued, and the patient was again given a bolus of lidocaine. While the bolus was being given, the patient had a grand mal seizure that responded to 10 mg of diazepam given intravenously. The seizure was followed by severe bradycardia with reduction of BP. The patient's BP and pulse responded to dopamine hydrochloride and atropine sulfate respectively. Intubation was performed. Shortly thereafter, the patient regained consciousness, and administration of dopamine and lidocaine was withdrawn.

Four and a half hours later, a second grand mal seizure occurred that responded to a total of 20 mg of diazepam given in 2.5 mg increments. Sodium phenobarbital was then given.

Thereafter, the patient remained stable; extubation was performed on the second hospital day, and the patient had no additional seizure activity. Neurologically, she was intact except for mild recent memory loss. Theophylline level 12 hours after admission was 96 μg/ml, at 30 hours it was 23.1 μg/ml, and at 64 hours 3.6 μg/ml.

The authors conclude that treatment of massive theophylline overdose remains confined to aggressive support of the cardiovascular system and control of seizure activity with diazepam. Unfortunately, the place hemoperfusion occupies, if any, is still not clear. The best advice is perhaps that given very recently by Park in the American Journal of Medicine (78[R]). He concludes that charcoal perfusion is indeed a useful procedure for the treatment of theophylline intoxication where plasma concentrations exceed 60 μg/ml at 4 hours after ingestion or where special risk factors are present (age over 60, significant liver or heart disease or a prolonged theophylline half-life). There is no evidence that hemoperfusion is of any benefit once complications of overdosage such as seizures have developed.

Sahney et al (48[CR]) described 4 patients with severe theophylline toxicity (blood levels 60–180 μg/ml). Three of them, with neurotoxic signs, were treated with hemoperfusion. Two of these were hemoperfused early after the onset of seizures; they recovered with no neurologic deficit. In the third patient hemoperfusion was delayed for 16 hours after uncontrolled seizures; severe brain damage resulted. The fourth patient, who had the highest peak theophylline level but no seizures, was successfully treated with conservative management and peritoneal dialysis. Based on their own experience and that of others the authors believe that hemoperfusion is a safe and effective method to remove the drug even in very young infants.

The efficacy of hemodialysis in the management of acute theophylline intoxication was also studied by Krishna et al (49[C]). They describe a patient presenting with theophylline-induced seizures managed successfully by hemodialysis.

Although fatal theophylline overdosage is well recognized, the clinical and biochemical features of *acute pancreatitis* have not previously been described in this situation. Burgan et al (50[C]) reported a case of fatal overdose from theophylline accompanied by the clinical picture of acute pancreatitis and appreciably raised serum amylase activity. Regardless of the source of the amylase in this case the authors suggest that it was a direct result of theophylline intoxication, and in view of the successful management of theophylline poisoning using resin or charcoal hemoperfusion it is important that this association should be borne in mind. The widespread prescribing of theophylline renders it liable to abuse in self-poisoning, and theophylline overdosage should be considered as a possible underlying cause of apparent pancreatitis in patients who also suffer from chronic obstructive airway disease.

Influence of influenza Last year Kremer et al (51) reported altered theophylline clearance in asthmatic patients during an influenza B outbreak. Walker and Middelkamp (52[C]) have now confirmed their observation that acutely ill children receiving theophylline can experience a sudden decrease in theophylline clearance. The authors described 2 asthmatic children who had a concomitant viral illness and 48% and 62% decrease of the body clearance of the drug from previous measurements when healthy. These data show that serum levels must be monitored and drug dosage adjusted to fit individual clearance rates to avoid theophylline toxicity during symptomatic viral illnesses.

The matter cannot however be regarded as settled; Fischer et al (53[C]) in 12 patients and Britton and Ruben (54[C]) in 5 others failed to demonstrate any influence of influenza vaccine on serum theophylline levels.

The influence of the patient's state The influence of the disorder treated as well as of concomitant diseases on pharmacokinetics and tolerance of theophylline was discussed in previous issues of SEDA (SEDA-4, 2; SEDA-7, 4). Since then LeGatt (55[C]) has published an observation of the toxic effects of the drug which was used in the usual therapeutic doses for the treatment of an elderly patient with congestive heart failure. The patient experienced toxic symptoms, and plasma concentrations were found to have reached 60.6 μg/ml; theophylline administration was subsequently discontinued. It would seem that plasma concentrations and toxicity of theophylline are unpredictable in patients with CHF because of the great variability in clearance. This case demonstrates the necessity for careful monitoring of theophylline plasma levels in such patients.

An interesting case of life-threatening theophylline intoxication in a hypothyroid patient was described by Aderka et al (56[C]). In this patient, who suffered also from chronic obstructive lung disease and mild congestive heart failure, treatment with 1 g/day theophylline administered orally was followed by a life-threatening theophylline intoxication manifested by repeated epileptic fits and ventricular fibrillation, successfully converted to sinus rhythm. The plasma theophylline was 34.7 μg/ml when the life-threatening arrhythmia occurred.

Pharmacokinetic studies conducted during the hypothyroid state revealed a markedly prolonged theophylline plasma half-life of 29.5 hr 2 months later; after reestablishment of an euthyroid state, theophylline plasma half-life was shortened to normal, i.e. 5.7 hr, and the theophylline plasma level was 13.5 μg/ml, while the daily intake was 1 g. The authors conclude that hypothyroidism may predispose to theophylline intoxication, probably because of the decreased activity of the hepatic microsomal drug-metabolizing enzymes responsible for the degradation of theophylline.

Interactions (59[CR]) Elimination of theophylline from the body occurs mainly (approx. 90%) by biotransformation followed by excretion of the metabolites. Drugs influencing microsomal enzyme systems in the liver, may therefore affect the elimination of theophylline, and thus the serum concentration of the drug. As a consequence, therapy with theophylline – a drug having a small therapeutic range – might be disturbed.

Some practical recommendations on the correction of theophylline doses during concomitant medication with other drugs have been presented by Jonkman et al (57[R]). Co-medication with *phenobarbital* may require an increase in the theophylline dose by about 30% and co-medication with *phenytoin* by as much as 75%. Concomitant therapy with *allopurinol, cimetidine, erythromycin, furosemide, isoprenaline* or *propranolol* may, on the other hand, require a decrease of the theophylline dose by about 20–30%; for *oleandomycin* the decrease should be about 50%. The data on the influence of *influenza vaccination* are conflicting.

As large interindividual variations in effect may occur, the correction of the dose should preferably be guided by serum theophylline determinations. In case of co-medication with a drug not yet known to interact with theophylline pharmacokinetics, the initial dosage regimen should be relatively low.

Shenfield (58[R]) in his review on combination bronchodilator therapy analyzed the data on the efficacy and toxicity of different combinations of anti-asthmatic drugs. Studies on *methylxanthines (usually theophylline) and adrenoceptor agonists* may be divided into two groups: those using ephedrine and those using more selective beta-adrenoceptor agonists. Ephedrine is a relatively ineffective bronchodilator and often fails to add any useful bronchodilatation to theophylline; it does not appear to synergize with it, whereas the more selective beta-adrenoceptor agonist drugs all appear to have an additive effect with the methylxanthines. In Shenfield's view it is often possible to achieve the same therapeutic effect with half doses of drugs from two different groups as with a full dose of one drug. This may sometimes, but not always, reduce side effects. There is evidence that giving two drugs by different routes is a useful therapeutic procedure; for example, the addition of an inhaled beta-adrenoceptor agonist may improve upon the maximal bronchodilatation achieved with intravenous theophylline. When theophylline is administered plasma levels of the drug should be monitored and it is possible that, when used in combination with a beta-adrenoceptor agonist, a therapeutic range lower than that normally recommended may apply.

A note of caution must be expressed with respect to Shenfield's views. Wilson and Sutherland have advanced the view that the increased rate of fatalities among younger asthma patients in New Zealand was due to this very combination of beta-agonists and methylxanthines (82[R]) though their view has in turn been challenged by others (83[r]).

A fatal case of theophylline intoxication involving *cimetidine* is presented by Anderson et al (60[C]). In this case a number of factors leading to a decrease in theophylline clearance and the patient's death may have been operative; these included advanced age, chronic lung disease, liver disease, and administration of cimetidine. Since early toxic effects of theophylline can mimic peptic ulcer disease, cimetidine might be prescribed for these gastrointestinal symptoms with subsequent worsening of theophylline poisoning.

The concurrent administration of theophylline and *erythromycin* to children may result in an increase in theophylline serum concentrations, but this increase has previously been reported only in patients above 2.5 years of age. Murray and Brown (61[C]) have now shown that the interaction may occur in even younger children.

They described a 1-year-old, 7 kg boy with a 6-month history of asthma who was admitted to the hospital with diagnosis of status asthmaticus and pneumonia. The patient received treatment with theophylline (administered as aminophylline) at a dosage 20–30 mg/kg/day i.v. for 3 days followed by oral aminophylline solution at a sufficient dosage required to maintain therapeutic level. Other medication included: erythromycin estolate suspension (50 mg orally every 6 hours) and sulfisoxazole suspension (525 mg initially followed by 260 mg every 6 hours). On the 5th day, 6 watery stools were noted. Increased irritability and poor feeding began on the following morning; diarrhea continued and the patient vomited. Serum theophylline concentrations greater than 20 μg/ml correlated with the development of these symptoms. One aminophylline dose was withheld and the dosage retitrated to produce more acceptable serum theophylline concentrations. The toxic symptoms rapidly resolved. The patient was discharged on the 10th day, and a chest X-ray before discharge showed a resolving pulmonary infiltrate.

The presence of pneumonia has been shown to reduce theophylline clearance; with resolution of the infection, theophylline clearance improves. Despite the resolving pneumonia, which one would expect to be associated with decreased serum theophylline concentrations, the *theophylline* concentrations rose at a dosage that was previously well tolerated, and this was probably a direct consequence of the concurrent use of erythromycin.

Brown et al (62[C]) draw attention to the fact that severe adverse reactions may result from interaction between certain new *cephalosporins* (including *moxalactam*) and the alcohol in theophylline elixir. They described a case of a 'disulfiram-like' reaction in a hospitalized patient receiving moxalactam and elixir of theophylline. In this patient the severest reactions were seen with the administration of larger amounts of alcohol. 300 mg of theophylline as an elixir (20% alcohol) will be accompanied by 11 g of alcohol; 60 ml of beer by contrast contains only 1.8 g of alcohol.

A very interesting report on a *ketamine*-aminophylline interaction has been presented by Hirshman et al (63[C]). During the past 9 years the authors have observed the occurrence of extensor-type seizures in 4 asthmatic patients receiving theophylline within minutes following induction of anesthesia with ketamine.

One of their patients, a 50-year-old, 50 kg woman, was scheduled for a vocal cord stripping operation. She had a history of alcohol abuse and chronic obstructive pulmonary disease with a marked bronchospastic component, for which she was being treated with 300 mg, q.i.d., of a long-acting theophylline preparation. The patient denied a history of seizures. Four previous general anesthesias were uncomplicated. Physical examination was unremarkable. Preoperative laboratory tests were normal.

90 min prior to surgery, an i.v. infusion of aminophylline (1 mg/kg/hr) was started and premedication of 5 mg diazepam was given i.m. Ketamine, 100 mg, was given i.v. over a 2-min period for induction of anesthesia. With the patient breathing spontaneously, 1.5% halothane in oxygen was started. The patient then developed random eye and limb movements. Approximately 2 to 3 min later, she became impossible to ventilate and developed a heart rate of 200 beats/min. Extensor spasm and opisthotonic posturing of the extremities, neck, and jaw ensued. Succinylcholine, 80 mg, was administered. Halothane was discontinued because of multifocal premature ventricular contractions (PVCs) and runs of ventricular tachycardia. The extensor seizures ceased. Ventilation via a mask became possible and intubation of the trachea was accomplished without difficulty. No wheezing was audible. Within minutes, ventilation again became impossible and the extensor spasms returned. Pancuronium 3 mg i.v. was given to facilitate controlled ventilation. Cardiac abnormalities continued despite 7.5 mg diazepam and 100 mg lidocaine. With continuous chest auscultation, 0.75 mg propranolol was given over a 5-min period, at which time heart rate decreased from 180 to 120 beats/min and PVCs resolved. Blood gases were normal. Serum theophylline level was 19 μg/ml (therapeutic level 10/20 μg/ml). Surgery was cancelled. The patient was transferred to the recovery room and mechanically ventilated. The patient was alert and the trachea was extubated without problems 2 hours later.

A subsequent study with theophylline and ketamine in mice confirmed a lowering of the seizure threshold with the concurrent use of both drugs. This report should serve to alert the anesthesiologist to the possible occurrence of seizures during concomitant use of ketamine and aminophylline. Perhaps ketamine should be avoided in some patients currently taking aminophylline, or anti-seizure premedication be instituted in patients at risk.

Effects of ethylenediamine Since the publication of Annual 7 several new reports on adverse reactions to aminophylline connected with *toxic effects of ethylenediamine* have appeared in the literature. Neumann (64[C]) reported the case of a 48-year-old man suffering from spastic bronchitis, who developed an urticarial rash during the injection of aminophylline. Test reactions were positive to ethylenediamine (ED) and negative to theophylline. Only few similar observations following systemic application of ED have been reported; contact dermatitis due to ED is however more frequent and its incidence has increased during the last years. Sensitizers are ED and in some cases several ED-derivatives, such as epoxy resin hardeners, coolant oils, piperazine and promethazine. No toxic effects of ED at customary doses are known and none are to be expected because of the minimal amount of ED in these preparations.

Two other cases of allergy to ethylenediamine were reported by Mohsenifar et al (65[C]). Both subjects developed erythroderma after receiving intravenous aminophylline. When these patients were given a preparation of pure theophylline, no adverse effects were noted. One of these patients had been treated in the past with intravenous aminophylline without the development of a skin rash, suggesting that the absence of reaction to a prior trial of aminophylline does not exclude this drug as the allergen.

Nierenberg and Glazener (66[C]) evaluated the case of a patient with severe bronchospasm and a history of extensive exfoliative dermatitis after prior exposure to aminophylline. It was concluded that the patient was sensitive only to ethylenediamine; when he was challenged with anhydrous theophylline, he tolerated this well, and his bronchospasm improved.

The development of severe exfoliative dermatitis in this latter patient after exposure to aminophylline recalls cases previously reported in the dermatological and industrial medicine literature, though not in the usual pharmacology reference sources. The authors concluded that whereas the incidence of aminophylline-induced exfoliative dermatitis seems to be quantitatively infrequent, it can be qualitatively severe when it occurs. Physicians confronted with this problem should be aware of the many medical preparations that contain or cross-react with ethylenediamine. Perhaps of greater importance, physicians should not deprive their aminophylline-sensitive asthmatic patients of theophylline itself, when ethylenediamine is responsible for the sensitivity reaction.

Mathewson (67[R]) noted that aminophylline is a valuable drug, but the seriousness of its side actions demands that it be used cautiously and under close surveillance. When i.v. aminophylline is given the risks are sufficient to indicate that it be administered only where monitoring equipment and personnel are at intensive care level.

Enprofylline

Enprofylline (3-propylxanthine) is a new compound which has proved to be a potent bronchodilator in man and animals. Laursen et al (68[cr]) have studied the bronchodilating effect of 2 doses of peroral enprofylline compared with placebo in 24 asthmatic patients. Enprofylline produced significantly greater bronchodilatation than placebo. Doses of 2 mg/kg and 4 mg/kg caused a mean maximal increase in FEV1 of 26% and 35% respectively. The degree and incidence of *headache* and *nausea* were estimated by means of a scoring system. Dose-related effects on both parameters were observed. Determinations of blood pressure and heart rate showed no differences between placebo and active treatment with enprofylline. Twelve patients complained of headache when given the low dose of enprofylline, 16 experienced headache after the high dose and 3 patients after the placebo. Five patients complained of nausea when given the low dose, 9 with the high dose and no patients experienced nausea after receiving placebo. One patient treated with the high dose vomited. One patient developed palpitations after taking the placebo, while 3 developed palpitations after 4 mg/kg. One patient experienced slight dizziness after 2 mg/kg of enprofylline.

ANORECTIC AGENTS

GENERAL

Douglas and Munro (69[CR]) have analyzed the current state of drug treatment of obesity including the evaluation of efficacy and adverse reactions to anorectic agents. Analysis of the commonly reported side effects to these anorectic agents reveals a striking frequency both to the active preparation and during placebo therapy (Table 2). This data was obtained from three reviews and eight representative original papers. Interrogation of patients previously treated with an antiobesity agent revealed that almost half of those receiving amphetamine reported an unpleasant side effect, as did 44% of those taking mazindol and 42% of subjects treated with phenmetrazine. The reported rates of adverse reactions with phentermine, fenfluramine and diethylpropion were 31%, 30% and 27% respectively.

The Dawn reports of 1973–75 and 1976 emphasized the potential for drug abuse among teenagers with amphetamine and, to a lesser extent, phenmetrazine (Tables 3 and 4). Both these drugs are now controlled in the U.K. by the Misuse of Drugs Act 1971 and by comparable regulations in some other countries. Although drug abuse is rarely found in the obese patient, the potential for abuse with amphetamine and phenmetrazine is such that neither should be prescribed for the treatment of obesity.

There is also a potential for drug abuse with phentermine and diethylpropion, and the latter may have been manufactured illegally for sale as a stimulant drug. However, abuse is rare and probably limited to those persons already addicted to other drugs. The lack of euphoriant effects with fenfluramine is such that the potential for abuse must be extremely low, though it is not entirely unknown.

ANORECTIC AGENTS AND HEAT-STROKE

Kew et al (70[C]) have reported a rare complication of treatment with anorectic agents. An 11-year-old girl taking two appetite-suppressant agents developed fatal heat-stroke while participating in a 'nature hike' in environmental conditions in which heat-stroke would not normally have been anticipated. The ambient temperature was 34°C. The other 107 participating children suffered no significant effects. The drugs involved were phentermine (30 mg per day) and propylhexedrine hydrochloride (50 mg twice a day). She was also taking a diuretic,

Table 2. *Percentage incidence of adverse drug effects at recommended dosage of antiobesity drugs (adapted from Bray and Greenway, 1976)*

Adverse effect	Amphetamine	Phenmetrazine	Phentermine	Diethylpropion	Mazindol	Fenfluramine	Placebo
Source	a, b	c, d	e, f, g	h, i	j, k, l	m	n
Insomnia	12	12	6	6	6	2	2
Nervousness	8	20	14	4	3	6	4
Lethargy	3	4	8	2	4	15	3
Depression	1	1	1	–	–	3	1
Dizziness	6	6	9	1	3	10	1
Dry mouth	22	10	17	5	7	6	3
Nausea	8	5	4	4	7	6	1
Constipation	8	6	8	6	3	–	4
Diarrhea	–	–	–	–	–	13	2
Palpitations (rapid pulse)	2	3	–	3	2	–	1

a. Seaton et al (1964)
b. Vernace (1974)
c. Poindexter (1960)
d. Schapiro and Brogan (1960)
e. Steel et al (1973)
f. Steel et al (1964b)
g. Truant et al (1972)
h. Noble (1971)
i. G.P. Research Group (1978)
j. G.P. Research Group (1978)
k. Vernace (1974)
l. Asher (personal communication)
m. Pinder et al (1975)
n. Steel et al (1973)

 For the publications referred to in the table the reader should consult the original paper.

Table 3. *Misuse of antiobesity drugs (Dawn Reports, 1973–1975) (Adapted from Carabillo, 1978)*

Drug	Reports per million prescriptions
Amphetamine	45.3
Phenmetrazine	5.7
Phentermine	1.7
Diethylpropion	1.3
Mazindol	0.7
Fenfluramine	1.6

Reprinted with permission from Douglas and Munro (69), 1982, Pergamon Press Ltd.

bumetanide (0.5 mg once a week). She had lost about 10 kg in weight and at the time of the hike was no longer significantly overweight.

The authors consider that heat intolerance was in this case connected with the sympathomimetic action of these anorectic drugs. Sympathomimetic amines used as appetite suppressants not only increase endogenous heat production as a result of their stimulatory effects on the central nervous system, but also impede the dissipation of heat from the body by producing peripheral vasoconstriction.

INDIVIDUAL ANORECTIC AGENTS

Fenfluramine

Although fenfluramine produces substantial weight loss, the patient usually regains weight after drug withdrawal. To determine whether or not recurrence of weight gain can be prevented by continuing to give fenfluramine, Douglas et al (71[c]) studied the effect of longer-term fenfluramine administration in a group of women who had successfully lost weight on the drug. Forty-two obese women who lost 6 kg after 26 weeks on fenfluramine tablets had their treatment changed to either an equivalent dose of a sustained-release preparation of fenfluramine or matching placebo in double-blind fashion. Of the 21 given placebo all but 2 regained weight over the following year. Of the 21 crossed over to fenfluramine, 8 maintained their weight loss, 7 regained weight, and 6 had to be withdrawn for reasons other than weight gain.

Side effects attributable to fenfluramine in this study were infrequent. This is not surprising because most patients known to be intolerant of fenfluramine had been excluded from the study. However, one subject became *depressed* in the presence of high plasma drug concentrations. A reversible *pulmonary hypertension* developed in another subject who had been on fenfluramine 120 mg daily for 35 weeks. This latter (potentially serious) adverse reaction which has been described with other anorectic drugs seems to be rare with fenfluramine but the risks may increase with longer term treatment or with repeated courses of therapy. The authors recommend that patients on long-term or repeated treatment should be advised to report immediately any increase in breathlessness on exertion. The possible hazards of prolonged use require further evaluation.

Gaul (72[c]) reported on another case of chronic pulmonary hypertension after fenfluramine intake. Here the first symptoms of exertional dyspnea appeared 3 months after completing an 8-month course of treatment. 3 years later she still complained of

Table 4. *Misuse of antiobesity drugs (Adapted from Carabillo, 1978)*

Dawn Reports* (1976) (99)	Antiobesity drug market (%)	Antiobesity drug misuse problem (%)	Stimulant effect (%)	Motives for misuse	
				Dependence state (%)	Other or unknown (%)
Phenmetrazine	13	50	31	53	16
Diethylpropion	44	31	75	1	24
Phentermine	24	12	55	4	41
Mazindol	10	1	47	7	46
Fenfluramine	9	6	67	2	31

*Excluding all other anorectic drugs.
Reprinted with permission from Douglas and Munro (69), 1982, Pergamon Press Ltd.

short syncopal attacks during exertion. Clinical examination showed a pulmonary artery pressure of 95/40 mm Hg, pulmonary artery resistance 899 $dyn \cdot s \cdot cm^{-5}$, mean wedge pressure 12 mm Hg and typical pulmonary vessel cut-off at pulmonary angiography.

The association of pulmonary hypertension (PH) and anorectic drugs in man is known with respect to aminorex fumarate, chlorfentermine and phenformin. The present evidence suggests that every available anorectic drug can potentially cause this complication.

The report of Pietrusko et al (73[c]) describes failure to replicate the findings of two earlier studies of a relationship between plasma levels of the appetite-suppressant fenfluramine (and of its metabolite norfenfluramine) and weight loss. Fenfluramine was here initiated with a dosage of 20 mg 3 times a day. Dosage was increased stepwise, as tolerated, to a maximum of 160 mg per day. Because of the occurrence of side effects, only 9 patients achieved this dosage level. The findings suggested that there was little or no correlation between the blood levels of fenfluramine (or its metabolite) and weight loss.

In all, 27 of the 36 patients reported side effects which prevented them from reaching the maximum dosage of 160 mg per day. The most common side effects, experienced by 25–35% of the group were drowsiness, dry mouth or diarrhea, while 8–10% reported headaches, feelings of chilliness or dizziness and 1 or 2 patients each reported difficulty in concentration, depression, nausea or nightmares. If weight loss is indeed not related to drug levels, as suggested by this report, there is no merit in increasing drug levels to tolerance as is the current practice; modest dosage to produce modest drug levels is indicated.

Phenylpropanolamine

Noble (74[C]) has contested earlier evidence that phenylpropanolamine in weight control preparations can produce increased blood pressure. In three large-scale investigations more than 400 obese patients were studied, using a dose of 50 mg 3 times daily (with or without 200 mg caffeine in slow-release form) tested against placebo. There was also a single blind trial of 75 mg phenylpropanolamine in controlled-release form.

In the group as a whole, no significant increase in blood pressure was found. 2 patients did experience noteworthy rises in blood pressure after treatment with 75 mg PPA, but these increases were felt not to be drug related. There was indeed in other patients a trend to a decline in blood pressure as their weight fell, which one might expect.

These data agree with those of a previously multi-center study (SED-5, 9). Nevertheless, it may be that in certain individuals hypertensive reactions to phenylpropanolamine can occur. Howrie and Wolfson (75[C]) have for example reported in detail on phenylpropanolamine-induced hypertensive seizures in an adolescent using for weight reduction a nonprescription diet product Dex-A-Diet II capsules, containing 75 mg PPA and 200 mg caffeine.

Phentaramine

Hamer and Phelps (76[C]) report an unusual case of inadvertent intra-arterial injection of a crushed Preludin tablet (phentaramine 75 mg) mixed in tap water. The patient was a 26-year-old woman who acknowledged an extensive drug abuse history. Severe hand pain, vasospasm, and ischemia occurred. Treatment with regional axillary block, intravenous dextran, intra-arterial prixcoline, and salicylate anticoagulation may have influenced the favorable outcome. Intimal damage, vasospasm, and various additive effects after intra-arterial injection can however in some cases have serious sequelae. Prompt diagnosis, vasodilatation, elevation and compression, pain relief and, in some cases, surgery appear to improve salvage of what is frequently a major extremity injury.

Jecht (77[C]) describes a 23-year-old woman who suffered from a painful cutaneovascular reaction. She was taking nikethamide and D-non-pseudoephedrine and was a heavy smoker (40 cigarettes per day). Her history and signs resembled those of ergotism, the disease being apparently due to a combined effect of the analeptic, the anorectic drug and the excessive smoking.

REFERENCES

1. Anon (1981) Phenylpropanolamine weight control products. *Natl Clgh Poison Control Cent. Bull., 25,* 16.
2. Sawyer DR, Conner CS et al (1982) Managing acute toxicity from nonprescription stimulants. *Clin. Pharm., 1,* 529.
3. Weesner KM, Denison M et al (1982) Cardiac arrhythmias in an adolescent following ingestion of an over-the-counter stimulant. *Clin. Paediatr., 21,* 700.
4. Bernstein E, Diskant BM et al (1982) Phenylpropanolamine: a potentially hazardous drug. *Ann. Emerg. Med., 11,* 311(43).
5. Anderson RJ, Reed WG et al (1982) History, epidemiology and medical complications of nasal inhaler abuse. *J. Toxicol. Clin. Toxic., 19,* 95.
6. Monroe RR, Drell HJ (1947) Oral use of stimulants obtained from inhalers. *J. Am. Med. Assoc., 135,* 909.
7. Anon (1959) Amphetamine inhalers regarded as prescription drug. *Fed. Regist., 24,* 956.
8. Marsden P, Sheldon J (1972) Acute poisoning by propylhexedrine. *Br. Med. J., 1,* 730.
9. Sturner WQ, Spruell FG, Garriott JC (1974) Two propylhexedrine associated fatalities: Benzedrine revisited. *J. Forensic Sci., 19,* 572.
10. DiMaio VJM, Garriott JC (1977) Intravenous abuse of propylhexedrine. *J. Forensic Sci., 22,* 152.
11. White L (1977) Pulmonary hypertension and sudden death associated with propylhexedrine abuse. *Forensic Sci. Gaz., 8,* 3.
12. Anderson RJ, Garza HR, Garriott JC et al (1979) Intravenous propylhexedrine (Benzedrex) abuse and sudden death. *Am. J. Med., 67,* 15.
13. Foerster E, Hatchett D et al (1978) A rapid comprehensive screening procedure for basic drugs in blood or tissue by gas chromatography. *J. Anal. Toxicol., 2,* 50.
14. Liggett SB (1982) Propylhexedrine intoxication: clinical presentation and pharmacology. *South. Med. J., 75,* 250.
15. Croft CH, Firth BG, Hillis LD (1982) Propylhexedrine-induced left ventricular dysfunction. *Ann. Intern. Med., 97,* 560.
16. Powers JM (1982) Decongestant-induced bleopharospasm and orofacial dystonia. *J. Am. Med. Assoc., 247,* 3244.
17. Eriksson M, Wibell L (1982) Haemorrhagic cerebral infarction associated with amphetamine abuse. *J. Neurosurg., 26,* 109.
18. Matick H, Anderson D, Brumlik J (1983) Cerebral vasculitis associated with oral amphetamine overdose. *Arch. Neurol., 40,* 253.
19. Shibahashi H, Hosaka Y et al (1982) Brain abscess in an addict to amphetamine: case report. *Neurol. Med. Chir. (Tokyo), 22,* 319.
20. Call TD, Hartneck J, Dickinson WA et al (1982) Acute cardiomyopathy secondary to intravenous amphetamine abuse. *Ann. Intern. Med., 97,* 559.
21. Scandling J, Spital A (1982) Amphetamine-associated myoglobinuric renal failure. *South. Med. J., 75,* 237.
22. Deveaugh-Geiss J, Pandurangi A (1982) Confusional paranoid psychosis after withdrawal from sympathiomimetic amines: two case reports. *Am. J. Psychiatry, 139,* 1190.
23. Djenderedjian A, Tashjian R (1982) Agoraphobia following amphetamine withdrawal. *J. Clin. Psychiatry, 43,* 248.
24. Rosen RA (1981) Angina associated with pseudoephedrine. *Ann. Emerg. Med., 10,* 93.
25. Loizou LA, Hamilton JG et al (1982) Intracranial haemorrhage in association with pseudoephedrine overdose. *J. Neurol. Neurosurg. Psychiatry, 45,* 471.
26. Haglund RMJ, Howerton LL (1982) Ritalin: Consequences of abuse in a clinical population. *Int. J. Addict., 17,* 349.
27. Chillar RK, Jackson AL, Alaan L (1982) Hemiplegia after intracarotid injection of methylphenidate. *Arch. Neurol., 39,* 598.
28. Cowart VS (1982) Stimulant therapy for attention disorders. *J. Am. Med. Assoc., 248,* 279.
29. Lowe TL, Cohen DJ, Detlor J et al (1982) Stimulant medications precipitate Tourette's syndrome. *J. Am. Med. Assoc., 247,* 1729.
30. Young JG (1981) Methylphenidate-induced hallucinosis: case histories and possible mechanisms of action. *Dev. Behav. Pediatr., 2,* 35.
31. Satterfield JH, Schell AM, Barb SD (1980) Potential risk of prolonged administration of stimulant medication for hyperactive children. *Dev. Behav. Pediatr., 1,* 102.
32. Singh BK, Singh A, Chusid E (1983) Chorea in long-term use of pemoline. *Ann. Neurol., 13,* 218.
33. Feldschuh J, Gambino R (1983) Extreme central acidosis from Abbott epinephrine. *Am. J. Med., 74,* 30.
34. Itil TM, Menon GN, Bozak M et al (1982) The effects of oxiracetam (ISF 2522) in patients with organic brain syndrome (a double-blind controlled study with piracetam) *Drug Dev. Res., 2,* 447.
35. Conrad KA, Blanchard J, Trang JM (1982) Cardiovascular effects of caffeine in elderly men. *J. Am. Geriatr. Soc., 30,* 267.
36. Dobmeyer DJ, Stine RA, Leier CV et al (1982) Arrhythmogenic effects of caffeine in man as determined by programmed electrical stimulation. *Clin. Res., 30,* 182A.
37. Benowitz NL, Osterloh J, Goldschlager N et al (1982) Massive catecholamine release from caffeine poisoning. *J. Am. Med. Assoc., 248,* 1097.
38. Worthington-Roberts B, Weigle A (1983) Caffeine and pregnancy outcome. *J. Obstet. Gynecol. Neonat. Nursing, 12,* 21.
39. Martin JC (1982) An overview: maternal nicotine and caffeine consumption and off-

spring outcome. *Neurobehav. Toxicol. Teratol.*, *4*, 421.
40. Smith FA (1981) Therapeutic drug monitoring of theophylline, salicylates, and acetaminophen. *Clin. Lab. Med.*, *1*, 559.
41. Hendeles L, Weinberger M (1983) Improved efficacy and safety of theophylline in the control of airways hyperreactivity. *Pharmacol. Ther.*, *18*, 91.
42. Flewellen EH, Nelson TE (1983) Is theophylline, aminophylline, or caffeine (methylxanthines) contraindicated in malignant hyperthermia susceptible patients? *Anesth. Analg. (Paris)*, *62*, 115.
43. Newth CJL, Newth CV, Turner JAP (1982) Comparison of nebulised sodium cromoglycate and oral theophylline in controlling symptoms of chronic asthma in pre-school children: a double blind study. *Aust. NZ J. Med.*, *12*, 232.
44. Cantani A, Businco E, Businco L et al (1983) Evaluation of long-term oral administration of theophylline. *Allergol. Immunopathol.*, *11*, 11.
45. Haddad ZH, Sakai R (1982) Massive accidental theophylline ingestion: linear first order elimination kinetics in an infant. *Ann. Allergy*, *48*, 178.
46. Nakada T, Kwee IL, Lerner AM et al (1983) Theophylline-induced seizures: clinical and pathophysiologic aspects. *West. J. Med.*, *138*, 371.
47. Dean LS (1982) Massive theophylline overdosage. *J. Am. Med. Assoc.*, *248*,
48. Sahney S, Abarzua J, Sessums L (1983) Hemoperfusion in theophylline neurotoxicity. *Pediatrics*, *71*, 615.
49. Krishna GG, Zahrowski JJ, Nissenson AR (1983) *Dialysis Transplant*, *12*, 40.
50. Burgan THS, Gupta I, Bate CM (1982) Fatal overdose of theophylline simulating acute pancreatitis. *Br. Med. J.*, *284*, 939.
51. Kraemer MJ, Furukawa CT, Koup JR et al (1982) Altered theophylline clearance during an influenza B outbreak. *Pediatrics*, *69*, 476.
52. Walker SB, Middelkamp JN (1982) Theophylline toxicity and viral infections. *Pediatrics*, *70*, 508.
53. Fischer RG, Booth BH, Mitchell DQ et al (1982) Influence of trivalent influenza vaccine on serum theophylline levels. *Can. Med. Assoc. J.*, *126*, 1312.
54. Britton L, Ruben FL, (1982) Serum theophylline levels after influenza vaccination. *Can. Med. Assoc. J.*, *126*, 1375.
55. LeGatt DF (1983) Theophylline toxicity – a consequence of congestive heart failure. *Drug Intell. Clin. Pharm.*, *17*, 59.
56. Aderka D, Shavit G, Garfinkel D et al (1983) Life-threatening theophylline intoxication in a hypothyroid patient. *Respiration*, *44*, 77.
57. Jonkman JHG, Koëter GH, Berg WC (1983) Geneesmiddelen met een therapeutisch belangrijke invloed op de farmacokinetiek van theofylline. *Pharm. Weekbl.*, *118*, 185.
58. Shenfield GM (1982) Combination bronchodilator therapy. *Drugs*, *24*, 414.
59. Jackson JE (1982) Effects of drugs and diet on theophylline pharmacokinetics. *Acta Paediatr. Jpn*, *24*, 124.
60. Anderson JR, Poklis A, Slavin RG (1983) A fatal case of theophylline intoxication. *Arch. Intern. Med.*, *153*, 559.
61. Murray MD, Brown BK (1982) Theophylline-erythromycin interaction in an infant. *Clin. Pharm*, *1*, 107 and 111.
62. Brown KR, Guglielmo BJ, Pons VG, Jacobs RA (1982) Theophylline elixir, moxalactam, and a disulfiram reaction. *Ann. Intern. Med.*, *97*, 621.
63. Hirshman CA, Kriegler W, Littlejohn G et al (1982) Ketamine-aminophylline-induced decrease in seizure threshold. *Anesthesiology*, *56*, 464.
64. Neumann H (1983) Allergische und toxische Nebenwirkungen von Ethylendiamin. *Allergologie*, *6*, 27.
65. Mohsenifar Z, Lehrman S, Carson SA, Tashkin D (1982) Two cases of allergy to aminophylline. *Ann. Allerg.*, *49*, 281.
66. Nierenberg DW, Glazener FS (1982) Aminophylline-induced exfoliative dermatitis: cause and implications. *West. J. Med.*, *137*, 328.
67. Mathewson HS (1982) Intravenous aminophylline: a dangerous therapeutic weapon. *Respir. Care*, *27*, 713.
68. Laursen LC, Johannesson N, Dirksen A et al (1983) Enprofylline – effects of a new bronchodilating xanthine derivative in asthmatic patients. *Allergy*, *38*, 75.
69. Douglas JG, Munro JF (1982) Drug treatment and obesity. *Pharm. Ther.*, *18*, 351.
70. Kew MC, Hopp M, Rothberg A (1982) Fatal heat-stroke in a child taking appetite-suppressant drugs. *S. Afr. Med. J.*, *62*, 905.
71. Douglas JG, Preston PG, Gough J et al (1983) Long-term efficacy of fenfluramine in treatment of obesity. *Lancet*, *1*, 384.
72. Gaul G, Blazek G, Deutsch E et al (1982) Ein Fall von chronischer pulmonaler Hypertonie nach Fenfluramineeinnahme. *Wien. Klin. Wochenschr.*, *94*, 618.
73. Pietrusko R, Stunkard A, Brownwell K (1982) Plasma fenfluramine levels, weight loss and side effects: a failure to find a relationship. *Int. J. Obesity*, *6*, 567.
74. Noble RE (1982) Phenylpropanolamine and blood pressure. *Lancet*, *1*, 1419.
75. Howrie DL, Wolfson JH et al (1982) Phenylpropanolamine-induced hypertension. *J. Pediatr.*, *102*, 143.
76. Hamer R, Phelps D (1981) Inadvertent intra-arterial injection of phentaramine: a complication of drug abuse. *Ann. Emerg. Med.*, *10*, 148 (45).
77. Jecht E (1983) Ergotismus-ähnliche Reaktion auf Arzneimittel- und Nikotinabusus. *Z. Hautkr.* *58*, 33.
78. Park GD et al (1983) Theophylline overdose. Treatment with charcoal haemoperfusion. *Am. J. Med.*, *74*, 961.
79. Clark JE, Devenport JK (1983) Theophylline

exacerbating spasticity. *J. Am. Med. Assoc., 250,* 485.
80. McEwen J (1983) Phenylpropanolamine-associated hypertension after the use of 'over-the-counter' appetite-suppressant products. *Med. J. Aust., 2,* 71.
81. Frewin DB (1983) Phenylpropanolamine. How safe is it? *Med. J. Aust., 2,* 54.
82. Wilson JD, Sutherland DC (1982) Combined beta agonists and methylxanthines in asthma. *N. Engl. J. Med., 307,* 1707.
83. Isles AF, Newth CJL (1983) Combined beta agonists and methylxanthines in asthma. *N. Engl. J. Med., 309* (letter to the editor).

Barry Blackwell

2 Antidepressant drugs

TRICYCLIC ANTIDEPRESSANTS

Sexual dysfunction

A review of the literature (1[R]) regarding sexual dysfunction due to antidepressant drugs in men draws a distinction between *erectile dysfunction, ejaculatory problems* and *changes in libido.* A complicating factor is the lack of information concerning the base rate of these problems due to depression itself. The review draws on both published findings and reports provided by the pharmaceutical manufacturers with regard to tricyclic antidepressants. Impotence due to loss of erectile function has been reported in at least 30 cases involving most of the commonly used tricyclic compounds in the low normal dose ranges. A recent review adds additional reports attributable to low dosage (75 mg daily or less) of clomipramine (2[C]).

Delayed and occasionally painful ejaculation appears to occur with a similar frequency across the same range of drugs. Both increased and decreased libido has been reported but it is virtually impossible to distinguish drug relatedness from the natural history of the condition. A small number of uncontrolled studies have reported therapeutic benefits due to antidepressant medication in patients with premature ejaculation or disturbed sexual function accompanied by clinical depression (3[C]).

The mechanism of action mediating the sexual dysfunction is controversial. One article (2[C]) discusses adrenergic mechanisms while another invokes the anticholinergic system and suggests (4[C]) taking physostigmine 15 mg 1 hour before intercourse to reverse ejaculatory dysfunction.

In addition to these reports of sexual dysfunction in men, delay of orgasm has also been reported in *women* (5[C], 2[C]). Similar reports of sexual dysfunction have occurred due to MAO inhibitors (SEDA-5, 19; 1[R]).

Skin

Skin rashes are so common that it is difficult to determine a cause and effect relationship to drug treatment. A choice must be made between waiting to see if the rash clears despite continued treatment or switching to a different compound and, if necessary, rechallenging the patient at a later date. Skin reactions to tricyclic antidepressants which have been reported include *cutaneous vasculitis, urticaria* and *photosensitivity.* The risk of allergic reactions is reported to be somewhat higher with amitriptyline than with imipramine.

Two case reports (6[C]) of skin rashes suggest that *cross allergenicity* does not necessarily occur to structurally related tricyclic compounds. One patient developed a pruritic maculopapular rash after 14 days treatment with desipramine 100 mg daily and was subsequently switched to thioridazine 100 mg daily without recurrence. A second patient was treated with amitriptyline 75 mg daily; after a few days she developed a pruritic maculopapular rash which cleared but reappeared when the patient was rechallenged a month later. As a result the patient was switched to imipramine 75 mg which she took for over 6 months with no dermatologic problems.

Hearing

Another example of an unwanted effect to appear after prolonged availability of a particular type of drug is the *tinnitus* recently reported to occur during treatment of tricyclic antidepressants. An early trial of imipramine (7[C]) reported 2 cases of transient deafness but in the subsequent 20 years no auditory manifestations were recorded. In 1980 a report appeared (8[Cr]) concerning

Side Effects of Drugs Annual 8
M.N.G. Dukes, editor

ISBN 0 444 90339 9
$0.80 per article per page (transactional system)
$0.20 per article per page (licensing system)

4 patients all treated with imipramine in daily dosages below 150 mg. Each patient complained of buzzing or ringing in the ears. In each case the symptoms improved or disappeared on dose reduction with maintenance of therapeutic benefit and in one instance the patient was switched to an equivalent dosage of desipramine without a recurrence.

A further case report (9[C]) concerned a patient treated with protriptyline 45 mg daily who developed ringing in both ears after 12 days of treatment. The symptom severity decreased with dosage reduction and disappeared entirely after desipramine (100 mg daily) was substituted. The authors of this report speculate on the possible mechanism and postulate a non-vibratory tinnitus originating from either neurological factors or changes in blood flow.

The possibility that changes in hearing are reflections of alterations in blood pressure and flow to the inner ear is discussed in a further case report (10[C]). A 42-year-old woman responded well to amitriptyline 100 mg daily. After 4 weeks she developed tinnitus in the right ear and otologic testing revealed hypacusis for low frequencies. Because blood pressure was low (100/60 mm Hg) she was given an infusion of volume-expanding low-molecular dextran. The symptom disappeared and her blood pressure returned to normal. Despite a reduction in dosage of amitriptyline to 75 mg the symptom recurred accompanied again by hypotension. Both were again successfully treated with dextran and the patient was switched to mianserin without any subsequent auditory symptoms or changes in blood pressure.

Another unusual disturbance of hearing has been reported in a child being treated with tricyclics. Auditory acuity was normal, but *discriminative ability for both clear and distorted speech* was depressed. The disorder cleared within some days of the withdrawal of the drug (11[C]).

Withdrawal

The evidence for a withdrawal syndrome due to abrupt discontinuation of tricyclic antidepressants is now more compelling (SEDA-5, 16). Its significance is heightened by the increasing tendency to prescribe such drugs either as 'maintenance' therapy or for 'prophylaxis' against future episodes. If withdrawal effects are a reality the distinction between dependency and prophylaxis may be difficult to draw.

A review of the previous literature (12[CR]) concludes that reports have involved both imipramine and doxepin. Symptoms occur as early as the morning following a missed dose (13[C]) but more often after 48 hours and up to 2 weeks following discontinuation. They include *anxiety, restlessness, diaphoresis, diarrhea, hot or cold flashes* and *piloerection*. A case of *delirium* following discontinuation has been reported (14[C]) as well as instances of *mania* (15[CR]).

The existence of a withdrawal syndrome was subjected to a controlled test (12[CR]) in 7 patients who had been maintained on chronic administration of amitriptyline (up to 250 mg daily), imipramine (200 mg daily) or desipramine (250 mg daily). After 4 weeks of supervised drug taking, a placebo was substituted under double blind conditions for between 10 and 21 days. There were *increases in both plasma and urine MHPG levels* beginning within 36 hours and reaching a peak 3 weeks after discontinuation which averaged 74% above the baseline. Despite this pronounced neurochemical change there were no alterations in pulse rate or heart beat and only 2 patients experienced clear increases in anxiety.

This report indicates that there is clearly a need for larger controlled studies to determine the incidence and severity of withdrawal effects following cessation of tricyclic treatment. Based on uncontrolled observations it has been suggested that the incidence varies from under a quarter to over a half of patients.

A report of 3 cases (16[Cr]) has suggested that central cholinergic overactivity is implicated and atropine sulfate (3 mg daily) or synthetic anticholinergic agents (benztropine mesylate 4 mg daily) were reported to successfully ameliorate withdrawal symptoms within a few hours. The authors suggest that this technique may be especially useful in patients who must be abruptly discontinued from tricyclics because the patient develops an allergic or idiosyncratic reaction to the drug.

Miscellaneous effects

Vasospasm The first case of vasospasm induced by imipramine has been reported in an adult (17[Cr]), though such incidents have been described earlier in children. A woman aged 37 who had responded inadequately to 50–150 mg amitriptyline daily was switched to imipramine in a dose of 150 mg daily. Within 10 days she noticed marked improvement in her depression, but her hands and feet became cold and turned blue several times a day, each episode lasting from 5 minutes to several hours; she also complained of severe pain radiating up both arms, and during these episodes her radial pulse was found to diminish. The causal link was confirmed by two periods of rechallenge with the drug, the latter in a 75 mg daily dose. There was recovery from the complications some weeks after final withdrawal of imipramine.

Treatment of overdosage Some doubt is thrown on the value of activated charcoal for the treatment of tricyclic overdosage by a report on 48 cases admitted for suspected tricyclic poisoning; 28 received only supportive care whilst the remaining 20 received in addition activated charcoal (18[C]). There was no difference in clinical benefit or the rate of fall of plasma drug concentration between the two groups. It is doubtful, however, whether this report provides sufficient justification for abandoning activated charcoal as an added measure in such cases, particularly since 18 of the patients were subsequently found not to have taken tricyclic antidepressants after all.

Second generation effects A report from Kuwait relates to a woman who had taken both clomipramine and chlordiazepoxide (as well as long acting penicillin) during a great part of her pregnancy (19[Cr]). She delivered a mentally retarded baby with microcephaly, strabismus and congenital hypothyroidism. Thyroid function in the mother was normal. The question as to whether tricyclic drugs may be teratogenic in a small proportion of births (SED-9, 28) remains unanswered; certainly no clear pattern of deformities has emerged and many cases are impossible to analyze because, as in this instance, various other drugs have been taken concurrently.

INTERACTIONS WITH TRICYCLIC ANTIDEPRESSANTS

Alcohol

Patients taking antidepressants are usually cautioned to avoid alcohol because of assumed *additive effects* on cognitive function. A recent review (20[R]) discusses studies performed on non MAOI antidepressants in normal volunteers using a variety of neuropsychological and performance tests. Included in these studies are four which have shown enhanced impairment due to alcohol. The drugs involved have included imipramine (50 mg dose), amitriptyline (up to 75 mg daily), nortriptyline (up to 25 mg daily) and clomipramine (25 mg daily) and doxepin. A recent study (21[C]) compared single doses of placebo, zimeldine (200 mg) or amitriptyline (75 mg) in 6 normal volunteers given ethanol (50 g). The combination of amitriptyline and ethanol produced a marked increase in body sway suggesting additive effects. Zimelidine showed no changes alone or in combination with alcohol.

These adverse interactions have occurred in normal volunteers taking low dosages of drugs and relatively small amounts of alcohol. The risks are obviously higher in patients taking larger amounts whose attention and concentration may already be impaired by depression and some of whom may be at increased risk for alcohol ingestion.

A Japanese study (22[C]) reports the interaction of alcohol and single 20 mg doses of amitriptyline or imipramine in 6 healthy male volunteers. The levels of alcohol in blood and urine were slightly increased after imipramine but not amitriptyline with considerable variability between subjects. The serum concentrations of amitriptyline and its active metabolite were decreased while those of imipramine as its active metabolite were remarkably increased in 3 out of 5 subjects. This study highlights the complex nature of the problem. Not only may additive impairment occur (mediated at the receptor rather than plasma level) but alcohol may modify the metabolism of antidepressants in ways that could alter their therapeutic and toxic effects.

Other psychotropic drugs

Increasing evidence for non-therapeutic interactions between tricyclic compounds and other psychotropic drugs was reviewed previously (SEDA-7, 18). Further evidence has been added from other sources.

A study (23[C]) comparing 99 patients receiving amitriptyline or nortriptyline alone with 60 patients receiving one of these drugs in combination with *perphenazine* (mean dose 9.8 ± 3.2 mg/day) showed an increase in antidepressant plasma levels of up to 70%.

An analysis (24[C]) of adverse reactions in 84 patients taking desipramine (2.5 mg/kg) found that age over 60 and concurrent use of *antipsychotic medication* were significantly associated with major adverse reactions. The incidence was only 8% of those on desipramine alone compared to 32% (11 out of 34 patients) in those receiving antipsychotic medication (mostly perphenazine or haloperidol). In this study also the mean steady state plasma levels were almost double (227.7 ng/ml) in patients on a combination compared to those on desipramine alone (121.7 ng/ml).

Further evidence of a toxic interaction between *benzodiazepines* and tricyclic antidepressants is provided by an analysis of fatalities due to overdose (25[C]). Fifty deaths due to amitriptyline only were compared to 24 deaths due to combination of amitriptyline with a variety of benzodiazepines. In the absence of benzodiazepines 50% of the amitriptyline deaths were associated with blood levels up to 4.3 mg/l. In the presence of a benzodiazepine this concentration accounted for over 75% of deaths.

Sympathomimetic amines

We have previously reviewed the synergistic action of tricyclic antidepressants with a variety of sympathomimetic amines (SEDA-1, 11; SEDA-6, 19). Two further examples of this type of interaction have been reported.

Four patients undergoing nasal surgery (26[C]) who experienced massive vasodilation, significant intraoperative bleeding and rapid loss of anesthetic effect had all been taking low dosage tricyclic antidepressants (100 mg or less of imipramine or doxepin daily) for long periods (over 2 years). The authors speculate that these adverse effects are mediated by the action of tricyclic antidepressants in blocking the vasoconstrictor postsynaptic α_1 receptors thus allowing an unopposed, excessive vasodilatory effect of *adrenaline* in the local anesthetic on β_2 receptors. They recommend that tricyclic antidepressants be discontinued for 7 to 14 days prior to surgery. This conflicts with a previous suggestion (SEDA-3, 14) that it is always safer to continue tricyclic antidepressants in patients about to undergo general anesthesia. This recommendation should be modified to account for the nature of the surgery and the type of local anesthesia to be used.

Another related interaction has been reported with *levodopa* (27[C]). An 82-year-old woman was treated for Parkinson's disease with Sinemet 110 (levodopa 100 mg, carbidopa 10 mg) two tablets thrice daily. Imipramine 75 mg daily was added for depression and 2 days later the patient developed a pulse rate of 132, blood pressure of 210/110 mm Hg (previously 150/80 mm Hg); severe agitation, tremor and rigidity. Signs and symptoms disappeared within 24 hours of stopping imipramine but recurred when amitriptyline in the same dose was inadvertently administered. The author speculates that the tricyclic antidepressant sensitized peripheral receptors to the dopamine produced from the levodopa and that the amount of carbidopa in the combination was inadequate to block peripheral oxidative deamination of the amino acid.

SECOND GENERATION ANTIDEPRESSANTS

The end of zimelidine?

As of September 1983, the Astra company withdrew its antidepressant zimelidine worldwide; at that time it had been introduced in five European countries only and given to an estimated 200,000 patients (28[r]). Zimelidine, as pointed out in SEDA-7 (p. 22), appeared to have a markedly different adverse reaction profile to the tricyclic antidepressant drugs, though at that moment it still required further definition. By May

1983, the Swedish Adverse Drug Reactions Advisory Committee had issued a Bulletin drawing attention to the occurrence of hypersensitivity reactions, which had also been observed during the phase of clinical trials. They included fever, headache, muscle or joint pains and liver reactions; as a rule the reactions occurred within 4 weeks after the start of treatment.

As more information accumulated, it became clear that further complications could occur in such cases. To cite literally a statement issued by the Swedish National Board of Health and Welfare on September 16th 1983:

'Since that time more reports have been received about hypersensitivity reactions, some of which in a few cases have been connected with neurological complications like serious meningitis, polyradiculitis or isolated facial paralysis. Particularly serious are an increasing number of reports regarding polyneuropathies where 8 patients have developed polyradiculitis of the Guillain-Barré type with sensory loss and/or motorial loss. All 8 patients developed 'hypersensitivity' reactions 1 to 3 weeks after start of treatment and polyradiculitis about 2 to 14 days later' (29[R]).

At approximately the same time, the British Department of Health and Social Security was aware of 400 reports of adverse reactions to the drug, which in Great Britain had been the subject of an estimated 100,000 prescriptions (30[r]). Four patients had died, though causal links had not necessarily been established.

Zimelidine was first reviewed in these volumes as long ago as 1980 on the basis of early clinical work (SEDA-4, 19). The events of 1983 remind us with what rapidity, following the introduction onto the market, serious adverse events may emerge which lead to the withdrawal of a new compound and which had failed to be identified before that time despite extensive clinical studies; it is clear that the processes of investigation and regulation still can leave serious gaps in our knowledge of adverse events.

Amoxapine

A major review (31[R]) of this compound and its pharmacology concludes that it is similar in clinical efficacy and potency to standard tricyclic compounds with a sedative action intermediate between amitriptyline and imipramine. As previously noted in these volumes, however, (SEDA-4, 21; SEDA-5, 17) amoxapine has a tricyclic nucleus with a modified piperazine side chain and is closely related to the neuroleptic loxapine. In animal studies amoxapine has no antiserotoninergic properties and less anticholinergic activity than prototype drugs. Peak plasma levels are achieved in less than two hours and the half lives of the parent drug and its two active metabolites are 8, 6 and 30 hours.

Amoxapine is less potent than other tricyclic antidepressants with a therapeutic dose range of 75 to 600 mg daily (usual doses 200 to 400 mg daily). Clinical effects have not been consistently correlated with plasma levels but the compound shows comparable efficacy to other tricyclics in heterogenous populations of depressed patients. Controlled comparisons show its clinical profile to be very similar to imipramine (32[C]) and somewhat less sedative than amitriptyline (33[C], 34[C], 35[C]). In two of these studies (33[C], 35[C]) results confirmed the suggestion of a somewhat earlier onset of action.

Amoxapine appears to share the same commonly occurring side effects as other tricyclic compounds including those attributable to anticholinergic activity. Its structural similarity to the neuroleptic compounds however appears to confer an additional hazard of side effects usually found in that category of drugs such as galactorrhea and extrapyramidal disorders.

A 23-year-old woman treated with amoxapine for 2 weeks with up to 300 mg daily (36[C]) developed *galactorrhoea.* The symptoms subsided 2 weeks after the drug was withdrawn and the authors speculate that the effect is related to the compound's chemical relationship to the neuroleptic agents. A 29-year-old woman treated with amoxapine 300 mg daily (37[C]) developed *scanty menstruation* and secretion of breast milk after 2 weeks' treatment. Symptoms disappeared when the drug was stopped and reappeared when treatment was initiated following relapse. Serum prolactin levels increased towards the upper limits of normal during drug treatment and peaked well above the normal level following 100 mg of amoxapine (but not after two divided 50 mg doses). These observations suggest that the drug may have dopamine-blocking activity to the tuberoinfundibular pathway.

A typical *dystonic reaction* occurred in a 27-year-old man receiving 600 mg for 2 days and a possible malignant neuroleptic syndrome in a 45-year-old man treated with up to 400 mg amoxapine for over 2 weeks (38[C]). This second patient was also treated concurrently with haloperidol 10 mg daily, another potent antidopaminergic compound.

In a study of its potential neuroleptic properties (39[Cr]) amoxapine and its metabolite, 7-hydroxyamoxapine, were found to show potent neuroleptic activity using a radioreceptor assay both in vivo and using plasma drawn from patients receiving treatment with neuroleptics or antidepressants. Patients receiving amoxapine had comparable neuroleptic activity to those receiving loxapine while none of the other tricyclic antidepressants showed this property (amitriptyline, nortriptyline, imipramine and desipramine). The authors caution, as we have done, (SEDA-5, 17) about the potential for causing *tardive dyskinesia* with prolonged administration. The first such case has now been reported (40[C]). A 60-year-old woman with a major depressive disorder was treated initially with amoxapine 150 mg daily. After 3 months this dose was increased to 250 mg and maintained for a further 5 months. At this time she was noted to have a chronic buccolingual dyskinesia of 2 months duration which became somewhat less intense 5 months after cessation of treatment with amoxapine. There was no history of ever having received a neuroleptic.

The *cardiotoxicity* and *lethality in overdose* of amoxapine is still not fully defined. In carefully selected clinical trial populations it showed tachycardia and hypotension similar to other tricyclic compounds with no serious cardiac complications (31[R]).

In 3 earlier cases (31[R]) patients who took up to 2700 mg recovered but 2 had *epileptic seizures.* Two young women who ingested up to four g of amoxapine (41[C]) presented with *coma*, multiple seizures and *metabolic acidosis* with residual evidence of neurologic damage 1 to 3 months after overdose. It is unclear whether these effects are directly attributable to the drug or secondary to the severe acidosis and its management. A long term follow-up of one of these cases (42[C]) reports that the patient recovered from coma after 3 weeks and showed progressive neurologic recovery for a further 3 months. At this time there were still marked deficits in cerebellar, memory, and speech functions which presented until discharge from hospital after 7 months. Another 5 cases of overdose (43[C]) in patients taking 6 g of amoxapine all recovered without sequelae (including a 6-year-old child who took an undetermined amount). All 5 patients developed generalized seizures that were successfully controlled with intravenous diazepam or phenytoin sodium and all showed central nervous system depression. Except for sinus tachycardia the continuous ECG recordings revealed no evidence of serious cardiotoxicity.

The manufacturers report (44[c]) that 91 cases of overdose have occurred. Consistent with its lower potency the minimum lethal dose of 2.5 g is somewhat higher than the lethal dose of other tricyclic compounds. No instances of cardiotoxicity or of EKG changes (other than tachycardia) have occurred but epileptic seizures are reported in up to half the patients. *Renal toxicity* occurred in 9 patients (10%) of whom 2 died.

A case report (45[C]) provides details of a 39-year-old woman who ingested 5 g of amoxapine. Clinical details were scanty but urine output remained below 400 ml/day for 2 days. The presence of a serum creatinine phosphokinase of over 50,000 U led to a diagnosis of rhabdomyolysis and acute renal failure (although urine myoglobin was negative). Renal dialysis was instituted with full recovery. The authors speculate that muscle toxicity or renal damage may have been due either to a direct action of amoxapine or induced secondary to convulsions.

Overall amoxapine appears to have the major advantage over other tricyclic compounds of possible earlier onset of action and relative freedom from serious cardiotoxic effects. Its major drawbacks are its potential for inducing neuroleptic side effects, and in overdose a high incidence of seizures with the possibility of long term neurologic and renal damage.

Agranulocytosis What appears to be the first case of agranulocytosis due to amoxapine was reported in 1983 (46[C]) in a 42-year-old woman who received 50 mg amoxapine daily for 65 days before being hospitalized for signs and symptoms which proved to be due to a severe agranulocytosis with a white blood cell count of 200/mm^3. After withdrawal of the drug and intensive treatment recovery was complete. The nature of the symptoms strongly suggested an allergic mechanism.

Rx

Bupropion

Background *Bupropion is a compound synthesized and tested exclusively in the United States during the past 10 years and reported to be on the verge of approval by the F.D.A. Very little had been published on the compound until the recent appearance of a complete issue of the Journal of Clinical Psychiatry (May 1983, 5 (2)) which was devoted to reports from investigators and to the manufacturer's compilations of pharmacological, clinical and side effect data.*

Bupropion is a substituted chloropropriophenone of the amino ketone class with a single benzene ring and three carbon aliphatic side chains that give it a structure reminiscent of stimulant and anorectic drugs such as diethylpropion. The nature of the molecular substitutions is intended to provide the compound with antidepressant actions and protect it from undesirable stimulant properties (47[C]). In animal toxicology studies bupropion overdose conditions were associated with central nervous stimulation and convulsions, and chronic administration produced mild reversible hepatotoxicity and anemia (48[C]).

Preclinical pharmacologic testing in animal models revealed a profile of mild stimulant properties and a specific but atypical antidepressant effect with a selective action on dopamine uptake in rat brain synaptosomes compared to tricyclic compounds which preferentially inhibit noradrenaline and serotonin uptake. Unlike sympathomimetic amines, bupropion does not increase the release of catecholamines from synaptosomes. Animal testing also suggested absence of anticholinergic and weak cardiodepressant properties (49[C], 50[C]). Of particular interest is the fact that bupropion does not produce down regulation of postsynaptic β receptors, a mechanism recently invoked to explain antidepressant actions.

In animals and normal volunteers bupropion is rapidly absorbed with peak plasma concentrations within two hours (51[C]).

Clinical reports *Bupropion has been evaluated in doses ranging from 300 to 750 mg daily given in a 3 times daily regimen for periods of up to 6 months (52[R]). Plasma concentrations vary 10-fold in patients receiving the same dose and appear unrelated to dosage or age (53[C]). Antidepressant response was correlated with steady state bupropion levels in a curvilinear fashion with a narrow therapeutic window between 75–100 ng/ml of drug.*

In comparisons with placebo bupropion was significantly superior in 3 out of 5 studies analyzed separately (54[C]). There was a noticeable absence of sedation and the most frequent drug related side effect was dry mouth (13% of patients) with fewer patients also reporting constipation and blurred vision. Stimulant side effects (excitement, increased motor activity, toxic confusional state) occurred in about 3% of patients. The only other drug related side effects were nausea and vomiting (4%), faintness or dizziness (6.4%) and skin rashes (2.7%).

In an uncontrolled study of 380 depressed outpatients (55[C]) treated in general medical practice in dosages from 150 to 450 mg daily 41 patients (11%) dropped out with side effects. Dry mouth occurred in 25% of patients and constipation in 11%. Insomnia, agitation and decreased appetite and nausea occurred in about 15% of the population.

Given the absence of sedative actions, relatively low incidence of anticholinergic activity and mildly stimulant side effect profile, it is interesting that all except one comparative controlled study has been against amitriptyline which is among the most sedating and anticholinergic tricyclic compounds. This strategy has the effect of maximizing the allegedly 'unique' properties of bupropion but also restricts the generalizability of conclusions based on the comparison.

In a double blind controlled comparison of bupropion (450 to 750 mg daily) and amitriptyline (75 to 225 mg daily) in 40 depressed patients (56[C]) the tricyclic antidepressant was more effective at days 7 and 14 but not after 21 or 28 days suggesting a slower onset of action with bupropion. Despite the alleged freedom from anticholinergic activity constipation occurred with equal frequency in 41% and 39% of patients receiving bupropion and amitriptyline. Dry mouth occurred in 64% and 89% of the two groups respectively and blurred vision in 36% and 72%.

In contrast the CNS effects of the two compounds differed markedly. Amitriptyline produced sedation in 61% compared to 4% on bupropion. However, bupropion patients reported tremor (31%), agitation (14%)

and hallucinations (9%). The latter were tactile in nature.

In a 6 center study 124 depressed outpatients (57[C]) were treated with either amitriptyline 75 or 150 mg at night or bupropion 300 or 450 mg in divided doses. Despite the different drug regimens the two drugs showed comparable overall efficacy after 6 weeks (much or very much improvement in 74% of patients on bupropion and 79% of those on amitriptyline). However, after one week of treatment there were trends in favor of more rapid response to amitriptyline on all 6 rating scales used. Eight patients on bupropion (11%) dropped out of the study (compared to 7% on amitriptyline) with complaints of skin rash (4 patients), anorexia, dizziness, palpitations, numbness, ataxia and dry mouth.

Another multicenter study (58[C]) involved depressed inpatients and outpatients. In 118 outpatients 300 to 450 mg of bupropion in a divided schedule was compared with 75 to 150 mg of amitriptyline at night. These regimens are not equivalent, the dose ranges differ and the mean maximum dose of bupropion is comparatively higher. In addition 30% of bupropion patients required sedative hypnotics for anxiety and insomnia compared to only 17% of amitriptyline patients. Once again both drugs performed comparably well after 6 weeks but trends in favor of more rapid response to amitriptyline are present until then in all 6 rating scales.

In the inpatient part of the same study, 92 depressed patients were treated with either bupropion 300 to 750 mg daily or amitriptyline 75 to 225 mg daily for 6 weeks. The final outcome for both drugs was a comparable and significant decrease in depression but bupropion patients were consistently more depressed throughout the first 4 weeks and the early termination rates were significantly higher with 20% of bupropion patients dropping out compared to 8% of amitriptyline patients. Autonomic and anticholinergic side effects were quite frequent in both groups and one bupropion treated patient developed urinary retention. Agitation and excitement was common with bupropion and fatigue or tiredness with amitriptyline. Increase in appetite was commoner with amitriptyline and decrease or nausea with bupropion.

Two studies of bupropion have been completed in patients aged 55 or over. In one study (59[C]) 63 patients received either placebo, imipramine 25 mg daily, bupropion 150 mg daily or bupropion 300 mg daily. All active treatments produced similar and satisfactory clinical improvement after 4 weeks although the effects of low dose bupropion were slower in onset and less pronounced throughout. Imipramine produced significantly more nervousness, fatigue, tremor, dry mouth and constipation than either bupropion or placebo.

In another study (60[C]) 38 older patients were treated with either imipramine 75–200 mg daily, placebo, bupropion 150 mg daily or bupropion 300–450 mg daily for 4 weeks. Imipramine patients reported significantly less dry mouth than patients receiving low dose but not high dose bupropion.

Since the symposium at which these results were presented was held, there has been one other published report concerning bupropion (61[C]). Twelve hospitalized depressed patients who received bupropion at a mean daily dose of 561 mg (±120 mg) for 3–12 days were compared with 12 patients receiving conventional antidepressants (150 mg or more daily for 2 weeks) and 12 drug-free controls. Six patients on bupropion developed such severe perceptual changes that drug dosage had to be lowered or discontinued. The prominent subjective effects were alteration in time sense, increased sensitivity to sensory stimuli and vivid dreaming. The authors speculate that the mechanism involved may be related to bupropion actions on dopamine metabolism and they compare and contrast the changes with those attributed to L-dopa and LSD. It is interesting that although all patients met DSM-III criteria for affective disorders, the 3 who displayed the most disturbances had previously been diagnosed as schizophrenic.

Cardiotoxicity *A number of studies have been directed towards specific concerns that relate to the cardiotoxic and epileptogenic potential of bupropion which will be relevant to future overdose experience.*

Twelve patients who had previously developed orthostatic hypotension (62[C]) on tricyclic antidepressants (mean systolic drop of 32.4 mm Hg) were placed on bupropion 300 mg increasing progressively to 600 mg daily in a single blind fashion following a placebo baseline. Overall the group of patients showed no significant changes in pulse rate or falls in blood pressure compared to placebo but 3 individual patients developed systolic blood pressure decreases of 10, 14 and 33 mm Hg, the largest of which was associated with symptoms (headache and sweating). Another study (63[C]) compared the EKG profiles of 46 male patients half of whom were treated with bupropion (mean dose 552 mg) and the remainder with amitriptyline (mean dose 151 mg). Rhythm strips obtained from 1 to 3 times during 6 weeks of treatment were analyzed to define average values. Patients receiving amitriptyline showed significant increases compared to post treatment baseline in PR interval and QRS duration with decrease in QRS height. There were no significant changes in patients on bupropion. Finally the manufacturers have analyzed the cardiovascular profile of bupropion based on data in 700 patients including 5 patients who took overdoses (64[C]). Analysis of the large pool of patients showed no significant changes in pulse rate or blood pressure with either bupropion or amitriptyline. In the overdose sample the patients ingested between 900 and 3000 mg (up to 6 times the average therapeutic dose). No significant cardiovascular or other effects were noted and all 5 patients recovered. The manufacturers note that the substantial size of bupropion tablets (larger than 10 mm diameter) may deter patients from large overdoses.

Seizures *Ten patients treated with bupropion in clinical trials have developed epileptic seizures (65[C]). Four of these were on dosages of 750 mg or more daily, 5 on 600 mg daily and 1 on 450 mg daily. The clinical data is consistent with the animal toxicity (48[C]) suggesting that bupropion in high dosages will lower seizure threshold. In an extensive and useful analysis of the world literature on epileptic seizures in tricyclic antidepressants the authors (65[C]) conclude that the incidence is 1 in 200 for patients receiving over 200 mg daily and 1 in 1,000 to 2,000 for dose levels of tricyclic antidepressant below this level. The risks for bupropion appear comparable and are also dose related.*

Abuse risk *An obvious concern with bupropion has been its potential for amphetamine-like abuse. This concern is based on its chemical structure, its stimulant profile in animal and clinical studies and on findings in animals suggesting that bupropion substituted for amphetamine is a drug discrimination task and was self-administered intravenously by monkeys (66[Cr]). A study to evaluate this aspect was carried out on 13 male volunteers using the Addiction Research Center methodology and scales (66[Cr]). Subjects were given placebo, d-amphetamine 15 or 30 mg and bupropion 100, 200 or 400 mg in a double blind randomized schedule. Bupropion did not differ significantly from placebo in this study and was clearly discriminated from amphetamine. However, the data suggest a dose dependent increase in the tendency to identify bupropion as amphetamine as well as increases in the LSD and morphine-benzedrine scales. While these changes are small and not statistically significant they suggest that higher dosages of bupropion should be subjected to similar scrutiny. In another experiment (67[C]) in normal volunteers bupropion 100 mg abolished the drowsiness and vigilance impairment caused by diazepam 2.5 and 5 mg and produced a similar but less clearcut action in reversing the effects of alcohol. Comparisons with d-amphetamine (5 and 10 mg), amitriptyline (25 mg) and bupropion (50 and 100 mg) showed improvement in auditory vigilance and finger tapping with amphetamine, impairment with amitriptyline and no change with bupropion. Overall these results do suggest some stimulant action that is apparent against an obtunded baseline but it might require higher dose levels to reveal effects due to the drug alone.*

Weight loss *A final suggestion of stimulant properties is a consistent tendency across clinical trials to produce weight loss rather than the traditional weight gain experienced with tricyclic antidepressants. Data pooled from these studies and analyzed by the manufacturer (68[C]) reveal an average weight loss of between 1 and 2 pounds during 4 weeks or more of treatment with bupropion (50–750 mg daily) compared to an increase of 3 to 9 pounds during treatment for equivalent periods due to amitriptyline (75–225 mg daily). The authors suggest that this weight loss due to bupropion may be caused by a combination of subtle changes in decreased food intake, enhanced levels of basal metabolism or increased physical activity (compared to a decrease with sedative tricyclic compounds).*

Conclusion *Overall the data on bupropion suggest that it is an effective antidepressant but with several limitations. It appears to have a somewhat narrow dose range (300 to 750 mg daily) with a tendency to slower* *onset of action compared to amitriptyline. It is not suitable for once daily administration and the absence of sedative effects may require adjunctive hypnotic drug use in significant numbers of patients. Compared to amitriptyline it has fewer anticholinergic side effects but it is not free of these actions and only further studies compared to other less anticholinergic tricyclic compounds will elucidate this claim. Bupropion also causes stimulant effects such as agitation, excitement, insomnia and weight loss. Skin rashes and gastrointestinal disturbances may also occur. In high dosages (over 400 mg daily) one study reports dissociative experiences, especially in patients with a history of schizophrenia. In overdose bupropion has a reduced tendency to cause cardiotoxicity but is equivalent to tricyclic compounds in lowering seizure threshold.*

In its clinical and pharmacologic profile bupropion is quite similar to viloxazine (SEDA-1, 12; SEDA-2, 12; SEDA-3, 16), another compound which is structurally distinct from tricyclic antidepressants, has minimal sedative, anticholinergic or adrenergic effects and which seems to have some central stimulant actions that are possibly due to a selective action on dopaminergic neurones without all the undesirable or addictive potential of amphetamines. The clinical utility of such compounds may be somewhat narrow compared to the tricyclic drugs since viloxazine has been available in Britain for over 5 years but is not widely utilized compared to the older more sedative compounds; in many other countries it has not been licenced at all.

OTHER SECOND-GENERATION ANTIDEPRESSANTS

Femoxetine and Paroxetine These two structurally similar drugs are currently in the phase of research; both are serotonin-uptake inhibitors. It has been claimed that femoxetine will alleviate depression without causing sedation or anticholinergic side-effects. Unless wrongly quoted in the press, the licensee appears to have claimed that the drug has potential for producing cardiovascular side effects; one must assume that the original statement was the reverse of that ultimately printed! (69[r])

Nomifensine A recent report describes a lupus-like syndrome in a woman of 60 who had been taking 100 mg nomifensine daily for nine months. The condition responded to withdrawal of the drug and cortisone treatment (70[C]).

Mianserin The marked safety of mianserin in cases of severe overdosage again appears clear from a Norwegian report on four cases of attempted suicide who had taken doses ranging from 1.2 to 2.5 grams; all were women aged between 20 and 35, and all recovered uneventfully without experiencing serious changes in the level of consciousness, hypotension or ECG alterations (71[CR]).

REFERENCES

1. Mitchell JE, Popkin MK (1983) Antidepressant drug therapy and sexual dysfunction in men: A review. *J. Clin. Psychopharmacol., 3,* 76.
2. Quirk KC, Einarson TR (1982) Sexual dysfunction and clomipramine. *Can. J. Psychiatry, 27,* 228.
3. Renshaw DC (1975) Doxepin treatment of sexual dysfunction associated with depression. In: *Sinequan: A Monograph of Clinical Studies.* Excerpta Medica, Amsterdam.
4. Kraupel Taylor F (1972) Loss of libido in depression. *Br. Med. J., 1,* 305.
5. Sathananthan G, Gershon S (1973) Renal damage due to imipramine. *Lancet, 1,* 833.
6. Salem RB, Fischer RG, Horton M (1982) Lack of cross-allergenicity between tricyclic antidepressants. *South. Med. J., 75,* 1020.
7. Barker PA, Ashcroft GW, Binns JD (1960) Imipramine in chronic depression. *J. Ment. Sci., 106,* 1447.
8. Racy J, Ward-RAcy EA (1980) Tinnitus in imipramine therapy. *Am. J. Psychiatry, 137,* 854.
9. Evans DL, Golden RN (1981) Protriptyline and tinnitus. *J. Clin. Psychopharmacol., 1,* 404.
10. Fleischhauer J (1982) Acute hypacusis of the inner ear as a result of reduced blood pressure by amitriptyline. A rare complication of the therapy with amitriptyline. *Int. Pharmacopsychiatry, 17,* 123.
11. Smith KE, Reece CA, Kauffman R (1972) Ototoxic reaction associated with use of nortriptyline hydrochloride, case report. *J. Pediatr., 80,* 1046.
12. Charney DS, Heninger GH, Steinberg HL (1982) Abrupt discontinuation of tricyclic

antidepressant drugs: Evidence for noradrenergic activity. *Br. J. Psychiatry, 141,* 377.
13. Stern SL, Mendels J (1980) Withdrawal symptoms during the course of imipramine therapy. *J. Clin. Psychiatry, 41,* 66.
14. Santos AB, McCurdy L (1980) Delirium after abrupt withdrawal from doxepin: Case report. *Am. J. Psychiatry, 137,* 239.
15. Mirin SM, Schatzberg AF, Creasey DE (1981) Hypomania and mania after withdrawal of tricyclic antidepressants. *Am. J. Psychiatry, 138,* 87.
16. DiSalver SC, Feinberg M, Greden JF (1983) Antidepressant withdrawal symptoms treated with anticholinergic drugs. *Am. J. Psychiatry, 140,* 249.
17. Appelbaum PS, Kapoor W, (1983) Imipramine-induced Vasospasm: a case report. *Am. J. Psychiatry, 140,* 913–5.
18. Crome P et al (1983) Tricyclic antidepressant overdose. *Human Toxicol., 2,* 205.
19. Anon (1983) Report on Clomipramine HCl. *Kuwait Univ. Drug Adverse React. Ser., 2,* 14.
20. Thompson PJ, Trimble MR (1982) Non-MAOI antidepressant drugs and cognitive functions: a review. *Psychol. Med., 12,* 539.
21. Scott DB, Fagan D, Tiplady B (1982) Effects of amitriptyline and zimeldine in combination with ethanol. *Psychopharmacology, 76,* 209.
22. Watanabe N, Moroji T, Tada K et al (1982) Interaction of alcohol and tricyclic antidepressants in human. *Jpn. J. Alcohol Drug Depend., 17,* 129.
23. Linnoila M, George L, Guthrie S (1982) Interaction between antidepressants and perphenazine in psychiatric inpatients. *Am. J. Psychiatry, 139,* 1329.
24. Nelson JC, Jatlow PI, Bock J et al (1982) Major adverse reactions during desipramine treatment. *Arch. Gen. Psychiatry, 39,* 1055.
25. King LA (1982) Synergistic effect of benzodiazepines in fatal amitriptyline poisonings. *Lancet, 2,* 982.
26. Schechter GL, Brase DA, Powell J (1982) Adverse effects of tricyclic antidepressants during nasal surgery. *Otolaryngol. Head Neck Surg., 29,* 233.
27. Edwards M (1982) Adverse interaction of levodopa with tricyclic antidepressants. *Practitioner, 226,* 1447.
28. Anon (1983) Astra withdraws Zelmid worldwide. *Scrip, 831,* 1.
29. Anon (1983) Information about withdrawn registration of Zelmid (zimelidine). National Board of Health and Welfare, Uppsala, Sweden, September 16.
30. Anon (1983) Astra's Zelmid statement. *Scrip, 832,* 5.
31. Jue SG, Dawson GW, Brogden RN (1982) Amoxapine: a review of its pharmacology and efficacy in depressed states. *Drugs, 24,* 1.
32. Bagodia VN, Shah LP, Pradan PV, Gada MT (1979) A double-blind controlled study of amoxapine and imipramine in cases of depression. *Curr. Ther. Res., 26,* 417.
33. Sethi BB, Sharma I, Singh H, Metha VK (1979) Amoxapine and amitriptyline: A double-blind study in depressed patients. *Curr. Ther. Res., 25,* 726.
34. Fruensgaard K, Hansen CE, Korsgaard S et al (1979) Amoxapine vs amitriptyline in endogenous depression. *Acta Psychiatr. Scand., 59,* 502.
35. Kaumeier HS, Haase HJ (1980) A double-blind comparison between amoxapine and amitriptyline in depressed patients. *Int. J. Clin. Pharmacol., 18,* 177.
36. Jaffe K, Zisook S (1979) Galactorrhea in a patient treated with amoxapine. *J. Clin. Psychiatry, 39,* 821.
37. Gelenberg AJ, Cooper DS, Doller JC, Maloof F (1979) Galactorrhea and hyperprolactinemia associated with amoxapine therapy. *J. Am. Med. Assoc., 242,* 1900.
38. Steele TE (1982) Adverse reactions suggesting amoxapine induced dopamine blockade. *Am. J. Psychiatry, 139,* 1500.
39. Cohen BM, Harris PQ, Alterman RI, Cole JO (1982) Amoxapine: neuroleptic as well as antidepressant? *Am. J. Psychiatry, 139,* 1165.
40. Lapierre YD, Anderson K (1983) Dyskinesia associated with amoxapine antidepressant therapy: a case report. *Am. J. Psychiatry, 140,* 493.
41. Goldberg MJ, Spector R (1982) Amoxapine overdose: report of two patients with severe neurologic damage. *Am. Intern. Med., 96,* 463.
42. Brown JL, Perry PJ (1982) Amoxapine neurotoxicity: a case report with long term follow up. *Drug Intell. Clin. Pharm., 16,* 404.
43. Kulig K, Rumark BH, Sullivan JB et al (1982) Amoxapine overdose. Coma and seizures without cardiotoxic effects. *J. Am. Med. Assoc., 284,* 1092.
44. Bishop MP, Kilte H (1983) Neurotoxicity and amoxapine overdose: a more reasonable perspective. *Drug Intell. Clin. Pharm., 17,* 131.
45. Abpres K, Shelp WD, Kosseff A, Thomas S (1982) Amoxapine-associated rhabdomyolysis and acute renal failure: case report. *J. Clin. Psychiatry, 43,* 426.
46. Christensen BC (1983) A granulocytosis associated with amoxapine. *Am. J. Psychiatry, 140,* 921.
47. Mehta NB (1983) The chemistry of bupropion. *J. Clin. Psychiatry, 44 (Sec. 2),* 56.
48. Tucker WE Jr (1983) Preclinical toxicology of bupropion: an overview. *J. Clin. Psychiatry, 44 (Sec. 2),* 60.
49. Soroko FE, Maxwell RA (1983) The pharmacologic basis for therapeutic interest in bupropion. *J. Clin. Psychiatry, 44 (Sec. 2),* 67.
50. Ferris RM, Cooper BR, Maxwell RA (1983) Studies of bupropion's mechanism of antidepressant activity. *J. Clin. Psychiatry, 44, (Sec. 2),* 74.
51. Lai AA, Schroeder DH (1983) Clinical phar-

macokinetics of bupropion: a review. *J. Clin. Psychiatry, 44 (Sec. 2)*, 82.

52. Shopsin B (1983) Bupropion: A new clinical profile in the psychobiology of depression. *J. Clin. Psychiatry, 44 (Sec. 2)*, 140.
53. Preskorn SH (1983) Antidepressant response and plasma concentrations of bupropion. *J. Clin. Psychiatry, 44 (Sec. 2)*, 137.
54. Zung WWK (1983) Review of placebo-controlled trials with bupropion. *J. Clin. Psychiatry, 44 (Sec. 2)*, 104.
55. Kirksey DF, Harto-Truax N (1983) Private practice evaluation of the safety and efficacy of bupropion in depressed outpatients. *J. Clin. Psychiatry, 44 (Sec. 2)*, 143.
56. Davidson J, Miller R, Van Wyck Fleet J et al (1983) A double-blind comparison of bupropion and amitriptyline in depressed inpatients. *J. Clin. Psychiatry, 44 (Sec. 2)*, 115.
57. Mendels J, Amin MM, Chouinard G et al (1983) A comparative study of bupropion and amitriptyline in depressed outpatients. *J. Clin. Psychiatry, 44 (Sec. 2)*, 118.
58. Chouinard G (1983) Bupropion and amitriptyline in the treatment of depressed patients. *J. Clin. Psychiatry, 44 (Sec. 2)*, 121.
59. Branconnier RJ, Cole JO, Ghazvinian S et al (1983) Clinical pharmacology of bupropion and imipramine in elderly depressives. *J. Clin. Psychiatry, 44 (Sec. 2)*, 130.
60. Kane JM, Cole K, Sarantakos S et al (1983) Safety and efficacy of bupropion in elderly patients: preliminary observations. *J. Clin. Psychiatry, 44 (Sec. 2)*, 134.
61. Becker RE, Dufresne RL (1983) Perceptual changes with bupropion, a novel antidepressant. *Am. J. Psychiatry, 139*, 1200.
62. Farid FF, Wenger TL, Tsai SY et al (1983) Use of bupropion in patients who exhibit orthostatic hypotension on tricyclic antidepressants. *J. Clin. Psychiatry, 44 (Sec. 2)*, 170.
63. Wenger TL, Cohn JB, Bustrack J (1983) Comparison of the effects of bupropion and amitriptyline on cardiac conduction in depressed patients. *J. Clin. Psychiatry, 44 (Sec. 2)*, 174.
64. Wenger TL, Stern WC (1983) The cardiovascular profile of bupropion. *J. Clin. Psychiatry, 44 (Sec. 2)*, 176.
65. Peck AW, Stern WC, Watkinson C (1983) Incidence of seizures during treatment with tricyclic antidepressant drugs and bupropion. *J. Clin. Psychiatry, 44 (Sec. 2)*, 197.
66. Griffith JD, Carranza J, Griffith C, Miller LL (1983) Bupropion: clinical assay for amphetamine-like abuse potential. *J. Clin. Psychiatry, 44 (Sec. 2)*, 206.
67. Peck AW, Hamilton M (1983) Psychopharmacology of bupropion in normal volunteers. *J. Clin. Psychiatry, 44 (Sec. 2)*, 202.
68. Harto-Truax N, Stern WC, Miller LL et al (1983) Effects of bupropion on body weight. *J. Clin. Psychiatry, 44 (Sec. 2)*, 183.
69. Anon (1983) B-M licenses Ferrosan antidepressant. *Scrip, 832*, 15.
70. Garcia-Morteo O, Maldonado-Cocco JA (1983) Lupus-like syndrome during treatment with nomifensine (Letter). *Arthr. Rheum., 26*, 936.
71. Sirnes PA, Moe TJ, Offergaard S (1983) Fire tilfelle av overdosering med mianserin (Tolvon). *Tidsskr. Nor. Laegeforen, 103*, 1819.

3

Mogens Schou

Lithium

GENERAL

In principle, side effects are those effects of a treatment, usually unwanted, which occur in addition to the wanted effect or effects. In practice the term is often used more loosely by patients and physicians, frequently as a designation for whatever troubles or complaints that may develop during the treatment period and which cannot be indubitably ascribed to the disease. This is particularly relevant in connection with long-term treatment of a chronic or recurrent disease. A recent study (1[C]) compared the prevalence of subjective 'side effects', recorded through completion of a check-list, in 258 control subjects, 65 drug-free depressed in-patients, and 94 lithium-treated out-patients. The drug-free depressed patients reported significantly more side effects (poor memory, dry mouth, drowsiness) than did both the control subjects and the lithium-treated patients. The side effect score was not higher for the patients in lithium treatment than for the controls, and the side effects that did occur in the patients were related to their affective morbidity and personality variables. Patients on lithium complained significantly less of headache and migraine than did control subjects. It may be remembered that lithium administration has been used as a treatment for various kinds of periodic headache.

The findings of that study are somewhat at variance with experiences from another clinic (2[C], 3[C]), where side effects were quite frequent in lithium-treated patients. However, as pointed out in one of the reports (3[C]), this may be related to the lower serum lithium concentrations employed in the former than in the latter clinic (where doses and serum lithium levels have later been reduced). Also other surveys report fairly frequent side effects but at the same time emphasize the usually positive benefit/cost ratio of the treatment (4[C]–6[C]).

A review on somatic side effects of long-term lithium treatment (7[C]) points out that these adverse reactions usually can be prevented, ameliorated or treated through careful selection of patients, employment of lowest effective doses, and close monitoring of the patients. Elderly persons should not be deprived of well indicated lithium treatment, but certain special precautions must be taken in order to avoid unpleasantness and risk (8[R], 9[R]).

Side effects of lithium treatment are dealt with in considerable detail in recently published guidelines for physicians (10[R]) and for patients and relatives (11[R]).

EFFECTS ON ORGANS AND SYSTEMS

Cardiovascular system

A patient with severe lithium poisoning developed reversible first degree atrioventricular block, intraventricular conduction delay, and prolonged Q-T interval (12[C]), but in general lithium does not affect the heart to a clinically significant extent. Patients without heart disease showed appropriate QTPK-interval shortening with exercise (13[C]). An episode of reversible respiratory failure was observed in a patient with stable chronic obstructive lung disease who was given lithium treatment for manic-depressive illness (14[C]).

A review on cardiovascular side effects of lithium treatment (15[R]) concludes that flat or negative T-waves as well as U-waves lack clinical significance. Alteration of impulse formation and conduction, e.g. sick sinus node syndrome, can occur in cases of lithium overdosage but may be found also at therapeutic serum lithium levels. Sick sinus node syndrome may require implantation of

Side Effects of Drugs Annual 8
M.N.G. Dukes, editor

ISBN 0 444 90339 9
$0.80 per article per page (transactional system)
$0.20 per article per page (licensing system)

a pacemaker before lithium treatment is started. Lithium-induced AV-block as well as bundle-branch block are very rare. Collaboration of psychiatrist and cardiologist is necessary when cardiac patients are treated with lithium.

Neuromuscular system

Hand tremor, the most frequent neurological side effect of lithium, can usually be controlled quite effectively with beta-blocking drugs, but patients with asthma may not tolerate some of these. Two patients with a history of bronchospasm had their lithium-induced tremor treated successfully with metoprolol, a cardio-selective beta-blocker, without suffering respiratory problems (16[C]). In one patient this treatment was ineffective in relieving the tremor (17[C]). In a non-blind study on 7 patients, lithium-induced tremor seemed to be reduced by administration of essential fatty acids (18[C]).

After 14 months on lithium (serum lithium 0.7–0.9 mmol/l) plus amitriptyline a 50-year-old patient developed constructional dyspraxia with difficulty in finding words in conversation and memory impairment. One month after discontinuation of lithium the symptoms had disappeared (19[C]). Another patient showed a somewhat similar picture at serum lithium values of 0.4–0.8 mmol/l (20[C]), but that patient had additional signs of general neurotoxicity (21[C]).

Two reports suggest that the red blood cell/plasma lithium ratio is better correlated with neurotoxicity than plasma lithium alone (22[C], 23[C]). The reviewer feels that evidence is still tenuous as regards the *predictive* value of this ratio.

Lithium exacerbated interictal aggressiveness in a patient with temporal lobe spike activity (24[C]) and accentuated extrapyramidal signs in 5 out of 6 patients with Alzheimer's dementia (25[C]).

Mind

Psychological effects and psychological side effects of lithium treatment are not always easy to distinguish, and it has been suggested (26[C], 27[C]) that certain psychological effects of lithium, which manifest themselves during the patients' otherwise symptom-free intervals, may be part of, and a prerequisite for, the prophylactic effect of the treatment. In patients on long-term lithium treatment, temporary placebo substitution may induce impairment as well as improvement of subjective well-being and performance tasks (28[C], 29[C]). Some lithium-induced changes in performance tests are associated with the left-hemisphere asymmetry as revealed by EEG (27[C], 30[C]).

Psychological problems involved in long-term treatment with lithium (and other drugs) go far beyond the question of 'side effects'. These complicated issues play a role for the patients' life quality during prophylactic lithium treatment and are of primary importance for compliance (27[C], 31[C], 32[C]). There seems to be a growing awareness that for a number of patients psychological support and appropriate psychotherapy may be decisive adjuncts to long-term lithium administration (33[C]).

Endocrine and metabolic

The endocrine and metabolic effects of lithium treatment have recently been reviewed (34[R]). A *hypoglycemic action* of lithium (35[C]) may in patients with diabetes mellitus lead to relief of this disease during lithium treatment (36[C]). A non-pregnant woman started to *lactate* when given lithium (37[C]). Lithium seems to stimulate humoral auto-antibodies, particularly the *antithyroidal,* during long-term treatment (38[C]).

Thyroid Lithium effects on thyroid size and function, on serum TSH concentration, and on response to TRH continue to be reported (39[C]–41[C]). The occasional report of hyperthyroidism developing during lithium treatment appeared also this year (42[C]). A cross-sectional study of 237 patients in long-term lithium treatment (43[C]) revealed that 10 patients had very high TSH values and abnormal concentrations of T_3 and T_4. 'Overt hypothyroidism' was found in 7% of the patients, about 10 times more frequently than would be expected in a control population. Lithium was discontinued in 3 patients; one of them still needed replacement treatment 1.5 years later. On the basis of a high prevalence of goiter among lithium-treated patients coming from an endemic area in Italy (44[C]), the authors suggest that such patients should be given thyroid hormone prophylactically concurrently with lithium.

A study on 47 lithium-treated patients

(46% with goiter as compared with 7% in a control group) failed to reveal any association between elevated TSH values and changes in cognitive functions (45[C]).

In 2 cases a solitary thyroid nodule developed during lithium treatment (46[C], 47[C]), possibly representing aggravation of a pre-existing nodule through lithium-induced TSH 'bombardment'.

Various observations suggest a connection between the type of disease course in manic-depressive illness on the one hand and elevation of serum TSH on the other. TSH-elevation was significantly more frequent among lithium-treated 'rapid cyclers' than among lithium-treated manic-depressive patients with a more protracted disease course (48[C]). It has been hypothesized that patients with pre-existing, subclinical hypothyroidism may be at particular risk of developing affective disturbances (49[C]–51[C]). More factors than those mentioned in general endocrinological textbooks may be at work to determine whether a patient in lithium treatment does or does not develop thyroid abnormality.

Parathyroid Twelve patients in long-term lithium treatment showed significantly higher serum total calcium, ionized calcium and parathyroid hormone than age- and sex-matched controls (52[C]), but the biochemical changes were not associated with subjective complaints, and the authors conclude that mild hypercalcemia in the absence of complications should not lead to discontinuation of lithium. They also point out that chronic overstimulation of the parathyroid glands may produce independently functioning adenomas; this has been reported during lithium treatment. A single patient (53[C]) showed marked elevation of serum calcium and serum parathyroid hormone accompanied by abdominal pains. Lithium was discontinued, and there was a rapid fall of both variables, although slight elevation of both serum calcium and serum parathyroid hormone remained after 6 months. The authors suggest that their patient may have had pre-existing slight hyperparathyroidism.

Hematological

Although further case reports have appeared of leukemia developing during lithium treatment (54[C]–57[C]), an epidemiologic study involving a population of 173,000 persons yielded negative results. Computer research revealed 187 patients suffering from leukemia; 13 of these had been seen by a psychiatrist, but none had been given lithium (58[C]). These British findings accord with a similarly negative American survey (59[C]). If lithium treatment does, indeed, occasionally cause or precipitate leukemia, this must be a rare occurrence.

The well-known leukocytosis produced by lithium and the employment of lithium as a treatment for neutropenic states are outside the scope of this review.

Gastrointestinal

Loose stools and defecation urge, rather than diarrhea as such, were experienced by about one-fifth of 237 patients in long-term lithium treatment (2[C], 3[C]). It was not associated with such patient and treatment variables as age, sex, treatment duration, serum lithium concentration, or – unexpectedly – treatment regimen (number of daily doses, conventional or slow-release tablets). Loose stools were significantly less frequent in patients given tricyclic antidepressants concurrently, probably due to the anticholinergic action of the latter. Remedies recommended against lithium-induced loose stools include antispasmodic drugs (60[C]) and the substitution of lithium citrate for lithium carbonate (61[C]). The etiological role played by lithium in a single case of 'acute abdomen' with intestinal vasculitis seems debatable (62[C]).

Subjective peptic ulcer complaints were significantly less frequent among 91 manic-depressive patients treated with lithium than among 76 manic-depressive patients not given this treatment (63[C]). All the patients were in an interval between affective episodes at the time of examination.

Lithium affects salivation rate much less than do the antidepressant drugs, but one case of sialorrhea has been reported (64[C]). Another patient developed chronic submandibular sialadenitis which required excision (65[C]). In a population of Australian children the concentration of spontaneously occurring lithium in saliva was inversely associated with caries development (66[C]).

Urinary system

There is a continuing stream of publications about the effect of long-term lithium treatment on kidney function, an outcome of the studies started by what has been called 'the kidney scare' (67[R]). These publications have not changed the general picture or the conclusions drawn in Annuals 4–7. Whereas the glomerular filtration rate is affected little or not at all by lithium treatment, even when this is given for many years, the urinary concentrating ability becomes lowered in many patients (68[C]–75[C]). A slight reduction of glomerular filtration rate in patients with markedly lowered concentrating ability may be explained through a mild constant underhydration (75[C]).

Not all lithium-treated patients with a renal concentrating defect show polyuria/polydipsia, and the concentrating ability is not impaired in all polyuric/polydipsic patients. Primary polydipsia may play a certain role (76[C], 77[C]), but lowered renal response to the antidiuretic hormone is presumably a central factor in most cases. Baseline plasma vasopressin levels are higher in lithium-treated patients than in controls, somewhat higher in patients without and much higher in patients with polyuria, and water deprivation leads to a further rise (78[C], 79[C]). Production of antidiuretic hormone is therefore neither blocked nor inhibited during lithium treatment, but the kidneys respond less readily to the hormone. The patients who develop polyuria may be those with the greatest resistance to vasopressin.

Thiazide treatment has usually some beneficial effect on lithium-induced polyuria (80[C]), but this is obviously a therapy involving risk. Amiloride may be a safer choice (81[C]).

Whereas previously it was commonly believed that a treatment regimen with wide variations of the serum lithium course during the day was associated with fewer side effects than a regimen with less wide variations, some evidence has been presented indicating that lithium-induced polyuria may be less frequent with the former than with the latter regimen (82[C]–84[C]). However, opposite observations have also been reported (75[C]), and it is the reviewer's opinion that definitive conclusions as regards the superiority of a treatment regimen with more constant serum values must await within-clinic trials with random allocation of treatment regimens and with assessment of not only side effects but also therapeutic and prophylactic effects of the treatment.

Two reports have appeared about the development of transitory nephrotic syndromes during lithium treatment (85[C], 86[C]).

Comparisons of lithium-treated patients with control persons showed in one study slightly higher urinary excretion of the renal enzyme β-hexosaminidase in the former group (87[C]), and in another study no difference between the groups as regards urinary excretion of N-acetyl-β-glucosaminidase (88[C]). Such determinations are technically easy, but their value for screening or prediction remains unproven.

Although rat data cannot be applied directly to humans, the observation of marked functional and structural changes in the kidneys of newborn rats exposed to lithium via their mothers' milk (89) may suggest caution about breast-feeding during lithium treatment.

Eyes

Apart from a report of photophobia during lithium poisoning (90[C]), lithium administration does not seem to affect vision or have any other effect on the eyes, as revealed by examination of 73 patients in long-term treatment (91[C]). Although a few cases of retinal changes possibly associated with lithium use are available in the National Registry of Drug-Induced Side Effects in the United States, the Registry does not consider this to provide clear evidence that lithium causes retinal changes (92[C]).

Skin and hair

Development or aggravation of acne and psoriasis during lithium treatment continue to be reported sporadically (93[C], 94[C]); acneiform eruption in 8 out of 18 patients is an unusually high frequency (95[C]). Tetracycline treatment of acne may interfere with renal lithium elimination and lead to lithium poisoning (96[C]). Sarantidis and Waters (152) conclude from their own preliminary material that cutaneous side effects are more prone to occur in women.

Single case reports include a lupus-like syndrome (97[C]) and increased growth of a wart (98[C]). Diffuse or localized hair loss was observed in 7 cases (99[C]) and in 12 cases (100[C]). Regrowth of hair took place after withdrawal of lithium or even during continued treatment. A review on dermatological reactions to lithium (101[R]) suggests that they may occur more commonly than previously documented. The authors estimate that with the exception of some psoriatic cases, management is usually possible without the need for lithium discontinuation.

Sexual function

Sexual dysfunction during lithium treatment is an occasional complaint which might be revealed more often if asked for specifically. It is not always clear, however, whether the trouble is due to the lithium treatment as such or to the underlying disease. A case report dealt with 2 patients with loss of libido and impairment of erection ability (102[C]). One patient received a blind placebo substitution and the dysfunction disappeared rapidly. In the other patient the symptoms remitted spontaneously in spite of continued lithium treatment.

Second generation effects

A newborn child presented lithium intoxication, extreme hypotonia, goiter, and signs of congenital heart disease. Cardiac catheterization and angiocardiography revealed elevated pulmonary vascular resistance (103[C]). It has been suggested that patients who are treated with lithium during early pregnancy should be subjected to echocardiographic screening before 20 weeks' gestation in order to detect Ebstein's anomaly in the fetus (104[C]).

Poisoning

Lithium poisoning may be developed after intake of an acute overdose with suicidal intent (105[C]–106[C]), as a result of complications (drug interactions!) which lower the lithium clearance (107[C]–112[C]), or owing to wrong dosage caused by a pharmaceutical error (113[C]). The central nervous system, the renal function, and the fluid/electrolyte balance are primarily affected, but occasionally more unusual reactions are seen: action myoclonus (106[C]), allergic erythema (105[C]), delirium with EEG changes (109[C], 114[C]), glucosuria (111[C]), electrocardiographic changes (110[C]), and rhabdomyolysis (107[C]). Severe poisoning is usually treated with hemodialysis, which may be monitored not only with serum lithium determinations but also with determinations of lithium in whole blood and in the dialysate (115[C]). Forced diuresis may be of value in patients with a normal renal function (116[C]).

Most patients survive lithium poisoning without after-effects, but there are some who die of the poisoning and others who survive with long-lasting or permanent sequelae, mostly of cerebellar nature but sometimes with peripheral neuropathy or parkinsonism (107[C], 117[C], 121[C]). One patient died of heart failure 3 years after a lithium intoxication with neurological sequelae and was subjected to necropsy (122[C]). This revealed extensive damage to granulae and Purkinje cells in the cerebellum; gliosis in the dentate nucleus, the inferior olives, and the nucleus ruber; cytoplasmic inclusions in various nerve cells of the cranial nerve nuclei; and cytoplasmic vacuoles, especially in the cells of the supraoptic nucleus.

Interactions

Interaction of lithium with drugs, with other treatments, and with certain risk situations was the subject of a Special Review in last year's Annual; reviews have also been published by others (123[R]–124[R]).

Lithium interaction with neuroleptics may be seen despite 'therapeutic' serum lithium levels, but the symptoms are usually mild and transitory unless large doses of neuroleptics are used (125[C]–130[C]). The combination occasionally leads to elevated serum lithium levels (131[C], 132[C]). Higher red blood cell/plasma lithium ratios in patients given the combination than in those given lithium alone may indicate that lithium is distributed differently across the cell membrane under the former circumstances (133[C]). EEG monitoring under combined treatment with lithium and neuroleptics failed to predict interaction (134[C]).

Combined treatment with antidepressant drugs led to significantly more tremor than did treatment with lithium alone (135[C]).

Elderly manic-depressive patients may find themselves in a situation when they need continuous lithium treatment for manic-depressive illness and in addition require treatment for rheumatism. Since non-steroid, non-salicylate anti-inflammatory drugs (indomethacin, etc.) reduce the renal elimination of lithium and may give rise to lithium poisoning (105^C, 136^C), it is fortunate that aspirin has been shown not to raise serum lithium levels (137^C).

Case reports of possible interaction of lithium with other drugs have included carbamazepine (138^C), marijuana (139^C), piroxicam (140^C), sulfamethoxazole (141^C), metronidazole (142^C), and mefenamic acid (143^C).

Electric convulsive treatment given concurrently with lithium may occasionally lead to confusion and disorientation (144^C). These reactions may not be strong enough, or sufficiently documented, to warrant general proscription of the combination (145^C), but it is unclear whether the combined treatment offers advantage (146^C). Discontinuation of lithium 2–3 days before the start of ECT may be advisable.

During lithium treatment some patients may develop diseases that require surgical intervention and anesthesia, and it is important that surgeons and anesthesiologists are aware of the particular risks and precautions attendant to this situation (147^C–149^C). Lithium treatment should be discontinued 2–3 days before major surgery and not resumed until kidney function and fluid/electrolyte balance are again normal. The interruption should be as brief as possible in order to avoid the risk of manic or depressive relapse. Many of the patients are unable to concentrate urine maximally and are therefore at risk of dehydration. Fluid should be administered parenterally if patients are forbidden oral fluid intake pre-operatively, if they are unconscious for many hours, or if they vomit massively (150^C, 151^C).

REFERENCES

1. Abou-Saleh MT, Coppen A (1983) Subjective side-effects of amitriptyline and lithium in affective disorders. *Br. J. Psychiatry, 142,* 391.
2. Vestergaard P, Amdisen A, Schou M (1980) Clinically significant side effects of lithium treatment: A survey of 237 patients in long-term treatment. *Acta Psychiatr. Scand., 62, 193.*
3. Vestergaard P (1983) Clinically important side effects of long-term lithium treatment: a review. *Acta Psychiatr. Scand., 67 (Suppl. 305),* 1.
4. Beloncle M, Martin A, Masson J-M, Voisinet C (1982) Le lithium dans les psychoses périodiques: Bilan de 10 ans chez 34 sujets. *Ann. Méd. Psychol., 140,* 369.
5. Duncavage MB, Nasr SJ, Post RM (1983) Subjective side effects of lithium carbonate: A longitudinal study. *J. Clin. Psychopharmacol., 3,* 100.
6. Lyskowski J, Nasrallah HA, Dunner FJ, Buchner K (1982) A longitudinal survey of side effects in a lithium clinic. *J. Clin. Psychiatry, 43,* 284.
7. Grof P, O'Sullivan K (1983) Somatic side effects of long-term lithium treatment. In: Ayd FJ (Ed), *Affective Disorders Reassessed.* Ayd Med. Comm., New York (to be published).
8. Jefferson JW (1983) Lithium and affective disorder in the elderly. *Compr. Psychiatry, 24,* 166.
9. Murray N, Hopwood S, Balfour DJK et al (1983) The influence of age on lithium efficacy and side-effects in out-patients. *Psychol. Med., 13,* 53.
10. Jefferson JW, Greist JH, Ackerman DL (1983) *Lithium Encyclopedia for Clinical Practice.* American Psychiatric Press, USA.
11. Schou M (1983) *Lithium Treatment of Manic-Depressive Illness: A Practical Guide, 2nd Revised Ed.* Karger, Basel.
12. Mateer JR, Clark MR (1982) Lithium toxicity with rarely reported ECG manifestations. *Ann. Emerg. Med., 11,* 208.
13. Johnson RE, Ware JD, Moffitt SS et al (1982) Response to exercise in patients taking psychotropic drugs: arrhythmias and the QT interval (QT wave peak). *Arch. Intern. Med., 142,* 755.
14. Weiner M, Chausow A, Wolpert E et al (1983) Effect of lithium on the responses to added respiratory resistances. *N. Engl. J. Med., 308,* 319.
15. Kirchmair H, Kirchmair W (1982) Kardiovaskuläre Nebenwirkungen unter Lithium-Therapie. *Neuropsychiatr. Clin., 1,* 59.
16. Gaby NS, Lefkowitz DS, Israel JR (1983) Treatment of lithium tremor with metoprolol. *Am. J. Psychiatry, 140,* 593.
17. North DS, Roering JL (1982) Ineffectiveness of metoprolol in controlling lithium-induced tremor. *Clin. Pharm., 1,* 264.
18. Lieb J, Horrobin DF (1981) Treatment of lithium-induced tremor and familial essential tremor with essential fatty acids. *Prog. Lipid Res., 20,* 535.
19. Worrall EP, Gillham RA (1983) Lithium-induced constructional dyspraxia. *Br. Med. J., 286,* 189.
20. McGovern GP (1983) Lithium induced constructional dyspraxia. *Br. Med. J., 286,* 646.
21. Worrall EP (1983) Lithium induced constructional dyspraxia. *Br. Med. J., 286,* 984.
22. Gay C, Olié JP, Dupin T et al (1983) Intérêt de l'étude cinétique du lithium intraérythrocytaire dans la recherche de corrélations bio-cliniques chez les sujets intolérants. *Encéphale,*

9, 37.

23. Elizur A, Yeret A, Segal Z, Graff E (1982) Lithium and electrolyte plasma/RBC ratio and paradoxical lithium neurotoxicity. *Prog. Neuro-Psychopharmacol. Biol. Psychiatry, 6,* 235.
24. Schiff HB, Sabin TD, Geller A et al (1982) Lithium in aggressive behavior. *Am. J. Psychiatry, 139,* 1346.
25. Kelwala S, Pomara N, Stanley M, Sitaram N (1983) Lithium induced accentuation of extrapyramidal signs in Alzheimer's dementia. *Soc. Biol. Psychiatry,* 182 (Abstr.).
26. Müller-Oerlinghausen B, Kropf D (1979) Effects of lithium on normal experience and behaviour: Conditional and descriptive approach to the structure of its action. In: Schou M, Stromgren E (Eds), *Origin, Prevention and Treatment of Affective Disorders,* p. 41. Academic Press, London.
27. Müller-Oerlinghausen B (1982) Psychological effects, compliance, and response to long-term lithium. *Br. J. Psychiatry, 141,* 411.
28. Greil W, Broucek B, Klein HE, Engel-Sittenfeld P (1982) Discontinuation of lithium maintenance therapy: Reversibility of clinical, psychological and neuroendocrinological changes. In: Emrich HM et al (Eds), *Basic Mechanisms in the Action of Lithium,* p. 235. Excerpta Medica, Amsterdam.
29. Kropf D (1981) Wirkungen von Lithium auf normale psychische Funktionen als Bedingungen für die Prophylaxe. *Bibl. Psychiatr., 161,* 141.
30. Ulrich G, Scheuler W, Müller-Oerlinghausen B (1982) Zur visuell-morphologischen Analyse des hirnelektrischen Verhaltens bei Patienten mit manisch-depressiven und schizo-affektiven Psychosen unter Lithiumprophylaxe. *Fortschr. Neurol. Psychiatr., 50,* 24.
31. Jamison KR (1982) Psychological issues in lithium therapy. In: Jamison KR (Ed), *Lithium: Clinical Considerations,* p. 11. Excerpta Medica, Amsterdam.
32. Vestergaard P, Amdisen A (1983) Patient attitudes towards lithium. *Acta Psychiatr. Scand., 67,* 8.
33. Jamison KR, Goodwin FK (1983) Psychotherapeutic treatment of manic-depressive patients on lithium. In: Greenhill MH, Gralnick A (Eds), *Psychopharmacology and Psychotherapy,* p. 53. Free Press, New York.
34. Lazarus JH (1982) Endocrine and metabolic effects of lithium. *Adverse Drug React., 1,* 181.
35. Nasr S, Shah J, Leon-Jones F, De Schickler R (1983) Glucose tolerance test in lithium-treated patients. *Soc. Biol. Psychiatry,* 145 (Abstr.).
36. Saran AS (1982) Antidiabetic effects of lithium. *J. Clin. Psychiatry, 43,* 383.
37. Ohishi K, Higashimura T (1982) A case of manic state associated with lithium induced lactation. *Folia Psychiatr. Neurol. Jpn, 36,* 199.
38. Albrecht J, Hopf U (1982) Influence of lithium on humoral auto-immune phenomena: A study of thyroidal autoantibodies in manic-depressive patients. *Arzneim. Forsch., 32,* 886.
39. Broucek B, Greil W, Klein H (1982) Unterbrechung einer chronischen Lithium-Therapie: Einfluss auf psychopathologische und neuroendokrinologische Parameter. *Arzneim. Forsch., 32,* 885.
40. Höschl C (1981) Effect of lithium on the TRH-test. *Act. Nerv. Super. (Praha), 23,* 276.
41. Wasilewski B (1982) Stan tarxzycy przy przewlekłym stosowaniu soli litu w celach profilaktycznych u osób z chorobami afektywnymi. *Psychiatr. Pol., 16,* 113.
42. Jaubert D, Chagnon A, Camillieri G et al (1982) Hyperthyroïdie au lithium (une nouvelle observation). *L.M.M. Méd. Sud-Est, 18,* 5918.
43. Amdisen A, Andersen CJ (1982) Lithium treatment and thyroid function: a survey of 237 patients in long-term lithium treatment. *Pharmacopsychiatria, 15,* 149.
44. Martino E, Placidi GF, Sardano G et al (1982) High incidence of goiter in patients treated with lithium carbonate. *Ann. Endocrinol., 43,* 269.
45. Grønfeldt IZ, Jørgensen PB (1982) Lithiumbehandling af stemningssygdomme: Virkning på thyreoideafunktion, psykisk status og psykisk funktionsevne. *Nord. Psykiatr. Tidsskr., 36,* 231.
46. Chee YC, Ong TC (1982) Lithium and the solitary thyroid nodule – a case report. *Singapore Med. J., 23,* 285.
47. Close P, Nagel M, Unger J (1982) Thyroglobuline et lithium: A propos d'un cas d'hyperthyroglobulinémie et de goitre suite de la prise prolongée de lithium. *Acta Clin. Belg., 37,* 318.
48. Cowdry RW, Wehr TA, Zis AP, Goodwin FK (1983) Thyroid abnormalities associated with rapid-cycling bipolar illness. *Arch. Gen. Psychiatry, 40,* 414.
49. O'Shanick GJ, Ellinwood EH (1982) Persistent elevation of thyroid-stimulating hormone in women with bipolar affective disorder. *Am. J. Psychiatry, 139,* 513.
50. Loosen PT, Tipermas A (1983) Thyroid hormones in manic-depressive disorders. *Am. J. Psychiatry, 140,* 511.
51. Ellinwood EH, O'Shanick GJ (1983) Thyroid hormones in manic-depressive disorders. *Am. J. Psychiatry, 140,* 512.
52. Franks RD, Dubovsky SL, Lifshitz M et al (1982) Long-term lithium carbonate therapy causes hyperparathyroidism. *Arch. Gen. Psychiatry, 39,* 1074.
53. Pedersen KK, Pedersen KE (1982) Svær hyperkalcæmi i forbindelse med lithiumbehandling. *Ugeskr. Læg., 144,* 3841.
54. Giustolisi R, Di Raimondo F, Guglielmo P et al (1982) Lithium and acute myeloid leukemia. *Haematologia (Pavia), 67,* 944.
55. Sethi BB, Prakash R, Sethi N (1982) Chronic myeloid leukemia during lithium therapy: Case

report. *J. Clin. Psychiatry, 43,* 296.

56. Tosato G, Whang-Peng J, Levine AS (1978) Acute lymphoblastic leukemia followed by chronic myelocytic leukemia. *Blood, 52,* 1033.
57. Witz F, Rigon JL, Lederlin P et al (1983) Lithium et leucémie aiguë myéloïde. *Sem. Hôp. Paris, 59,* 559.
58. Resek G, Olivieri S (1983) No association between lithium therapy and leukaemia. *Lancet, 1,* 940.
59. Lyskowski J, Nasrallah HA (1981) Lithium therapy and the risk for leukemia. *Br. J. Psychiatry, 139,* 256.
60. Hollister LE (1982) Lithium-induced diarrhea. *J. Am. Med. Assoc., 248,* 236.
61. Vasile RG, Shelton RP (1982) Alleviating gastrointestinal side effects of lithium carbonate by substituting lithium citrate. *J. Clin. Psychopharmacol., 2,* 420.
62. Cannon SR (1982) Intestinal vasculitis and lithium carbonate associated diarrhea. *Postgrad. Med. J., 58,* 445.
63. Jepsen PW, Jensen E, Plenge P, Rafaelsen OJ (1983) Peptic ulcer complaints in lithium-treated and non-lithium-treated manic-depressive patients. *Acta Psychiatr. Scand., 67,* 358.
64. Donaldson SR (1982) Sialorrhea as a side effect of lithium: A case report. *Am. J. Psychiatry, 139,* 1350.
65. Forrest DV, Schvey MH, Cooper TB (1983) Salivary Lithiolith? *J. Clin. Psychiatry, 44,* 161.
66. Agus HM, Schamschula RG (1983) Lithium content, buffering capacity and flow rate of saliva and caries experience of Australian children. *Caries Res., 17,* 139.
67. Schou M, Vestergaard P (1981) Lithium and the kidney scare (Editorial). *Psychosomatics, 22,* 92.
68. Amsterdam J, Cox M (1983) A prospective study of lithium-induced nephropathy. *Soc. Biol. Psychiatr.,* 157 (Abstr.).
69. Kampf D, Müller-Oerlinghausen B, Albrecht J, Kessel M (1983) Lithium-Prophylaxe: Nephrotoxizität und therapeutische Konsequenzen. *Internist, 24,* 110.
70. Khandelwal SK, Chugh KS, Sakhuja V et al (1983) Renal function in long-term lithium prophylaxis. *Indian J. Med. Res., 77,* 107.
71. Ostrow DG, Coe FL, Wolpert EA (1982) A study of renal function in patients treated with a flexible dose lithium regimen. *J. Psychiatr. Treatm., 4,* 269.
72. Tyrer SP, Schacht RG, McCarthy MJ et al (1983) The effect of lithium on renal haemodynamic function. *Psychol. Med., 13,* 61.
73. Vaamonde CA, Millan N, Magrinat G et al (1983) Preservation of normal glomerular filtration rate after 7.7 years of continued lithium therapy. *Kidney Int., 23,* 139.
74. Walker RG, Davies BM, Holwill BJ et al (1982) A clinico-pathological study of lithium nephrotoxicity. *J. Chronic Dis., 35,* 685.
75. Wallin L, Alling C, Aurell M (1982) Impairment of renal function in patients on long-term lithium treatment. *Clin. Nephrol., 17,* 23.
76. Conte G, Canton A, dal Caserta D et al (1982) La polidipsia primitiva quale causa de poliuria in pazienti in trattamento cronico con carbonato di litio. *Minerva Nefrol., 29,* 177.
77. Gold PW, Robertson GL, Post RM et al (1983) The effect of lithium on the osmoregulation of arginine vasopressin secretion. *J. Clin. Endocrinol., 56,* 295.
78. Hansen HE, Pedersen EB, Ørskov H et al (1982) Plasma arginine-vasopressin, renal-concentrating ability and lithium excretion in a group of patients on long-term lithium treatment. *Nephron, 32,* 125.
79. Morgan DB, Penney MD, Hullin RP et al (1982) The responses to water deprivation in lithium-treated patients with and without polyuria. *Clin. Sci., 63,* 549.
80. Lauriers AD, Lassays C, Jouvent R (1982) Lithium et diabète insipide: Aspects théoriques et pratiques; intérêt thérapeutique des thiazidiques. *Sem. Hôp. Paris, 58,* 703.
81. Kosten TR, Forrest JN (1982) Treatment of severe lithium-induced nephrogenic diabetes insipidus with amiloride. *Clin. Res., 30,* 540A.
82. Perry PJ (1982) Lithium nephrotoxicity. *Drug Intell. Clin. Pharm., 16,* 740.
83. Plenge P, Mellerup ET, Bolwig TG et al (1982) Lithium treatment: Does the kidney prefer one daily dose instead of two? *Acta Psychiatr. Scand., 66,* 121.
84. Schou M, Amdisen A, Thomsen K et al (1982) Lithium treatment regimen and renal water handling: The significance of dosage pattern and tablet type examined through comparison of results from two clinics with different treatment regimens. *Psychopharmacology (Berlin), 77,* 387.
85. Depner TA (1982) Nephrotic syndrome secondary to lithium therapy. *Nephron, 30,* 286.
86. Singer L, Imbs JL, Danion JM et al (1982) Sels de lithium et syndrome néphrotique. *Thérapie, 37,* 587.
87. Thysell H, Hultberg B, Regnell G (1982) Urinary β-hexosaminidase excretion in patients treated with lithium, thymoleptic and/or neuroleptic drugs. *Acta Psychiatr. Scand., 66,* 486.
88. Garvey MJ, Tuason VB, Blomquist CH, Hwang S (1982) Use of renal enzymes to evaluate nephrotoxicity in lithium treated patients. *Br. J. Psychiatry, 141,* 420.
89. Christensen S, Ottosen PD, Olsen S (1982) Severe functional and structural renal changes caused by lithium in the developing rat kidney. *Acta Path. Microbiol. Scand., Sect. A, 90,* 257.
90. Caplan RP, Fry AH (1982) Photophobia in lithium intoxication. *Br. Med. J., 285,* 1314.
91. Hiroz C-A, Assimacopoulos T, Cuendet J-F et al (1981) Les effets secondaires du lithium en ophtalmologie. *Encéphale, 7,* 123.
92. Fraunfelder FT (1983) Lithium carbonate

therapy and senile macular degeneration. *J. Am. Med. Assoc.*, *249*, 2389.

93. Lambert D, Beer F, Gisselmann R et al (1982) Manifestations cutanées des thérapeutiques par le lithium. *Ann. Dermatol. Venéréol.*, *109*, 19.

94. Pincelli C, Coppini M, Zucchi M, Zanini M (1982) Psoriasi e carbonato di litio. *G. Ital. Dermatol. Venereol.*, *117*, 113.

95. Lee K (1980) Acneiform eruption in lithium-treated patients. (In Korean.) *Neuropsychiatry (Seoul)*, *19*, 6.

96. Heng MCY (1982) Lithium carbonate toxicity: Acneiform eruption and other manifestations. *Arch. Dermatol.*, *118*, 246.

97. Shukla VR (1982) Lithium and lupuslike syndrome. *J. Am. Med. Assoc.*, *248*, 921.

98. White SW (1982) Lithium and warts. *Int. J. Dermatol.*, *21*, 107.

99. Dawber R, Mortimer P (1982) Hair loss during lithium treatment. *Br. J. Dermatol.*, *107*, 124.

100. Orwin A (1983) Hair loss following lithium therapy. *Br. J. Dermatol.*, *108*, 503.

101. Deandrea D, Walker N, Mehlmauer M, White K (1982) Dermatological reactions to lithium: A critical review. *J. Clin. Psychopharmacol.*, *2*, 199.

102. Blay SL, Ferraz MPT, Calil HM (1982) Lithium-induced male sexual impairment: Two case reports. *J. Clin. Psychiatry*, *43*, 497.

103. Filtenborg JA (1982) Persistent pulmonary hypertension after lithium intoxication in the newborn. *Eur. J. Pediatr.*, *138*, 321.

104. Allan LD, Desai G, Tynan MJ (1982) Prenatal echocardiographic screening for Ebstein's anomaly for mothers on lithium therapy. *Lancet*, *2*, 875.

105. Perrot D, Bouffard Y, Roux H et al (1982) Intoxication aiguë volontaire au lithium. *J. Toxicol. Méd.*, *2*, 49.

106. Rosen PB, Stevens R (1983) Action myoclonus in lithium toxicity. *Ann. Neurol.*, *13*, 221.

107. Unger J, Decaux G, L'Hermite M (1982) Rhabdomyolysis, acute renal failure, endocrine alterations and neurological sequelae in a case of lithium selfpoisoning. *Acta Clin. Belg.*, *37*, 216.

108. Demers RG, Rivenbark JF (1982) Lithium intoxication and its clinical management. *South Med. J.*, *75*, 738.

109. Depaulo JR, Folstein MF, Correa EI (1982) The course of delirium due to lithium intoxication. *J. Clin. Psychiatry*, *43*, 447.

110. Dieryck J (1983) Lithiumintoxicatie: Zeldzaam maar gevaarlijk. *Tijdschr. Geneeskd.*, *39*, 269.

111. Poussel JF, Chauplannaz G, Trillet M, Valentin C (1982) Coma hyperosmolaire et lithium. *Lyon Méd.*, *247*, 545.

112. Vogl G, Emrich HM (1982) Pathophysiological aspects of lithium intoxication. In: Emrich HM et al (Eds), *Basic Mechanisms in the Action of Lithium*, p. 215. Excerpta Medica, Amsterdam.

113. Nam J-H (1979) A study of toxic symptoms due to lithium overdosage. (In Korean.) *Neuropsychiatry (Seoul)*, *18*, 266.

114. Norris MS, Mathew RJ, Webb WW (1983) Delirium associated with lithium-induced hypothyroidism: A case report. *Am. J. Psychiatry*, *140*, 355.

115. Clendeninn NJ, Pond SM, Kaysen G et al (1982) Potential pitfalls in the evaluation of the usefulness of hemodialysis for the removal of lithium. *J. Toxicol. Clin. Toxic.*, *19*, 341.

116. O'Connor J, Gleeson J (1982) Acute lithium intoxication: Peritoneal dialysis or forced diuresis. *NZ Med. J.*, *95*, 790.

117. Apte SN, Langston JW (1983) Permanent neurological deficits due to lithium toxicity. *Ann. Neurol.*, *13*, 453.

118. Grandjean EM, Schira JC, Cavanese JC et al (1982) Séquelles neurologiques après intoxication au lithium: rôle possible d'un déficit en thiamine. *Schweiz. Med. Wochenschr.*, *112*, 1014.

119. Muff S, Meienberg O (1983) Irreversible neurologische Schäden durch Lithiumtherapie. *Dtsch. Med. Wochenschr.*, *108*, 663.

120. Pamphlett RS, MacKenzie RA (1982) Severe peripheral neuropathy due to lithium intoxication. *J. Neurol. Neurosurg. Psychiatry*, *45*, 656.

121. Singh SV (1982) Lithium carbonate/fluphenazine decanoate producing irreversible brain damage. *Lancet*, *2*, 278.

122. Peiffer J (1981) Clinical and neuropathological aspects of long-term damage to the central nervous system after lithium medication. *Arch. Psychiatr. Nervenkr.*, *231*, 41.

123. Amdisen A (1982) Lithium and drug interactions. *Drugs*, *24*, 133.

124. De Flines EW (1982) Lithium en neuroleptica, een gevaarlijke combinatie? *Pharm. Weekbl.*, *117*, 1132.

125. Hollister LE (1982) Polypharmacy: Which drug combinations make sense? *Hosp. Commun. Psychiatry*, *33*, 433.

126. Jefferson JW, Greist JH, Baudhuin M (1981) Lithium: Interactions with other drugs. *J. Clin. Psychopharmacol.*, *1*, 124.

127. Salem RB (1982) A pharmacist's guide to monitoring lithium drug-drug interactions. *Drug Intell. Clin. Pharm.*, *16*, 745.

128. Menes C, Burra P, Hoaken PCS (1980) Untoward effects following combined neuroleptic-lithium therapy: Cardiac arrhythmias and seizure. *Can. J. Psychiatry*, *25*, 573.

129. Prakash R, Kelwala S, Ban TA (1982) Neurotoxicity with combined administration of lithium and a neuroleptic. *Compr. Psychiatry*, *23*, 567.

130. Rosenbaum A (1982) Administering lithium carbonate and haloperidol. *Hosp. Commun. Psychiatry*, *33*, 186.

131. Guern G, le Segalen F, Boucher Y et al (1982) Intoxication par le lithium associé à des

neuroleptiques. *Cah. Anesthiol., 30,* 955.
132. McGennis AJ (1983) Hazards of lithium and neuroleptics in schizo-affective disorder. *Br. J. Psychiatry, 142,* 99.
133. von Knorring L, Smigan L, Perris C, Oreland L (1983) Lithium and neuroleptic drugs in combination: Effect on lithium RBC/plasma ratio. *Int. Pharmacopsychiatry, 17,* 287.
134. Prakash R, Manov G (1982) EEG during combined administration of lithium and neuroleptics. *Acta Psychiatr. Scand., 66,* 336.
135. Perényi A, Rihmer Z, Bánki CM (1983) Parkinsonian symptoms with lithium, lithium-neuroleptic and lithium-antidepressant treatment. *J. Affect. Dis., 5,* 171.
136. Danion JM, Singer L, Imbs JL et al (1982) Sels de lithium et rein: interactions médicamenteuses. Effets rénaux indésirables. *J. Méd. Strasbourg, 13,* 431.
137. Reimann IW, Diener U, Frölich JC (1983) Indomethacin but not aspirin increases plasma lithium ion levels. *Arch. Gen. Psychiatry, 40,* 283.
138. Chaudry RP, Waters BGH (1982) Lithium and carbamazepine interaction: possible neurotoxicity. *J. Clin. Psychiatry, 44,* 30.
139. Ratey JJ, Ciraulo DA, Shader RI (1981) Lithium and marihuana. *J. Clin. Psychopharmacol., 1,* 32.
140. Kerry RJ, Owen G, Michaelson S (1983) Possible toxic interaction between lithium and piroxicam. *Lancet, 1,* 418.
141. Desvilles M, Sevestre P (1982) Effet paradoxal de l'association Lithium et sulfaméthoxazol-triméthopine. *Nouv. Presse Méd., II,* 3267.
142. Brinkley JR (1982) Metronidazole-induced lithium intoxication. *Int. Drug Ther. Newslett., 17,* 15.
143. Honey J (1982) Lithium-mefenamic acid interaction. *Int. Drug Ther. Newslett., 17,* 16.
144. Martin BA, Kramer PM (1982) Clinical significance of the interaction between lithium and a neuromuscular blocker. *Am. J. Psychiatry, 139,* 1326.
145. Martin BA, Kramer PM (1983) Lithium-ECT interactions. *Am. J. Psychiatry, 140,* 666.
146. Albala AA, Rioux P (1983) Lithium-ECT interactions. *Am. J. Psychiatry, 140,* 666.
147. Boileau S, Laxenaire MC (1981) Médicaments neuropsychiatriques interférant avec la conduite de l'anesthésie générale. *Ann. Méd. Nancy l'Est, 20,* 725.
148. Janowsky EC, Risch C, Janowsky DS (1981) Effects of anesthesia on patients taking psychotropic drugs. *J. Clin. Psychopharmacol., 1,* 14.
149. Pottecher T, Galani M, Otteni JC (1982) Lithium et intervention chirurgicale. *J. Méd. Strasbourg, 13,* 363.
150. Schou M, Hippius H (1983) Lithium-råd for kirurger og narkoselæger. *Nord. Med., 98,* 106.
151. Schou M (1981) Lithium treatment and preoperative fluid deprivation. *Br. Med. J., 283,* 1253.
152. Sarantidis D, Waters B (1983) A review and controlled study of cutaneous conditions associated with lithium carbonate. *Br. J. Psychiatry, 143,* 42.

Carl Salzman and Alan I. Green

4 Social drugs

The abuse of various drugs, many of which have no current medical use, continues to be widespread. This year's chapter will review certain general effects of drug abuse: renal toxicity, infection and flashback. In addition, a number of specific agents will be discussed in some detail.

Renal toxicity

Abused street drugs such as heroin, amphetamines, phencyclidine, pentazocine and codeine are known to cause renal damage (1[R]). *Acute renal failure*, associated with rhabdomyolysis, has been described, although the exact etiology is unknown (1[R]). Some investigators have suggested it might be due to nephrotoxicity of myoglobin. Hypotension-based acute renal failure has been reported in heroin addicts. A recent paper described 2 cases of acute renal failure following phencyclidine (PCP) intoxication thought to be due to hyperuricemic nephropathy (2[C]). The authors suggest that blood uric acid be measured in all patients with major PCP intoxication. All these forms of acute renal failure carry a good prognosis if proper management, including hemodialysis (when necessary), is employed.

Acute renal insufficiency, secondary to bacterial endocarditis and viral hepatitis, has been described in drug addicts. The renal toxicity is a glomerulonephritis thought to be secondary to circulating immune complexes; it tends to clear with the underlying condition (1[R]). Immune complexes were thought to be involved in the pathogenesis of 3 cases of membranoproliferative glomerulonephritis type I following 2- to 3-year histories of parenteral pentazocine abuse (3[C]). All patients developed the nephrotic syndrome with hypertension and hematuria. The authors postulated that the drug itself, additives used in the drug preparation or microorganisms might have been related to the immune complex development.

Chronic renal failure has been reported to occur as a result of subcutaneous or intravenous drug abuse (1[R]). In heroin addicts, it may be due to a focal sclerosis involving some of the glomeruli. In such cases, the prognosis is poor, unless the heroin use ceases; some patients with a mild condition have had an improvement in renal function with a switch to oral methadone. With intravenous amephetamine use, a systemic vasculitis or polyarteritis may cause the renal failure. In this case as well, renal function can stabilize after amphetamine use stops. When heroin or amphetamine is abused subcutaneously ('skin popping'), the abusers may be at risk for developing the nephrotic syndrome due to induction of amyloidosis.

Infection

Intravenous drug use is often complicated by various infections: cellulitis, abscesses, septic arthritis, osteomyelitis, endocarditis, hepatitis, pneumonia and malaria have all been reported (4[C]). Ophthalmologic complications have been described as well, including septic retinitis, talc emboli, retinal neovascularization and metastatic endophthalmitis (5[C]). The cases of endophthalmitis have generally been caused by *Candida albicans.* One recent report implicated *Aspergillus flavus* in metastatic endophthalmitis found in an intravenous cocaine user (7[C]). *Aspergillosis* endophthalmitis is usually thought to have a poor prognosis. In this case, however, when the patient was treated with vitrectomy and antifungal agents, useful vision was restored. A second report described a case of focal submacular septic choroiditis, secondary to an embolus, resulting in permanent monocular loss of central vision in a heroin and phenmetrazine abuser (5[C]).

Side Effects of Drugs Annual 8
M.N.G. Dukes, editor

ISBN 0 444 90339 9
$0.80 per article per page (transactional system)
$0.20 per article per page (licensing system)

Necrotizing fasciitis, an infection of subcutaneous and fascial tissues, has been reported in 2 i.v. cocain abusers (4[C]). The infection, which at first resembled a cellulitis, caused severe local disease, as well as systemic toxic symptoms. The pathogens were a mixture of anaerobes and aerobes. The authors speculated that the infection was caused by the accidental subcutaneous intramuscular injection of cocaine, a vasoconstrictor. Their successful therapy employed antimicrobials effective against both types of pathogens.

Some drug abuse related infections result from non-parenteral use. A report from the Centers for Disease Control described an outbreak of enteritis caused by *Salmonella meunchen* traced to contaminated marijuana samples (6[C]). The authors suggested that the salmonella infection was caused by hand to mouth or cigarette to mouth contact.

Flashback

A recent article summarized the literature on flashback phenomena and reported on an in-depth study of one case (8[R]). Flashback phenomena are defined as a return of hallucinogenic effects after the immediate drug effect has worn off. They are often reported as visual intrusions, but other sensory modalities may also be involved, as may distortions in time sense, self-image or reality sense. Typical flashback effects include: perceptual distortions, depersonalizations, anxiety, disorientation, 'union with the world', various bodily sensations, and spontaneous and recurring images (8[R]).

Flashbacks have been estimated to occur in approximately 23% of a drug-using population (8[R]). The rate of their occurrence may be daily or nearly so (21% in one sample), 2 or 3 times monthly (18%), or every month or so (43%) (8[R]). Most individuals seem to have decreasing frequency of experiences, but 18% may have an increase (9[C]). Some individuals continue to experience flashbacks for years. Continued marijuana use following the hallucinogen use is thought to be related to their existence; alcohol, stress and even pleasurable thoughts have been implicated as well (8[R]).

Very little is known about the etiology of flashback phenomena. Theories include psychological, organic or social deficits. Psychological studies of individuals with flashbacks have provided conflicting data. Some subjects seem to have normal character structure while others have an obsessive-compulsive or hysterical make-up; some are characterized as frivolous, spontaneous, outspoken, or active, while others are described as regressive, immature, maladjusted, vulnerable, passive or thought disordered (8[R]). The careful study of one case seemed to detect some organic abnormalities on neurophysiological, EEG and blood flow measures (8[R]). The authors called for careful neurophysiologic and neuropsychologic assessment of individuals with flashback phenomena.

Cannabis and pregnancy *(SEDA-4, 26; SEDA-5, 28; SEDA-6, 32; SEDA-7, 39)*

As noted in previous reviews teratogenic effects of marijuana have been searched for, but the resulting data is equivocal. Although the cannabinoids may increase in utero fetal loss, the effects on viable offspring are uncertain (10[R]). In the male, testosterone levels are decreased in users, and sperm motility and concentration may be lowered; there is no proof, however, that fertility is affected. There is one report that tetrahydrocannabinol may have deleterious effects on the primary oocytes of young female mice; the clinical significance for humans is unknown (10[R]). In a study of pregnant women, marijuana use was associated with a shorter gestation period and less maternal weight gain. No effect on birth weight, length of labor or labor difficulty was found (11[C]). Yet, in another study, labor itself was found to be more hazardous and the newborns exhibited more meconium staining in the marijuana users than in non-users (12[C]). When neonatal behavior was examined, babies born to heavy marijuana users had increased tremors, startles and altered visual responsiveness at 2 to 4 days of age. These symptoms were attenuated by day 30, and at 1 year of age no developmental abnormalities were noted (11[C]).

Pentazocine and tripelennamine *(SEDA-7, 39)*

As reported previously, drug users inject oral preparations of pentazocine (Talwin) and tripelennamine (Pyribenzamine). Some users employ the combination when heroin is not available; others seem to prefer it (13[C]). On the streets, the combination is known as T's and Blues (or B's). The 'T' is a pentazocine hydrochloride tablet; 'Blue' is a tripelennamine tablet. The user crushes the tablets in water, filters the mixture and injects the filtrate intravenously. Toxic effects have been described: Annual 7 discussed resulting pulmonary lesions; dermatologic complications have been seen as well (14[c]). A recent article reported on neurological effects of the combination (15[C]). Seizures, thought to be due to either emboli or toxic effects of the tripelennamine, were seen in half of the patients studied. A number of patients had strokes or CNS infections. The strokes were probably the result of foreign body emboli. The CNS infections were quite serious – in one case leading to death, in the others to permanent destruction of brain tissue. The cultured organisms included *aspergillus, nocardia, streptococcus* and *pseudomonas.*

Heaney and Gotlieb have described a case of granulocytopenia which developed in a man known to be an intravenous user of T's and Blues (24[C]). The granulocyte count began to recover by the fourth hospital day. The authors speculated that the abuse of T's and Blues was a 'highly probable' cause of the complication (24[C]).

Phencyclidine

Phencyclidine (PCP) abuse continues to be a major medical problem. Several investigators have recently reported on the intoxication syndrome. One group attempted to classify the syndrome in terms of major and minor patterns of symptoms (16[C]). Major patterns included one of the following symptoms: acute brain syndrome, toxic psychosis, catatonia or coma. Minor patterns included lethargy or stupor, and some mixture of violence, agitation, euphoria and bizarre behavior in an alert and oriented patient. The authors found that patients with major patterns had greater need for hospitalization and more medical complications than those with minor patterns. The most common medical complication seen was rhabdomyolysis, which in some cases led to acute renal failure (see Renal toxicity, above) (16[C], 17[c]). Another group noted the insensitivity of routine gas chromatography with flame ionization detection (GC-FID) for PCP assay in the urine (18[C]). If gas chromatography with nitrogen detection (GC-N2), which is much more sensitive, is used as a standard, GC-FID misses more than 80% of the PCP positive urines.

Cocaine *(SEDA-7, 38)*

A rise in cocaine use (along with a similar increase in the complications from its use) has been noted since the early 1970's. A recent review described the toxicity reaction, which results from adrenergic stimulation of the central nervous, cardiovascular, and respiratory systems (19[R]). Symptoms may include: tachycardia, tachypnea, hypertension, euphoria and hyperactivity. Hyperpyrexia and a paradoxical respiratory depression may be observed following high doses. Death may result from cardiac or respiratory collapse. A recent report described a serious pulmonary edema that developed in a 36-year-old man shortly after injecting 'freebase' cocaine intravenously (20[C]). ('Freebase' is a purified form of cocaine prepared by solvent extraction. It is usually smoked or inhaled.) Despite vigorous intensive care treatment, the man died from the pulmonary edema within 3 hours. In other reported fatal overdoses, convulsions and death have usually occurred quickly (within minutes). Most patients who have survived for the first 3 hours after the overdose have been likely to recover. Treatment of the toxicity reaction includes respiratory and cardiovascular resuscitative measures. Short-acting barbiturates, benzodiazepines and propranolol have all been used with some success (19[R]).

Miscellaneous social drugs

Volatile nitrites As described in Annual 7 (p. 39), amyl nitrite and butyl nitrite are inhaled to produce stimulant and aphrodisiac effects. Such use, however, is known to be associated with toxicity. A recent report suggests that if taken orally, amyl nitrite may produce a life-threatening form of methemoglobinemia (21[C]). In the case described, successful treatment involved resuscitation and the administration of methylene blue.

Caffeine-containing street drugs A letter described 2 cases of toxicity after taking caffeine-containing street drugs (22[C]). In both cases, severe abdominal cramping, vomiting, tachycardia, tachypnea and anxiety were found. One patient was combative and hostile.

'New synthetic heroin' In parts of California, a mixture of MPTP (1-methyl-4-phenyl-1,2,5,6-tetrahydropyridine) with trace amounts of MPPP (1-methyl-4-phenyl-4-propionoxypiperidine) – a meperidine analog of which MTPT is a byproduct – has been sold on the streets under the name of 'new synthetic heroin'. There have been 4 case reports of the striking development of parkinsonism within 1 week of the intravenous use of this mixture (23[C]). All the patients responded to L-dopa and carbidopa, but 5 months later they all continued to require it. The authors suspected that MPTP was the offending agent, and that it caused actual loss of cells in the substantia nigra. They recommended the evaluation of the drug for the production of an animal model of Parkinson's disease.

REFERENCES

1. Levitan D (1982) Effects of drug abuse on the kidney. *Dialysis Transplant., 11,* 885.
2. Patel R (1982) Acute uric acid nephropathy: A complication of phencyclidine intoxication. *Postgrad. Med. J., 58,* 783.
3. Stachura S, Jayakumar S, Pardo M (1983) Talwin addict nephropathy. *Clin. Nephrol., 19,* 147.
4. Jacobsen JM, Hirschman SZ (1982) Necrotizing fasciitis complicating intravenous drug abuse. *Arch. Intern. Med., 142,* 634.
5. Limaye SR, Goldberg MH (1982) Septic submacular chorodial embolus associated with intravenous drug abuse. *Ann. Ophthalmol., 14,* 518.
6. Taylor DN, Wachsmuth IK, Shangkuan Y et al (1982) Salmanellosis associated with marijuana. *N. Engl. J. Med., 306,* 1249.
7. Michelson SB, Freedman SD, Boyden DG (1982) Aspergillus endophthalmitis in a drug abuser. *Ann. Ophthalmol., 14,* 1051.
8. Alarcon RD, Dickinson WA, Dohn HH (1982) Flashback phenomena: Clinical and diagnostic dilemmas. *J. Nerv. Ment. Dis.,* 217.
9. Matefy RE, Hayes C, Hirsch J (1978) Psychedelic drug flashbacks; subjective reports and biographical data. *Addict. Behav., 3,* 165.
10. Morishima A (1982) Drugs of abuse: their effects on embryos and fetuses. *Acta Pediatr. Jpn, 24,* 36.
11. Fried PA (1982) Marijuana use by pregnant women and effects on offspring: an update. *Neurobehav. Toxicol. Teratol., 4,* 451.
12. Greenland S, Staisch KJ, Brown N et al (1982) Effects of marijuana on human pregnancy, labor, and delivery. *Neurobehav. Toxicol. Teratol., 4,* 447.
13. Showalter CV (1980) T's and Blues. *J. Am. Med. Assoc., 244,* 1224.
14. Padilla RS, Becker L, Hoffman H et al (1979) Cutaneous and venous complications of pentazocine abuse. *Arch. Dermatol., 115,* 975.
15. Caplan LR, Thomas C, Banks G (1982) Central nervous system complications of addiction to 'T's and Blues'. *Neurology, 32,* 623.
16. McCarron MM, Schulze BW, Thompson GA et al (1981) Acute phencyclidine intoxication: clinical patterns, complications and treatment. *Ann. Emerg. Med., 10,* 290.
17. Barton CH, Sterling ML, Vaziri ND (1981) Phencyclidine intoxication: clinical experience in 27 cases confirmed by urine assay. *Ann. Emerg. Med., 10,* 243.
18. Fallis RJ, Amitine A, Werner LP et al (1982) Massive phencyclidine intoxication. *J. Nerv. Ment. Dis., 170,* 217.
19. Gay GR (1982) Clinical management of acute and chronic cocaine poisoning. *Ann. Emerg. Med., 11,* 562.
20. Allred RJ, Ewer S (1981) Fatal pulmonary edema following intravenous 'freebase' cocaine use. *Ann. Emerg. Med., 10,* 441.
21. McGrath RB, Perry SM (1982) The production of methemoglobin by amyl nitrite. *Resp. Care, 27,* 959.
22. May DC, Long T, Madden R et al (1981) Caffeine toxicity secondary to street drug ingestion. *Ann. Emerg. Med., 170,* 549.
23. Langston JW, Ballard P, Tetrud JW et al (1983) Chronic parkinsonism in humans due to a product of meperidine-analog synthesis. *Science, 219,* 979.
24. Heaney RM, Gotlieb N (1983) Granulocytopenia after intravenous abuse of pentazocine and terpelennamine ('T's and Blues'). *South. Med. J., 76,* 654.

T.C. Jerram

5 Hypnotics and sedatives

The benzodiazepines fill the greater part of this chapter in two ways, the increase in the number of benzodiazepines being promoted and investigated being only equalled by the realization that they can have serious dependence problems. Particularly in view of the latter, several substances which at one time appeared to have been superseded are now discussed. No further information has appeared about any possible links between malignant disease and minor tranquilizers.

BENZODIAZEPINES

General

Dependence and withdrawal symptoms Many further reports have been published of withdrawal symptoms from benzodiazepines. Relatively little of this is new information, but it does confirm that withdrawal symptoms occur quite widely and with most, if not all, of these drugs. The clinical picture is now clearly established (SEDA-7, 44; 57[R]). In mild cases general symptoms of anxiety are common (apprehension, dizziness, headache, muscular tension and pain) with more specific features such as metallic taste and an increased sensitivity to light and noise. More severe symptoms occur: these include vomiting, tremor, sweating, muscular cramps and postural hypotension. More rarely, hyperthermia, frank seizures, or psychotic symptoms can occur. Those patients with underlying cardiovascular disorders may be at risk during these periods (1[R]). The time course of these symptoms is believed to vary with the agent and to be influenced by its metabolic half-life. Symptoms may be prolonged and may change their nature over the withdrawal period. Mellor and Jain (2[C]) studied diazepam withdrawal in 10 patients whose daily dosage had been 60–120 mg. They found that symptoms continued for about 6 weeks but that different symptoms occurred at different times. Tremor, anxiety and insomnia were fairly constant throughout the study period while tachycardia, clouding of consciousness and hallucinations occurred in the first 10 days. They then found that perceptual changes and ataxia were maximal after 3 weeks and suggest that these may be related to a bi-exponential elimination curve for desmethyldiazepam (3[c]). Their patients were all in-patients and therefore presumably more ill. Laughren et al (4[C]) studied 24 middle-aged men as out-patients and compared the effects of continued maintenance, abrupt withdrawal and gradual withdrawal of diazepam. They found little difference between the groups on self-report measures of anxiety and withdrawal symptoms although anxiety was increased in the abrupt withdrawal group at 4 weeks. Their study, incidentally, shows some of the difficulties of investigating these patients, in that one third of them did not complete the protocol. The authors also argue that 'withdrawal from chronic diazepam use does not result in any rapid recurrence of anxiety or prominent withdrawal symptoms in most patients' and point out that physicians must consider 'what alternative treatments are available to this large, chronically anxious population'. One possible reason for this failure to find many withdrawal symptoms was the relatively low dose (mean 17 mg/day) that their patients were taking. However, Hallstrom and Lader (5[c]) observed a small number of patients who claimed to be dependent on a high dose (mean 135 mg/day) or a low dose (mean 20 mg/day) of diazepam or its equivalent and found little difference either on symptoms or EEG changes between the two groups.

The same authors also attempted to assess the incidence of benzodiazepine dependence

Side Effects of Drugs Annual 8
M.N.G. Dukes, editor

ISBN 0 444 09339 9
$0.80 per article per page (transactional system)
$0.20 per article per page (licensing system)

in long-term users of the drugs (6[c]). This is not a proper epidemiological study as such in that the users were self-selected (in response to a newsletter) and suffered mainly from phobias. Of 71 responders, 58 had tried to reduce or stop their medication at some time and all but 5 had noticed a return of symptoms. Nearly half the subjects also reported new symptoms and if two or more new symptoms can be regarded as a 'withdrawal syndrome' then this occurred in 14 subjects. The authors also point out that the respondents were predominantly middle-aged, married and in employment and so did not conform to the usual stereotype of drug abusers. In the meantime Tyrer et al (22[C]) have noted that 44% of their series of patients gradually withdrawn from diazepam experienced true withdrawal symptoms, including reduced sleep, depersonalization and sadness. However, pseudo-withdrawal complaints could also be induced in patients who merely thought their drug was being reduced.

Withdrawal effects have also been noted after brief (3 weeks) use of halazepam and oxazepam (8[c]). In future, clinical trials of new benzodiazepines should include observations on the patients after the end of the active treatment to detect such effects.

The mechanism for dependence is unclear, but it is assumed to be related to the presence of specific receptors in the central nervous system. This is a rapidly developing area as further receptor sites are established both centrally and peripherally (9[R]), for which no specific function is yet known. Generally, sedative drugs are believed to act by enhancing γ-aminobutyric acid (GABA) transmission. Should tolerance occur to this mechanism, withdrawal of sedative would then lead to an acute reduction in GABA function which may cause symptoms. Cowen and Nutt (10[R]) have suggested that this may be a mechanism common to many sedatives including benzodiazepines, alcohol and barbiturates.

So far, the management of withdrawal symptoms is not clearly established. Mellor and Jain (2[c]) saw no effects from chlorpromazine or hydroxyzine and in a General Practice study a variety of benzodiazepines were withdrawn over a period of up to 6 weeks without too much difficulty (14[c]). With a fairly simple controlled program two-thirds of patients were abstinent at follow-up 3 to 5 months later.

Other effects The effects of benzodiazepines on *pregnancy and labor* have been comprehensively reviewed (11[R]). As the benzodiazepines are lipophilic and undissociated agents they cross the placenta rapidly and are taken up by the fetus, this process being facilitated in later pregnancy by changes in the placenta itself and in uterine circulation. The pharmacokinetics also change in pregnancy, due to changes in drug disposition with total plasma clearance remaining the same but terminal half life being prolonged. In the normal infant hydroxylation is very limited and other pathways (demethylation and conjugation reactions) are also limited in premature babies.

Dement et al have reviewed the effects on daytime *alertness and insomnia* (12[R]). They argue that up till now, sleep laboratory investigations have concentrated upon measures of sleep, particularly EEG recordings, with relatively little emphasis on daytime performance. In their view, insomnia itself only rarely requires treatment and most patients seek help for what they regard as the effects of insomnia – daytime drowsiness, depression and irritability. They have devised a measure of sleepiness which can be repeatedly estimated – the multiple sleep latency test (MSLT). Preliminary results show that long-acting benzodiazepines such as flurazepam increase daytime sleepiness whereas it is decreased by short-acting ones. However, if the drug is too short-acting early morning or terminal insomnia may occur, as has been reported with midozolam and triazolam (13[c]).

An important negative finding was reported (19[c]). In view of the possibility that benzodiazepines might cause *cerebral atrophy* the authors carried out computerized tomographic brain scans on 28 benzodiazepine users and compared them to normals and to alcoholics. All radiological indices of brain size were normal both for benzodiazepine dependents and normals.

Public health aspects Skegg et al (15[C]) identified 79 admissions to hospital for deliberate *overdose.* A psychotropic drug was taken in 53 episodes, the most common ones being diazepam and nitrazepam. These cases were then studied by a record linkage study involving a total population of 34,870. This showed that although psychotropic drugs featured heavily as a proportion of overdoses, the number of people actually prescribed psychotropics who subsequently overdosed was very low – 3 per 1000. A further study has appeared assessing the effect of two benzodiazepines – temazepam and flurazepam – on *driving ability* in volunteer women (16[c]). On testing, flurazepam subjects hit significantly more obstacles than under placebo conditions. Although the subjects did not drive fast or misjudge whether the vehicle could pass through a gap, on both drugs they hit the sides of the gap significantly more often. This suggested carelessness rather than an increase in risk-taking behavior or diminution in judgment.

Interactions King (17[c]) has produced evidence from fatal poisonings that *amitriptyline* overdose was more lethal when combined with a benzodiazepine. In 50 cases involving amitriptyline only, the post-mortem amitriptyline levels were higher than in 24 cases where two drugs were taken. As the levels of benzodiazepine were often within the therapeutic range, a synergistic effect cannot be discounted. The complex relationship between *ethanol* and the benzodiazepines has been fully reviewed (18[R]). Kinetically, acute ethanol use delays benzodiazepine metabolism by demethylation or hydroxylation, but chronic use accelerates it. There also appears to be some synergism as regards the sedative and psychomotor effects of the combination.

INDIVIDUAL BENZODIAZEPINES

Diazepam

Parenteral use Further investigations have been reported on the various sequelae of intravenous use of diazepam (20[C]). This was a very thorough study with a prolonged follow-up (up to 12 weeks if necessary). It was found that two-thirds of patients experienced sequelae of one sort or another, the majority progressing to *thrombophlebitis*. The incidence did not appear to be influenced by any of the following variables; vein diameter, pain on injection, dose of diazepam or volume of solution injected. The main variable that did distinguish between those who developed complications and normals was that blood flow velocity was higher in normals; furthermore when complications did ensue they were resolved more satisfactorily in veins with higher initial blood flow velocities, suggesting that where possible, fairly large veins should be used. A further unusual experience was reported (45[c]). A healthy 26-year-old male developed phlebitis from intravenous diazepam, which resolved in 2 days with symptomatic treatment. However, 3 days later he took diazepam 10 mg orally and some hours later tenderness and erythema recurred along the original vein site. The authors suggest that diazepam may have interfered with a subclinical healing process but do not appear to have considered whether there was an allergic mechanism. The danger that i.v. diazepam may cause excessive *sedation* was highlighted by Allen and Gough (46[c]) who used intravenous doxapram in an attempt to reverse this sedation. The study was subsequently criticized, particularly for the dose of diazepam used which was regarded as excessive (47[r]). Intravenous diazepam is often the treatment of choice for status epilepticus. 7 cases were reported of children who suffered respiratory depression as a result of such conventional treatment (48[C]). In 5 of them there was evidence of raised intracranial pressure and it is possible in such circumstances that the respiratory centre is more sensitive.

Oral use A direct association between diazepam and hepatitis was described in one patient (49[cr]). A 45-year-old male was admitted with chest pain. Although there were signs of possible liver damage (raised SGOT and excessive whiskey ingestion) he was given diazepam 5 mg t.d.s. 4 days later isoniazid was added but the following day his liver enzymes had risen and both drugs were stopped. Rechallenge with diazepam 11 days later caused an increase in SGOT and a subsequent liver biopsy showed 'focal necrosis with necrotic hepatocytes being replaced by neutrophils and eosinophils. Intracellular cholestasis was also present'. Sedative drugs are potentially dangerous in liver disease. Rivett and Benatar report on a woman who developed viral hepatitis and encephalopathy (50[c]). She was treated with single doses of hydroxyzine, diazepam and clothiapine but subsequently died. From the information given it is not possible to state whether any drug was causative or if so, which.

Triazolam

A sleep laboratory study has confirmed the hypnotic effects of triazolam 0.5 mg (51[cR]). The usual phenomena were found – especially a highly significant reduction in stage 4 sleep, similar to that found with flurazepam. Generally subjects performed well on cognitive tests the next morning and 'rebound insomnia' was not seen. However there was some *impairment of memory* and the authors discuss the possible reasons for this. They feel that their data may be best explained by a non-specific effect upon arousal, but point out that triazolam had acute effects on performance, arousal threshold and memory when subjects were woken from sleep. Insomniac patients treated with triazolam may therefore not respond to signals (such as smoke detectors) or recall night-time activities such as telephone calls or taking medicines.

Midazolam

Midazolam is an imidazobenzodiazepine which is short-acting and has the advantage of being water-soluble. Its intravenous use as a sedative prior to gastroscopy was reported in 40 patients (52[c]). A standard dose was used (0.07 mg/kg) and although this was effective in patients aged over 60 years, there was considerable variation over-all. Local venous complications were not seen. Midazolam also appears to be effective as an induction agent in children (53[c]). Despite its very brief half-life the drug has been used as a hypnotic. A South American study of 6 patients took place in a sleep laboratory (54[c]). Midazolam appeared to be an effective hypnotic with the usual benzodiazepine effects. Side effects that were noted were headache, muscular weakness and dizziness, although the dosage used (30 mg) was rather high. A more conventional dose (15 mg) was compared to flunitrazepam 1 mg, and placebo in normals who suffered from midwinter insomnia in the Arctic Circle (67[c]). Despite the difference in elimination half-lives the two active drugs appeared to be equally effective.

Flurazepam

Contradictory views have been expressed on this drug. Mendelson et al (55[c]) studied 11 chronically insomniac patients for 28 nights followed by 7 nights of withdrawal. EEG measures of total sleep time and sleep efficiency were improved but the changes in sleep latency and nocturnal wakings were insignificant. The main changes occurred in the first 2 nights when subjective benefits were noted and when cognitive impairment was maximal. Metabolic products (desalkylflurazepam) accumulated and plasma drug concentrations did not correlate with sleep measures. On the other hand Kales and Kales (56[R]) summarized their results with temazepam, triazolam and flurazepam. They favor the last drug as it is effective in initiating sleep, its effects continue for up to 4 weeks and rebound insomnia does not occur. Their report also emphasizes other factors in the treatment of insomnia including general advice, specific counseling and psychotherapeutic techniques and appropriate antidepressant treatment. Flurazepam appears to be particularly prone to cause problems in the elderly including confusion, disorientation and effects upon respiration (57[R]).

Other benzodiazepines

Temazepam and nitrazepam were studied in 71 elderly in-patients (58[C]). This study shows the problems of investigating such a group of patients – 13 dropped out, many found difficulty in completing some of the tests involved and there was wide variation in base-line levels. However both drugs accumulated in the plasma over 7 days and reaction time was slowed over the same period. Individual differences were important – patients with low scores on basic intelligence tests (Raven's progressive matrices and the Mill Hill vocabulary score) did badly.

Ketazolam in an open study of 35 patients was reported (59[c]). Although there were many methodological errors, Deberdt reported that 8 of the patients experienced side effects including the usual drowsiness. However one patient experienced weight change and one an allergic reaction of which no further details are given.

Chlordiazepoxide in a possible *interaction* with levodopa has been reported (60[c]). A 66-year-old female had Parkinson's disease which had been well controlled by levodopa, benztropine and diphenhydramine. She took part in a clinical trial in which she took chlordiazepoxide 10 mg t.i.d. for 2 weeks. She became drowsy and ataxic: when reviewed at the clinic she had tremor and rigidity which resolved when the chlordiazepoxide was stopped.

Bromazepam has been used in several open trials in a variety of out-patient and in-patient settings (61[c], 62[c]). The effects, both wanted and unwanted, seem similar to other benzodiazepines but loss of libido, tremor and excitement were recorded.

Newer benzodiazepines

As has been noted in previous years, new forms of the benzodiazepine molecule continue to appear, this year being no exception. Generally the side effects which are noted are similar to those of the longer established drugs; the newer drugs are reported here either because of an unusual reaction or indication, or for the sake of completeness.

Estazolam is a triazolo-benzodiazepine (cf. triazolam and alprazolam) which is marketed as a hypnotic in Denmark. Lingjaerde had previously observed that this drug had an effect upon *auditory hallucinations* and has now reported (21[C]) a multi-center study in which 51 schizophrenic patients took part in a double-blind trial in which estazolam 6 mg/day was compared to placebo with particular interest being shown in any effect on hallucinations. The protocol was slightly unusual in that, while the design was of a cross-over trial, half of the patients received two courses of the active drug. Both groups improved in the first study period, regardless of the medication, but this improvement was maintained better on the group who then began active treatment. Unfortunately, for many of the symptoms the results showed this trend but did not reach statistical significance. Side effects were few, particularly since the dose was fairly high and neuroleptics were continued, but 2 patients dropped out because of heavy sedation and 1 because of a skin eruption; headache and restlessness were also observed.

Halazepam is a fluoridated 1,4-benzodiazepine with a median half-life of excretion of 14 hours, but is rapidly metabolized to N-desmethyldiazepam and is thus little different from many other benzodiazepines. Drowsiness and dry mouth seem to occur commonly with its use and in elderly patients motor coordination is impaired (23[R]).

Quazepam is a trifluoroethyl benzodiazepine. Its effects were studied in 60 elderly insomniac patients (24[c]). Although its effects appeared similar to those of other such drugs, there did not appear to be any advantages, as drowsiness, anorexia, asthenia, headache and pruritus were all noted. Quazepam has a long elimination half-life and shares a metabolic pathway with flurazepam; a dose of 30 mg appeared to be as effective as flunitrazepam 1 mg or 2 mg in a series of patients given a single-dose hypnotic prior to surgery (25[c]).

Alprazolam is the first triazolobenzodiazepine to be marketed in the United States and in Canada. A comprehensive review is available (26[R]) which describes the pharmacokinetic data and the earlier clinical trials with the drug. The former suggests that elderly males may be more susceptible to side effects. Although it appears to have no significant advantages over other benzodiazepines as regards the usual side effects, considerable discussion has taken place as to whether it has any antidepressant activity. This may only be in the sense of sharing with more orthodox antidepressants an effect in panic attacks or panic disorder (27[r]) rather than in more formal depressive illness itself. The U.K. Data sheet on alprazolam does not include a warning that depression may follow its use and considerable play is made of this in promotional material: however, Fawcett and Kravitz (26[R]), in summarizing the adverse reactions from many studies, suggest that 10% of patients on alprazolam report depression. If alprazolam does have an effect upon mood, this may be significant – in an addendum to Fawcett and Kravitz's review Gelenberg suggests that there is anecdotal evidence that the well-known 'paradoxical reaction' may be occurring quite frequently in alprazolam-treated patients. An amino-alkyl derivative, adinazolam is also undergoing preliminary clinical investigation.

Prazepam is yet another precursor of desmethyldiazepam whose use has been reported (28[c]).

Brotizolam has been compared to flurazepam in hospitalized elderly patients (29[c]).

Metaclazepam Mallach and Schmidt (30[C]) have studied the interaction between alcohol and metaclazepam in 125 normals. It appears that when alcohol is ingested the plasma concentration of metaclazepam is higher than when the drug is taken alone: the combination causes dizziness, ataxia, prolonging of the effects of alcohol and fatigue.

Loprazolam appears to have no advantages or disadvantages when compared to nitrazepam (65[c]).

OTHER DRUGS

Chlormezanone

With the realization that the benzodiazepines as a group suffer from several disadvantages, attention has been turned to alternative sedatives, some of which have been available for several years. For instance Ghosh (31[c]) has reported a 4-week open study in which chlormezanone 200 mg was used as night sedation in 32 patients admitted to a geriatric ward: he found that duration and quality of sleep was improved and there was no deterioration on a test of mental agility. *Drowsiness/lethargy* was the only side effect noticed. A larger dose (400 mg) was used on younger patients in a sleep laboratory study (34[c]). Chlormezanone increased total sleep time and decreased wakefulness but did not reduce sleep latency. A case of chlormezanone *overdose* has also been described (32[c]). A 36-year-old woman took 7 g of the drug: although she was comatose on admission she regained consciousness over the next 15 hours and had no further complaints. However, even drugs such as this one are not without problems as is shown by a case history of drug abuse (33[c]).

A 37-year-old man developed neck pain radiating to the occiput and into the arms: initially diazepam was effective, but in 1974 this was replaced by chlormezanone which was equally effective. In 1979 it was observed that his intake of the drug had increased but attempts to limit his use failed and he is now taking approximately 25 tablets daily. Although, if deprived of treatment he tries to obtain it from other physicians, he shows no other behavior of an addictive nature.

In the discussion the authors point out that while chlormezanone abuse has not been reported before, this may be due to its relatively limited use.

Other effects of chlormezanone include headache, skin rashes, dryness of the mouth and cholestatic jaundice.

Chlormethiazole

Chlormethiazole has previously been implicated in the development of *dysphagia* (SEDA-7, 53). A further case has been reported in which a 55-year-old woman receiving treatment for delirium tremens and suspected pancreatitis complained of severe retrosternal pain 4 hours after taking chlormethiazole (35[c]). Endoscopy was done 2 days later and extensive irregularly shaped ulcers were seen in the esophagus. Although repeat endoscopy 1 week later showed satisfactory healing, pressures found on manometry were still abnormal one month later.

Glutethimide

An unusual complication was ascribed to withdrawal of glutethemide (36[c]) in a man being admitted to hospital following a suspected overdose. He subsequently developed *catatonia* which was treated conservatively and which cleared spontaneously after 10 days in hospital. As it is recognized that catatonia can occur with metabolic and toxic conditions including various drugs, it would probably be prudent to include glutethimide as a possible precipitant.

Thalidomide

The use of thalidomide is now mainly restricted to dermatology. Tomas et al (37[c]) reported on 4 years experience of treating 18 patients with giant aphthous ulcers or Behcet's disease. They did not observe any neurotoxicity and 2 patients could not tolerate the drug because of gastrointestinal symptoms; generally speaking the results of treatment were considered to be similar to that of other drugs such as corticosteroids and immuno-suppressants. It is possible, in fact, that thalidomide works in these conditions by immuno-suppression (38[R]). However, symptoms of polyneuritis occurred in one quarter of 60 patients with chronic lupus erythematosus (39[c]): although the treatment was successful, the authors suggest that alternative treatments such as anti-malarials or local steroids should be used first.

Paraldehyde

Paraldehyde is now rarely used. An alcoholic male underwent aorto-femoral bypass with lumbar sympathectomy (40[cR]). Two days later he developed delirium tremens and received 23 ml of paraldehyde parenterally over a 10-hour period. Following his last injection he became apneic, cyanotic and hypotensive. He subsequently recovered but in the meantime non-cardiac pulmonary edema was established. Mountain and his colleagues suggest that paraldehyde was responsible and that it may have a direct effect on the alveolar-capillary membrane.

Didropyridin

Three cases of agranulocytosis following exposure to Didropyridin were noted over a period in Berlin (41[c]). Two of the patients responded well to treatment but the third continued to have a low white cell count.

Fenobam

A further report has appeared on fenobam (42[c]). This is a drug whose chemical structure is different from other psychotropics. In this study 29 patients took part in a double-blind trial comparing this agent to diazepam and placebo. Although the patient groups were small and all three groups improved, both the active groups fared better than the placebo group. Side effects noted in the fenobam group included nausea, insomnia, agitation, drowsiness, anorexia and bed-time derealization.

Tracazolate

Preliminary findings have been reported on a further non-benzodiazepine substance, tracazolate (44[r]). Animal experiments indicate that it may have a wider separation between anxiolytic and ataxic effects and that it may not potentiate other CNS depressants. It is now being subjected to investigation in human volunteers.

Barbiturates

Barbiturates remain a public health problem. McCarron et al (63[C]) studied 609 consecutive cases of short-acting barbiturate intoxication over a 5-year period and reviewed case notes of a further 531 cases. They suggest that there is usually a fairly good correlation between level of intoxication and plasma levels of barbiturate; and that if these are dissonant this is either because some other condition is present as well or because the patient is habituated to barbiturates. They found the usual complications of hypoglycemia, aspiration pneumonia, pulmonary edema and skin lesions: cardiac arrhythmia, GI tract hemorrhage and rhabdomyolysis also occurred. A further hazard of phenobarbital (used as an anticonvulsant) is that it can decrease the blood level and therefore the effectiveness of metronidazole (64[c]). A patient with trichomoniasis finally responded only when double the usual dose of metronidazole was given. High-dose phenobarbital when given as a bolus intravenously may cause venous thrombosis (65[c]).

Misuse

An astonishing danger of many psychotropic drugs was reported from Australia (43[c]). Apparently scuba divers ingest sedatives to enhance the euphoria of the nitrogen narcosis that is experienced during diving. In the case reported the patient became unconscious and was brought to the surface rapidly. On his regaining consciousness after 48 hours, it transpired that he had developed 'the bends'. While treatment was successful, the author warns that this was to an extent fortuitous.

REFERENCES

1. Mackinnon GL, Parker WA (1982) Benzodiazepine withdrawal syndrome: a literature review and evaluation. *Am. J. Drug Alcohol Abuse*, *9*, 19.
2. Mellor CS, Jain VK (1982) Diazepam withdrawal syndrome: its prolonged and changing nature. *Can. Med. Assoc. J.*, *127*, 1093.
3. Tognoni G, Gomeni R, De Maio D et al (1975) Pharmacokinetics of N-desmethyldiazepam in patients suffering from insomnia and treated with nortriptyline. *Br. J. Clin. Pharmacol.*, *2*, 227.

4. Laughren TP, Battey Y, Greenblatt DJ et al (1982) A controlled trial of diazepam withdrawal in chronically anxious outpatients. *Acta Psychiatr. Scand., 65,* 171.
5. Hallstrom C, Lader M (1981) Benzodiazepine withdrawal phenomena. *Int. Pharmacopsychiatry, 16,* 235.
6. Hallstrom C, Lader M (1982) The incidence of benzodiazepine dependence in long-term users. *J. Psychiatr. Treat. Eval., 4,* 293.
7. Schöpf J (1983) Withdrawal phenomena after long-term administration of benzodiazepines: a review of recent investigations. *Pharmacopsychiatry, 16,* 1.
8. Pecknold JC, McClure DJ, Fleuri D et al (1982) Benzodiazepine withdrawal effects. *Prog. Neuropsychopharmacol. Biol. Psychiatry, 6,* 517.
9. Richards JG, Möhler J, Haefely W (1982) Benzodiazepine binding sites – receptors or acceptors? *Trends Pharmacol. Sci., 3,* 233.
10. Cowen PJ, Nutt DJ (1982) Abstinence symptoms after withdrawal of tranquillising drugs: is there a common neurochemical mechanism? *Lancet, 2,* 360.
11. Kanto JH (1982) Use of benzodiazepines during pregnancy, labour and lactation with particular reference to pharmacokinetic considerations. *Drugs, 23,* 354.
12. Dement W, Seidel W, Crskadon M (1982) Daytime alertness insomnia and benzodiazepines. *Sleep, 5,* S28.
13. Kales A, Soldatos CR, Bixler EO et al (1983) Early morning insomnia with rapidly eliminated benzodiazepines. *Science, 220,* 95.
14. Hopkins DR, Sethi KBS, Mucklow JC (1982) Benzodiazepine withdrawal in general practice. *J. R. Coll. Pract., 32,* 758.
15. Skegg K, Skegg DCG, Richards SM (1983) Incidence of self poisoning in patients prescribed psychotropic drugs. *Br. Med. J., 286,* 841.
16. Betts TA, Birtle J (1982) Effect of two hypnotic drugs on actual driving performance next morning. *Br. Med. J., 285,* 852.
17. King LA (1982) Synergistic effect of benzodiazepines in fatal amitriptyline poisonings. *Lancet, 2,* 982.
18. Sellers EM, Busto U (1982) Benzodiazepines and ethanol: assessment of the effects and consequences of psychotropic drug interactions. *J. Clin. Psychopharmacol., 2,* 249.
19. Poser W, Poser S, Roscher D et al (1983) Do benzodiazepines cause cerebral atrophy? *Lancet, 1,* 715.
20. Glaser JW, Blanton PL, Thrush WJ (1982) Incidence and extent of venous sequelae with intravenous diazepam utilizing a standardized conscious sedation technique. *J. Periodontol., 53,* 700.
21. Lingjaerde O (1982) Effect of the benzodiazepine derivative estazolam in patients with auditory hallucinations. *Acta Psychiatr. Scand., 65,* 339.
22. Tyrer P, Owen R, Dawling S (1983) Gradual withdrawal of diazepam after long-term therapy. *Lancet, 1,* 1402.
23. Fann WE, Pitts WM, Whelass JC (1982) Pharmacology, efficacy and adverse effects of Halazepam, a new benzodiazepine. *Pharmacotherapy, 2,* 72.
24. Martinez JT, Serna CT (1982) Short-term treatment with quazepam of insomnia in geriatric patients. *Clin. Ther., 5,* 174.
25. Wickstrom E, Allgulander C (1983) Comparison of quazepam, flunitrazepam and placebo as single-dose hypnotics before surgery. *Eur. J. Clin. Pharmacol., 24,* 67.
26. Fawcett JA, Kravitz HM (1982) Alprazolam: pharmacokinetics, clinical efficacy, and mechanism of action. *Pharmacotherapy, 2,* 243.
27. Snaith RP (1983) Panic Disorder. *Br. Med. J., 286,* 1376.
28. Elens P (1982) Klinische studie van prazepam bij gehospitaliseerde psychiatrische patienten. *Ars Med., 2,* 850.
29. Martinez JS, Palos JL (1982) Estudio comparativo de dos distintos hipnogenos en pacientes geriatricos. *Invest. Med. Int., 9,* 66.
30. Mallach HG, Schmidt V (1982) Examination to assess the interaction between alcohol and a new 1,4 benzodiazepine (Metaclazepam). *Blutalkohol, 19,* 416.
31. Ghosh AK (1982) Four-week tolerance study of chlormezanone for the treatment of insomnia in the elderly. *J. Int. Med. Res., 10,* 431.
32. Armstrong D, Braithwaite RA, Vale JA (1983) Chlormezanone poisoning. *Br. Med. J., 286,* 845.
33. Kirkeby OJ, Risoe C, Veel T (1982) Et tilfelle av klormazanonmisbruk. *Tidsskr. Nor. Laegeforen., 102,* 1863.
34. Anonymous (1983) Chlormezanone: from sedative to hypnotic? *Drug Ther. Bull., 21,* 32.
35. Rohner Von HG, Berges W, Wienbeck M (1982) Clomethiazol tablets induce ulcers in the esophagus. *Z. Gastroenterol., 20,* 469.
36. Campbell R, Schaffer CB, Tupin J (1983) Catatonia associated with glutethimide withdrawal. *J. Clin. Psychiatry, 44,* 32.
37. Torras H, Lecha M, Mascaro JM (1982) Le talidomina en al tratamiento de las aftosis y enfermedad de Behcet. *Med. Cutanea Ibero-Lat.-Am., 10,* 103.
38. Hunziker T, Krebs A (1983) Thalidomid in der Dermatologie. *Hautarzt, 34,* 66.
39. Knop J, Bonsmann G, Happle R et al (1983) Thalidomide in the treatment of sixty cases of chronic discoid lupus erythematosus. *Br. J. Dermatol., 108,* 461.
40. Mountain R, Ferguson S, Fowler A et al (1982) Noncardiac pulmonary edema following administration of parenteral paraldehyde. *Chest, 82,* 371.
41. Schleusner A (1982) Agranulozytose durch Benedorm (Didropyridin). *Folia Haematol., 109,* 443.
42. Pecknold JC, McClure DJ, Appeltauer L et

al (1982) Treatment of anxiety using fenobam (a nonbenzodiazepine) in a double-blind standard (diazepam) placebo-controlled study. *J. Clin. Psychopharmacol.*, *2*, 129.

43. Unsworth IP (1982) Spinal decompression sickness while scuba diving under the influence of drugs. *Med. J. Austr.*, *1*, 543.

44. Anon (1982) ICI's tracazolate: less CNS depression. *Scrip*, *688*, 16.

45. Brandstette RD, Gotz VP (1983) Recurrence of intravenous-diazepam-induced phlebitis from oral diazepam. *Drug Intell. Clin. Pharm.*, *17*, 125.

46. Allen CJ, Gough KR (1983) Effect of doxapram on heavy sedation produced by intravenous diazepam. *Br. Med. J.*, *286*, 1181.

47. Lake APJ, Houston T (1983) Effect of doxapram on heavy sedation produced by intravenous diazepam (letter). *Br. Med. J.*, *286*, 2061.

48. Gatrad AR (1982) Dangers of intravenous diazepam in controlling fits in patients with raised intracranial pressure. *Br. J. Clin. Pract.*, *36*, 189.

49. Tedesco FJ, Mills LR (1982) Diazepam (Valium) hepatitis. *Dig. Dis. Sci.*, *27*, 470.

50. Rivett K, Benatar SR (1982) The danger of sedative drug administration in liver disease. *S. Afr. Med. Tijdskr.*, *61*, 649.

51. Spinweber CL, Johnson LC (1982) Effects of triazolam (0.5 mg) on sleep, performance, memory and arousal threshold. *Psychopharmacology*, *76*, 5.

52. Brophy T, Dundee JW, Heazelwood V et al (1982) Midazolam, a water-soluble benzodiazepine, for gastroscopy. *Anaesth. Intensive Care*, *10*, 344.

53. Holloway AM, Jordaan D, Brock-Utne JG (1982) Midazolam for the intravenous induction of anaesthesia in children. *Anaesth. Intensive Care*, *10*, 340.

54. Monti JM, Debellis J, Gratadoux E et al (1982) Sleep laboratory study of the effects of midazolam in insomniac patients. *Eur. J. Clin. Pharmacol.*, *21*, 479.

55. Mendelson WB, Weingartner H, Greenblatt DJ et al (1982) A clinical study of flurazepam. *Sleep*, *5*, 350.

56. Kales A, Kales JD (1983) Sleep laboratory studies of hypnotic drugs: efficacy and withdrawal effects. *J. Clin. Psychopharmacol.*, *3*, 140.

57. Guilleminault C, Silvestri R (1982) Aging, drugs and sleep. *Neurobiol. Aging*, *3*, 379.

58. Cook PJ, Huggett A, Graham-Pole R et al (1983) Hypnotic accumulation and hangover in elderly inpatients: a controlled double-blind study of temazepam and nitrazepam. *Br. Med. J.*, *286*, 100.

59. Deberdt R (1982) Utilisation du Ketazolam comme anxiolytique dans la medecine generale: étude ouverte, menée par des medicine généralistes. *Ars Med.*, *37*, 1326.

60. Yosselson-Superstine S, Lipman AG (1982) Chlordiazepoxide interaction with levadopa. *Ann. Intern. Med.*, *96*, 259.

61. Kress JJ, Maheo M, Cledes A et al (1982) Essai clinique du bromazepam en psychiatrie hospitalière. *Nouv. Presse Méd.*, *11*, 1735.

62. Horseau C, Brion C (1982) Essai clinique du bromazepam. *Nouv Presse Méd.*, *11*, 1741.

63. McCarron MM, Schulze BW, Walberg CB et al (1982) Short-acting barbiturate overdosage. *J. Am. Med. Assoc.*, *248*, 55.

64. Mead PB, Gibson M, Schentag JJ et al (1982) Possible alteration of metronidazole metabolism by phenobarbital. *N. Engl. J. Med.*, *306*, 1490.

65. DeNicola LK, Hays DP (1983) Thrombophlebosis due to high dose barbiturates. *Drug Intell. Clin. Pharm.*, *16*, 880.

66. Salkind MR, Silverstone R (1983) The clinical and psychometric evaluation of a new hypnotic drug, loprazolam, in general practice. *Curr. Med. Res. Opin.*, *8*, 368.

67. Lingjaerde O, Bratlid T, Westby OC et al (1983) Effect of midazolam, flunitrazepam and placebo against midwinter insomnia in northern Norway. *Acta Psychiatr. Scand.*, *67*, 118.

E.A. Babayan, G.M. Rudenko and V.K. Lepakhin

6 Neuroleptics and antipsychotics

Antipsychotic drug therapy and sexual dysfunction

Sexual side effects associated with antipsychotic drug therapy may frequently go unrecognized, either because patients treated with these drugs do not mention the development of sexual dysfunction or physicians fail to inquire about it. The available data suggest that when information is sought, such problems are frequently found.

Sexual dysfunction in men

Mitchell and Popkin (1[R]) have recently reviewed the literature of male sexual dysfunction associated with antipsychotic drug treatment. They point out that the available clinical information on this side effect of neuroleptics consists primarily of individual case reports or small series of patients. Unfortunately, important data have frequently been omitted; not uncommonly, authors will report one type of problem, such as ejaculatory dysfunction, and fail to mention changes in other sexual functions as well as such relevant factors as the use of other medication (psychotropic or nonpsychotropic) and a history of earlier sexual dysfunction.

One must also remember that many patients receiving antipsychotic drugs may have impaired sexual dysfunction which is not attributable to the medications they receive but may be a symptom of their illness. In a recently published study Nestros and Lehmann (2[C]) come to the (hardly surprising) finding that male schizophrenic patients report less frequent sexual ideation and activity, both before and during the period of their illness, than do nonpsychotic control subjects.

The categories of drug-induced sexual dysfunction dealt with in the review by Mitchell and Popkin included problems with erectile function, changes in the quality of orgasm, ejaculatory dysfunction, change in libido, and priapism. Of these, erectile and ejaculatory disturbances have been the most frequently reported.

Most reported cases of erectile dysfunction indicate appearance of the problem shortly after the initiation of antipsychotic therapy, not uncommonly within 24 hours. To date, most cases reported have involved young men. The problem appears to recede fairly soon after the antipsychotic drug is withdrawn.

Impotence or erectile dysfunction have been reported in association with several phenothiazine tranquilizers. The agent most frequently mentioned is thioridazine. Kotin et al (3[C]) interviewed 87 sexually active patients taking a neuroleptic; they excluded patients with medical problems known to predispose the individual to sexual difficulties. Sixty percent of the subjects receiving thioridazine reported sexual dysfunction, whereas only 25% of the patients taking other neuroleptics reported such problems. Of the patients taking thioridazine, 44% reported difficulty in achieving erection and 35% difficulty in maintaining erection. For patients taking other antipsychotic drugs, the corresponding figures were 19% and 11%.

Thioridazine is also the drug most commonly associated with ejaculatory dysfunction. Blair and Simpson (4[C]) estimated that 30% of one group of patients taking thioridazine experienced ejaculatory dysfunction. In their comparative study Kotin et al (3[C]) noted that 28 of 57 patients who had taken (or were taking) thioridazine reported changes in ejaculatory orgasm, while 9 reported a decreased amount of ejaculate.

The lowest daily dose reported to have been associated with this problem is 30 mg (5[C]).

Side Effects of Drugs Annual 8
M.N.G. Dukes, editor

ISBN 0 444 90339 9
$0.80 per article per page (transactional system)
$0.20 per article per page (licensing system)

Isolated cases of ejaculatory dysfunction have also been reported with the following drugs and minimum doses: chlorpromazine, 400 mg/day (6[C]) and 50–75 mg/day (7[C]); chlorprothixene, 300 mg/day (8[C]); piperacetazine, 100 mg/day (9[C]); and mesoridazine, 60 mg/day (10[C]).

Spontaneous ejaculation *The first report of spontaneous ejaculation associated with the therapeutic use of psychotropic drugs was recently described by Keitner and Selub (11[C]).*

A 46-year-old man with major depression had previously received thioridazine but on admission his only medication was acetaminophen, and he had no active physical disorder.

On the 4th day of hospitalization, he was started on trifluoperazine, 20 mg at bedtime, which was increased to 30 mg on the 7th day but lowered again to 20 mg on the 8th day and to 5 mg on the 9th day. That day he reported his first spontaneous ejaculation and orgasm. A second spontaneous ejaculation occurred on the 10th hospital day.

Due to inadequate clinical response and continued complaints of side effects, he was switched to thiothixene 10 mg on day 15 with an increase to 20 mg on day 16. The patient reported his third spontaneous ejaculation on that same day and the fourth and last one, on day 17.

In all, he had four episodes of spontaneous ejaculation with orgasms while on neuroleptics alone. All occurred during the day in the company of women, although in nonsexual context. Each began with warm preorgasmic penile sensations; ejaculation followed within 20 to 60 seconds and was accompanied by a pleasurable feeling akin to coital orgasm. He maintained that he had made no attempt at self-stimulation and that he had either no erection or only a partial erection.

The patient had no history of sexual dysfunction, spontaneous or premature ejaculations, even while on thioridazine, during his previous hospitalization. However, he had not had sexual intercourse for the past 2 years.

One possible explanation for this effect is postsynaptic receptor supersensitivity. Another mechanism may be the neuroleptic effect on presynaptic dopamine receptors. It is interesting to note that spontaneous ejaculation also occurs in opiate addiction withdrawal (12[R]).

Effect on orgasm *Some authors have reported normal orgasmic function in men despite ejaculatory disturbance secondary to thioridazine treatment (13[C], 14[C], 15[C]). Others have noted a disturbance in the quality of orgasm (16[C], 17[C]). Kotin et al (3[C]) noted that 8% (6 of 77) of the patients in their series reported a change in the quality of orgasm. Four were receiving thioridazine, and 2 were taking other neuroleptics. Two of the patients taking thioridazine reported painful orgasm; the same occurred in a patient initially receiving 10 mg/day of trifluoperazine and, later, 5 mg/day of haloperidol (18[C]).*

Effect on libido *Changes in libido associated with antipsychotic drug therapy have not been systematically studied. Discussion of libido has usually been omitted from case reports of sexual dysfunction, perhaps because changes in libido are particularly difficult to interpret. Patients with other forms of sexual dysfunction may secondarily develop decreased libido. When mentioned in reports of sexual dysfunction secondary to antipsychotics, libido has generally been found to be decreased (19[C], 20[C]).*

Priapism *One of the most serious sexual adverse reactions to neuroleptics is priapism – a prolonged painful erection of the penis. This condition frequently requires surgical intervention (21[C]). Mitchell and Popkin (1[R]) found 19 cases of priapism in which an antipsychotic drug was considered to be involved. In 6 cases patients were taking thioridazine (minimum dose, 100 mg/day), in 1 case in combination with triflupromazine (22[C], 23[C]). A single case of priapism associated with mesoridazine at a dose of 400 mg/day has been reported (24[C]). Six case reports have involved patients taking chlorpromazine at a daily minimum dose of 100 mg (25[C], 26[C], 27[C], 28[C]). One case report involved a man who developed priapism after a single intramuscular injection of 25 mg of chlorpromazine (29[C]). In the other 4 cases the specific phenothiazine was not identified (30[C]). In an additional series of 46 patients with priapism, medications 'such as phenothiazine drugs or heparin' were believed to be involved in 7 of the cases (31[R]). One case of frequent prolonged erection has been reported with molindone. Illberg (32[C]) reported priapism in association with perphenazine treatment.*

Impotence *Impotence in association with the use of pimozide was described by*

Ananth (34[C]). That the patient's impotence was a side effect of pimozide was confirmed by the fact that it occurred while he was taking this drug, disappeared when the medication was discontinued and occurred again after renewal of the treatment with pimozide.

Sperm motility *The effects of chlorpromazine, diazepam, phenytoin and phenobarbitone on human sperm motility were investigated in vitro by Hong et al (35[CR]). Only chlorpromazine inhibited human sperm motility and the concentration which decreased sperm motility by 50% of control was 0.22 mM. The authors conclude that the clinical implication of such reduced motility awaits further evaluation. It is of interest that chlorpromazine, which markedly inhibits sperm motility in vitro has not been reported to have such effects in vivo, while on the other hand, phenytoin reduces sperm motility in vivo, but not in vitro. It is also worth noting that human plasma levels of chlorpromazine rarely exceed 0.001 mM.*

Sex differences

As pointed out above, there is generally little firm information available on the relative frequency of neuroleptic-induced sexual disturbances as between the sexes. However, Ghadirian et al (33[CR]) have evaluated the incidence and severity of sexual dysfunction in both male and female schizophrenic patients on long term antipsychotic treatment and examined the relationship of sexual dysfunction to plasma prolactin levels. In female patients, menstrual disorders were included as part of sexual dysfunction. A random sample of 55 schizophrenic outpatients, 26 men and 29 women, treated with neuroleptics was selected from the long-term follow-up clinic; patients rated their current sexual function on specially designed scales. The results of the study are shown in Table 1.

The results of this study suggest that antipsychotic drugs induce sexual dysfunction more readily in male than in female patients. One possible explanation could be that women possess a higher level of estrogens than men. Estrogens have antidopaminergic properties that could render the dopamine receptors in female patients more tolerant to the antidopaminergic properties of antipsychotic medication. These authors suggest that plasma prolactin level measurements may help to assess sexual dysfunction in men though not in women. Neuroleptics appear to induce a high incidence of menstrual disorders which may possibly be related to high plasma prolactin levels.

Sexual dysfunction in women

While studies abound on male sexual dysfunction secondary to major tranquilizer use little information is available concerning the sexual effects of neuroleptics in women. The focus instead has been on reproductive function, including amenorrhea, menstrual irregularity, false-positive pregnancy test, breast engorgement, and lactation. The incidence of disturbed sexual function in women secondary to use of neuroleptics is uncertain, though some data will be presented later in this review.

Degen (36[CR]) reported 2 cases of women who developed orgastic inhibition (delay of orgasm) while taking neuroleptics.

A 29-year-old woman had developed symptoms of schizophrenia at the age of 20 and had had three psychiatric hospitalizations in the past 9 years. She had been free of psychotic episodes for 1 year, and was taking trifluoperazine 15 mg/day, at the time of her visit. She wished to stop the treatment because of orgastic inhibition, claiming that it was taking her about 10 times as long to reach orgasm as it did before she took trifluoperazine. She subsequently began taking diazepam (5 mg) before intercourse, or to smoke marijuana. Either or both of these treatments prior to coitus provided some relief, but she continued to believe that discontinuation of trifluoperazine would be preferable.

She was then persuaded to switch to another neuroleptic and received a prescription for loxapine succinate, 20 mg/day; one week later she reported that the length of time it took her to reach orgasm had returned almost to what was normal for her (about 15 min). As she remained free of psychotic symptoms, loxapine was gradually lowered to 5 mg/day. The patient maintained this regimen for the next year without recurrence of her psychotic symptoms and with normal sexual function. She no longer took diazepam and/or marijuana to facilitate orgasm.

Another case of orgastic inhibition was associated with the use of thioridazine.

The psychosexual history of a 27-year-old schizophrenic woman revealed that she had never had a sexual partner. However, she masturbated regularly 3 or 4 times a week. Since she had begun

*Table 1. Results of a sexual dysfunction questionnaire**

	% of positive cases	*Mean score ± SD for positive cases*
Male patients (N = 26)		
1. Difficulty in achieving erection	*38*	*5.0 ± 1.6*
2. Difficulty in maintaining erection	*42*	*4.6 ± 1.6*
3. Decreased ability to achieve orgasm	*58*	*4.1 ± 1.8*
4. Changes in quality of orgasm	*58*	*3.9 ± 1.6*
5. Decreased quantity of ejaculate	*46*	*4.2 ± 1.6*
6. Current difficulty in sexual functioning	*54*	*4.7 ± 1.9*
Total score	*81*	
Female patients: sexual dysfunction (N = 27)		
1. Changes in quality of orgasm	*33*	*4.4 ± 1.7*
2. Pain during orgasm	*7*	*2.5 ± 0.7*
3. Decreased ability to achieve orgasm	*22*	*3.5 ± 1.8*
4. Current difficulty in sexual functioning	*30*	*3.9 ± 2.1*
Total score	*44*	
Female patients: menstrual disorders (N = 23)		
1. Increased irregularity of menstruations	*78*	*3.7 ± 1.5*
2. Change in quantity of menses	*78*	*3.7 ± 1.3*
Total score	*91*	

**In each case, the patient was asked to rate on a 7-point scale (1 to 7) any changes in functioning since beginning to take antipsychotic medication.*

taking thioridazine, it was taking her longer to climax and she often became fatigued and was not able to continue. This made her feel frustrated and tense. She knew from past experience that either stopping thioridazine or continuing thioridazine with the addition of diazepam and/or doxepin and/or alcohol would relax her sexually, and she would be able to reach orgasm within 20 min. With this history thioridazine was discontinued and she was then placed on fluphenazine decanoate 12.5 mg i.m. every 2 weeks, which controlled her psychotic symptomatology and produced no sexual difficulties. She continued this treatment for a year with no complaints of side effects. There have been no more requests for diazepam or doxepin.

The case of a female schizophrenic who developed an anorgasmic episode while on thioridazine was presented by Shen and Park (37[CR]). She regained orgasmic capacity after thioridazine was discontinued. The authors suggest that thioridazine-induced inhibition of female orgasm does occur and that the problem may be underreported or overlooked. They draw attention to the fact that nonorgasmic women may experience frustrations in a variety of ways, including pelvic complaints, lower abdominal pain, itching, vaginal discharge as well as increased tension, irritability and fatigue.

The sexual dysfunction in women receiving neuroleptics is potentially serious and has to date received little attention in the psychiatric and medical literature. It is important to elicit a sexual history by careful questioning in all patients receiving neuroleptics, since sexual dysfunction during their use by women is easily missed. Physicians should assure patients that this disturbance is temporary, and that sexual function will be regained once the causative medication is withdrawn. Attention to this problem may improve the rate of medication compliance among patients.

Extrapyramidal side effects

The different types of extrapyramidal side effects and in particular the tardive dyskinesia (TD) induced by neuroleptics were thoroughly discussed in previous Annuals (SEDA-6, 46; SEDA-7, 56). During the last year many new papers on this topic have appeared in the literature. Goetz et al in their review summarize the data on epidemiology, neuropathology and pharmacological therapy of TD; they consider that treatment of TD with neuroleptics themselves is treatment with the presumed offending agents and should be avoided. Such therapy may temporarily diminish the symptoms of the condition, but in fact aggravate the underlying defect.

Simpson et al (38[R]) provide a valuable

overview of the various approaches to the treatment of TD (Table 2) but they stress that none is entirely satisfactory and that prevention of this side effect must be the primary aim. Above all, clinicians should carefully evaluate the indication for neuroleptic drugs, and avoid their use in conditions which may be treated with more benign agents. Another review of the management of TD, with broadly similar conclusions is that by Goetz et al (39[R]).

The preliminary results of a double-blind study of the *effect of propranolol* on TD were presented by Schrodt et al (40[C]). They found no evidence of a short-term dose-dependent effect. However, a long-term treatment response was observed in 2 of 4 patients. Recent research has demonstrated

Table 2. *Drugs used in treatment of tardive dyskinesia (38[R])*

Neurotransmitter affected	Agent type	Mechanism	Examples of drugs used	Expected result on tardive dyskinesia symptoms
Dopamine	Dopamine blockers (antagonists)	Block dopamine postsynaptic transmission	Haloperidol* Thioridazine Clozapine* Oxiperomide, sulpiride (new D_2 blockers) Pimozide* Thiopropazate*	Temporary improvement but may result in further worsening
	Dopamine-depleting drugs	Deplete dopamine from vesicles	Reserpine Tetrabenazine* α-Methyl-para-tyrosine Oxypertine α-Methyldopa	Improvement may be temporary
	Dopamine agonists	Facilitate dopamine transmission (to reverse antagonist-induced hypersensitivity)	Levodopa d-Amphetamine Apomorphine Amantadine Methylphenidate Bromocriptine Hydergine	Conflicting results, moderate improvement with some agents
Acetylcholine	Cholinergics	Stimulate anticholinergic transmission	Physostigmine* Deanol Choline Lecithin	Improvement with IV physostigmine, but a useful oral agent has not been validated yet
	Anti-cholinergics	Block anti-cholinergic transmission	Scopolamine Biperiden Benztropine Trihexyphenidyl	Worsens tardive dyskinesia
γ-Aminobutyric acid (GABA)	GABA agonists	Stimulate GABA transmission	Valproic acid Baclofen Clonazepam Diazepam Muscimol γ-Acetylenic GABA	Moderate improvement, but results are not clear
Norepinephrine	Norepinephrine	Increase norepinephrine	Fusaric acid Disulfiram	Uncontrolled reports; too little data to comment further
Serotonin	Serotonin	Increase 5-HT	l-Tryptophan	Conflicting results from controlled studies

*Success confirmed by double-blind study(ies).

that long-term propranolol use can alter the synaptic transmission process. Designers of future studies should take these findings into account and allow adequate time for detection of treatment effects.

Jeste et al (41[C]) performed an investigation to explore the possibility of *abnormal neuroleptic metabolism* in TD patients. Using a liquid chromatographic assay, they measured serum neuroleptic concentrations in 8 female patients with TD and 8 controls. All 16 patients were receiving either thioridazine or mesoridazine at stable doses. TD patients were found to have a significantly higher ratio of serum concentration to daily dose of neuroleptics as compared with controls. A 1-year follow-up revealed that this ratio did not change appreciably in those patients who continued to receive neuroleptics. Of the various thioridazine metabolites, sulforidazine (which is reportedly the most potent in terms of its affinity for dopaminergic and α-noradrenergic receptors) seemed to be significantly elevated in the serum of TD patients as compared with non-TD patients. This data suggest a need for further pharmacokinetic investigations to study neuroleptic metabolism in patients with TD.

Hausner (42[C]) draw attention to the problem of differential diagnosis between neuroleptic-induced parkinsonism and Parkinson's disease. True Parkinson's disease can occur in psychotic individuals, yet such a patient on antipsychotic medication who develops parkinsonian signs may automatically be diagnosed as (and treated for) neuroleptic-induced parkinsonism. Idiopathic parkinsonism and pseudoparkinsonism are different conditions with differing causes and treatments. Clinically significant criteria which may aid in proper diagnosis include the clinical course, time and age of onset, nature of tremor, unilaterality of signs, and response to anticholinergic medication. Appropriate diagnosis is essential, as treatment approaches differ for the two disorders.

Four cases of idiopathic parkinsonism in psychiatric patients originally misdiagnosed as having pseudoparkinsonism, are presented in this same paper by Hausner. The danger of ascribing parkinsonian signs to neuroleptic treatment rather than to Parkinson's disease proper was noted by Hollister 20 years ago and now appears to be an even greater problem: there are increasing numbers of antipsychotics available, as well as widespread usage of more potent agents that have a higher incidence of extrapyramidal side effects. With increasing recognition of the criteria for differential diagnosis, treatment should proceed more effectively.

Some difficulties in diagnosing TD have been discussed by Faheem et al (43[C]), who present a case of dyskinetic symptoms limited to the diaphragm and laryngeal muscles. Mild respiratory and speech symptoms in the absence of classical orobuccal or body dyskinesia were for many years misinterpreted as a manifestation of the patient's psychiatric illness. This could have been a costly mistake with potentially life-threatening complications. Progressive onset of dyskinesia after 1.5 years of neuroleptic use, with the dyskinesia becoming worse after reduction of dose and later withdrawal of neuroleptics, points to the possibility of tardive dyskinesia in this patient.

Emotional arousal and drug-induced dystonia

Sovner and McGorrill (44[C]) reported in 1982 on the results of their retrospective review of the association between the presence of emotional arousal and the onset of drug-induced dystonia. 6 out of 167 inpatients treated with neuroleptics were identified as having developed a dystonic reaction in the context of an intense, negative emotional experience (Table 3). In 3 of the 6, the reaction was immediate. The authors concluded that emotional arousal should be considered as a factor in determining the onset of dystonic muscle spasms in susceptible individuals. The recognition that drug-induced dystonia can be precipitated by emotional arousal should help in differential diagnosis of this side effect.

Similarly, the role of emotional factors in the development of drug-induced oculogyric crises has been examined by Bumpass and Knoll (45[CR]). The authors review the literature on cases of oculogyric crisis attributable to neuroleptics. This often dramatic side effect is usually controlled by adjusting the dosage, changing the neuroleptic, or adding antiparkinson medication. These traditional methods failed to control the symptom in the authors' patient, and it became apparent that emotional factors

Table 3. Description of six emotionally precipitated dystonic reactions (44C)

Drug/days of treatment	*Emotionally precipitating event (PE)*	*Dystonic reaction (DR)*	*Time interval (PE to DR)*	*Time of day*
HPL/1*	*Group therapy hearing emotion-laden statements)*	*Eyes rolled back with rapid blinking, thick tongue, difficulty speaking*	*Immediate onset*	*1:15 PM*
TFZ/1*	*Family meeting*	*Difficulty swallowing and speaking, neck and arms rigid*	*Immediate onset*	*6:30 PM*
FPZ/3*	*Notice by social worker that children might be taken away*	*Neck extended, tonic spasm of tongue, neck, and back*	*2 hours*	*1:15 PM*
HPL/1*	*Family visit (during which patient appeared tremulous and was mute)*	*Diagnosed by psychiatrist (ordered I.M. diphenhydramine)*	*2½ hours*	*10:30 PM*
HPL/1*	*Group therapy (patient confronted by group about intellectualizing)*	*Thick tongue, difficulty speaking*	*1 hour*	*2:45 PM*
PPZ/1*	*Patient present during phone call and argument between his psychiatrist and college professor*	*Patient became highly distraught (Psychiatrist ordered prn diphenhydramine to offset 'EPS')*	*Immediate onset*	*2:00 PM*

**Abbreviations: FPZ = fluphenazine hydrochloride; HPL = haloperidol; PPZ = perhenazine; TFZ = trifluoperazine.*

were significant and had to be considered if treatment was to be successful.

The patient was a 21-year-old woman receiving trifluoperazine, trihexyphenidyl and flurazepam; the phenothiazine was later replaced by thioridazine. In the presence of an increased state of emotional arousal and/or a reduction in the ability of the neuromuscular system to compensate (e.g. because of fatigue) oculogyric crises occurred. A treatment programme was devised focusing on three areas: (a) reduction of neuropharmacological factors that could result in a tendency for deviant direction of the eyes (adjust dosage, change neuroleptic, or add antiparkinson drugs); (b) minimalization of factors reducing the effectiveness of the compensating mechanisms mediated through the neuromuscular system (avoid fatigue, limit alcohol, correct underlying metabolic disorders); and (c) avoidance of states of emotional arousal that overwhelm the patient's adaptive skills. In this patient, prolonged improvement occurred only after all the above measures had been included in the patient's therapeutic program.

Emotional factors also played a role in a case of TD in a non-psychiatric patient during short-term use of the combined neuroleptic/anticholinergic drug Stelabid, reported by Chouinard et al (46C).

Stelabid, a compound primarily used to treat gastrointestinal disorders, contains 5 mg of isopropamide (an anticholinergic drug) and 2 mg of trifluoperazine (a neuroleptic phenothiazine). There have been a few reports of neuroleptic-induced TD in nonpsychiatric patients. In this case Stelabid was prescribed to a 58-year-old man for the treatment of heartburn and stomach pains. He took 1 tablet orally 3 times a day for 4 months. Seven weeks after termination of this treatment continuous movements of the patient's face, lips and tongue appeared. His tongue was partially protruded and he constantly twisted it from side to side while smacking his lips and moving his jaws from side to side with chewing movements of large amplitude; his mouth was open. The extremities and the trunk were not involved. Because the patient had no previous psychiatric history and because an experience suggested that some reversibility of severe TD is possible, it was decided against suppressing the TD with neuroleptics. Instead, since anxiety can exacerbate TD, he received 10 mg of diazepam to be taken orally 3 times a day. The symptom ratings showed a gradual decrease: the total score for dyskinesia, which was 17 at the time of admission, had been reduced to 10. However, the patient remained markedly disabled by abnormal movements of the jaw and tongue.

Miscellaneous adverse effects

Dysphagias Neuroleptic-associated dysphagia could be a potentially fatal adverse reaction to the pharmacotherapy of schizophrenia. Moss and Green (47[CR]) describe a case of neuroleptic-associated dysphagia in which manometry was used to document changes in esophageal motility during manipulation of the patient's medication. Upper esophageal dystonia was the etiology most consistent with the manometric findings.

The possible association between psychotropic drugs and disorders of swallowing was also studied by Craig and Richardson (48[C]). Unlike the patient described by Moss and Green most of their patients who exhibited an impaired gag reflex or actually choked to death had no earlier history of swallowing dysfunction, suggesting that many more patients may be at risk of sudden fatal choking than is readily apparent on cursory examination. These findings suggest the need for periodic examination of the gag reflex, especially among patients with TD who are receiving anticholinergic drugs.

Catatonia The catatonic state with obtundation and fever has been found to be a potentially fatal complication of phenothiazine treatment, especially at high doses of potent neuroleptics. Nakra and Hai-Gho Hwu (49[C]) present a case with two discrete episodes of severe catatonic state, altered consciousness, and urinary incontinence, but without fever, after moderate doses of haloperidol and fluphenazine decanoate in an elderly patient. Both episodes were reversible after drug discontinuation. The episode after fluphenazine decanoate was more severe.

Tongue protrusion An unusual complication of a phenothiazine drug thioridazine was described by Miglets et al (50[C]) in a 34-year-old female treated for a depressive state. The rhythmic protrusion of her tongue had been noted for several days prior to its entrapment; this resulted in venous engorgement, edema, and finally necrosis of the undersurface of the tongue. Spasm of the muscles of mastication was very severe. She was treated successfully with intravenous diphenhydramine to relieve muscular spasm. Sixty seconds after receiving 50 mg of diphenhydramine her muscles relaxed and her jaws could be easily opened with digital pressure. Intramuscular diphenhydramine was given on a regular schedule for 2 days. Within 3 days her tongue was still swollen but she could close her mouth. Healing progressed rapidly. Three months later she was asymptomatic with no permanent sequelae.

Hepatotoxicity Hepatotoxicity associated with chlorpromazine is well described in the medical literature. Jones et al (51[CR]) present new results from two databases available to the US Food and Drug Administration: a computerized file of spontaneous reports of suspected adverse drug reactions, and drug-diagnosis record linkage data from the 1980 Medicaid Records of Michigan and Minnesota. Spontaneous reports of suspected adverse drug reactions were reported to the FDA by industry and the medical community. A total of 542 reports of suspected phenothiazine-induced hepatotoxicity have been accumulated since 1969. On the basis of the data analyzed the authors suggest that hepatotoxicity may be as frequent with piperidine and piperazine phenothiazine compounds as with chlorpromazine, despite previous literature suggestions that the toxicity of these compounds is less. In order to establish rates, the 1980–1981 record-linkage database of all drugs dispensed was utilized, and diagnosis by date of service covering the 1.4 million Michigan and Minnesota Medicaid recipients for a period of 18 months. Table 4 summarizes the rates for the mutually exclusive categories of phenothiazines by state, age, and sex categories.

The authors found evidence of significant hepatotoxic effect for the phenothiazines and for persons under age 50, but not over 50, relative to comparable population control. They suggest that immunological or hormonal mechanisms play a substantial role in the medication of phenothiazine hepatotoxicity.

The frequency of disturbances of the liver function in patients on clozapine in comparison with perazine and haloperidol in 478 patients was investigated by Bauer and Gaertner (52[CR]) using case histories recor-

Table 4. *Rates of specified hepatic diagnosis in patients on phenothiazines and controls, Medicaid 1980–1981, by age, sex, and state (51[R])*

	Minnesota			Michigan		
	Cases	No. at risk	Rate 1000	Cases	No. at risk	Rate 1000
Female						
under 50						
Phenothiazine	7	700	10.0	101	2273	44.4
No phenothiazine	266	55088	4.8	2692	197464	13.6
	Rate ratio: 2.0 (0.9–4.9)*			Rate ratio: 3.3 (2.7–3.9)		
50 and over						
Phenothiazine	1	1394	0.7	63	3409	18.8
No phenothiazine	32	13106	2.4	744	39257	19.0
	Rate ratio: 0.3 (0.0–303)			Rate ratio: 1.0 (0.7–1.4)		
Male						
under 50						
Phenothiazine	4	518	7.7	52	1583	32.8
No phenothiazine	243	37404	6.5	1212	124117	9.8
	Rate ratio: 1.2 (0.2–15.7)			Rate ratio: 3.3 (2.5–4.4)		
50 and over						
Phenothiazine	2	536	3.7	27	1225	22.0
No phenothiazine	26	6480	4.0	338	15433	21.9
	Rate ratio: 0.0 (0.6–1.6)			Rate ratio: 1.0 (0.8–1.2)		

*Ninety-five percent confidence interval.

ded at the psychiatric clinic of Tübingen over a 4-year period. During the period of the investigation no case of jaundice occurred; however non-symptomatic increases of the liver values could be observed. The three drugs did not differ in this respect.

Disturbances of leukopoiesis Bauer and Gaertner in their study found no cases of agranulocytosis among 478 patients treated with clozapine, perazine or haloperidol. Only 1 leukopenia occurred on clozapine, 1 on perazine and 6 on haloperidol.

Pisciotta (53[R]) has reviewed the literature on drug-induced agranulocytosis. He points out that cases of this complication described in medical papers and relating to chlorpromazine and its derivatives point to toxic effects of the drugs on marrow precursors. Patients sensitive to chlorpromazine show a proliferative defect in the final phase of DNA synthesis. While this defect might be genetic in origin, no evidence to support such a hereditary abnormality has yet been found.

Lupus erythematosus A case of paresthesiae peripheral neuropathy, pericardial and pleural effusions, and other changes consistent with systemic lupus erythematosus associated with the use of moderately high doses of chlorprothixene was described by Mcnevin and Mackay (54[C]). There have earlier been single case reports of a syndrome resembling systemic lupus erythematosus resulting from the use of the other neuroleptics, but not previously with chlorprothixene.

A 29-year-old woman with a history of psychiatric problems was treated with 950 mg of chlorprothixene per day. The patient appears to have developed the following problems: ascending peripheral neuropathy of a mixed sensorimotor type, pleural effusion, and pericardial effusion, perhaps with an associated myocarditis. These changes halted and then reversed as the drug was withdrawn.

One important implication of this case is that many of the peripheral neuropathies earlier reported may in fact have had associated but undetected drug-induced connective tissue disorders.

Canoso and Sise (55[CR]) undertook a study to determine the frequency of the lupus anticoagulant, its association with immunological abnormalities and clinical findings in psychiatric patients treated with chlorpromazine, other phenothiazines and a control group. The lupus anticoagulant, also referred to as a non-specific inhibitor to coagulation, was originally described in patients with systemic lupus erythematosus. This inhibitor was later demonstrated in a variety of disorders and in drug induced lupus-like syndromes.

70 hospitalized males with psychiatric conditions were entered consecutively in the study. The control group consisted of 53 patients in long-term care wards who had never received phenothiazines. The anticoagulant was present in 11 of 30 patients receiving chlorpromazine, in none of 17 patients who had been off phenothiazine therapy for over a year and in none of 53 controls. It was also seen in 5 of 13 patients who had been switched from chlorpromazine to another phenothiazine even after several years off chlorpromazine. The anticoagulant was characterized by prolongation of the partial thromboplastin time, thromboplastin dilution test, and Russell's viper venom time. Washed frozen platelets partially corrected the abnormality induced by the anticoagulant. In all but one case the anticoagulant was associated with positive antinuclear antibody test and/or increased serum IgM. 6 of 16 patients also had decreased complement levels, and 2 had a positive direct Coombs' test. None of these patients manifested bleeding, hemolysis, splenomegaly, or other clinical features of systemic lupus erythematosus.

Cutaneous reactions Two new reports on photosensitive dermatitis due to phenothiazines have appeared since publication of Annual 7. Toriruki et al (56[C]) have described a 74-year-old man who had eczematous eruptions on sun-exposed areas. Photopatch tests were positive to chlorpromazine and promethazine, and the action spectrum for the photosensitivity was in the long-wave ultraviolet light range. It was concluded that the chronic photosensitive dermatitis was due to phenothiazines.

Von Ertle (57[C]) has presented a case of contact and photodermatitis in a farmer due to chlorpromazine. This farmer specialized in pig-breeding and showed acute dermatitis of his hands, forearms and face after using chlorpromazine for the sedation of pigs. Epicutaneous and photo-patch tests showed positive reactions to chlorpromazine. Further tests with other occupational materials were negative. This observation shows that in cases of contact dermatitis in farmers, besides antibiotics, vitamins and other feeding additives, sedatives of the phenothiazine-type should not be forgotten.

A case of thiothixene-induced skin lesions reported by Matsuoka et al (58[C]). Cutaneous reactions due to this drug are rare. A 31-year-old woman was seen for an asymptomatic 'rash' involving her palms. The cutaneous lesions developed a few days following initiation of the treatment with 40 mg of thiothixene. This patient's palmar erythema and telangiectasias appear to be manifestations of drug sensitivity. The skin lesions resolved when the dosage of the drug was decreased and exacerbated in response to rechallenge with a high dose. The antinuclear antibody test was positive and was associated with the skin lesions.

General anesthesia after neuroleptic malignant syndrome One of the most serious and potentially lethal complications of therapy with neuroleptics is the malignant syndrome, described in previous Annuals (SEDA-4, 37; SEDA-6, 49; SEDA-7, 62). Similarly, one of the most dangerous complications of general anesthesia is malignant hyperthermia. For both these syndromes, i.e. neuroleptic malignant syndrome and malignant hyperthermia, a common pathophysiology has been postulated. The two syndromes may also be clinically indistinguishable from 'acute lethal catatonia' which is characterized by fever, muscular hypertonicity, and stupor. Lotstra et al (59[CR]) reported the very interesting case of a patient in whom the neuroleptic malignant syndrome appeared following treatment with levomepromazine 50 mg/day and diazepam 20 mg/day. After remission from the malignant syndrome, the patient underwent general anesthesia 9 times for electroconvulsive therapy without ill effect. This case suggests that neuroleptic malignant syndrome and malignant hyperthermia in fact have different pathogenetic mechanisms.

Interactions There are further reports on the interaction of neuroleptics and other psychoactive drugs with other substances. Wootton (60[C]) reported the death of a 40-year-old white female, attributed to the combined effects of thioridazine, and clonidine with *frusemide.*

The victim had been treated over a period of several months for menopausal changes and depression. She was prescribed clonidine and amitriptyline but stopped taking the amitriptyline after 6 weeks because of adverse effects. A recurrent weight problem induced her to restrict her diet severely and to take large quantities of unprescribed diuretics and food supplements. On the evening prior to her death, she complained of feeling unwell, which she attributed to mild sunstroke. She went to bed at 21.30 hours and was found dead at 06.00 the following morning. Laboratory investigation revealed the presence of thioridazine, frusemide and clonidine in various tissues. It was surmised at the inquest that the hypokalemia induced by the diuretic, together with the myocardial effects of the clonidine and the thioridazine, precipitated the death of the victim.

The case of a young woman who had an acute neurotoxic reaction while on oral *lithium carbonate* and intramuscular fluphenazine decanoate is described by Singh (61[C]). Despite withdrawal of all medication she remained dysarthric for the next 2 years. The development of a fine postural hand tremor after the addition of fluphenazine decanoate was the first indication of the neurotoxic reaction in this case, and this may be a useful warning sign. Close monitoring of neurological status and plasma lithium levels is advisable in patients receiving such a drug combination.

REFERENCES

1. Mitchell JE, Popkin MK (1982) Antipsychotic drug therapy and sexual dysfunction in men. *Am. J. Psychiat., 139,* 633.
2. Nestros JN, Lehmann HE (1979) Neuroleptics and male sexual dysfunction. *Int. Drug Therapy Newsletter, 14,* 21.
3. Kotin J, Wilbert DE, Verburg D (1976) Thioridazine and sexual dysfunction. *Am. J. Psychiat., 133,* 82.
4. Blair JH, Simpson GM (1966) Effect of antipsychotic drugs on reproductive functions. *Dis. Nerv. Syst., 27,* 645.
5. Heller J (1961) Another case of inhibition of ejaculation as a side effect of Mellaril. *Am. J. Psychiat., 118,* 173.
6. Greenberg H (1971) Inhibition of ejaculation by chlorpromazine. *Nerv. Ment. Dis., 152,* 364.
7. Boleloucky Z (1965) Chlorpromazine inhibition of ejaculation. *Acta Nerv. Super. (Praha), 7,* 245.
8. Ditman KS (1964) Inhibition of ejaculation by chlorprothixene. *Am. J. Psychiat., 120,* 1004.
9. Jeffries JJ (1974) Piperacetazine-induced failure to ejaculation. *Can. Psychiat. Assoc. J., 19,* 322.
10. Shader RI (1972) Sexual dysfunction associated with mezoridazine besylate (Serentil). *Psychopharmacologia (Berlin), 27,* 293.
11. Keitner GI, Selub S (1983) Spontaneous ejaculations and neuroleptics. *J. Clin. Psychopharmacol., 3,* 34.
12. Ray O (1978) *Drugs, Society, and Human Behavior.* CV Mosby, St. Louis; p. 325.
13. Freyhan FA (1961) Loss of ejaculation during Mellaril treatment. *Am. J. Psychiat., 118,* 171.
14. Clein L (1962) Thioridazine and ejaculation. *Br. Med. J., 2,* 548.
15. Greenberg HR, Carrillo C (1968) Thioridazine-induced inhibition of masturbatory ejaculation in an adolescent. *Am. J. Psychiat., 124,* 991.
16. Haider I (1966) Thioridazine and sexual dysfunction. *Int. J. Neuropsychiat., 5,* 255.
17. Datshkovsky J (1961) Mellaril: ejaculation disorders. *Am. J. Psychiat., 118,* 564.
18. Berger SH (1979) Trifluoperazine and haloperidol: sources of ejaculatory pain? *Am. J. Psychiat., 136,* 350.
19. Witton K (1962) Sexual dysfunction secondary to Mellaril. *Dis. Nerv. Syst., 23,* 175.
20. Bartholomew AA (1967) Experience of two years' use of a long-acting phenothiazine: fluphenazine enanthate. *Med. J. Aust., 2,* 66.
21. Moloney PJ, Elliott GB, Johnson HW (1975) Experiences with priapism. *J. Urol., 114,* 72.
22. Dorman BW, Schmidt JD (1976) Association of priapism in phenothiazine therapy. *J. Urol., 116,* 51.
23. Dahl DS, Middleton RG (1974) Comparison between cavernosaphenous and cavernospongiosum shunting in the treatment of idiopathic priapism: a report of 5 operations. *J. Urol., 112,* 614.
24. Gottlieb JI, Lustberg T (1977) Phenothiazine-induced priapism: a case report. *Am. J. Psychiat., 134,* 1445.
25. Bastecky J, Gregova L (1974) Priapism as a possible complication of the chlorpromazine treatment. *Acta Nerv. Super. (Praha), 16,* 175.
26. Meiraz D, Fishelovitch J (1969) Priapism and largactil medication. *Isr. J. Med. Sci., 5,* 1254.
27. Dawson-Butterworth K (1969) Idiopathic priapism associated with schizophrenia. *Br. J. Clin. Pract., 23,* 125.
28. Dawson-Butterworth K (1970) Priapism and phenothiazines. *Br. Med. J., 2,* 118.
29. Merkin TE (1977) Priapism as a sequela of chlorpromazine therapy. *JACEP, 6,* 367.
30. Nelson JH, Winter CC (1977) Priapism: evolution of management in 48 patients in a 22-year series. *J. Urol., 117,* 455.
31. Larocque MA, Cosgrove MD (1974): Priapism: a review of 46 cases. *J. Urol., 112,* 770.
32. Illberg P (1964) The use of perphenazine in the treatment of drug resistant schizophrenia. *Am. J. Psychiat., 120,* 810.
33. Ghadirian AM, Chouinard G, Annable L (1982) Sexual dysfunction and plasma prolactin levels in neuroleptic-treated schizophrenic

outpatients. *J. Nerv. Ment. Dis., 170,* 463.

34. Ananth J (1982) Impotence associated with pimozide. *Am. J. Psychiat., 139,* 1374.
35. Hong CY, Chaput de Saintonge DM, Turner P (1982) Effects of chlorpromazine and other drugs acting in the central nervous system on human sperm motility. *Eur. J. Clin. Pharmacol., 22,* 413.
36. Degen K (1982) Sexual dysfunction in women using major tranquilizers. *J. Acad. Psychosom. Med., 23,* 959.
37. Shen WW, Park S (1982) Thioridazine-induced inhibition of female orgasm. *Psychiat. J. Univ. Ottawa, 7,* 249.
38. Simpson GM, Pi EH, Sramek JJ (1982) Management of tardive dyskinesia: Current update. *Drugs, 23,* 381.
39. Goetz CG, Weiner WJ, Nausieda PA, Klawans HL (1982) Tardive dyskinesia: pharmacology and clinical implications. *Clin. Neuropharm., 5,* 3.
40. Schrodt GR, Wright JH, Simpson R et al (1982) Treatment of tardive dyskinesia with propranolol. *J. Clin. Psychiat., 43,* 328.
41. Jeste DV, Liniola M, Wagner RL, Wyatt RJ (1982) Serum neuroleptic concentrations and tardive dyskinesia. *Psychopharmacology, 76,* 377.
42. Hausner RS (1983) Neuroleptic-induced parkinsonism and Parkinson's disease: differential diagnosis and treatment. *J. Clin. Psychiat., 44,* 13.
43. Faheem A, Brightwell DR, Burton GE, Struss A (1982) Respiratory dyskinesia and dysarthria from prolonged neuroleptic use: tardive dyskinesia? *Am. J. Psychiat., 139,* 517.
44. Sovner R, McGorrill S (1982) Stress as a precipitant of neuroleptic-induced dyskinesia. *Psychosomatics, 23,* 707.
45. Bumpass ER, Knoll JL (1982) Single case study. Emotional factors in oculogyric crisis. *J. Nerv. Ment. Dis., 170,* 366.
46. Chouinard G, Boisvert D, Bradwejn J (1982) Tardive dyskinesia in a nonpsychiatric patient due to short-term use of a neuroleptic/anticholinergic combination drug. *CMA Journal, 126,* 821.
47. Moss HB, Green A (1982) Neuroleptic-associated dysphagia confirmed by esophageal manometry. *Am. J. Psychiat., 139,* 515.
48. Craig TJ, Richardson MA (1982) Swallowing, tardive dyskinesia, and anticholinergics. *Am. J. Psychiat., 139,* 1083.
49. Nakra BRS, Hai-Gho-Hwu (1982): Catatonic-like syndrome during neuroleptic therapy. *Psychosomatics, 23,* 769.
50. Miglets AW, Racey G, Hoffer JL (1983) Phenothiazine induced lingual trauma. *Laryngoscope, 93,* 108.
51. Jones JK, Van de Carr SW, Zimmerman H, Leroy A (1983) Hepatotoxicity associated with phenothiazines. *Psychopharmacol. Bull., 19,* 24.
52. Bauer D, Gaertner HJ (1983) Wirkungen der Neuroleptica auf die Leberfunktion, des blutbildende System, den Blutdruck und die Temperaturregulation. *Pharmacopsychiat., 16,* 23.
53. Piscota AV (1982) Drug-induced agranulocytosis. *Haematologica, 67,* 292.
54. Mcnevin S, Mackay M (1982) Chlorprothixene-induced systemic lupus erythematosus. *J. Clin. Psychopharmacol., 2,* 411.
55. Canoso RT, Sise HS (1982) Chlorpromazine-induced lupus anticoagulant and associated immunologic abnormalities. *Am. J. Hematol., 13,* 121.
56. Torinuki W, Kumai N, Miura T (1982) Chronic photosensitive dermatitis due to phenothiazines. *Tohoku J. Exp. Med., 138,* 223.
57. Von Ertle T (1982) Beruflich bedingte Kontakt- und Photokontaktallergie bei einem Landwirt durch chlorpromazin. *Dermatosen, 30,* 120.
58. Matsuoka LY (1982) Thiothixene drug sensitivity. *J. Am. Acad. Dermatol., 7,* 405.
59. Lotstra F, Linkowski P, Mendlewicz J (1983) General anesthesia after neuroleptic malignant syndrome. *Biol. Psychiat., 18,* 243.
60. Wootton DG (1982) A fatality due to drug synergism. *Med. Sci. Law, 22,* 220.
61. Singh SV (1982) Lithium carbonate/fluphenazine decanoate producing irreversible brain damage (letter). *Lancet, 2,* 278.

G.A.B. Davies-Jones

7 Anticonvulsant drugs

GENERAL TOPICS

Osteopathia antiepileptica *(SED-10, SEDA-7, 74)*

The precise mechanism(s) responsible for this complication is not known but there is evidence for increased excretion of 25-OH-D, the immediate precursor of 1,25-$(OH)_2$D, the active form of vitamin D in bone and intestine, and also of 1,25-$(OH)_2$D itself. Deficiency of 24,25-$(OH)_2$D seems to be a fairly constant accompaniment of anticonvulsant osteomalacia and this may play an important role (SED-10; 1[R]).

Anticonvulsants and cognitive function

Impairment of cognitive function by anticonvulsant medication is recognized (SED-10). Thompson and Trimble (2[R]) have recently shown that the reduction in polypharmacy and the use of carbamazepine both had beneficial effects on cognitive function and mood.

Plasma biotin

The mean plasma biotin levels in epileptics treated with phenytoin, carbamazepine and primidone in various combinations were significantly lower than in controls (3[R]). Treatment with either of these drugs singly also produced lower plasma biotin levels. Single drug therapy with valproate did not produce levels as low as those found with any of the other drugs when used singly. Dermatitis and ataxia are clinical manifestations of an inborn error of biotin-dependent enzymes, and are also well-known side effects of anticonvulsants with the exception of sodium valproate.

Side Effects of Drugs Annual 8
M.N.G. Dukes, editor

ISBN 0 444 90339 9
$0.80 per article per page (transactional system)
$0.20 per article per page (licensing system)

Serum zinc and vitamin E concentrations

Higashi et al (4[R]) found evidence of vitamin E deficiency and zinc deficiency in children on long-term treatment with phenytoin and phenobarbitone.

Anticonvulsant peripheral neuropathy

Shorvon and Reynolds (5[R]) undertook an electrophysiological study of sensory nerve function during and after exposure to high serum levels of phenytoin, a clinical and electrophysiological study of previously untreated epileptic patients who had been carefully monitored prospectively on phenytoin or carbamazepine monotherapy for 1–5 years, and a clinical and electrophysiological study of chronic epileptic patients on treatment with barbiturates alone. In the 51 patients on phenytoin or carbamazepine they found no clinical evidence of neuropathy. 18% of those on phenytoin and none on carbamazepine had mild abnormalities of sensory action potentials or sensory conduction. The electrophysiological changes in the phenytoin-treated patients were possibly related to previous exposure to high phenytoin or low folate levels or both. In 10 chronic epileptic patients reversible slowing of sensory nerve conduction during phenytoin intoxication was observed. In 6 patients on chronic barbiturate monotherapy clinical evidence of neuropathy was found in 2 and electrophysiological abnormalities in 5, including reversible slowing of sensory conduction during intoxication in 1. The results suggested the possibility that permanent neuropathy due to phenytoin (and perhaps barbiturates) may result from prolonged or repeated episodes of intoxication or folate deficiency. The predominant electrophysiological change in patients taking phenytoin within therapeutic levels was a reduction in amplitude of sensory nerve action potential with relative preservation of the conduction velocity. This contrasts with the moderate slowing of sensory nerve conduction velocity among patients with phenytoin toxicity.

INDIVIDUAL DRUGS

Sodium valproate

Acute valproate intoxication results in coma (SED-10). Mortensen et al (9[c]) observed a 20-year-old female comatose for several days after ingesting 75 g sodium valproate. She was successfully treated with hemodialysis, hemoperfusion, i.v. glucose and intensive care. A peak level of 2120 mg/ml of sodium valproate was registered 8.5 hours after ingestion of the drug. No evidence of thrombocytopenia or hepatic insufficiency was seen. There was slight increase in serum amylase, glycine, plasma ammonia and serum propionate, transient proteinuria and increased urinary excretion of adipic and suberic acid. There was a transient decrease in serum calcium.

Immune thrombocytopenia secondary to sodium valproate is well recognized (SED-10) and Barr et al (10[R]) found immune-mediated thrombocytolysis in 15 of 45 children with epilepsy and transient neutropenia in 12. They did not find any difference in serum valproic acid levels between patients with or without thrombocytopenia, and there was a significant inverse correlation between platelet associated IgG and platelet count. *Hepatotoxicity* due to valproate may merely consist of transient elevation of liver enzymes or result in fulminant hepatic necrosis and death (SED-10). Zimmerman and Ishak (11[R]) analysed 23 fatal cases of valproate induced hepatic injury. Ages ranged from 1 to 28 years and all but 3 were less than 20 years old. Convulsions, facial edema, lassitude and vomiting were prominent features. Hypoglycemia was observed in 6 and transaminase levels were modestly elevated in most cases. Histologically the liver showed characteristic microvesicular steatosis usually accompanied by hepatocellular necrosis, and probably secondary to an idiosyncratic metabolic cause. They postulated a metabolite responsible for the steatosis and a different one for the necrosis.

Zafrani and Berthelot (12[R]) also described the typical histological features of microvacuolar fatty metamorphosis of small lipid droplets filling the cytoplasm of the hepatocytes leaving the nucleus in a central position. The *steatosis* was predominantly centro- and midlobular except in one case where periportal hepatocytes were mainly involved. Necrosis was limited to the centrizonal areas in most cases and it was submassive in 4 of the 31 fatal cases. Cirrhosis was found in 1 patient. Valproate hepatotoxicity occurs within a few months of starting treatment. Zafrani and Berthelot also commented on blood coagulopathy found in some of the patients and disseminated intravascular coagulation (DIC) was suspected in 7. Although characteristically occurring in young people 2 cases of reversible but histologically typical valproate hepatotoxicity were recorded by Thygesen and Boesen (13[c]) in women of 24 and 73 years of age.

Reduced plasma and carnitine levels and *hyperammonemia* were found in patients treated with valproic acid as compared with untreated epileptic patients and controls (14[R]). A similar reduction in serum carnitine was found by Böhles et al (15[c]) in a 3-year-old girl with Reye syndrome due to sodium valproate and they suggested that hypocarnitinemia may be important in the pathogenesis of valproate induced liver disease. Asymptomatic hyperammonemia was found in 29 of 55 patients receiving valproic acid by Murphy and Marquardt (16[R]). Elevations of plasma ammonia as high as 140 μmol/l were well tolerated. On this evidence hyperammonemia alone is not an indication for reducing or stopping valproic acid treatment and symptoms as well as the other indices of hepatic dysfunction should be used to determine whether to discontinue the drug.

Sodium valproate and *congenital anomalies*, particularly neural tube defects, is a controversial topic (17[r], 18[r]). Although not proven this is probably a true association, but further studies are awaited. The conclusions reached in SED-10 must remain for the present, and particularly that all anticonvulsants should be regarded as potentially teratogenic. A hypothesis that congenital defects associated with valproate might be due to zinc deficiency (since the drug binds zinc) deserves further study (41[r]).

Overdosage Karlsen et al (42[C]) have described a 16-year-old girl who took a 30 g overdose of valproate. She became soporous and serum bilirubin rose to 23 μmol/l. She was discharged in good condition by the 3rd day and serum bilirubin had fallen to a normal 7 μmol/l by the 7th day.

Interactions Sodium valproate increases serum levels of *phenytoin, phenobarbitone* and *primidone* (SED-9, 78). Unlike other anticonvulsant drugs sodium valproate is not an inducer of metabolism. It appears to have non-specific inhibition of drug metabolism in relation to phenytoin, phenobarbitone and primidone (6[R], 7[R]), thereby resulting in raised serum levels. Valproate also displaces phenytoin from its binding with albumin resulting in the increase in free phenytoin. No definite interaction between valproate and *carbamazepine* has been described. Various conflicting reports have appeared in the literature, but in an 'in vitro' study of the interaction between valproic acid and carbamazepine Mattson et al. (8[R]) showed that valproate competes with carbamazepine for plasma protein binding sites resulting in significantly increased free carbamazepine.

Diphenylhydantoin

Gingival hypertrophy is a frequent side effect of phenytoin treatment, characterized by accumulation of connective tissue substance within the gingiva propria. Kantor and Hassell (19[R]) found that fibroblasts from phenytoin-hypertrophied human gums synthesize and secrete elevated amounts of sulfated glycosaminoglycans in vitro in the absence of phenytoin in the culture medium. If this phenomenon occurs in vivo it may account for the accumulation of excess ground substance in hypertrophied gingiva.

Subcutaneous thickening and *coarsening of the facial features* are well known effects of phenytoin. Trunnell and Waisman (20[c]) now describe *hypertrophic retroauricular folds* due to fibrous tissue proliferation as a result of phenytoin treatment. They suggest that its pathogenesis is similar to that responsible for the subcutaneous thickening and gingival hypertrophy.

Phenytoin-induced hypersensitivity reactions may involve most systems (SED-10). Not surprisingly *necrotizing vasculopathy* has been reported (21[c]) but this is rare.

Immunological effects of phenytoin have been reported (SED-9, 77). Recently Bardana et al (22[R]) studied prospectively changes in serum immunoglobulins, complement and antinuclear antibody in 118 patients over 5 years. 27 patients had idiopathic epilepsy, 50 secondary epilepsy, 41 had neurological syndromes without epilepsy and 83 were normal volunteers. Studies were undertaken before treatment and at 6-month intervals. Before treatment patients with idiopathic epilepsy had a higher than expected incidence of low serum IgA. Patients with secondary epilepsy and neurological disorders without epilepsy had a greater than expected incidence of high serum IgA. Phenytoin treatment was associated with further decreases in serum IgA in patients with idiopathic and secondary epilepsy. Total serum IgE concentrations also decreased significantly during treatment with phenytoin in all patient categories. Minor decreases in serum IgG and IgM were noted, but serum IgD and complement were not affected. Antinuclear antibodies were observed with the same frequency before and after phenytoin treatment.

Arthralgia and arthritis as part of idiosyncratic reactions to phenytoin have been mentioned rarely in the past but Stalnikowicz (23[c]) described a patient in whom acute arthritis was the major sign. Harney (43[C]) described a case of *myopathy* together with a hypersensitivity reaction marked by *hepatitis* and a *raised serum creatine kinase.*

Palm and Hallmans (24[R]) studied the effect of phenytoin on the metabolism of zinc and copper and postulated that the drug may cause a relative *zinc deficiency* through a chelate binding between zinc and phenytoin and/or an increased absorption and accumulation of copper.

Phenytoin clearance is increased in *pregnancy* but the metabolism of the drug decreases in the first few postpartum months and plasma levels rise. Puckett et al (25[c]) studied the metabolism of phenytoin during lactation. Stable phenytoin blood levels were found until the 6th month postpartum when the frequency and intensity of breast feeding decreased and the level of phenytoin in the plasma increased, implying a decrease in phenytoin clearance with cessation of lactation.

A paper by Levine suggests that a viral influenza-like infection can result in a temporary rise in phenytoin levels to toxic concentrations (44[c]).

Interactions *Salicylate* increases serum phenytoin levels but according to Inoue and Walsh (26[c]) the interaction is a little more complex. They found biphasic fluctuations of serum phenytoin level when aspirin was added to chronic phenytoin therapy for an epileptic patient. Initially the serum phenytoin level decreased but after 4 months on aspirin and phenytoin serum levels of phenytoin increased and was associated with mild nystagmus and serum folate deficiency. A biphasic response in the primidone-phenytoin interaction has also been described (27[c]), the net effect being an enhanced increase in plasma phenobarbitone levels. Marquis et al (28[c]) found that phenytoin given for 10–15 days in dosage that produced plasma levels in the usual therapeutic range decreased the half life of *theophylline* and increased its clearance by approximately two fold. Phenytoin increases the metabolism of *quinidine* by hepatic enzyme induction. Urbano (29[c]) pointed out the possibility of precipitating "malignant ventricular ectopy" when phenytoin is added to quinidine treatment by reducing the serum quinidine level. If phenytoin is thought to be required in addition to quinidine careful serum monitoring of the drug levels is necessary and appropriate adjustment of the dosage made. A decrease in *disopyramide* serum concentration was found in 2 patients with concurrent administration of phenytoin (30[c]). The serum concentration of another antiarrhythmic agent – *mexiletine,* useful in the control of ventricular arrhythmias – is lowered after phenytoin administration, probably due to hepatic enzyme induction (31[c]). *Metronidazole* has in several patients been shown to raise blood phenytoin to toxic levels (45[c]).

Primidone

Sher et al (47[c]) observed a hallucinatory psychosis in a severely retarded woman who had been receiving 250 mg primidone t.i.d. for 7 years. After 4 days of hallucinations she became decidedly schizophrenic. She was found to have been taking phenobarbitone in addition, though this was denied by the family. After reduction of the primidone dose to 25 mg/o.d. and treatment with neuroleptics the psychosis receded, though phenobarbitone levels were still high.

Carbamazepine

As reported in SEDA-10 carbamazepine increased the production of porphyrin in chick embryo hepatocyte culture. Laiwah et al (32[c]) have now described a case of non-hereditary acute porphyria, similar to acute, intermittent porphyria, following the treatment of epilepsy with carbamazepine. They thought that carbamazepine exerted a direct suppressant effect on uroporphyrin-1 synthase in addition to its indirect enzyme-inducing properties. Rideout et al (46[c]) have since suggested that this effect may be due to depression of ALA-D levels rather than reduced HMB-S activity.

Carbamazepine-associated toxic epidermal necrolysis and exfoliative dermatitis were reported by Breathnach et al (33[c]) and Reed et al (34[c]), respectively.

Isoniazid is known to interact with phenytoin to produce elevated phenytoin levels and toxicity. Recently a double drug interaction between carbamazepine and isoniazid has been reported (35[c]). Isoniazid resulted in a large increase in serum carbamazepine concentration most probably due to decreased hepatic clearance. Isoniazid-induced hepatotoxicity was also observed, possibly by carbamazepine, a known inducing agent, producing increased formation of a reactive intermediate which is itself hepatotoxic.

One of the major advantages of carbamazepine is believed to be not only its freedom from behavioral side effects but its beneficial effect on *mood and cognitive function.* However Silverstein et al (36[R]) identified 7 among 200 children in whom introduction of the drug was followed by acute adverse behavioral changes.

Warren and Steinbook (37[c]) describe the occurrence of *reticulocytosis* due to carbamazepine. This was not due to hemolysis or anemia and blood loss, but was probably an idiosyncratic reaction. No record of carbamazepine induced thrombocytopenia has appeared before, but 2 cases have now been reported (38[c]), 39[c]). This resolved on stopping the drug. In 1 patient IgG antiplatelet antibodies due to carbamazepine were detected (39[c]).

The effect of carbamazepine on *serum immunoglobulin concentrations* were described by Gilhus et al (40[R]). Serum IgA, IgG and IgM concentrations were determined in 30 patients with partial epilepsy before and during carbamazepine therapy. No patient had received anticonvulsant drugs before the study. During the first month of treatment the IgA and IgM concentrations decreased significantly, but no further decrease occurred over the following 3 months. 15 patients were followed for 8–30 months. The IgA concentrations remained low, while the IgM concentrations tended to increase but not to the pretreatment level.

Carbamazepine had no effect on IgG serum concentration. The serum levels of IgA and IgM were unrelated to the serum carbamazepine levels.

REFERENCES

1. Zerwekh JE, Homan R, Tindall R et al (1982) Decreased serum 24,25-Dihydroxyvitamin D concentration during long term anti-convulsant therapy in adult epileptics. *Ann. Neurol., 12,* 184.
2. Thompson PJ, Trimble MR (1982) Anticonvulsant drugs and cognitive functions. *Epilepsia, 23,* 531.
3. Krause K-H, Berlit P, Bonjour JP (1982) Impaired biotin status in anticonvulsant therapy. *Ann. Neurol., 12,* 485.
4. Higashi A, Ikeda T, Makoto M et al (1982) Serum zinc and Vitamin E concentrations in handicapped children treated with anticonvulsants. *Dev. Pharmacol. Ther., 5,* 109.
5. Shorvon SD, Reynolds EH (1982) Anticonvulsant peripheral neuropathy: a clinical and electrophysiological study of patients on single drug treatment with Phenytoin, Carbamazepine or barbiturates. *J. Neurol. Neurosurg Psychiatry, 45,* 620.
6. Levy RH, Koch KM (1982) Drug interactions with Valproic Acid. *Drugs, 24,* 543.
7. Haraguchi H, Minoru H, Egoshi N et al (1982) Drug interaction in vivo between Phenobarbital and Valproic Acid. *Jpn. J. Neuro/Psycho/Pharmacol, 4,* 177.
8. Mattson GF, Mattson RH, Cramer JA (1982) Interaction between Valproic Acid and Carbamazepine: an in vivo study of protein binding. *Ther. Drug Monitoring, 4,* 181.
9. Mortensen PB, Hansen HE, Pedersen B et al (1983) Acute Valproate intoxication: biochemical investigations and hemodialysis treatment. *Int. J. Clin. Pharmacol. Ther. Toxicol., 21,* 64.
10. Barr RD, Copeland SA, Stockwell ML et al (1982) Valproic Acid and immune thrombocytopenia. *Arch. Dis. Childh., 57,* 681.
11. Zimmerman HJ, Ishak KG, (1982) Valproate induced hepatic injury. Analyses of 23 fatal cases. *Hepatology, 5,* 591.
12. Zafrani ES, Berthelot P (1982) Sodium valproate in the induction of unusual hepatotoxicity. *Hepatology, 5,* 648.
13. Thygesen J, Boesen F (1982) Two cases of reversible liver lesion induced by Valproate. *Acta Neurol. Scand., 66,* 396.
14. Ohtani Y, Endo F, Matsuda I (1982) Carnitine deficiency and hyperammonaemia associated Impaired biotin status in anticonvulsant therapy.
15. Böhles H, Richter K, Wagner-Thiessen E et al (1982) Decreased serum carnitine in valproate induced Reye syndrome. *Eur. J. Pediatr., 139,* 185.
16. Murphy JV, Marquardt K (1982) Asymptomatic hyperammonaemia in patients receiving Valproic Acid. *Arch. Neurol., 39,* 591.
17. Jeavons PM (1982) Sodium Valproate and neural tube defects. *Lancet, 2,* 1282.
18. Macrae KD (1982) Sodium Valproate and neural tube defects. *Lancet, 2,* 1283.
19. Kantor ML, Hassell JM (1982) Increased accumulation of sulfated glycosaminoglycans in cultures of human fibroblasts from Phenytoin induced gingival overgrowth. *J. Dent. Res., 62,* 383.
20. Trunnell TN, Waisman M (1982) Hypertrophic retroauricular folds attributable to diphenylhydantoin therapy. *Cutis, 30,* 207.
21. Yermakov VM, Hitti JF, Sutton AL (1982) Necrotising vasculitis associated with diphenylhydantoin: Two fatal cases. *Hum. Pathol., 13,* 182.
22. Bardana EJ, Gabrourel JD, Davies GH et al (1983) Effects of phenytoin on Man's immunity. Evaluation of changes in serum immunoglobulins, complement and antinuclear antibody. *Am. J. Med., 74,* 289.
23. Stalnikowicz R, Mosseri M, Shalev O (1982) Phenytoin induced arthritis. *Neurology, 32,* 1317.
24. Palm R, Hallmans G (1982) Zinc and copper metabolism in phenytoin therapy. *Epilepsia, 23,* 453.
25. Puckett JB, Butler WM, McFarland JA (1982) Phenytoin and lactation. *Arch. Neurol., 39,* 457.
26. Inoue F, Walsh RJ (1983) Folate supplement and phenytoin salicylate interaction. *Neurology, 33,* 115.
27. Porro MG, Kupferberg HJ, Porter RJ et al (1982) Phenytoin: an inhibitor and inducer of primidone metabolism in an epileptic patient. *Br. J. Clin. Pharmacol., 14,* 294.
28. Marquis JF, Carruthers SG, Spence JD et al (1982) Phenytoin-theophylline interaction. *N. Engl. J. Med., 307,* 1189.
29. Urbano AM (1983) Phenytoin-quinidine interaction in a patient with recurrent ventricular tachyarrhythmias. *N. Engl. J. Med., 308,* 225.
30. Kessler JM, Keys PW, Stafford RW (1982) Disopyramide and Phenytoin interaction. *Clin Pharmacol, 1,* 263.

31. Begg EJ, Chinwah PM, Webb C et al (1982) Enhanced metabolism of mexiletine after phenytoin administration. *Br. J. Clin. Pharmacol., 14,* 219.
32. Laiwah AACY, Thompson GG, Philip M et al (1983) Carbamazepine induced non-hereditary acute porphyria. *Lancet, 1,* 790.
33. Breathnach SM, McGibbon DH, Ive FA et al (1982) Carbamazepine (Tegretol) and toxic epidermal necrolysis: report of three cases with histopathological observations. *Clin. Dermatol., 7,* 585.
34. Reed MD, Bertino JS, Blumer JL (1982) Carbamazepine associated exfoliative dermatitis. *Clin. Pharmacol., 1,* 78.
35. Wright JM, Stokes EF, Sweeney VP (1982) Isoniazid induced Carbamazepine toxicity and vice versa. *A double drug interaction.* N. Engl. J. Med., 307, 1325.
36. Silverstein FS, Parrish MA, Johnston MV (1982) Adverse behavioural reactions in children treated with Carbamazepine (Tegretol). *J. Pediatr., 101,* 785.
37. Warren JA, Steinbook RM (1983) Case report of Carbamazepine induced reticulocytosis. *Am. J. Psychiatr., 140,* 247.
38. Schoenfeld Y, Baruch NB, Livni E et al (1982) Carbamazepine (Tegretol) induced thrombocytopenia. *Acta Haematol., 68,* 74.
39. Kornberg A, Kobrin I (1982) IgG antiplatelet antibodies due to Carbamazepine. *Acta Haematol., 68,* 68.
40. Gilhus NE, Strandjord RE, Aarli A (1982) The effect of Carbamazepine on serum immunoglobulin concentrations. *Acta Neurol, Scand., 66,* 172.
41. Hurd RW, Wilder BJ, Van Rinsvelt HA (1983) Valproate, birth defects, and zinc. *Lancet, 1,* 181.
42. Karlsen RL et al (1983) Sodium valproate overdose: transient increase in serum bilirubin. *Acta Med. Scand, 213,* 405.
43. Harney J, Glasberg MR (1983) Myopathy and hypersensitivity to phenytoin. *Neurology, 33,* 790.
44. Levine M, Jones MW (1983) Toxic reaction to phenytoin following a viral infection. *Canad. Med. Assoc. J., 128,* 1270.
45. Picard EH (1983) Side effects of metronidazole. *Mayo Clin. Proc., 58,* 401.
46. Rideout JM, Wright DJ, Lim CK et al (1983) Carbamazepine-induced non-hereditary acute porphyria. *Lancet, 2,* 464.
47. Sher A et al (1983) Primidone: psychosis. *Drug Intell. Clin. Pharm., 17,* 551.

Thomas H. Bewley and A. Hamid Ghodse

8 Opioid analgesics and narcotic antagonists

OPIATES

Morphine, heroin, methadone *(33[R], 46[R])*

Kaiko et al (51[R]) have recently reviewed the use of *narcotics in the elderly*. Demographic and analgesic data were surveyed following 1103 doses of morphine in 715 patients. The assays were double-blind cross-over studies and pharmacokinetic studies were also carried out. They found an age-related increase in analgesic effectiveness, with particularly aged patients responding to morphine as though they had received 3–4 times more than young adult patients. This appears to be primarily a function of an increase in duration, rather than an increase in peak analgesic effects, consistent with the finding of decreased morphine clearance with age. By contrast Mitchell et al (66[C]) studied the *risks to young children* given sedative premedication so that they remain motionless for computed tomographic (CT) head scans. They determined rates and risk factors for serious adverse reactions among 106 hospitalized children monitored by an intensive drug surveillance program. Reactions occurred in 13 patients (13%), including 4 cases of life-threatening cardiorespiratory depression or arrest after narcotic premedication. Other reactions included CNS depression, behavior changes, voiding problems and vomiting. The risk of reaction was elevated in subjects who received high doses of a premedication drug (relative risk 5.2) and in those who received 4 or more premedication drugs (relative risk 3.7). All life-threatening reactions occurred among infants younger than 3 months, and 2 of these followed medication, with only morphine sulfate, in the recommended dose. Risks of adverse reactions from premedication should be considered by physicians who order CT scans for hospitalized children who may have a CNS disease that predisposes them to adverse reactions from premedication.

Fell et al (28[Cr]) *compared* controlled-release *morphine sulfate tablets with intramuscular morphine* in 50 patients undergoing hysterectomy or cholecystectomy. Controlled-release morphine sulfate produced comparable pain relief with that of intramuscular morphine, and depression of respiratory function after operation was similar with the 2 analgesic regimens. The mean total dose of drug per patient given over 48 hours to patients undergoing hysterectomy was 115 mg for morphine sulfate and 53 mg for morphine. Patients undergoing cholecystectomy received 130 mg morphine sulfate or 76 mg morphine. The frequency of nausea and dizziness was similar for both analgesic regimens but morphine sulfate tablets appeared to make patients much more sleepy than intramuscular morphine. Both regimens proved equally acceptable to patients.

Ceriello et al (14[Cr]) studied the effect of protracted morphine administration on *carboxyhydrate metabolism* in 27 male addicts. They were found to have increased glycosylated hemoglobin A, indicating an intolerance to ingested carbohydrates. A clinical guide to the diagnosis and treatment of heroin-related *sexual dysfunction* has been developed by Smith et al (95[R]) from 3 separate studies of sexual function in heroin addicts, using standardized questionnaires and 500 brief sex histories of heroin addicts entering into treatment. Data is presented about sexual dysfunction in 42 male and 16 female heroin addicts, but in this paper only those por-

Side Effects of Drugs Annual 8
M.N.G. Dukes, editor

ISBN 0 444 90339 9
$0.80 per article per page (transactional system)
$0.20 per article per page (licensing system)

tions of the studies relating to specific clinical guidelines are discussed. McLean et al (61[cr]) describe a case in which narcotic-induced spasm of the *sphincter of Oddi*, clearly demonstrated in an operative cholangiogram, was reversed by a narcotic antagonist. The spasm was thus distinguished from obstruction of the distal common bile duct and exploration of the duct was indeed unnecessary. Chapman et al (15[c]) report a case of *toxic-shock syndrome* related to intravenous heroin use. Although *Staphylococcus aureus* was not cultured from the patient, there was a rapid rise in antibody titre to enterotoxin F, suggesting the possibility of direct intravenous inoculation of toxin at the time of heroin injection. Brashear (7[R]) has reviewed the effects of heroin, morphine, methadone and propoxyphene on the *lung*. Respiratory depression, hypoxemia, and pulmonary edema (permeability type) are the major pulmonary complications of the abuse of these drugs. Pulmonary granulomatosis is also described. There have been 3 reports of rhabdomyolysis in addicts after an opiate overdose (23[c], 25[cr], 48[c]), and in each case other complications have also developed. The patient described by Cuvillier et al (23[c]) suffered from acute pulmonary edema; the patient described by Kathrein et al (52[cr]) developed *acute renal failure* which was reversed after hemodialysis and decompression fasciotomy of the affected muscles. *Rhabdomyolysis* in the patient reported by Jacome (48[c]) was associated with neurogenic bladder and lumbo-sacral plexus neuropathy. Pullan et al (83[c]) measured serum cortisol and ACTH in 10 chronic methadone addicts and 5 ex-addicts. Although there was no significant difference in cortisol levels between the two groups ACTH was higher in those taking methadone. The authors suggest that in chronic methadone addicts a state of "compensated" primary hypoadrenalism exists in which a partial block of cortisol secretion in the adrenal cortex is compensated for by increased plasma ACTH (due to lack of negative feedback).

Codeine, dihydrocodeine

Ponte (80[c]) has described a case of *erythema multiforme* in a 2-year-old child who had been treated with Acifed-C expectorant containing codeine for a suspected viral upper respiratory tract infection. The rash was characteristic of erythema multiforme, but with no involvement of mucous membranes. As the rash abated rapidly when drug therapy was discontinued, Ponte suggests that it was caused by codeine although it might, as he admits, have been due to a viral insult.

Seymour et al (93[Cr]) set out in a double-blind, randomised, placebo-controlled trial to assess the efficacy of single doses (25 mg and 50 mg) of intravenous dihydrocodeine in 24 patients who had undergone dental surgery. After both doses of dihydrocodeine, patients reported significantly more pain ($p < 0.05$) than after placebo. The hyperalgesia after 50 mg dihydrocodeine was greater and of longer duration than after 25 mg dihydrocodeine.

Pethidine

The introduction of the technique of continuous monitoring of fetal heart rate has enabled accurate observations to be made on the effects of drugs administered to the mother in labor. Ron et al (86[CR]) reported fetal *bradycardia* lasting up to 7 min in 53 fetuses out of 1910 (2.7%) following the administration of 75 mg pethidine (meperidine) and 25 mg promethazine intravenously to the mothers during labor. Bergman et al (5[C]) also studied the effect of pethidine 75 mg with promethazine 25 mg administered during active labor. These analgesic drugs are known to affect uterine contractions by enhancing both amplitude and frequency, but are thought to affect uterine tone minimally. Twenty cases of uterine hypertonia resulting in fetal bradycardia were monitored in a period of 6 months in women receiving these drugs during labor (4% of women receiving these drugs). In all cases, the uterine hypertonia appeared shortly after the drug administration. The uterine hypertonus as well as the fetal bradycardia were self-limited and no intervention was undertaken. Epstein et al (26[c]) reported a single case of sinusoidal *fetal heart rate* (FHR) pattern in association with maternal intrapartum administration of pethidine with promethazine, although the patient had also received oxytocin. The sinusoidal pattern was reversed after maternal intrapartum administration of naloxone. These authors agree with Bergman et al (5[C]) that fetal bradycardia is self-limited and that conservative management is appropriate. Oliva et al (73[cr]) evaluated fetal heart rate and uterine contractions during analgesia in labor and found that pethidine produces strong and prolonged loss of cyclic variation of fetal heart rate and inhibition of myometrial contractility. Similar changes of less degree were induced by pentazocine. They concluded that both pethidine and pentazocine should be used carefully and only in the absence of fetal hypoxia.

Rooth et al (87[Cr]) studied the effects of maternal pethidine (100 mg i.m.) administration on the pH and pCO_2 of *cord blood and neonatal arterial blood* in 150 infants at 1–2 hours after birth; 95 infants whose mothers had not received pethidine served as a control group. Pethidine administration showed no effect on pH or pCO_2 of cord blood and neonatal arterial blood at 1–2 hours after birth if the time interval between pethidine administration and delivery was less than 1 hour. However, when the interval was more than 1 hour, umbilical vein blood pCO_2 was higher; neonatal arterial blood pCO_2 was higher; neonatal baseline heart rate was higher, although long-term variability was similar; the percentage time spent crying was considerably reduced compared with the corresponding values in the control group. The authors point out that the long-term effects of pethidine are unknown but the adverse neonatal factors, particularly if the time interval between administration of the drug and delivery is more than 1 hour, should be kept in mind.

Levy and Rockoff (58[c]), while recognizing that *anaphylactic reactions* to narcotics are very rare, report a case in a 2.5-year-old girl that occurred within moments of the i.v. administration of pethidine. The diagnosis was confirmed later by the demonstration of IgE antibody specific to pethidine.

Hershey (41[r]) has reviewed the *central neurotoxic effects* of pethidine which may cause agitation, tremor, myoclonus or seizures: in fact these excitatory side effects correlated better with plasma levels of the metabolite normeperidine than with meperidine itself. Renal failure may predispose certain patients to neurotoxicity.

Fentanyl

The occurrence of *respiratory depression*, which may be delayed for several hours, is a well recognised side effect of fentanyl and Nilsson and Roseberg (72[c]) have reported another case. They comment that this potentially very dangerous effect is explained in pharmacokinetic studies by a mobilization of fentanyl from tissue stores. Fentanyl *pharmacokinetics* have been studied in some detail by Lehmann et al (57[CR]). Plasma fentanyl was poorly correlated to $paCO_2$ indicating great intra- and interindividual differences in the response to the analgesic. Prediction of pharmacodynamic fentanyl effects from plasma pharmacokinetic data therefore seems to be difficult, if at all possible. The importance of additional factors (vigilance, analgesia, relaxation) must not be underestimated when postoperative respiratory depression after fentanyl is discussed. Postoperative truncal rigidity following fentanyl anesthesia has been reported in 3 cases by Christian et al (18[cr]) who attribute it to a secondary peak of fentanyl in the circulation. They point out that it could seriously compromise the mechanically ventilated patient particularly when hypothermia is superimposed. However they found that treatment with naloxone or neuromuscular blockers was effective in attenuating the rigidity.

Convulsions are also an unusual response to fentanyl administration and Tadikonda et al (103[c]) report 2 cases (out of 5 that they have encountered) of generalized seizures during the rapid intravenous administration of fentanyl. In 1 patient an arterial blood sample during the convulsions had a plasma level of fentanyl of 620 ng/ml and the authors believed that similar blood levels were achieved in the other 4 patients who developed seizures. They also point out that premedicant doses of diazepam or lorazepam did not apparently attenuate the convulsions.

The effect of *high dose fentanyl infusion in open heart surgery*, and in particular on undesirable *hypertensive episodes* was investigated by Townsend et al (105[c]). They found that a loading dose of fentanyl 75 μg/kg followed by an infusion of 0.75 μg/kg/min provided a more hemodynamically stable anesthetic with fewer additional pharmacological interventions when compared to a loading dose alone. Higher mean plasma fentanyl concentrations resulted in lower mean renin values. This strongly suggests that hypertension encountered during aortocoronary bypass surgery in patients under fentanyl anaesthesia is not due to the renin-angiotensin system. Crone et al (22[Cr]) also found that high dose fentanyl anesthesia did not provide hemodynamic stability in 8 of their 12 male patients who were given fentanyl (75–100 μg/kg) anesthesia with oxygen during elective aortocoronary bypass operations.

According to McCammon and Madura (60[C]) reversal of fentanyl induced spasm of the sphincter of Oddi, occurring in the course of cholecystectomy, can be attained by glucagon as effectively as by naloxone.

Dextropropoxyphene

Two unusual side-effects of dextropropoxyphene have been reported. Weiss (110[c]) described the case of an 18-year-old woman who suffered *cardiac arrest* and became comatose after ingesting a large amount of propoxyphene and salicylates. Six days after admission, her pupils, initially miotic, became fixed and dilated. On the 7th day disc edema developed apparently due to optic neuritis from acute propoxyphene overdose; within 8 weeks the disc edema resolved into a pale white atrophy with severe loss of vision. The author claims that this is the first reported case of *optic atrophy* after propoxyphene overdose but acknowledges that acidosis, hypokalemia, or hypoxia may have been contributory factors.

Vincens et al (107[c]) have reported 4 cases of *necrotizing anorectitis* and 4 cases of *proctitis* in 28- to 87-year-old women, and attributed this to long-term administration (2–24 months) of dextropropoxyphene plus paracetamol suppositories (Diantalvic), because of systemic pain (generally related to arthrosis). The gravity of the clinical findings, the close clinical, histological, and evolutive relationship between these observations are underlined, as is the difficulty of diagnosis with an anorectal localisation of Crohn's disease. The mechanism is unknown, but pharmacodependence seems certain in several patients who continue to use suppositories in spite of clear medical warnings, only to see their lesions reappear. The authors believe that these facts justify some restrictive measures concerning the utilization of these suppositories.

Possible dysmorphogenic effects of dextropropoxyphene

Although the neonatal opiate withdrawal syndrome resulting from maternal dependence on opiates during pregnancy has been described many times (SED-9, 104; SEDA-5, 67; SEDA-6, 73; SEDA-7, 87; SED-10), opiates are not usually considered to be teratogenic. Their safety in this respect however, like that of many other drugs "tried and tested" by years of use, has been very much taken for granted rather than proven by the application of the stringent tests to which newer drugs are subjected.

Dextropropoxyphene is a mild (i.e. less potent than codeine) analgesic derived from methadone. It is popular and widely used and indeed in the U.S.A. more prescriptions for propoxyphene (USP equivalent of dextropropoxyphene) are dispensed in retail pharmacies than any other drugs (65[R]). Any complacency about its safety in pregnancy, however, has been disturbed by the report by Golden, King, Robert et al (37[CR]) suggesting that dextropropoxyphene and paracetamol (acetaminophen USP) in combination may be teratogenic. On the face of it, this seems extremely unlikely. Indeed the manufacturers of paracetamol give it the rare accolade that "there is epidemiological evidence" of its safety in pregnancy (2[R]); the manufacturers of dextropropoxyphene merely comment in the ritual way, that its safety in pregnancy has not been established. The British National Formulary (8[R]), without mentioning it specifically in its list of drugs to be avoided or used with caution in pregnancy, perhaps includes it in the "etc" of narcotic analgesics but again there is no hint that it may cause congenital malformations. Indeed in the first case of neonatal withdrawal symptoms associated with maternal use of dextropropoxyphene, described by Tyson (106[C]), in which the mother had taken only dextropropoxyphene in pregnancy, the infant had no congenital malformations. Golden et al (37[CR]) describe a male infant born to a 28-year-old mother who had taken 6–10 tablets of the combination dextropropoxyphene 50 mg and paracetamol 325 mg daily throughout pregnancy for chronic orthopedic pain, together with phenobarbitone 32 mg, rarely, for sleep. A few hours after birth the baby manifested symptoms of drug withdrawal attributable to his antenatal exposure to dextropropoxyphene. Of more interest in relation to the teratogenic effect of dextropropoxyphene were his physical characteristics which include absence of left forearm and radial two digits, syndactyly of ulnar three digits, hypoplastic left femur, syndactyly of left fourth and fifth toes. Golden et al (37[CR]) also describe 3 other malformed infants born to women who used dextropropoxyphene during pregnancy. One infant was born to a mother who had also taken benzodiazepine. Her baby had widely spaced sutures, a beaked nose, micrognathia, and a bifid uvula. The fourth and fifth toes of his left foot were long, overlapping and curved medially. Another infant, whose mother had also taken meprobamate, had omphalocele, defective anterior abdominal wall defect in the diaphragm, congenital heart disease with partial ectopic cordis secondary to sternal cleft, and dysplastic hips. In the third case, described by Barrow and Souder (4[c]), the mother was dependent on dextropropoxyphene and consumed 20–36 capsules (65 mg each) daily. During the first 3 months of pregnancy she took numerous other medications, including antinausea preparations and diphenylhydantoin in addition to her usual dextropropoxyphene. The infant, born by Caesarean section during the 9th month, weighed only some 2 kg, had Pierre Robin syndrome and arthrogryposis. Later he was found to be severely retarded in growth and mentality. They also summarize the results of animal experiments with dextropropoxyphene which was found to cause congenital malformations of the central nervous system when injected into pregnant hamsters, but had no effect on rabbit, rat or mouse (35[C]).

In their discussion Golden et al (37[CR]) point out that all four infants suffered micrognathia and limb abnormalities and put forward the suggestion that, in the case that they describe, "the antepartum intake of dextropropoxyphene in association with paracetamol and/or phenobarbitone may have been teratogenic". As they point out paracetamol is not known to be teratogenic, phenobarbitone has been associated with congenital deformities (cleft lip and palate) only with massive drug intake "but the presence of several drugs may affect the path or rate at which each is metabolized leading to the production and accumulation of metabolite toxic to the fetus". There is indeed some evidence from adults, albeit scanty and indirect, that this may occur with dextropropoxyphene and other drugs (1[cr]). Golden et al (37[CR]) stress that the abnormalities may have occurred by chance alone but their report must be taken seriously, if only because the dextropropoxyphene and paracetamol combination (Distalgesic in U.K., Darocet in U.S.A.) has achieved a vast popularity, unwarranted according to many double-blind studies (25[R]). Nevertheless they are so widely available, so much a part of every day vocabulary, that they are likely to be taken complacently during many pregnancies, whether prescribed by doctors or "borrowed" from friends. Even a short delay in recognizing a teratogenic potential might be very serious.

Tramadol

Tramadol is a synthetic opioid introduced for the treatment of acute pain. It was investigated in a dosage of 1.5 mg/kg body weight i.v. with regard to changes in *hemodynamic parameters and blood gases.* The hemodynamic parameters generally remained stable; all changes were statistically not significant. There were no signs of respiratory depression (76[Cr]). Muller et al (68[CR]) also investigated the hemodynamic effects of i.v. tramadol at a dose of 1.5 mg/kg body weight as in the previous study and at a dose of 0.75 mg/kg body weight. They concluded that while during conventional pain therapy no hemodynamic and respiratory side effects of tramadol could be demonstrated, the typical qualities of opiates (postoperative ventilatory embarrassment) and unspecified adrenergic effects have to be taken into account after their use in high doses for anaesthetic purposes.

In a more recent paper, Rothe and Brather (90[c]) reported postoperative *depression of respiration* which they tentatively attributed to infusion anesthesia with tramadol. In 2 cases this occurred directly after the end of anesthesia, and in a 3rd case 6 hours later.

Alfentanil

Alfentanil is a new ultrashort-acting, potent, synthetic narcotic. Nauta et al (1982) (70[Cr]) have evaluated it as an anesthetic induction agent in 20, unsedated patients premedicated with atropine about to undergo general surgical operations with halothane-nitrous oxide anesthesia (Group I) and in 22 patients premedicated with lorazepam and atropine (9 with mitral valvular disease) (Group II), and 13 with coronary artery disease (Group III), about to undergo open-heart surgery with alfentanil-oxygen anesthesia. Alfentanil resulted in a transient small decrease in systolic arterial blood pressure with loss of consciousness in Groups II and III but no change in right atrial and mean pulmonary arterial pressure or cardiac output throughout the study period. Patients in Group I had no change in any cardiovascular variable measured. The only significant undesirable side effect was *chest wall rigidity,* which occurred in 50% of Group I and 22% and 31% of Groups II and III respectively. No patient remembered any aspect of laryngoscopy, endotracheal intubation, or surgery and only one thought the anesthetic induction was unpleasant. The authors concluded that rapid infusion with alfentanil results in a rapid, pleasant anesthetic induction with little change in cardiovascular dynamics and a minimum of side effects. Sebel et al (92[Cr]) tested it in 30 patients undergoing cardiac surgery. In the majority, there were no significant changes in cardiovascular measurements throughout the study, although 2 received sodium nitroprusside for the control of hypertension, and in 1 patient hypertension was so severe that the method of anesthesia was abandoned. Transient hypotension occurred on induction in 1 patient. 26 patients required alfentanil supplementation before bypass. Helmers et al (40[Cr]) also concluded that side effects were minor and infrequent when alfentanil was compared with fentanyl in a double-blind study of 90 female patients undergoing laparoscopic sterilization.

Opioid peptides

Metkephamid acetate is an analog of the naturally-occurring pentapeptide metenkephalin and is more resistant to enzymatic degradation. Its analgesic efficacy and side effects in a single parenteral dose of 70 mg were compared with those of pethidine (meperidine) hydrochloride 100 mg and placebo in a double-blind, randomised, controlled clinical trial (12[CR]). The time-effect curves of summated pain measures and analyses of derived measures all indicated that the analgesic activity of metkephamid 70 mg was significantly greater than that of placebo and not less than that of pethidine 100 mg. The metkephamid group had a greater incidence of side effects than the other two treatment groups, and the spectrum of side effects, similar to those reported in healthy volunteers receiving metkephamid, suggested that its pharmacological properties are different from those of standard narcotic analgesics. Side effects unique to metkephamid were a sensation of heaviness in the extremities, a sensation of burning at the injection site, fatigue, dry mouth, nasal congestion. All side effects were temporary, none lasting until the end of the 6-hour observation period.

The effect of a stable metenkephalin analog, FK 33-824 and other opioid or putative neurotransmitter peptides on histamine-induced itch and flare responses was studied in humans after intradermal injection (32[CR]). Significant enhancement of the histamine responses was induced by FK 33-824, β-endorphin and morphine. The potentiation induced by FK 33-824 did not seem to be due to histamine release or to prostaglandin formation and the mechanism of the effect remains to be shown. The specific morphine antagonist naloxone did not inhibit the potentiation by FK 33-824, which might indicate that ordinary opiate receptors were not involved. The results support the idea that pain and itch are qualitatively separate processes and suggest possible mechanisms of morphine-induced pruritus. The findings are of particular interest in view of recent reports on the presence of methionine-enkephalin in Merkel cells.

Zagon et al (112[R]) have prepared a comprehensive bibliography of the literature of the last hundred years concerned with opiates, endorphins, and the developing organism.

Epidural and extradural administration of opiates

The use of extradural and to a lesser extent intrathecal opiates remains a subject of great research interest and the Swedish Society of Anaesthetists has conducted a nationwide retrospective survey of clinical experience with these techniques (38[Cr]). Special interest was focused on the frequency and type of ventilatory depression. Up to May 1981 extradural morphine had been given to approximately 6000–9150 patients, extradural pethidine to 220–450 and intrathecal morphine to 90–150 patients. *Ventilatory depression* requiring treatment with naloxone was reported in 23 patients treated with extradural morphine (0.25–0.40%) and in 6 given intrathecal morphine (4–7%). In 22 patients the administration of extradural morphine was considered as a major contributory factor for the occurrence of ventilatory depression. Only 2 of these 22 patients experienced ventilatory depression later than 6 hours after the last dose of opiates (s.c., i.m., i.v., or extradural). Patients aged 70 years or more, those receiving thoracic extradural puncture and those with reduced ventilatory capacity seemed to be over-represented. Steppe and Camu (102[C]) also emphasize in the light of their own work the inherent dangers of ventilatory depression of high dose (10 mg) thoracic epidural morphine treatments in elderly patients. An important degree of sedation was also observed. A similar point is made by Palitzsch (75[CR]), who found that after epidural injection of 3 mg morphine, pCO increases of between 43 and 47 mm Hg (5.7–6.3 kPa) occurred together with a decrease of pO_2 in 7 out of 50 patients. Respiratory depression, he concluded, may occur particularly in older patients and in patients with increased intrathoracic or intra-abdominal pressure and requires a reduced dosage for epidural morphine analgesia. He suggested that the analgesic effect of epidural morphine occurs after diffusion of the morphine into the intrathecal space by occupation of specific spinal receptors in the substantia gelatinosa of the spinal cord. After cranial spread towards the fourth ventricle, supraspinal centers may be influenced depending on the applied dosage and on pathological changes of the epidural space.

Delay in the onset of respiratory depression is reported by many authors (27[CR], 44[c], 49[c], 53[r], 102[C]; and careful observation and monitoring is recommended, not only for the duration of the analgesia but for 12–24 hours thereafter and especially when administrations are repeated (44[c], 49[c], 53[r]). Eriksen and Jensen (27[CR]) comment that the frequency of this side effect appears to depend on positioning of the patient, form of administration, the dosage and volume of the opiate. Jensen et al (49[c]) recommend prolonged observation in order to detect late respiratory depression. The efficacy of naloxone in reversing the respiratory depression is clear (44[c], 49[c]).

Stokes-Adams attacks after the administration of extradural morphine have been reported by Christensen and Brandt (17[c]). They postulate that the attacks were probably caused by increased parasympathetic stimulation of the dorsal nucleus of the vagus. The delayed onset of the last attack, 15 hours after the last morphine injection, is in accordance with that reported for respiratory depression (which was not observed in this patient) suggesting, according to the authors, the same pharmacodynamic mode of action.

Torda and Pybus (104[C]) however reported no effects of clinical importance on heart rate, respiratory frequency or arterial pressure, after extradural injections of morphine sulfate 6 mg, methadone 6 mg, pethidine 60 mg, and fentanyl 60 mg in 24 postoperative patients. Arterial systolic pressure decreased after morphine and pethidine and pethidine also caused a statistically significant reduction in diastolic pressure. Other side effects reported after epidural morphine include nausea, vomiting, fatigue and headache (56[Cr], 64[Cr]); *disturbances* of micturition occur frequently, sometimes causing urinary retention (27[CR], 56[Cr], 64[Cr]). Petersen et al (78[CR]) examined the incidence of *urinary retention* during intramuscular and extradural morphine analgesia in the postoperative period of 56 healthy patients undergoing cholecystectomy or operations for duodenal ulcer, who received, in a randomized order, i.m., 'high level' or 'low level' extradural morphine. 35% of the i.m. group, 33% in the high-level group and 50% in the low-level group suffered urinary retention, in all cases within the first 24 h. *Pruritus* is still a commonly reported side effect although Eriksen and Jensen (27[CR]) found its frequency was considerably reduced when opiates without preservatives were employed. The possible mechanisms underlying it have been discussed by Scott and Fischer (31[r], 91[R]) who pointed out that facial pruritus associated with spinal opiate analgesia in man is thought to result either from release of histamine or from imbalance of sensory modulation secondary to spread of opiate to the medulla or fourth ventricle. An alternative possibility put forward by the authors is that the sensory imbalance may be secondary to rostral spread of opiate effect by nervous transmission. Evidence is adduced in support of possible anatomical pathways, and in support of a medullary 'itching centre' in man.

In contrast to the plethora of reports about side effects of epidural morphine, Jacobson et al (47[CR]) found in their comparison of extradural versus intramuscular diamorphine that extradural diamorphine provided safe and effective analgesia of rapid onset, with no specific undesirable side effects.

A surprising paucity of side effects was recorded by Moller and Eriksen (67[c]) who report on a case in which a very high dose (16 mg, 5 times daily) of extradural morphine was administered accidentally (160 mg within 48 hours). The patient had been treated for 6 months for painful metastases and had presumably become tolerant to the drug so that 4 hours after the last dose his respiration was unaffected although catatonic twitchings in his extremities developed. The concentration of free morphine in serum and cerebrospinal fluid was at this time 62 nmol/l and 10.9 nmol/l respectively.

An unusual complication is reported by Wenningsted-Torgard et al (111[c]) who described a case of *Staphylococcus aureus spondylitis* following epidural analgesia. Their patient was diabetic and also received injections of corticosteroids, which may have promoted the infection but the route of infection was probably from the skin through or along the catheter to the epidural space and then either directly or through lymphatic or blood vessels to the spine.

Buprenorphine is also being used as an epidural analgesic, both alone and in conjunction with the local anesthetic bupivacaine; no respiratory depression was reported although older patients receiving both drugs were characterised by pronounced sedation (59[CR]). Zinck and Fritz (114[cr]), however, in a case of epidural application of buprenorphine hydrochloride noted a reduction of arterial pO_2 4–6 hours after the injection. They felt that this could not be explained as a respiratory depression due to buprenorphine, because immediately after a repeat epidural application of the drug the pO_2 rose again and suggested that reduced pO_2 a long time after buprenorphine is a result of hypoventilation caused by increased pain. Christensen and Andersen (16[c]) reported on adverse reaction to extradural buprenorphine in 2 women with terminal cancer who developed tolerance to extradural morphine. Their medication was changed to extradural buprenorphine 0.3 mg which was injected 12 hours after the last dose of morphine. Exactly 2 hours later both patients developed signs of shock; pale and cold skin, low arterial pressure (90/60 mm Hg) and an average heart rate of 110 beats/min. The patients remained in this condition for nearly 2–3 hr, whereafter the symptoms disappeared spontaneously. No treatment (including i.v. naloxone) was successful. The pain was then treated with extradural morphine, but a smaller dose than previously was necessary to secure complete pain relief. The changed morphine sensitivity and the lack of effect of naloxone were presumably caused by the agonist/antagonist effect of buprenorphine. The injection of buprenorphine was given 12 hr after the last extradural morphine, so an interaction between buprenorphine and morphine may be excluded.

The treatment of chronic pain by the use of *meptazinol* administered into the epidural space was assessed by Budd et al (10[Cr]). They found that it produced excellent analgesia in 23 patients suffering from spinal and back pain. The extent and duration of analgesia were dose-dependent, but were appreciable with a single dose of 30 mg. At doses of 30 and 60 mg, side effects were infrequent but at the 90 mg level, nausea, vomiting and dizziness were severe. No significant changes were seen in any patient in cardiovascular or respiratory parameters.

Intrathecal opiates are used much less frequently than epidural opiates. However, 30 women, in labor, for whom an epidural injection using local anesthesia was hazardous (deformed spine) or contraindicated (allergic to local anesthetic agents) received an injection of 0.008 mg/cm of morphine chlorhydrate intrathecally (6[Cr]). After half an hour there was only a simple ache which was well tolerated right up to the time of delivery. Uterine action was not changed, which allowed 27 labors to be completed vaginally, of which 23 were without forceps. There was no hemodynamic change or respiratory depression, either immediately or later, in the mother nor in the infant (there were 26 Apgar scores of 9 or more). The ratio of plasma concentrations of morphine between the mother and the fetus using radioimmunological assays was inverted as time passed. These were at 6 ng/ml or less which explains the medullary characteristic of the analgesia and the absence of general repercussions. The authors concluded that the safety that is offered by the poor diffusion of substance between the fetus and the mother and the ability to prevent secondary effects (pruritus and headache) are features that make intrathecal analgesia an interesting alternative to a conduction block in labor.

Drug dependence in pregnancy

The neonatal abstinence syndrome is included in Hutchings review (45[R]) of the behavioral effects in human and animal offspring of methadone and heroin taken during pregnancy.

Among other major reviews on this topic is that of Finnegan (29[R]) who concludes that if pregnant drug-dependent women are maintained with low dosage of methadone and are given adequate prenatal care and counselling, complications of pregnancy and childbirth can be minimized. Furthermore, morbidity and mortality during pregnancy, the neonatal period, and in childhood should be substantially reduced. Kreek (54[R]) has also carried out an extensive review of opioid disposition and effects during chronic exposure in the perinatal period in man. As she points out a specific problem encountered when animal models are used to delineate opioid effects in the perinatal period is that the pharmacokinetic properties of most opioids are profoundly different in animals and in man. Amato et al (3[cr]) also studied the relationship between maternal abuse of methadone and neonatal signs of withdrawal.

Johnson and Rosen (50[CR]), as part of an ongoing longitudinal study of the developmental effects of prenatal methadone exposure, evaluated at 6 months of age, 41 children born to methadone-maintained mothers and 23 children from matched backgrounds but with a negative maternal history of drug abuse. Each child received physical and neurological examinations and a battery of behavioral assessments. The groups did not differ significantly in frequency of suspect-abnormal neurological signs or in mean scores on the three behavioral measures. Despite the great within-group variances, performance on the behavioral measures was not related to maternal or neonatal characteristics. There were significantly more low PDI scores (predictors of developmental difficulties) among methadone subjects particularly among methadone vs comparison males. These findings corroborate other studies that have shown: (1) delayed motor development in methadone-exposed infants, (2) greater vulnerability of males to adverse environmental conditions, and (3) correlation between early methadone exposure and behavioral abnormalities in adult male rats. The significance of prenatal methadone exposure as a risk factor is discussed.

In a second paper, the same authors (88[CR]) have reported on the somatic and neurobehavioral findings of children in the first 18 months of life born to methadone-maintained mothers and to a matched drug-free comparison group of mothers. Findings during the neonatal period were: (1) a 75% incidence of moderate-to-severe narcotic abstinence syndrome, (2) a significant incidence of head circumferences below the third percentile, and (3) elevated systolic blood pressure. In follow-up, the methadone children had: (1) significantly higher incidence of otitis media, (2) a significant incidence of head circumference below the third percentile, (3) neurologic findings of tone discrepancies, developmental delays, and poor fine motor coordination, (4) a high incidence of abnormal eye findings, and (5) significantly lower scores on the Bayley mental and motor developmental indices. The authors suggest that these neurobehavioral findings in children of methadone-treated mothers at 18 months of age may be predictors of later learning and behavioral problems.

Dirghangi and Ansari (24[cr]) described another hazard of drug abuse; they reported an unusual case of *ruptured mycotic aneurysm* of the right external iliac artery in a pregnant woman who was a heroin addict. In the third trimester, she developed a large hematoma that resulted in intrauterine fetal death, premature labor, and hypovolemic shock.

Smith (96[c]) in a valuable reminder about the potential transmission of drugs in breast milk described a case of codeine-induced bradycardia in a breast-fed infant.

The mother had ingested a single 30 mg codeine tablet for pain control following a minor surgical procedure 6 days prior to the time the child was seen in the clinic. The infant's only nourishment was from maternal breast-feeding. The infant's heart rate normalized within 24 hours and remained in the 130–145 range on repeated visits during the next month. The infant's birth and neonatal history revealed meconium staining of the amniotic fluid, a birth weight of 3345 g and normal Apgar scores. He developed neonatal unconjugated hyperbilirubinemia, total bilirubin reaching 16.1 mg/dl. He received phototherapy and was discharged from hospital at 5 days of age. Since codeine is metabolized in the liver, it is possible that excessive amounts remained in the infant's circulation because of immature hepatic enzyme systems, resulting in the depressive effect on the heart.

NARCOTIC ANTAGONISTS

Naloxone and naltrexone

Although naloxone and naltrexone are usually considered "pure" narcotic antagonists there has been some discussion about the possible dangers of naloxone use, and in particular about its routine administration to unconscious patients to elucidate the cause of coma. Gilman (36[r]) has reviewed reports of a *hypertensive effect* of naloxone and believes that the patient's condition should be assessed before naloxone is administered. Kulig (55[r]) however points out that the reported complications occurred postoperatively after the administration of large amounts of narcotics and multiple other agents and that no adverse effects other than the possible precipitation of opiate withdrawal have been reported when naloxone has been administered to unconscious patients in the emergency room. Furthermore massive doses of naloxone (up to 4 mg/kg) have been given to human volunteers with no serious side effects. The use of naltrexone as an effective adjunct in the rehabilitation of opiate addicts has been reviewed (43[r]).

Buprenorphine

Cook et al (20[CR]) carried out a controlled comparison of i.m. morphine and buprenorphine for analgesia after abdominal surgery. The two drugs were equally effective as analgesics at the doses used. Five in the buprenorphine group and none in the morphine group were excluded because of respiratory depression. Four of these had received opiates during operation. The remainder of the buprenorphine group developed progressively slower respiration rates after 12 hr. The results indicate that buprenorphine has a synergistic respiratory depressant effect with fentanyl and phenoperidine and may have a cumulative effect when given regularly on a 6-hourly regimen.

Sublingual buprenorphine (0.2 mg) was investigated for the treatment of cancer pain in 67 patients by Zens et al (113[CR]). The induction time was quite long (60 min) but effective pain relief was obtained even in final stages of cancer. The mean daily dose of buprenorphine was 1.2–1.7 mg, the mean duration of analgesia being 6–8 hours with a single dose of 0.2–1.0 mg buprenorphine. Typical opiate-side-effects were registered but were well tolerated after some days' treatment. There was no respiratory depression. Murray (69[c]) however reported a case of acute urinary retention associated with sublingual buprenorphine in a 68-year-old man with no previous symptoms of urinary outflow obstruction. Urodynamic assessment carried out when the patient was no longer taking buprenorphine was also normal. Rossano et al (89[CR]) compared i.m. and sublingual administration of buprenorphine (111 and 40 patients, respectively) and were able to confirm its prolonged analgesic action. The difference between the two modes of administration was not significant even though i.m. administration presented a statistically higher duration of action. Although the sublingual tablets had a higher frequency of nausea than the i.m. formulation, the authors considered sublingual administration preferable for the treatment of chronic pain in hospitalized patients, and suggested using a sublingual tablet at a lower dosage (0.2 mg).

Butorphanol

Butorphanol is an analgesic with both agonist and narcotic antagonist properties. Its value as an anesthetic agent was compared by Quam (84[CR]) with that of fentanyl, meperidine, and enflurane in 120 healthy women undergoing pelvic surgery. Subsequently, butorphanol was compared with meperidine for adequacy of pain relief postoperatively. Stability of blood pressure and pulse were similar in all anesthetic agents. Slight respiratory depression was noted in 17% of patients given butorphanol intraoperatively but did not increase with increased dosages. Butorphanol caused less nausea and emesis than the other agents. The chief side effect of butorphanol when used for postoperative analgesia, was drowsiness, observed in 20% of subjects. In another study of postoperative analgesia, dezocine, a relatively new mixed agonist/antagonist analgesic, was compared in a double-blind study with butorphanol and placebo (30[C]). A single intramuscular injection of dezocine was found to be at least as effective as butorphanol in the management of patients with moderate to severe postoperative pain and the most common side effects in those receiving active medication were nausea, vomiting, sedation and dizziness.

Stambaugh (101[C]) compared the analgesic efficacy of single oral doses of placebo, butorphanol, acetaminophen, and combined butorphanol/acetaminophen in a double-blind complete cross-over study in 20 hospitalized patients with moderate to severe pain due to metastatic carcinoma. It was concluded, that the combination provided greater analgesia than either drug alone or placebo without corresponding additive side effects.

Nalbuphine

Nalbuphine, a narcotic agonist/antagonist was compared in a double-blind study with morphine for the management of chronic pain associated with advanced malignancy in 37 patients (100[Cr]). Nalbuphine was found to be as effective an analgesic in long-term use as morphine, with less toxicity. Side effects of nalbuphine and morphine recorded in this study were indistinguishable with the exceptions of euphoria, psychotomimetic effects and constipation which were noted for morphine but not for nalbuphine. In long-term dosing there was less development of tolerance with nalbuphine compared to morphine, and six patients, previously on narcotic analgesic therapy, experienced withdrawal-like symptoms when given nalbuphine. Nalbuphine was found to be an effective analgesic with narcotic antagonist activity and appeared to be a good alternative to morphine in the management of chronic cancer pain.

Nalbuphine has also been used to reverse narcotic-induced respiratory depression in 15 patients after a nitrous oxide, narcotic, relaxant technique (62[C]). Arterial carbon dioxide tensions following administration of 0.1 mg/kg of nalbuphine were essentially the same as those previously reported with nalbuphine alone within five minutes. No patient verbalized the reversal of analgesia following administration of nalbuphine, nor did any patient renarcotize postoperatively. Nalbuphine's long duration of action and its ability to reverse morphine-type induced respiratory depression, appear to provide a safe option in terminating high dose narcotic techniques. Magruder et al (62[C]) point out that additional caution is warranted in patients with severe cardiovascular disease as emergence from most anaesthetics is associated with a pressor response. The pressor response of nalbuphine is moderate and pulse and pressure have not exceeded that observed in the pre-anesthetic state.

Hofmann and Weiler (42[CR]) used parenteral nalbuphine in combination with lorazepam as premedication for 30 local anaesthetic ophthalmic surgery cases. Clinical responses followed the known responses, and adverse side effects were minimal.

Pentazocine

There have been further case reports of *dependence* on pentazocine (11[cr]) and Mann et al (63[cr]) report a patient with pentazocine-induced cutaneous ulceration and chronic panniculitis after self-administration of the drug for 12 years. This appears to be the first report of such changes induced by pentazocine in the British literature. The possible mechanisms involved are discussed, including ischaemia, repeated needle trauma, chronic infection and "chemical irritation". The addition of tripelennamine to pentazocine (T's and Blues) for intravenous abuse causes particular problems (13[CR]) and is discussed in Chapter 4.

Stahl and Kasser (99[cr]) have described a case of pentazocine overdose. Their patient ingested 1.5 g pentazocine and developed status epilepticus, coma, respiratory depression, acidosis, profound hypotension, and ventricular arrhythmias. Although this patient survived after institution of general supportive measures, she did not respond to usual doses of naloxone and the authors suggest that pentazocine overdose may require higher doses of naloxone (5–20 mg) than are customarily used for narcotic overdoses. Poklis and Mackell (79[cr]), however, described the toxicological findings in 2 cases of fatal suicidal ingestion of pentazocine and compared them with findings in cases published earlier. Pentazocine blood and liver concentrations in the presented cases were 3.3 and 9.2 mg/l, and 34 and 43 mg/kg respectively. Blood and liver concentrations in reference cases ranged from 0.8–38 mg/l and 3–197 mg/kg, respectively.

Meptazinol

Meptazinol, an opioid antagonist drug with analgesic properties has been the subject of several studies in a general practice setting (77[Cr], 81[Cr], 82[C], 108[C], 109[CR]). Price and Latham (82[C]) described the side effect profile of oral meptazinol (200 mg) in comparison to placebo. Complaints were concerned primarily with the *gastrointestinal tract* probably because of the frequency of usage of other analgesics and nonsteroidal anti-inflammatory drugs also used by the patients who were complaining of acute or chronic musculo-skeletal pain. There was no evidence of any deleterious interaction between meptazinol and other medications taken during the course of the trial and no evidence of relationship between the incidence of side effects and age. In a double-blind study against placebo lasting for 14 days, Parker and Langrick (77[Cr]) found no significant difference in the incidence of adverse effects reported by patients in either treatment groups. Similarly, Wade and Ward (108[C]) in a double-blind comparison of meptazinol versus paracetamol and placebo reported that the frequency of adverse effects reported was low and similar in all three treatment groups although the same authors found that the side effect profile was better for meptazinol than Distalgesic (109[CR]).

Price and Latham (81[CR]) in their double-blind comparison of meptazinol (200 mg) and dextropropoxyphene/paracetamol found no significant difference in frequency of side effects in the two groups. Those side effects reported most frequently were nausea (12% + 11%) and giddy feelings (11% + 15%) for meptazinol and dextropropoxyphene/paracetamol, respectively.

The use of meptazinol as a *premedication* for surgical patients has been studied by Broadley et al (9[C]) in a randomized, double-blind trial involving 101 surgical patients, when a meptazinol-hyoscine mixture was compared with Omnopon-hyoscine. Blood pressure and respiratory rate were significantly reduced to a similar extent by both premedicant combinations. The two mixtures produced a similar degree of sedation, and both were associated with a useful inhibition of salivary secretion. Side effects were reported in 25% patients in the meptazinol group, and in 28% of those receiving Omnopon, although a number of these effects may be attributable to hyoscine. There was no difference in the pattern of postoperative analgesic requirements between the two groups, and no unfavorable interaction was noted with any anesthetic. Church (19[CR]) compared continuous infusion of meptazinol with pethidine in the relief of postoperative pain and found that although both drugs provided effective analgesia, and no patients exhibited clinically significant respiratory depression or sleep apnea, high ($>$ 6 Kpa) end-tidal pCO_2 values were significantly more frequent in the pethidine than in the meptazinol group ($P < 0.01$). This suggests a greater margin of safety with the use of meptazinol and might make it especially appropriate for administration by continuous infusion. Harmer et al (39[CR]) assessed intramuscular on demand analgesia in a double-blind controlled trial of pethidine (50 mg), buprenorphine (0.15 mg), morphine (5 mg) and meptazinol (50 mg). Significant differences were found between drugs in dizziness (pethidine produced the worst score) but not with other side effects (e.g. nausea, drowsiness).

The use of meptazinol has also been assessed in cases of trauma (21[C]). In 19 trauma patients, meptazinol (100 mg) provided effective analgesia and no cardiovascular or respiratory depression was observed. Meptazinol had no effect on pupil diameter.

Another potential use for meptazinol is in the treatment of the pain of *myocardial infarction/unstable angina* (97[c]). A pilot study showed that meptazinol was effective in 15 of 22 subjects. There were no adverse hemodynamic effects nor respiratory depression. Nausea and/or vomiting occurred with administration of the drug but these symptoms may occur in patients with myocardial infarction who have not received any analgesia.

Meptazinol has also been compared with pethidine in a double-blind study for use *in labor* (71[Cr]). 28% of patients experienced side effects after meptazinol compared with 35% after pethidine. The commonest were nausea and vomiting. Significantly more babies whose mothers had received meptazinol had an Apgar score of 8 at 1 min after birth.

Ciramadol

In an open investigation Oosterlinck and Minnaert (74[C]) assessed the effect of different doses of intravenous ciramadol, a partial opioid agonist, in patients experiencing renal colic. Vomiting and nausea occurred in 9 patients and several patients felt a dizziness or a sensation of a "warm head" during the injection and immediately afterwards. These adverse effects were apparently related to standing and walking following the ciramadol injection although no changes in blood pressure or pulse rate were recorded. Some patients also experienced slight drowsiness. In a double-blind study Fragen and Caldwell (34[Cr]) compared 3 doses (20, 40 and 60 mg) of oral ciramadol and placebo for the treatment of moderate to severe postoperative pain. The highest dose used for moderate pain, 40 mg, was statistically more effective than placebo as measured by pain intensity differences and pain relief scores. The higher doses used to treat severe pain, 60 mg, was also more effective statistically than placebo and the lower doses of ciramadol at certain points during the 6-hour observation period. Drowsiness was minimal, and side effects were infrequent and mild in intensity. No clinically significant changes occurred in blood pressure, respiratory rate or heart rate and the authors concluded that 40 mg ciramadol for moderate postoperative pain and 60 mg ciramadol for severe postoperative pain would be the minimal oral doses to compare with standard analgesics in future studies.

Propiram

Propiram fumarate is a new oral analgesic with weak narcotic antagonist activity. Its use in treating postoperative ocular pain was assessed by Sloan Wilson and Landers (94[C]) in 50 patients after retinal surgery. Most patients received total daily doses of 50 to 100 mg for 1–2 days. Only 1 patient complained of any side effects of nausea and perspiration.

REFERENCES

1. Abernethy DR, Greenblatt DJ et al (1982) Impairment of hepatic drug oxidation by propoxyphene. *Ann. Int. Med.*, *97*, 223.
2. ABPI Data Sheet Compendium (1983–1984) Dataphars Publications Ltd., London.
3. Amato M, Frei H, Buhlmann U (1982) Drogentzugssyndrom beim Neugeborenen. *Schweiz. Med. Wochenschr.*, *112*, 442.
4. Barrow HV, Souder DE (1971) Propoxyphene and congenital malformations. *J. Am. Med. Ass.*, *217*, 1551.
5. Bergman A, Eckstein N, Yedwab G, David MP (1982) Fetal distress due to intravenous administration of pethidine (meperidine) with promethazine during labour. *Austr. N.Z. J. Obstet. Gynaecol.*, *22*, 215.
6. Bonnardot JP, Colau JC, Maillet M et al (1982) Intrathecal injection of morphine in labour. *J. Gynecol. Obstet. Biol. Reproduct.*, *11*, 619.
7. Brashear RE (1980) Effects of heroin, morphine, methadone, and propoxyphene on the lung. *Sem. Respir. Med.*, *2*, 59.
8. British National Formulary No. 5 (1983) British Medical Association and The Pharmaceutical Society of Great Britain, London.
9. Broadley J, Wilson T, Robson P (1982) The use of meptazinol as a premedication for surgical patients. *J. Int. Med. Res.*, *10*, 225.
10. Budd K, Robson PJ, Brown PM (1983) The treatment of chronic pain by the use of meptazinol administered into the epidural space. *Postgrad. Med. J.*, *59 (Suppl. 1)*, 68.
11. Bulfoni A (1982) Tossicodipendenza da pentazocine. *Gazz. Med. Ital.*, *141*, 673.
12. Calimlim JF, Wardell WM, Striwatanakul K (1982) Analgesic efficacy of parenteral metkephamid acetate in treatment of postoperative pain. *Lancet*, *1*, 1374.
13. Caplan LR, Chinnamma T, Banks G (1982) Central nervous system – complications of addictions to 'T's and Blues'. *Neurology*, *32*, 623.
14. Ceriello A, Giugliano D, Russo PD et al (1982) Increased glycosylated haemoglobin A_1 in opiate addicts: Evidence for hyperglycaemic effect of morphine. *Diabetologia*, *22*, 379.
15. Chapman RL, Colville JM, Lauther CB (1982) Toxic-shock syndrome related to intravenous heroin use. *N. Engl. J. Med.*, *307*, 820.
16. Christensen FR, Andersen LW (1982) Adverse reaction to extradural buprenorphine. *Brit. J. Anaesth.*, *54*, 476.
17. Christensen P, Brandt MR (1982) Extradural

morphine and Stokes-Adams attacks. *Brit. J. Anaesth., 54,* 363.

18. Christian CM, Waller JL, Moldenhauer CC (1983) Postoperative rigidity following fentanyl anesthesia. *Am. Soc. Anesthesiol., 58,* 275.
19. Church JJ (1983) Continuous infusion of meptazinol and pethidine in the relief of postoperative pain. *Postgrad. Med. J., 59 (Suppl. 1),* 41.
20. Cook PJ, James IM, Hobbs KEF et al (1982) Controlled comparison of i.m. morphine and buprenorphine for analgesia after abdominal surgery. *Brit. J. Anaesth., 54,* 285.
21. Copeland SA (1983) Preliminary evaluation of the use of meptazinol in trauma. *Postgrad. Med. J., 59 (Suppl. 1),* 64.
22. Crone LA, Wilson N, McSee J et al (1982) Haemodynamic and plasma vasopressin responses with high-dose fentanyl anaesthesia during aorto-coronary bypass operations. *Canad. Anaest. Soc. J., 29,* 525.
23. Cuvillier P, Gomez J, Dupont Th et al (1982) A propos d'une observation de rhabdomyolyse aigue lors d'une intoxication par morphinomimétiques. *Larc Méd., 11,* 947.
24. Dirghangi JK, Ansari MR (1982) Rupture of mycotic aneurysm during pregnancy. Another hazard of drug abuse. *Henry Ford Hosp. Med. J., 30,* 93.
25. Edit (1983) Distalgesic and its equivalents: Time for action. *Drugs Therapeut. Bull., 21,*
26. Epstein H, Waxman A, Gleicher N et al (1982) Meperidine-induced sinusoidal fetal heart rate pattern and reversal with naloxone. *Obstet. Gynecol., 59,* 22S.
27. Eriksen HO, Jensen FM (1982) Side-effects of epidural and spinal opiates. *Ugeskr. Laeg., 144,* 2627.
28. Fell D, Chmielewski A, Smith G (1982) Postoperative analgesia with controlled-release morphine sulphate: comparison with intramuscular morphine. *Br. Med. J., 285,* 92.
29. Finnegan LP (1982) Outcome of children born to women dependent upon narcotics. *Adv. Alcohol. Subst. Abuse, 1,* 55.
30. Findcane BT, Floyd JB, Petro DJ et al (1982) A double blind comparison of dezocine, butorphanol and placebo for postoperative pain relief. *Canad. Anaesth. Soc. J., 29,* 500.
31. Fischer HBJ, Scott PV (1982) Spinal opiate analgesia and facial pruritus. *Anaesthesia, 37,* 777.
32. Fjellner B, Hägermark Ö (1982) Potentiation of histamine-induced itch and flare responses in human skin by the enkephalin analogue FK 33-824, B-endorphin and morphine. *Arch. Dermatol. Res., 274,* 29.
33. Foley KM (1982) The practical use of narcotic analgesics. Symposium on Clinical Pharmacology of Symptom Control. *Med. Clin. N. Am., 66,* 1091.
34. Fragen RJ, Caldwell NJ (1982) Comparison of three doses of oral ciramadol and placebo for the treatment of moderate to severe postoperative pain. *J. Clin. Pharmacol., 22,* 459.
35. Geber WF, Schramm LC (1975) Congenital malformations of the central nervous system produced by narcotic analgesics in the hamster. *Am. J. Obstet. Gynecol., 123,* 785.
36. Gilman MA (1982) Possible dangers of naloxone use. *J. Am. Med. Assoc., 248,* 2972.
37. Golden NL, King EC, Robert J, Sokol NI (1982) Propoxyphene and acetaminophen. *Clin. Pediatr. 21,* 752.
38. Gustafsson LL, Schildt B, Jacobsen K (1982) Adverse effects of extradural and intrathecal opiates: Report of a nationwide survey in Sweden. *Br. J. Anaesth., 54,* 479.
39. Harmer M, Slattery PJ, Rosen M, Vickers MD (1983) Intramuscular on demand analgesia: double blind controlled trial of pethidine, buprenorphine, morphine and meptazinol. *Br. Med. J., 286,* 680.
40. Helmers JH, Leeuwen LV, Adam AA et al (1982) *Acta Anaesthesiol. Belg., 33,* 13.
41. Hershey LA (1983) Meperidine and central neurotoxicity. *Ann. Intern. Med., 98,* 548.
42. Hofmann RF, Weiler HH (1983) Lorazepam and nalbuphine as local anesthetic ophthalmic surgery premedications. *Ann. Ophthalmol., 15, 64.*
43. Edit (1982) Naltrexone – an investigational narcotic antagonist. *Hosp. Pharm., 17,* 687.
44. Husegaard HC, Hasselstrom L (1982) Tardiv respirationsdepression hos et barn efter morfin epiduralt. *Ugeskr. Laeg., 144,* 2652.
45. Hutchings DE (1982) Methadone and heroin during pregnancy: a review of behavioral effects in human and animal offspring. *Neurobehav. Toxicol. Teratol., 4,* 429.
46. Inturrisi L (1982) Narcotic drugs. *Med. Clin. N. Am., 66,* 1061.
47. Jacobsen L, Phillips PD, Hull CJ et al (1983) Extradural versus intramuscular diamorphine. *Anaesthesia, 38,* 10.
48. Jacome DE, (1982) Neurogenic bladder, lumbosacral plexus neuropathy and drug associated rhabdomyolysis. *J. Urol., 127,* 994.
49. Jensen FM, Christensen FR, Guldager H (1982) Late respiratory depression (SRD) following epidural morphine. *Ugeskr. Laeg., 144,* 2651.
50. Johnson HL, Rosen TS (1982) Prenatal methadone exposure: effects on behavior in early infancy. *Pediatr. Pharmacol., 2,* 113.
51. Kaiko RF, Wallenstein SL, Rogers AG (1982) Narcotics in the elderly. Symposium on Clinical Pharmacology of Symptom Control. *Med. Clin. N. Am., 66,* 1079.
52. Kathrein H, Kirchmair W, Konig P et al (1983) Rhabdomyolysis with acute renal failure after heroin poisoning. *Deutsche Med. Wochenschr., 108,* 464.
53. Knill RL, Lam AM, Thompson WR (1982) Epidural morphine and ventilatory depression. *Anesthesiology, 56,* 486.
54. Kreek MJ (1982) Opioid disposition and

effects during chronic exposure in the perinatal period in man. *Adv. Alcohol. Subst. Abuse, 1,* 21.

55. Kulig K, Rumack BH, Duffy JP et al (1982) Letter. *J. Am. Med. Assoc., 248,* 2973.
56. Lanz B, Theiss D, Riess W, Sommer U (1982) Epidural morphine for postoperative analgesia: a double-blind study. *Anesth. Analg., 61,* 236.
57. Lehmann KA, Freier J, Daub D (1982) Fentanyl pharmacokinetics and postoperative respiratory depression. *Anaesthetist, 31,* 111.
58. Levy JB, Rockoff MA (1982) Anaphylaxis to meperidine (clinical reports). *Anesth. Analg., 61,* 301.
59. Louis C, Freye E, Hartung E, Haag W (1982) Buprenorphine for peridural anaesthesia – A comparative study with and without bupivacaine. *Anästh. Intensivther. Notfallmed., 17,* 341.
60. McCammon RL, Madura JA (1983) Reversal of fentanyl induced spasm of the sphincter of Oddi. *Surg. Gynecol. Obstetr., 156,* 329.
61. McLean ER, Widmann WD, Small HS (1982) Cholangiographic demonstration of relief of narcotic-induced spasm of the sphincter of Oddi. *Am. Surg., 48,* 134.
62. Magruder MR, Delaney RD, Difazio CA (1982) Reversal of narcotic-induced respiratory depression with nalbuphine hydrochloride. *Anesthesiol. Rev., 9,* 34.
63. Mann RJ, Meacock DJ, Gostelow BE, Kennedy CTC (1982) Pentazocine ulcers. *J. Roy. Soc. Med., 75,* 903.
64. Mihic, DN, Binhert B, Hess PA (1982) Peridural morphine in the treatment of postoperative pain. *Reg. Anaesth, 5,* 42.
65. Miller RR, Feingold A, Paxinos J (1970) Propoxyphene hydrochloride – a critical review. *J. Am. Med. Assoc., 213,* 996.
66. Mitchell AA, Louik C, Lacouture P et al (1982) Risks to children from computed tomographic scan premedication. *J. Am. Med. Assoc., 247,* 2385.
67. Moller TW, Eriksen J (1982) Accidental high-dose extradural morphine. *Br. J. Anaesth., 54,* 1237.
68. Muller H, Stoyanov M, Brahler A, Hempelmann G, (1982) Effects of tramadol on haemodynamics and respiration during N_2O-O_2-ventilation and in the postoperative period. *Anaesthesist, 31,* 604.
69. Murray K (1983) Acute urinary retention associated with sublingual buprenorphine. *Br. Med. J., 286,* 763.
70. Nauta J, DeLange S, Koopman D et al (1982) Anesthetic induction with alfentanil: a new short-acting narcotic analgesic. *Anesth. Anal., 61,* 267.
71. Nicholas ADG, Robson PJ (1982) Double-blind comparison of meptazinol and pethidine in labour. *Br. J. Obstet. Gynaecol., 89,* 318.
72. Nilsson C, Roseberg B (1982) Recurrence of respiratory depression following neurolept analgesia. *Acta Anaesthesiol. Scand., 26,* 240.
73. Oliva GC, Marchetti P, Di Maggio A et al (1980) Effetti della meperidine e della pentazocina sul feto e sull'attivita contrattile uterina. *Ann. Ostetr. Ginecol. Med. Perinat., 101,* 67.
74. Oosterlinck W, Minnaert H (1982) An open comparative trial of three doses of ciramadol used intravenously in renal colic. *Curr. Med. Res. Opinion., 8,* 290.
75. Von Palitzsch J (1982) Respiratory effects of epidural morphine analgesia. *Anaesthesiol. Reanimat., 7,* 355.
76. Paravicini D, Zander J, Hansen J (1982) Wirkung von Tramadol auf Hämodynamik und Blutgase in der frühen postoperativen Phase. *Anaesthesist, 31,* 611.
77. Parker CE, Langrick AF (1982) A double-blind comparison of meptazinol and placebo in patients with acute and chronic pain presenting to the general practitioner. *J. Int. Med. Res., 10,* 408.
78. Petersen TK, Husted SE, Rybro L et al (1982) Urinary retention during i.m. and extradural morphine analgesia. *Br. J. Anaesth., 54,* 1175.
79. Poklis A, Mackell ML (1982) Toxicological findings in deaths due to ingestion of pentazocine: a report of two cases. *Forens. Sci. Int., 20,* 89.
80. Ponte CD (1983) A suspected case of codeine-induced multiforme. *Drug Intell. Clin. Pharm., 17,* 128.
81. Price RKJ, Latham AN (1982) Double-blind comparison of meptazinol (200 mg) and dextropropoxyphene/paracetamol in a multi-centre, general practice setting. *Curr. Med. Res. Opinion, 8,* 54.
82. Price RKJ, Latham AN (1982) Meptazinol: a side-effect profile compared to placebo in general practice. *J. Int. Med. Res., 10,* 219.
83. Pullan PT, Watson FE, Seow SSW, Rappeport W (1983) Methadone-induced hypoadrenalism. *Lancet, 1,* 714.
84. Quam SR (1982) Comparison of butorphanol with other anesthetic and analgesic agents. *J. Am. Osteopath. Assoc., 81,* 837.
85. Robson PJ (1983) Clinical review of parenteral meptazinol. *Postgrad. Med. J., 59 (Suppl. 1),* 85.
86. Ron M, Menashe M, Scherer D, Palti Z (1982) Fetal heart rate decelerations following the administration of meperidine-promethazine during labour. *Int. J. Gynaecol. Obstetr., 20,* 301.
87. Rooth G, Lysikiewicz A, Huch R, Huch A (1983) Some effects of maternal pethidine administration on the newborn. *Br. J. Obstetr. Gynaecol., 90,* 28.
88. Rosen TS, Johnson HL (1982) Children of methadone-maintained mothers: follow-up to 18 months of age. *J. Pediatr., 101,* 192.
89. Rossano C, De Luca LF, Firetto V et al (1982) Activity and tolerability of buprenorphine after parenteral and sublingual administration. *Clin. Ther., 5,* 61.
90. Rothe KF, Brather R (1983) Postoperative depression of respiration because of infusion

anaesthesia with tramadol? *Anaesthesist, 32,* 88.

91. Scott PV, Fischer HBJ (1982) Spinal opiate analgesia and facial pruritus: a neural theory. *Postgrad. Med. J., 58,* 531.

92. Sebel PS, Bovill JG, Van Der Haven A (1982) Cardiovascular effects of alfentanil anaesthesia. *Br. J. Anaesth., 54,* 1185.

93. Seymour RA, Rawlins MD, Rowell FJ (1982) Dihydrocodeine-induced hyperalgesia in postoperative dental pain. *Lancet, 1,* 1425.

94. Sloan Wilson R, Landers JH (1982) Use of a new oral analgesic, propiram fumarate, in treating postoperative ocular pain. *Ann. Ophthalmol., 14,* 1172.

95. Smith DE, Moser C, Wesson DR et al (1982) A clinical guide to the diagnosis and treatment of heroin-related sexual dysfunction. *J. Psychoactive Drugs, 14,* 91.

96. Smith JW (1982) Codeine-induced bradycardia in a breast-fed infant. *Clin. Res., 30,* 259A.

97. Sonecha T, Besterman EMM, Abdel-Hadi O, Kidner PH (1983) Initial assessment of meptazinol in the treatment of the pain of myocardial infarction/unstable angina. *Postgrad. Med. J., 59 (Suppl. 1),* 57.

98. Spielberg SP (1980) Acetaminophen toxicity in human lymphocytes in vitro. *J. Pharmacol. Exp. Ther., 213,* 395.

99. Stahl SM, Kasser IS (1983) Pentazocine overdose (case report). *Ann. Emergency Med., 12,* 28.

100. Stambaugh JE (1982) Evaluation of nalbuphine: efficacy and safety in the management of chronic pain associated with advanced malignancy. *Curr. Ther. Res., 31,* 393.

101. Stambaugh JE (1982) Additive analgesia of oral butorphanol/acetaminophen in patients with pain due to metastatic carcinoma. *Curr. Ther. Res., 31,* 386.

102. Steppe J, Camu F (1982) Epidural morphine for postoperative analgesia following abdominal surgery in elderly patients. *Acta Anaesthesiol. Belg., 33,* 43.

103. Rao, TLK, Mummanen, N, El-Etr AA (1982) Convulsions: An unusual response to intravenous fentanyl administration. *Anesth. Analg., 61,* 1020.

104. Torda TA, Pybus DA (1982) Comparison of four narcotic analgesics for extradural analgesia. *Br. J. Anaesth., 54,* 291.

105. Townsend JE, Wynands DG, Whalley D et al (1982) High dose fentanyl infusion and renin response in open heart surgery. *Canad. Anaesth. Soc. J., 29,* 511.

106. Tyson HK (1974) Neonatal withdrawal symptoms associated with maternal use of propoxyphene hydrochloride (Darvon). *Ped. Pharmacol. Ther., 85,* 684.

107. Vincens M, Ganansia R, Puy-Montbrun T et al (1982) Anites et ano-rectites necrosantes chez des malades ayant utilise au long cours des suppositoires associant dextropropoxyphene et paracetamol. *Thérapie, 37,* 321.

108. Wade AG, Ward PJ (1982) A double-blind comparison of meptazinol versus paracetamol and placebo in acute and chronic painful conditions presenting to the general practitioner. *Curr. Med. Res. Opinion, 8,* 191.

109. Wade AG, Ward PJ (1982) A double-blind comparison of meptazinol versus distalgesic in acute or chronic pain presenting to the general practitioner. *J. Int. Med. Res., 10,* 104.

110. Weiss IS (1982) Optic atrophy after propoxyphene overdose: Report of a case. *Ann. Ophthalmol., 14,* 586.

111. Wenningsted-Torgard K, Heyn J, Willumsen L (1982) Spondylitis following epidural morphine. A Case Report. *Scand. Soc. Anaesthesiol., 26,* 649.

112. Zagon IS, McLaughlin PJ, Weaver DJ, Zagon E (1982) Opiates, endorphins and the developing organism: A comprehensive bibliography. *Neurosci. Biobehav. Rev., 6,* 439.

113. Von Zens M, Piepenbrock S, Tryba M et al (1983) Sublingual buprenorphine in chronic treatment of cancer pain. *Fortschr. Therapie, 101,* 191.

114. Zinck B, Fritz KW (1982) Respiratory depression by epidural application of buprenorphine hydrochloride. *Anaesth. Intensivther. Notfallmed., 17,* 345.

J. Vaněček

9 Antipyretic analgesics

Analgesic nephropathy and urinary tumors

Although one would think that the time had come to quietly forget the issue of phenacetin's role in analgesic nephropathy and give the drug a decent burial, it would seem that, where it has continued to be sold, it has also continued to be abused. Between 1979 and 1980, the incidence of phenacetin abuse in autopsies of adult inhabitants of Basle during the last 2 years of the last decennium was 3.87%. The *incidence of abuse* varied considerably in different age groups, with a maximum of 16% in women in the age group of 50–59 years, but if the total figure is correct it means that 1500–3000 inhabitants of Basle are abusers of phenacetin-containing analgesics (1[C]). An even higher incidence of phenacetin abuse was detected pathologically in autopsies from the Kanton Hospital in St. Gallen (5.6%) (2[C]).

Other work from the same Swiss group shows that some 18% of phenacetin abusers have *gastric ulcers* (presumably as a consequence of the presence of aspirin in most compound analgesics); phenacetin abusers also tend to exhibit low body weight, brownish pigmentation of the skin, and hypertension (observed in 50–70% of patients). The hypertension is probably secondary to the analgesic nephropathy (3[C]).

Another working group from Basle designed a study to ascertain the *incidence of analgesic nephropathy* in apparently healthy women in the age of 30 to 49 years who took phenacetin-containing analgesics regularly, compared with a group who took such analgesics less regularly, or not at all. The two groups, consisting each of some 620 working women, showed significant differences in overall mortality, with 39 vs 13 deaths ($P < 0.001$), due to urinary tract disorders ($P = 0.033$) and cardiovascular diseases ($P = 0.008$) (4[CR]).

Again in Switzerland, calcium metabolism was compared in two groups of patients with chronic interstitial nephritis, in the first group due to phenacetin-containing analgesics, in the second due to exposure to other causes. It was found that, given a comparable degree and duration of renal failure, patients using phenacetin have lower blood calcium and consequently higher parathyroid hormone levels and alkaline phosphatase activities, suggesting more severe osteodystrophy (5[C]).

A publication from South Africa makes note of brownish *discoloration of the bladder mucosa* on cystoscopy, especially on the trigone as a sign of analgesic-associated nephropathy, in a patient not suspected of drug abuse previously. This phenomenon may help to establish the diagnosis of analgesic-associated nephropathy even where phenacetin abuse is denied by the patient (6[C]). The same authors found in a prospective study that analgesic nephropathy is responsible for approximately 13% of all cases of the *end-stage renal disease* treated in their renal unit (7[C]), and another South African center cited a figure of 20% (9[C]); the drug has now been withdrawn in that country.

Changes of renal disease mortality in Finland after *phenacetin restriction* have been studied by Sillanpää et al (8[CR]). Both an epidemiologic survey of the mortality from nephropathy and the autopsies showed clear and strong correlations with increased phenacetin consumption and with its discontinuation. The banning of phenacetin led within 2–4 years to a decline in the mortality from nephropathy to its pre-phenacetin level. The findings recall those earlier noted in Denmark and Sweden (SED-9, 33).

In New Zealand, since the ban of phenacetin in 1974 there has similarly been a decrease in the number of patients with analgesic nephropathy entering dialysis-

Side Effects of Drugs Annual 8
M.N.G. Dukes, editor

ISBN 0 444 90339 9
$0.80 per article per page (transactional system)
$0.20 per article per page (licensing system)

transplant programs, from 8% to 2–3% (10[C]).

Of the 50 *urinary tract tumors* in Swiss phenacetin abusers, 52% occurred in the bladder, 6% in the ureter, and 42% in the renal pelvis. The induction time for tumors of the urinary bladder was about 27 years, and for tumors of the renal pelvis about 20 years. Analgesic nephropathy was not always an accompanying disease (11[C]).

In West Berlin 83 out of 113 patients with tumors of the renal pelvis were examined with regard to phenacetin abuse known from case histories. On the average 5.6 kg had been taken over 24 years (12[c]).

In New South Wales a retrospective study based on interviews with 67 patients with carcinoma of the renal pelvis (40 women, 27 men) revealed a 10-fold relative risk of renal pelvic cancer in women consuming analgesics regularly, whereas men showed a risk ratio of 4–8 (13[C]).

ACETYLSALICYLIC ACID AND RELATED COMPOUNDS

Allergy and intolerance Aspirin allergy has a population frequency of about 4% when the diagnosis is made from the history, but positive reactions can be elicited in up to 20% of individuals if oral challenge tests with spirometry are performed. Four recent review articles have discussed the occurrence of respiratory reactions in adults (14[R]–17[R]).

Only a few reports concerning aspirin-caused *bronchial obstruction in children* have been published. When pulmonary function tests were performed in 52 Turkish asthmatic children (mean age 12.6 yr), the result indicated 14% intolerance. The authors suggest that aspirin intolerance is not rare among asthmatic children and can be detected by pulmonary function tests before clinical symptoms appear (18[C]). Tolerance evoked by daily administration of aspirin is able to bring clinical improvement in some cases (19[C]).

In a recent publication (20[R]) the prevalence of *non-immunological intolerance phenomena* was determined in 100 patients with chronic relapsing urticaria by oral tests to aspirin and food additives: 39 patients avoiding drugs strictly and on an additive-free diet exhibited intolerance phenomena to aspirin (23%), tartrazine (15%), indigotin and patent blue (13%), cholin yellow and yellow orange (8%), sodium benzoate and potassium sorbate (8%).

In another study of 386 patients with *chronic urticaria* 25% appeared to have a positive oral provocation test to aspirin, the highest percentages were found in patients with idiopathic urticaria, delayed pressure urticaria and cholinergic urticaria. Aspirin intolerance was not found in any of the forty-three patients with cold urticaria (21[c]).

Two cases of *purpura* evoked by aspirin, and diagnosed with the sequential vascular response test were described in Italy (22[C]). The authors suggest, that this symptom can be added to the many manifestations of aspirin intolerance. Nine more cases of supposed drug-induced *toxic epidermal necrolysis* (*Lyell's syndrome*), 2 of them caused by aspirin, have been published (23[C]).

Very unusual is the case of a 13-year-old boy with bursitis of the right knee, who was treated prior to surgical intervention with water-soluble aspirin tablets to relieve local pain (24[C]). The authors consider a slight *eosinophilia* (7%) and perioral *fixed drug eruption* to be an expression of hypersensitivity response elicited by aspirin, and suggest that the unexpected epithelioid cell granulomata, observed inside the neoplastic fibrous stroma of the non-ossifying fibroma of the distal metaphysis of the right femur, had their origin in this hypersensitivity.

Central nervous system Aspirin produces in some persons a substantial *decrease in speech understanding during noise,* even though there may not be a decrease in pure-tone sensitivity or speech discrimination in quiet. The effect could be elicited by administering a mere 3–4 tablets every 4–5 hours during 24 hours (25[C]).

Aspirin in a single dose of 1.95 g affected the quantitative *EEG, 'symptom self reports'*, and *cognitive functions* as compared to placebo. The effects of 0.65 g were similar in direction and pattern, but failed to attain measurable significance (26[C]).

Respiratory Salicylate intoxication is a recognized cause of the adult respiratory distress syndrome, but even small doses have an effect. A dose of 16 mg/kg (equivalent to a dose of 4 standard 325-mg aspirin tablets taken by an 81-kg person) has been found to induce a small but statistically significant reduction in both lung mucociliary clearance and tracheal mucociliary transport rate, as measured in healthy volunteers (27[C]). It seems that aspirin has a comparable effect on mucus transport in both the trachea and the intrapulmonary airways. Prostaglandins may play a part in the control of airway secretion.

Aspirin, salicylates and Reye's syndrome; the continuing story

(SEDA-7, 94)

Reye's syndrome is considered to be a multisystem disease that usually follows a viral or viral-like illness. In the United States over the past several years between 200 and 500 cases annually have been reported under a voluntary surveillance system; US Centers for Disease Control estimate the true annual frequency as lying between 600 and 1200 cases, but higher figures have been cited (SEDA-7, 95). Estimates of case-fatality rates range from 22 to 42% (28[R]).

Since the review in the 1983 Annual discussing the possible causative role of salicylates, new material has continued to appear. In all, 4 case-control studies of salicylate use and the etiology of Reye's syndrome have appeared, identified by their location as Arizona (29[C]), Ohio (30[C]) and Michigan 1 and 2 (31[C]). The Ohio study is the largest and the most sophisticated in design and analysis, the other three are based on small numbers of subjects. Each of the four studies demonstrate a statistically significant association of Reye's syndrome with aspirin administration during the prodromal illness. In total, all but 4 children with Reye's syndrome were reported to have received aspirin, compared to 151 of 247 control children. The evidence of these four studies was sufficiently strong to warrant a provisional warning to physicians in 1982 by the American Academy of Pediatrics (SEDA-7, 95).

Opposition to the theory of aspirin or salicylate causation has been spearheaded by a critical review by Daniels et al (32[R]). It is a fact that the symptoms of Reye's syndrome and salicylism have many parallels, and that in some cases these two entities may be indistinguishable.

The pathology of Reye's syndrome – intrahepatocytic microvesicular fat, hepatic glycogen depletion, absence of significant hepatic inflammation or necrosis, and non-inflammatory cerebral edema – has been well described, but little has been published on the pathology findings in salicylate-induced death.

Starko and Mullick (33[CR]) therefore have analyzed the histology or necropsy records of 13 children with salicylate intoxication for the presence of hepatic and cerebral pathology findings characteristic of Reye's syndrome. Liver sections showed intrahepatic microvesiculation and absence of significant inflammation or necrosis in 83% of cases. Intrahepatocytic microvesicular fat, with nuclei distributed either diffusely throughout the lobule or more prominently in the lobular periphery, was present in all the 6 available specimens. Liver tissue showed complete absence of stainable glycogen in 83% of specimens, 75% of children had cerebral edema. The light-microscopy hepatic findings and the gross cerebral findings for the majority of these children with salicylate intoxication were thus indistinguishable from the well known findings of children with Reye's syndrome (33[CR]).

These findings are non-specific; nevertheless, few disorders, all uncommon, are characterized by microvesicular fatty liver; they comprise tetracycline hepatotoxicity, idiopathic fatty liver of pregnancy, Jamaican vomiting sickness, diseases due to inborn errors of the Krebs urea cycle enzymes, and Reye's syndrome. A major difference is that patients with Reye's syndrome apparently take only therapeutic doses of salicylate and have only moderate levels of salicylates in their blood at the time of hospitalization; the salicylate level does not correlate with the severity of their illness at the time of admission. The authors suspect either a prodromal illness or a pharmacogenetic factor which may increase sensitivity to salicylate at therapeutic doses.

It should be pointed out that Daugherty et al have quite recently expressed their disagreement with the conclusion of Starko and Mullick that the liver histology in salicylate intoxication is so similar to that of Reye's syndrome; they consider that Reye's syndrome is a morphologically and clinically distinct entity which can be identified on the basis of hematoxylin and eosin sections of liver alone only if the comparison is limited to cases dying primarily of salicylate toxicity (34Cr).

The Reye's Syndrome Working Group of the Aspirin Foundation of America concluded in 1972 that 'the only responsible statements that can be made in relation to Reye's syndrome at this time are those that pertain to early recognition of Reye's syndrome and to prudent use of all medications in children' (35R). Similar conclusions have been expressed by well known European drug health policy commentators (37R): 'More evidence is needed to confirm or refute the association between salicylates and the syndrome. In the interim period the use of aspirin or other salicylates cannot be advised with safety in children suffering from influenza or chickenpox; until such time as other studies clarify the position, the use of alternative analgesics and antipyretics would be a sensible precaution' (36R).

Gastrointestinal The risk of aspirin-caused gastrointestinal bleeding is universally known, but the intensity is so variable that risk factors continue to be studied (38C). Recently published findings of increased gastrointestinal ulcer development in O blood group types, confirm previous publications; in patients having other blood groups, ulcers did not develop (39r).

An Australian case control study of patient histories over the 6 months before exacerbation of their chronic peptic ulcer (40C) shows that smoking in all patients and heavy analgesic ingestion in female patients are risk factors for chronic gastric ulcer. No significant risks were found for alcohol. Previous studies in this matter failed to differentiate gastric from duodenal ulcer and failed to use adequate epidemiological techniques.

In 10 healthy young adults aspirin doses of 2.6 g daily for 5 days consistently produced obvious endoscopic damage. There was a significant reduction ($P < 0.01$) in the prostaglandin E content of the gastric juice and the antral and duodenal mucosa, but no correlation was found between the severity of the mucosal damage and the degree of reduction in prostaglandin E. The authors concluded that aspirin damages the human gastric mucosa by at least two distinct mechanisms one of which is inhibition of protective prostaglandins (41C). In a double-blind study performed on 20 healthy male volunteers to determine the effect of prostaglandin E_2 tablets on aspirin-induced blood loss, 1 tablet (0.5 mg) of PGE_2 4 times daily prevented fecal blood loss, as measured using the radioactive (^{51}Cr) technique (42C).

The possibility that a proportion of patients who bleed take aspirin to relieve *indigestion associated with their hemorrhage* has been examined (43C). Comparison of 346 patients suffering from acute upper gastrointestinal hemorrhage with community controls showed that both aspirin and paracetamol intake were more common in patients than in controls, but the association for aspirin was stronger and was apparent with both recent and habitual intake, whereas the association for habitual intake was not detectable for paracetamol. This suggests that analgesic drugs are in part taken because of symptoms associated with bleeding.

A systematic endoscopic evaluation of the effect of aspirin administration (2.6 g/day) on the gastric mucosa in 12 healthy male volunteers (44C) revealed *gastric adaptation.* The damage present after 7 days of aspirin administration was significantly less than after 1 day of therapy and the period needed for resolution of the damage was also greater after 1 day than after 1 week of therapy.

In Czechoslovakia the case histories of 2 boys (6 and 5 years) with hemorrhage after several days administration of acetylsalicylic acid in therapeutic doses was published. In the first case X-ray examination revealed gastric ulcer, in the other showed a coarser outline of the mucosa in the oral portion of the stomach which together with clinical symptoms led to the diagnosis of erosive gastritis (45c).

Prevention of gastric damage by buffering is far from complete. A recent blind endoscopic study in normal volunteers (46C) showed that both plain aspirin and 'Bufferin' (with 1.5 mmol buffering capacity per tablet) produced multiple gastric and duodenal lesions when given over 24 hours. Paracetamol did not do so.

In a prospective investigator-blind crossover study the fecal blood loss caused by two differently *microencapsulated acetylsalicylic acid preparations* in patients with rheumatoid arthritis was determined (47C). 18 male patients with rheumatoid arthritis received microencapsulated acetylsalicylic acid 3 g daily – either with time-dependent or with pH-dependent release. With the exception of one patient only moderate bleeding was observed, which was less with pH-dependent release (4.2 ml/day) than with time-dependent release (5.3 ml/day).

Second generation effects Aspirin is known to cross the placenta after ingestion by the mother and has been associated with *abnormalities of hemostasis* in both the full-term and premature infant. Most published studies are based mainly on the mother's history. In a recent study by Stuart et al (48[C]), the history of aspirin intake was checked by evaluation of platelet malondialdehyde formation, which also allows exact timing of previous aspirin ingestion. Only 1 of 34 control maternal-neonatal pairs had hemostatic abnormalities. In the group of 10 maternal-neonatal pairs in which aspirin (5–10 g) had been ingested by the mother within 5 days before delivery, 6 of 10 mothers had an abnormal fall in hemoglobin levels post partum; in 4 of these 6 women there was also evidence of abnormal blood loss (hematoma, intraoperative bleeding or postpartum hemorrhage). 9 of the 10 infants in this group had a bleeding tendency (petechiae, cephalhematoma, subconjunctival hemorrhage, bleeding from a circumcision site or microscopic hematuria). In a third group where aspirin had been taken 6 to 10 days before delivery, no hemostatic abnormalities were noted. In the fourth group of 7 mothers who had received aspirin within 12 hours post partum, 4 of 7 mothers had a marked fall in hemoglobin levels, which was associated with considerable post-partum uterine bleeding in 2. The authors concluded that aspirin should be avoided during pregnancy, and that if ingestion has occurred within 5 days of delivery, the neonate should be evaluated for the presence of bleeding.

Overdosage Salicylate intoxication is common and carries a high mortality (50[R]). A recent study draws attention to the fact that *non-cardiogenic pulmonary edema,* a potentially lethal disorder, develops most commonly in persons who are middle-aged, smoke cigarettes, and have salicylate intoxication from chronic use of aspirin compounds (49[CR]). Forced alkaline diuresis, which is often employed in salicylate intoxication in order to enhance renal excretion and to induce a state of mild alkalemia, could conceivably worsen pulmonary edema (51[C]), especially in cases of adult respiratory distress syndrome. Hemodialysis removes carbon dioxide from the blood and through this mechanism may cause hypoventilation and worsen hypoxemia. Both forced diuresis and hemodialysis may be associated with hypophosphatemia, hypokalemia, and other metabolic alterations which may cause or worsen respiratory failure. It seems likely that crystalloid infusion and hemodialysis may each contribute to deterioration of the patients status (52[C]).

The evaluation of 112 cases (65 acute vs 47 chronic) of salicylate poisoning in children admitted to hospital showed that hyperventilation, dehydration, and severe central nervous system manifestations occurred more frequently in the chronic group (53[C]).

In a study of 44 patients with uncomplicated aspirin overdosage the *value of alkali treatment* was confirmed. Alkali alone was at least as effective and possibly more effective than forced alkaline diuresis in enhancing salicylate removal. Unlike diuresis regimens it did not cause fluid retention or biochemical disturbances. Renal excretion of salicylate depended much more on urine pH than flow rate, and forced diuresis alone had little useful effect (54a[C]).

Benorylate is the acetylsalicylic ester of paracetamol. When drug levels are to be measured, both salicylate and paracetamol should be assayed. Measuring salicylate levels alone, as recommended by the manufacturers, will not exclude toxic levels of paracetamol.

A 3-year-old boy with cystic fibrosis disliked taking aspirin for his juvenile chronic polyarthritis and the treatment was changed to benorylate suspension 4 g twice daily. He improved over 2 weeks after which his condition suddenly deteriorated. The serum salicylate was 39 mg/dl without clinical evidence of salicylate toxicity. However, the paracetamol level was very high at 11 mg/dl, and fatal liver damage ensued. Necropsy revealed changes typical of acute hepatocellular damage due to paracetamol poisoning (54b).

ANILINE DERIVATIVES

Paracetamol

Hematological *Agranulocytosis* has only exceptionally been verified with this drug (SEDA-6, 69), but some authors nevertheless suspect that paracetamol is responsible for up to 10% of cases of drug induced agranulocytosis. A recent report describes this complication in a 74-year-old man, treated for 3 years with 1.5 g of pure paracetamol daily as sole medication for coxarthrosis. So far all but one of the documented cases of agranulocytosis were seen in French patients (55[C]).

Liver The safety of paracetamol in therapeutic doses (4.0 g for 5 days) in the presence of chronic liver disease was evaluated in 6 subjects. Although the mean half-life of paracetamol was 3.43 hr, there was no evidence of drug cumulation or hepatotoxicity. In a double-blind, two-period crossover study on 20 subjects with stable chronic liver disease paracetamol was given at a dose of 4.0 g daily for 13 days and was well tolerated. This work suggests that there is no contraindication to the use of paracetamol in therapeutic doses in the presence of stable chronic liver disease (56[C]).

Nephrotoxicity Reversible acute renal failure was observed in 2 patients after taking paracetamol in therapeutic doses (one took 3 tablets of 250 mg, the other 2 tablets of 325 mg). In the first patient oliguria lasted 6 days, in the second anuria was observed over 48 hours. At renal biopsy healing of acute tubular necrosis was found in both patients without any other abnormality. There was no deposition of immunoglobulins or complement components (57).

Two cases of capillarosclerosis of the mucosal capillaries in the lower urinary tract were found in a series of 98 unselected hospital autopsies in northern Finland. A clinical history of phenacetin abuse could not be elicited in either case.

One of them, a diabetic with severe arteriosclerosis and metastatized carcinoma of the thyroid, had died of wound infection complicating amputations of the lower extremities. She had used paracetamol 1350 mg daily for 3 months during her last illness. The other, who died of subacute bacterial endocarditis, received cyclophosphamide 50 mg daily for 1 month followed by 125 mg daily for 3 months because of suspected Henoch-Schönlein nephropathy (58[C]).

Skin and appendages Necrotizing anorectitis (3 cases) and proctitis (4 cases), in women of widely varying ages has been attributed to long-term administration (2–24 months) of dextropropoxyphene plus paracetamol suppositories (Diantalvic) used for analgesia in arthrosis. The clinical and histological findings and the evolution of the condition were closely similar in all these patients but one must recognise the difficulty of diagnosing the condition. The mechanism is unknown; local irritation based on pharmacodependence is suspected (59[C]).

Second generation effects Paracetamol is frequently used in pregnancy, but a dose damaging the fetus is not known. A case of overdosage in a pregnant woman, who took 22.5 g of paracetamol at the 36th week, has been reported; she was treated with acetylcysteine and the pregnancy went to term normally (60[C]).

Overdosage Although severe hepatotoxicity from overdosage occurs in adults (62[C]), paracetamol seems to have a wider margin of safety in *younger children.* This has been ascribed to altered pharmacokinetics in this age group.

A 7-week-old female infant received 0.3 ml of paracetamol drops every 4 to 5 hours for 6 to 8 days before admission; the blood drug level was 10.7 mg/l approximately 54 hours after the last known intake. Similarly a 6-week-old male infant had been receiving paracetamol drops (0.3 or 0.6 ml every 4 hours) for 2 days; the blood level was found to be 119 mg/l. Both infants received intravenous fluids and glucose, and the latter was also treated with acetylcysteine (61[C]).

Lethal intoxication with paracetamol has however been described in a 2-month-old child. The rectally administered dose was 16.5 times that recommended and phenobarbital had also been given. A fulminant hepatic insufficiency complicated with acute renal insufficiency resulted (63[C]).

Profound *lactic acidosis* was observed in a 56-year-old woman who swallowed about 75 g of paracetamol, presenting serious toxicity within hours. Neither lactic acidosis nor severe acid base disturbance has previously been recorded in the early stages of paracetamol poisoning (64[C]).

Over a 4-year period, 103 patients presented to St Vincent's Hospital, Melbourne, after poisoning themselves with paracetamol. There was severe liver damage in only 4 patients, all of whom presented (or were recognized) 24 hours or more after the ingestion of paracetamol. The absence of severe liver damage in the remaining 99 patients was attributed to early intervention with specific therapy (65[R]).

Because *paracetamol and propoxyphene* are combined in several proprietary products, intoxication with these two drugs has been of increasing concern in recent years. The symptoms of propoxyphene overdose appear rapidly and death can occur very soon after ingestion of the drug. Potentially fatal complications include seizures and cardiopulmonary toxicity due to direct cardiac damage or to hypoxia caused by respiratory depression. Treatment consists of administration of the narcotic antagonist naloxone and intensive supportive care. Biochemical and symptomatic evidence of paracetamol toxicity is usually delayed for several days (66[CR]).

A plea has been made for *cimetidine* (300 mg twice a day) as an additional tool in treating paracetamol intoxication. Because cimetidine can inhibit the cytochrome P_{450} mixed-function oxidase system, and the actual hepatotoxic mechanism of paracetamol is believed to be the formation of a toxic tissue arylating metabolite, cimetidine could be an effective antidote to be used in conjunction with acetylcysteine (67[CR]). Certainly, there is some practical evidence that cimetidine may provide protection against paracetamol hepatotoxicity (68[C]), and a toxicity study in mice also points to its efficacy.

Previous studies with human subjects have shown that *chronic alcohol consumption* increases the risk of hepatotoxic effects from an overdose of paracetamol (SEDA-5, 10; SEDA-6, 59). Recent studies in humans have shown, on the other hand, that an acute dose of alcohol inhibits the development of hepatotoxic effects from a paracetamol overdose (SED-9, 73) and a small dose of alcohol consumed over a period of 1 hour prior to the ingestion of paracetamol will lead to a reduction in paracetamol-mercapturic acid excretion (69[c]).

An unusual case in which *Chlamydia psittaci infection* may have potentiated paracetamol-induced hepatic damage has been reported (70[C]).

REFERENCES

1. Mihatsch MJ, Hofer HO, Kortweg E et al (1982) Phenacetinabusus V: Häufigkeit der Phenacetinabuser im Basler Autopsiegut 1978–1980. *Schweiz. Med. Wochenschr., 112,* 1245.
2. Gloor F (1982) Die Kapillarosklerose in den ableitenden Harnwegen bei Schmerzmittel-(Phenazetin)-Missbrauch. *Pathologe, 3,* 132.
3. Mihatsch MJ, Kernen R, Zollinger HU (1982) Phenacetinabusus unter besonderer Berücksichtigung extrarenaler Befunde. *Schweiz. Med. Wochenschr., 112,* 1383.
4. Dubach UC, Rosner B, Pfister E (1983) Epidemiologic study of abuse of analgesics containing phenacetin. *N. Engl. J. Med., 308,* 357.
5. Jaeger Ph, Buckhardt P, Wauters J-P et al (1982) Atteinte particulièrement sévère métabolisme calcique dans la néphropathie par abus d'analgésiques. *Schweiz. Med. Wochenschr., 112,* 1791.
6. Fourie JVH, Pauw FH, De Bruin B (1982) Bladder urothelium in analgesic-associated nephropathy – a valuable diagnostic aid. *J. Urol., 128,* 262.
7. Fourie JVH, Pauw FH, De Bruin B (1982) Analgesic nephropathy. *S. Afr. Med. J., 62,* 351.
8. Sillanpää M, Kasanen A, Elonen A (1982) Changes of panorama in renal disease mortality in Finland after phenacetin restriction. *Acta Med. Scand., 212,* 313.
9. Furman KI (1982) Paracetamol as a cause of analgesic nephropathy. *S. Afr. Med. J., 62,* 885.
10. Munn E, Lynn KL, Bailey RR (1982) Renal papillary necrosis following regular consumption of non-steroidal anti-inflammatory drugs. *N. Z. Med. J., 95,* 213.
11. Mihatsch MJ, Knüsli C (1982) Phenacetin abuse and malignant tumors. *Klin. Wochenschr., 60,* 1339.
12. Leistenschneider W, Nagel R, Steffens J (1983) Nierenbeckentumoren und Phenacetinabusus. *Akta Urol., 14,* 15.
13. McCredie M, Ford JM, Taylor JS et al (1982) Analgesics and cancer of the renal pelvis in New South Wales. *Cancer, 49,* 2617.
14. Aaron TH, Muttitt ELC (1982) Reactions to acetylsalicylic acid. *Canad. Med. Assoc. J., 126,* 609.
15. Baldocchi G, Vervloet D, Vellieux P et al (1982) Intolérance à l'aspirine. *Rev. Franç. Allergol. Immunol. Clin., 22,* 5.
16. Szczeklik A (1982) Aspirin and asthma. *Europ. J. Resp. Dis., 63,* 376.
17. Margolis M, Mohan KK (1982) Analgesics and asthma. *S. Med. J., 75,* 1239.
18. Saraclar Y, Tuncer A (1981) Study on aspirin-induced bronchial obstruction in children with bronchial asthma. *Turk. J. Ped., 23,* 15.
19. Grzelewska-Rzymowska I, Kowalski ML, Rozniecki J et al (1982) Watwarzanie tolerancji aspiryny u chorych na astme z nadwrazlivoscia na aspiryne. *Polsk. Tyg. Lek., 37,* 19.
20. Kirchhof B, Haustein U-F, Rytter M (1982)

Azetylsalizylsäure-Additiva-Intoleranzphänomene bei chronisch rezidivierender Urikaria. *Dermatol. Monatsschr.*, *168*, 513.

21. Doeglas HMG (1983) Chronic urticaria: intolerance for aspirin and food additives and relationship with atopy. *Br. J. Dermatol.*, *108*, 108.

22. Della Torre F, Bellani M, Meregalli M (1981) Sindrome purpurica indotta dall'acido acetilsalicilico: Due casi clinici. *Rass. Geriatr.*, *17*, 35.

23. Gérard A, Roche G, Presles O et al (1982) Syndromes de Lyell médicamenteux. *Thérapie*, *37*, 475.

24. Cozzutto C, Comelli A (1982) Epithelioid granulomata in a nonossifying fibroma. *Virchows Arch. A*, *397*, 61.

25. Young Jr LL, Wilson KA (1982) Effects of acetylsalicylic acid on speech discrimination. *Audiology*, *21*, 342.

26. Fink M, Irwin BA (1982) Central nervous system effects of aspirin. *Clin. Pharmacol. Ther.*, *32*, 362.

27. Gerrity TR, Cortomanes E, Garrard CS et al (1983) The effect of aspirin on lung mucociliary clearance. *N. Engl. J. Med.*, *308*, 139.

28. Mortimer Jr EA (1982) Reye syndrome and salicylates. *Int. J. Epidemiol.*, *11*, 314.

29. Starko KM, Ray CG, Dominguez BS et al (1980) Reye's syndrome and salicylate use. *Pediatrics*, *66*, 859.

30. Halpin TJ, Holtzhauer FJ, Campbell RJ et al (1982) Reye's syndrome and medication use. *J. Amer. Med. Assoc.*, *248*, 687.

31. Waldman RJ, Hall WN, McGee H et al (1982) Aspirin as a risk factor in Reye's syndrome. *J. Amer. Med. Assoc.*, *247*, 3089.

32. Daniels SR, Greenberg RS, Ibrahim MA (1983) Scientific uncertainties in the studies of salicylate use and Reye's syndrome. *J. Amer. Med. Assoc.*, *249*, 1311.

33. Starko KR, Mullick FG (1983) Hepatic and cerebral pathology findings in children with fatal salicylate intoxication: further evidence for a causal relation between salicylate and Reye's syndrome. *Lancet*, *1*, 326.

34. Daugherty CC, McAdams AJ, Parton JJ (1983) Aspirin and Reye's syndrome. *Lancet*, *2*, 104.

35. RS Working Group (1982) Reye syndrome and salicylates: a spurious association. *Pediatrics*, *70*, 158.

36. Offerhaus L (1983) Kinderaspirine en het syndroom van Reye: verdacht maar nog niet veroordeeld. *Ned. T. Geneesk.*, *127*, 68.

37. Darcy PF (1983) More about Reye's syndrome and aspirin: a controversy. *Pharm. Intern.* *4*, 37.

38. Semble E, Metcalf D, Turner R (1982) Genetic predictors of patient response and side effects in the treatment of rheumatoid arthritis with a high dose nonsteroidal antiinflammatory drug regimen. *Arthr. Rheum.*, *25*, 370.

39. Buckwalter JA (1956) Disease association of the ABO blood group. *Acta Genet.*, *6*, 561.

40. Piper DW, McIntosh JH, Greig M et al (1982) Environmental factors and chronic gastric ulcer. *Scand. J. Gastroent.*, *17*, 721.

41. Cohen MM, MacDonald WC (1982) Mechanism of aspirin injury to human gastroduodenal mucosa. *Prostagl. Leukotr. Med.*, *9*, 241.

42. Yik KY, Dreidger AA, Watson WC (1982) Prostaglandin E_2 tablets prevent aspirin induced blood loss in man. *Digest. Dis. Sci.*, *27*, 972.

43. Coggon D, Langman MJS, Spiegelhalter D (1982) Aspirin, paracetamol, and haematemesis and melaena. *Gut*, *23*, 340.

44. Graham DY, Lacey Smith J, Dobbs SM (1983) Gastric adaptation occurs with aspirin administration in man. *Digest. Dis. Sci.*, *28*, 1.

45. Šlárová J, Ochová A (1982) Haemorrhage into the gastrointestinal system as a complication of acylpyrin treatment. *Českosl. Ped.*, *37*, 578.

46. Hoftiezer JW, O'Laughlin JC, Ivey KJ (1982) Effects of 24 hours of aspirin, Bufferin, paracetamol and placebo on normal human gastroduodenal mucosa. *Gut*, *23*, 692.

47. Dirksen A, Rasmussen SN, Manthorpe R (1982) Fecal blood loss caused by two differently microencapsulated acetylsalicylic acid preparations in patients with rheumatoid arthritis. *Scand. J. Rheumatol.*, *11*, 129.

48. Stuart MJ, Gross SJ, Elrad H et al (1982) Effects of acetylsalicylic-acid ingestion on maternal and neonatal hemostasis. *N. Engl. J. Med.*, *307*, 909.

49. Heffner JE (1982) Noncardiogenic pulmonary edema: a complication of salicylate toxicity. *Resp. Care*, *27*, 1215.

50. Brenner BE, Simon RR (1982) Management of salicylate intoxication. *Drugs*, *24*, 335.

51. Leatherman JW, Drage CW (1982) Adult respiratory distress syndrome due to salicylate intoxication. *Minn. Med.*, *65*, 677.

52. Zimmerman GA, Clemmer TP (1981) Acute respiratory failure during therapy for salicylate intoxication. *Ann. Emerg. Med.*, *10*, 104.

53. Gaudreault P, Temple AR, Lovejoy Jr FH (1982) The relative severity of acute versus chronic sailcylate poisoning in children: a clinical comparison. *Pediatrics*, *74*, 566.

54a. Prescott LF, Balali-Mood M, Critchley JAJH et al (1982): Diuresis or urinary alkalinisation for salicylate poisoning? *Br. Med. J.*, *285*, 1383.

54b. Symon DNK, Gray ES, Hanmer OJ et al (1982) Fatal paracetamol poisoning from benorylate therapy in child with cystic fibrosis. *Lancet*, *2*, 1153.

55. Hirsch JF, Pichard S, Flottes P et al (1982) Agranulocytose et hyperbilirubinémie au décours d'un traitement prolongé par le paracétamol. *Thérapie*, *37*, 593.

56. Benson GD (1983) Acetaminophen in chronic liver disease. *Clin. Pharmacol. Ther.*, *33*, 95.

57. Gabriel R, Caldwell J., Hartley RB (1982) Acute tubular necrosis, caused by therapeutic doses of paracetamol? *Clin. Nephrol.*, *18*, 269.

58. Karttunen T, Autio-Harmainen H, Sutinen S (1982) Capillarosclerosis of the urinary tract associated with the use of paracetamol and cyclophosphamide. *Acta Pathol. Microbiol. Immunol. Scand., Section A, 90,* 391.
59. Vincens M, Ganansia R, Puy-Montbrun T et al (1982) Anites et ano-rectites nécrosantes chez des malades ayant utilisé au long cours des suppositoires associant dextropropoxyphène et paracétamol. *Thérapie, 37,* 321.
60. Byer AJ, Traylor TR, Semmer JR (1982) Acetaminophen overdose in the third trimester of pregnancy. *J. Amer. Med. Ass., 247,* 3114.
61. Greene JW, Craft L, Ghishan F (1983) Acetaminophen poisoning in infancy. *Amer. J. Dis. Child., 137,* 386.
62. Black M, Cornell JF, Rabin L et al (1982) Late presentation of acetaminophen hepatotoxicity. *Digest. Dis. Sci., 27,* 370.
63. Cabrera MAM, Velázques PA, Muniz MI et al (1982) Intoxicación mortal por acetaminofén. *Rev. Med., 20,* 293.
64. Zezulka A, Wright N (1982) Severe metabolic acidosis early in paracetamol poisoning. *Br. Med. J., 285,* 851.
65. Breen KJ, Bury RW, Desmond PV (1982) Paracetamol self-poisoning. *Med. J. Aust., 1,* 77.
66. Pond SM, Tong TG, Kaysen GA et al (1982) Massive intoxication with acetaminophen and propoxyphene: unexpected survival and unusual pharmacokinetics of acetaminophen. *J. Toxicol. Clin. Toxicol., 19,* 1.
67. Ruffalo RL, Thompson JF (1982) Cimetidine and acetylcysteine as antidote for acetaminophen overdose. *S. Med. J., 75,* 954.
68. Jackson JE (1982) Cimetidine protects against acetaminophen hepatotoxicity. *Life Sci., 31,* 31.
69. Banda PW, Quert BD (1982) The effect of mild alcohol on the metabolism of acetaminophen. *Res. Commun. Chem. Pathol. Pharmacol., 38,* 57.
70. Davis AM, Helms CM, Mitros FA et al (1983) Severe hepatic damage after acetaminophen use in psittacosis. *Amer. J. Med., 74,* 349.

A. Del Favero

10 Antiinflammatory analgesics and drugs used in rheumatoid arthritis and gout

NONSTEROIDAL ANTIINFLAMMATORY DRUG TOXICITY IN JUVENILE RHEUMATOID ARTHRITIS

As little information has been published on the toxicity of nonsteroidal antiinflammatory drugs (NSAID) in children with juvenile rheumatoid arthritis, recently published data on this subject are worthy of attention. Side effects occur frequently and can be serious.

In a retrospective survey (1[C]), 79 of 101 patients (22 males and 79 females; mean age at the onset of arthritis of 6.7 years) treated with various NSAID including acetylsalicylic acid (ASA), developed an adverse reaction of sufficient severity to warrant discontinuation of treatment. These 79 patients were subsequently treated with different NSAID, but 40 still experienced side effects with the new compounds, 25 of the same and 15 of a different type. In the 280 (65%) therapeutic courses with NSAID other than ASA (90 with tolmetin, 53 with naproxen, 46 with fenoprofen, 33 with ibuprofen and 58 with other compounds), the side effects that most frequently led to the interruption of treatment were abdominal pain (5% of courses), headache (4.3%), nausea and vomiting (2.5%), rash (2.5%) and mouth ulcers (2.1%). A few patients also complained of alopecia, dizziness, changes in personality, tinnitus, blurred vision, edema, constipation, diarrhea and easy bruising. Laboratory abnormalities that required treatment with these drugs to be discontinued were anemia (5% of courses), urinary abnormalities (4%), occult gastrointestinal bleeding (1.4%), increase in transaminase greater than 100 IU/l (1%) and prolonged PTT (1 patient). A similar range of side effects has been found with fenoprofen, ketoprofen, naproxen, diclofenac, pirprofen, tolmetin, meclofenamate and proquazone in other short term prospective trials (2[c]–9[c]) but the withdrawal rate for drug induced reactions was lower in these studies.

Number, type and severity of the adverse effects reported to be caused by various NSAID, with the possible exception of meclofenamate, are roughly comparable. The frequency of gastrointestinal, mainly diarrhea, and cutaneous side effects that caused discontinuation of therapy was, in fact, troublesome and much greater with this anthranilic acid derivative than usually found with other compounds (18% as compared to 0.3%). The percentage of patients who had to interrupt treatment because of clinically significant drug-related abdominal pain, tinnitus, decreasing hearing acuity, changes in personality and increased serum transaminase was lower for NSAID than for ASA treated patients. However, the tendency for children taking the newer NSAID to develop anemia associated with gradual and consistent decreases in the hemoglobin and hematocrit values, but without signs of blood loss, is worrying. Whether these drugs actually affect hematopoiesis, promote hemodilution (10) or cause anemia by some other mechanism remains to be determined.

In conclusion, the type and severity of adverse reactions due to NSAID in children with JRA are similar to those encountered in adults with rheumatoid arthritis treated with the same drugs, but the frequency and severity are less than with ASA treat-

Side Effects of Drugs Annual 8
M.N.G. Dukes, editor

ISBN 0 444 90339 9
$0.80 per article per page (transactional system)
$0.20 per article per page (licensing system)

ment. The apparent better tolerability of the new NSAID, however, requires confirmation in long-term studies.

Nephrotoxicity of NSAID

This problem has previously been reviewed (SEDA-5, 88) but in view of the growing number of reports on NSAID-induced nephrotoxicity (11^C–24^C) and the better understanding of the implications of prostaglandins (PG) in the regulation of renal function and their role in the immune response, an updating of present knowledge may be helpful (25^R–29^R).

It is now clear that sometimes severe deterioration in renal function as a consequence of NSAID therapy occurs more frequently than previously thought and that it may be expressed by a multiplicity of clinical syndromes which include acute intrinsic (ischemic) renal failure, acute intersititial nephritis (sometimes with minimal-change glomerulopathy), with or without nephrotic syndrome and, more rarely, direct tubular toxicity, papillary necrosis and obstructive nephropathy. Certain other kidney disturbances, not necessarily related to a decrease in renal function, including water retention, hyperkalemia due to hyporeninemic hypoaldosteronism, and resistance to diuretics and to antihypertensive drugs have also been attributed to these drugs. Acute intrinsic renal failure is probably the most frequently reported side effect and occurs in patients with disorders characterized by high dependence on the compensatory vasodilatory role of renal PGs such as mild renal insufficiency including that which occurs in old age, volume depletion, renovascular disease, nephrotic syndrome with salt depletion, cardiac failure, hepatic cirrhosis with ascites and systemic lupus erythematosus. Evidence which suggests that multiple myeloma (30^C), recent myocardial infarction (31^C) and concomitant therapy with beta-blockers or triamterene (32^C–35^C) are additional predisposing factors in some patients has been recently published.

Although the mechanisms involved are probably multiple, it is now clear that inhibition of PG synthesis by NSAID plays a central role in all these effects. In fact, not only can prostaglandins interact with renin-angiotensin, bradykinins and catecholamines, the three different but interrelated hormonal systems involved in the regulation of electrolyte homeostasis and the maintenance of normal glomerular filtration and renal blood flow but, in some patients, PG inhibition may also be involved in the pathogenesis of the cell-mediated immune mechanisms responsible for interstitial nephritis. Both PGE_2 and PGI_2 inhibit T-cell function and inflammation and if their synthesis were inhibited by NSAID during the course of a cell-mediated immune reaction the delayed hypersensitivity reaction would be able to proceed unchecked. One of the lymphokines released is a permeability factor which, in certain conditions, may be responsible for the development of massive proteinuria, a typical feature of NSAID-induced acute allergic interstitial nephritis (SEDA-5, 88; 24^C, 36^C, 37^C, 38^C). Although all NSAID can cause renal toxicity, this may vary from one compound to another. In fact, there is preliminary evidence to suggest that the potential of sulindac to induce acute intrinsic renal function deterioration mediated by inhibition of renal PGs (39^C) is lower than for other NSAID. Sulindac, although able to cause interstitial nephritis or minimal change glomerulopathy (40^C, 41^C), unlike most other NSAID appears not to decrease urinary PG excretion, not to interfere with antihypertensive action of thiazides and not to significantly decrease the glomerular filtration rate in either patients who are intolerant to other NSAID or subjects with chronic glomerular disease (42, 43, 44). The active metabolite, sulindac sulfide, is a potent inhibitor of renal PG synthesis in vitro, so the apparent renal sparing in vivo may be related to the in vivo distribution of this metabolite (45).

In all the clinical situations mentioned above where there is experimental and clinical evidence to suggest that PGs synthesis is an important compensatory mechanism, a logical approach to patients who require treatment with NSAIDs would demand that their renal function be monitored. Although at present sulindac may be the preferred drug for patients in these conditions, more experience must be accumulated before its potential sparing effect on renal PGs and renal function can be confirmed.

PHENYLBUTAZONE AND RELATED COMPOUNDS

The future of butazones is in some doubt, an acute debate having been ignited by the sudden release of data on the total number of adverse and fatal effects recorded with these drugs. The topic is discussed in the introductory Essay to this volume.

Azapropazone *(SED-9, 154; SEDA-5, 100; SEDA-7, 107)*

The capacity of azapropazone to reduce serum urate levels and prevent acute attacks of gout was compared with that of allopurinol in a 6-month parallel study carried out on patients already satisfactorily maintained on allopurinol. A considerably higher incidence of both clinical (mainly gastrointestinal and cutaneous) and laboratory (moderate increases in blood urea and creatinine levels) adverse effects were encountered in the azapropazone treated group (46[c]).

Acute interstitial nephritis has been described with this drug (11[C]).

Mofebutazone *(SED-9, 145)*

Monophenylbutazone is expected to have the same side effects as phenylbutazone. Administered for 4 weeks to 175 patients with various arthritic conditions, it caused mainly gastrointestinal side effects in 17.2% of the cases and led to interruption of treatment in 5.5% (47[c]).

Phenylbutazone *(SED-9, 142; SEDA-4, 64; SEDA-5, 100; SEDA-6, 93; SEDA-7, 107)*

Intramuscular injection of this drug can be dangerous (SEDA-1, 87). In a representative study of 1384 cases of suspected therapeutic misadventure by doctors in north-west Germany, 74 cases involved *embolia cutis medicamentosa* caused by injections of analgesic and antipyretic drugs (notably phenylbutazone) which frequently led to severe and permanent disability. As there are no good indications for the i.m. injection of this drug, most of the reactions could have been prevented (48[c]).

Pericarditis Pericarditis was the more severe manifestation reported in 5 out of 12 patients who presented a more generalized drug-induced syndrome that included salivary gland enlargement with fever in all cases. Varying combinations of pleurisy, conjunctivitis, rash and signs of hepatic involvement were also noted (49[C], 50[C], 51[C]). The drug-induced pericarditis, which displayed the typical features of severe acute pericarditis, was complicated by atrial fibrillation (3 cases) and cardiac tamponade (1 case). The majority of cases slowly resolved spontaneously on cessation of phenylbutazone, but corticosteroids were required in 2 patients.

Small bowel ulcerations A case of multiple ileal ulcers resulting in recurrent obstruction and chronic bleeding has been attributed to long-term phenylbutazone therapy. Similar cases are quoted by the authors (52[Cr]). This unusual complication is probably extremely rare.

Skin Generalized pustular psoriasis occurred after 10 days treatment with phenylbutazone in a woman with a long history of well-controlled plague psoriasis. Another woman developed pustular psoriasis after 3 doses of oxyphenbutazone and had had a similar reaction to phenylbutazone 7 years previously (53[c]).

INDOMETHACIN AND RELATED COMPOUNDS

Indomethacin *(SED-9, 147; SEDA-4, 65; SEDA-5, 101; SEDA-6, 93; SEDA-7, 108)*

Intramuscular indomethacin induced few side effects at the site of injection (redness, pain, induration) and had good systemic tolerability (54[c]).

Intravenous infusion of 50 mg indomethacin was successfully used in the treatment of ureteral colic and only produced a few mild, transient side effects. Slow rate infusion (5 min) achieves the same therapeutic effect and reduces side effects (55[c]).

Gastrointestinal In a gastroscopic study, indomethacin given for 10 days to 15 normal volunteers in *rectal suppositories* produced less gastric mucosal injury than when given as oral capsules (56[c]). Experimental data support these clinical findings indicating that there is a synergistic interaction between direct topical irritation or absorption of the drug and the inhibition of cyclo-oxygenase in the genesis of gastric damage following oral administration (57, 58).

Necrotizing enterocolitis An association between the use of indomethacin in premature babies and the occurrence of necrotizing enterocolitis is strongly suspected in some reports, but not confirmed by other studies (SEDA-6, 93). A case of necrotizing enterocolitis in a 3-month-old baby treated with indomethacin for Bartter's syndrome supports the hypothesis that this drug may cause that complication (59[C]).

Pregnancy *Hydrops fetalis and cardiac failure* promoted by premature closure of the ductus arteriosus due to the mother having been treated with indomethacin, have been described (SEDA-7, 106; 60[C], 61[C]).

Kidney Two cases of probable indomethacin-induced *renal papillary necrosis* have been described in patients with chronic juvenile arthritis (12[C]).

Skin A case of *toxic epidermal necrolysis* secondary to indomethacin administration therapy has been reported. This life-threatening adverse reaction would seem to be very rare with this drug (62[C]).

The West Midlands Centre for Adverse Drug Reaction Reporting in Britain has received 3 other reports of the development of oral lichenoid reactions in patients with indomethacin.

A 64-year-old man with rheumatoid arthritis had been taking indomethacin for 9 months when he developed soreness, white areas and ulceration of the buccal mucosa. There was no skin, ocular or genital involvement, and no clinical evidence of arthropathy-associated oral ulceration. Appearance was typical of erosive lichen planus, and this was confirmed by biopsy. Hematological and biochemical indices were normal. He was treated with systemic corticosteroids and symptoms resolved within 2 weeks of discontinuing indomethacin. Symptoms returned when he was rechallenged with indomethacin suppositories, and also when he was given ibuprofen, fenclofenac, diflunisal and flurbiprofen.

The Centre has also received similar reports to ibuprofen, fenbufen, sulindac and naproxen. These drugs are known to be associated with non-specific oral ulceration but oral lichenoid reactions have not been previously described.

Bleeding Indomethacin, like other NSAID, can be very effective in the control of pain after major abdominal surgery, but *postoperative bleeding* is significantly more frequent in indomethacin-treated patients than in control subjects; an expected finding if one takes the antiplatelet activity of this drug into account. Indomethacin should probably not be used postoperatively in patients at increased risk of bleeding (63[c]).

Osmosin: merits and risks of the osmotic pump

It is striking that several of the dramatic drug withdrawals which have taken place in recent years have involved non-steroidal anti-inflammatory agents. The phenomenon is probably not unconnected with the fact that the market for drugs of this type, despite intense competition, remains a vast and lucrative one for the pharmaceutical industry, and that risks tend to be where there is still some doubt as to their efficacy/safety balance. The case of benoxaprofen has been commented upon in detail earlier in this series (SEDA-7, 109), and the story of zomepirac is to be found elsewhere in this Chapter. A different but related series of events can be narrated with respect to osmosin (Indosmos), an osmotic pump version of indomethacin which after a brief career was withdrawn from the market, probably definitively, in the summer of 1982.

Indomethacin, as a potent nonsteroidal antiinflammatory agent, found itself at the beginning of the eighties facing heavy competition from a series of newer drugs which were about to be introduced in this area; all were still patented for many years to come, whereas some of the indomethacin patents were about to expire, which could lead to a substantial fall in prices; some (notably benoxaprofen and piroxicam) were suitable for use as a single daily oral dose, which provided at least a marketing advantage; several were claimed, rightly or wrongly, to be relatively well tolerated by the stomach. One possible answer to these problems seemed to be offered by developing an osmotic pump form of indomethacin; in this form, the drug could be released relatively slowly, perhaps prolonging its duration of action and improving its gastric tolerability.

In actual fact, the question as to whether this form of indomethacin really possessed these advantages has never been satisfactorily settled. The literature (64[c]–67[c]) does not appear to demonstrate a reduction in gastric adverse effects, at least not if one assesses the papers in question with the critical eye which one has learned to bring to bear on claims of this type. On the other hand, it is clear that if a drug which has a potentially irritant action on the gastrointestinal tract is put into a slow-releasing form, this might result in the displacement of tolerability problems from the stomach to the lower parts of the gastrointestinal tract.

In the course of 1982 serious suspicions arose that this was indeed happening. In August, the British Committee on Safety of Medicines stated that it had received 200 reports of adverse effects to the product, which was considered a relatively high reporting level for a new drug, though more than 400,000 prescriptions had been issued over the previous 7-month period. Many of the reports related to effects traditionally associated with indomethacin (such as headache and gastrointestinal problems) and these did not seem to be less frequent with the new system. Two of the reports were of intestinal perforation distal to the duodenum, an unusual site for damage by NSAI drugs. The CSM remarked that the release characteristics of the system might expose certain areas of the bowel to higher indomethacin concentrations than usual. In addition, it was noted that the formulation contained potassium bicarbonate, a known bowel irritant (68).

Up to the time of writing, only a few further casuistic reports have become available on these latter aspects, but it has become clear that a fair number of cases of intestinal irritation, bleeding, perforation, and probably even death have been attributable to the new formulation, and these facts have led to the product's withdrawal from the countries where it had already been introduced (personal communication to the editor).

A viable theory of what happened to the osmotic pump version of indomethacin is that the tablets may well in some cases have adhered to particular points on the intestinal wall (or become lodged in diverticula) resulting in a much higher local concentration of indomethacin and potassium than usual. This would indeed explain the occurrence of severe reactions at this level.

More generally the experience with osmosin reminds the student of adverse effects of the need for a very cautious approach to new delivery systems which whilst solving some problems may create others.

Finally, the case of osmosin reminds us once more of the need to study new and modified anti-rheumatic drugs very thoroughly indeed in the patients for whom they are intended, i.e. the (largely middle-aged and elderly) rheumatic population; only in this way can a realistic impression be gained of any advantages which these – often expensive – new or modified products may have, and of any risks which they may introduce.

Clometacin *(SED-9, 149; SEDA-4, 66; SEDA-5, 102; SEDA-6, 94; SEDA-7, 109)*

Kidney Two patients with preexisting moderate renal insufficiency suffered *acute intrinsic renal failure* (13[C], 69[C]). A woman with normal renal function developed acute intrinsic renal failure after treatment with clometacin together with ketoprofen (70[C]). These cases add another nonsteroidal anti-inflammatory agent to the list of those capable of inducing acute reversible renal failure.

Hepatitis This well-known side effect (SEDA-7, 109) may be *associated* with other disorders. *Acute interstitial nephritis* alongside hepatitis developed after a few doses in a patient who had previously been treated with clometacin without problems (71[C]); and another with mild *renal insufficiency* and hepatitis developed *acute thrombocytopenia* and deterioration of renal function (72[C]). The clinical findings normalized in both patients when the treatment was interrupted.

Proglumetacin (protacin) *(SEDA-5, 102)*

In a 3-month study, proglumetacin 300–450 mg/day seemed to be as well tolerated as naproxen (73[c]) and no gastric mucosa alterations were documented in an endoscopic study on 20 patients with symptoms of gastrointestinal disorders after a 3-week treatment (74[c]). This finding must however be accepted with great reserve. So long as virtually all drugs of this type continue to cause gastric complications in a proportion of cases, one must suspect that this type of finding reflects methodological failings and has little clinical significance.

Sulindac *(SED-9, 149; SEDA-4, 66; SEDA-5, 101; SEDA-6, 94; SEDA-7, 109)*

Liver The occasional reports on *jaundice* and *increased serum liver enzymes*, most often alkaline phosphatase, and new well documented cases of sulindac hepatotoxicity (75[C]–77[C]) suggest that this reaction may be more common than previously thought. In most of these patients the drug-induced jaundice was of the cholestatic hepatocanalicular type. It is worth noting that since sulindac came onto the market in the USA, the Drug Adverse Reaction Program (DARP) has received a total of 57 reports of adverse reactions, during a period of 28 months, suspected to be attributable to this drug and among them 6 cases of jaundice and 5 cases of isolated liver enzyme increases. However, it should be remembered that the information contained in the DARP report is raw information which has not been scientifically verified (78[C]).

The mechanisms of these reactions are unknown, but may be tentatively attributed to *hypersensitivity*. Sulindac is metabolized in the liver and is subjected to enterohepatic circulation (79) but the relevance of this finding to the hepatotoxicity is unknown.

Hypersensitivity A reaction characterized by *fever, erythema multiforme, general peripheral lymphadenopathy, splenomegaly, increase in liver enzymes and eosinophilia* has been described in a patient who had presented the same unrecognized reaction one year earlier after exposure to the drug (80[C]). Similar cases have been reported to the Australian Adverse Drug Reaction Advisory Committee (81[c]).

Overdose Acute extreme and rapidly reversible *granulocytosis* appeared in a patient who ingested 12 g of sulindac (82[C]).

ARYLALKANOIC ACID DERIVATIVES AND RELATED COMPOUNDS

Alclofenac *(SED-9, 152; SEDA-4, 67)*

Interstitial nephritis with nephrotic syndrome, probably due to this drug, was observed in a patient also treated with diclofenac (14[C]). Alclofenac, withdrawn from the market in many countries due to a high incidence of skin rashes, has been held responsible for other nephrotoxic effects (SEDA-1, 92; SEDA-3, 94).

Benoxaprofen *(SEDA-4, 68; SEDA-5, 103; SEDA-6, 95; SEDA-7, 109)*

Side effects encountered with this drug have been extensively dealt with in Annual 7 and editorial comments have appeared in many journals (83–86).

In the UK, Lilly, the manufacturer of benoxaprofen, has rejected the request of an 'Opren action committee' representing 450 people who claimed they were harmed by the drug, to set up a no fault compensation scheme. The company's solicitors have told the committee that Lilly denies that the drug 'was responsible for the ill-effects which have been attributed to it' (87). The drug has however been finally abandoned by the company.

Carprofen *(SEDA-6, 96)*

Concern is being expressed regarding the increasing frequency of reports on laboratory signs of *liver dysfunction* with this drug (88[c], 89[c]).

Photosensitivity Eight cases of photosensitivity have been reported. Eruptions occurred 4 days to 3 weeks after starting treatment (90[C]).

Diclofenac *(SED-9, 152; SEDA-5, 103; SEDA-6, 96; SEDA-7, 112)*

In Britain the West Midlands Centre for Adverse Drug Reporting has received two reports of probable allergic reactions to diclofenac (personal communication to editor).

A 27-year-old man was given a single intramuscular injection of diclofenac for myalgia. About a week later he developed a severe skin eruption on the face, hands and legs, with a high fever and pronounced systemic disturbance. Skin biopsy showed vasculitis, and lymphocyte transformation tests showed unequivocal sensitization to diclofenac. The reaction eventually responded to high dose prednisolone, but lymphocytes still showed sensitization when retested 6 weeks later. There was no known prior exposure to either diclofenac or alclofenac.

A 62-year-old woman was treated for joint pain with diclofenac at a daily dose of 150 mg. A few days after commencing therapy, she developed Stevens Johnson syndrome, with skin and oral lesions as well as renal involvement (urea 32 mmol/

l). Diclofenac was withdrawn, and prednisolone was given. The skin and oral lesions healed within a week, and the urea gradually decreased over 6 weeks to 12.2 mmol/l.

Fenbufen *(SEDA-4, 68; SEDA-5, 104; SEDA-6, 96; SEDA-7, 112)*

A number of studies have been published on long-term experience with this drug. Gastrointestinal disorders, including *peptic ulcers* and *gastrointestinal bleeding*, are the most commonly reported side effects, as well as the main reason for discontinuing treatment. The drop-out rate due to adverse reactions in these long-term studies varied from 12 to 22% (91[c]–95[c]). In contrast to previous reports (SEDA-6, 96) with the exception of a few cases of transitory elevation of liver enzymes, no case of overt *hepatotoxicity* has been reported. *Mucocutaneous reactions*, a well known effect of this drug, and fluid retention appear to be more frequent in elderly patients (96[c]). One case of Lyell's syndrome has been reported (97[C]). A case of *granulocytopenia*, which developed during the first month of treatment, has also been reported (93[c]).

Fentiazac *(SEDA-5, 104)*

As reports on reversible *hepatotoxicity* would appear to confirm the doubts already expressed, further investigations are required to establish the long-term safety of this drug (SEDA-5, 104; 98[c]).

Flurbiprofen *(SED-9, 151; SEDA-5, 104; SEDA-7, 112)*

Two cases of probable drug-induced *jaundice* have been reported (99[C]).

Ibuprofen *(SED-9, 150; SEDA-4, 66; SEDA-5, 105; SEDA-6, 97; SEDA-7, 113)*

Although a double-blind cross-over study designed to compare the effects of ibuprofen, naproxen, fenoprofen and tolmetin in 85 rheumatoid arthritis patients indicated ibuprofen in equi-effective doses to be the best tolerated of these drugs, patients' and physicians' preference ranked naproxen first and ibuprofen second (100).

CNS *Cognitive dysfunction* and *personality changes* are thought to be rare side effects of therapy with this and other NSAID (SED-9, 150), but recent reports (101[C], 102[C]) suggest that their occurrence is more frequent, particularly in elderly patients. Forgetfulness, lack of concentration, sleeplessness, irritability, depression and even paranoid ideation and psychosis are cited. The fact that elderly patients are reluctant to volunteer information on these symptoms means that physicians should question their patients very carefully about these problems in order not to miss them.

Kidney Three-day treatment with low doses of ibuprofen and glafenin precipitated *acute renal failure*. The combination of two potentially nephrotoxic drugs should always be avoided (103[C]).

Interaction A patient on *phenytoin* developed toxicity symptoms of cerebellar ataxia, nausea and headaches one week after beginning a treatment with ibuprofen. Blood phenytoin levels were raised (104[C]). Other NSAID can cause the same interaction (SEDA-3, 59; SEDA-7, 107).

Indoprofen *(SED-9, 151; SEDA-5, 105; SEDA-7, 113)*

A survey of adverse reactions based on a heterogeneous series of studies for a total of 6764 patients shows the same pattern of side effects as previously described for this drug (SEDA-5, 105; SEDA-7, 113; 105[c]).

Ketoprofen *(SED-9, 151; SEDA-4, 67; SEDA-5, 105; SEDA-6, 96)*

This compound should be added to the already long list of NSAID that induce *acute interstitial nephritis* (22[C]).

Lonazolac

Reading the few published studies, one gets the impression that this arylacetic derivative causes the same pattern of side effects as those found with other NSAID. The majority of adverse reactions reported are *gastrointestinal* (nausea, vomiting, epigastric pain), followed by *headaches, dizziness, and skin reactions* (106[R], 107[c], 108[c]).

Two cases of *cholestatic hepatitis* have also been reported (109[c]).

Naproxen *(SED-9, 152; SEDA-4, 67; SEDA-5, 106; SEDA-6, 97; SEDA-7, 113)*

Local tolerance of i.v. naproxen was good in 65% of 26 subjects. The most frequent side effect (20% of patients) was a burning sensation along vein. This, however, was not the case if the drug was injected slowly (5 min) (110[c]).

Kidney A patient with rheumatoid arthritis developed the unusual association of interstitial nephritis and membranous glomerulonephritis with *renal failure* while on concurrent treatment with naproxen and penicillamine (111[C]).

Lung Acute *eosinophilic interstitial pneumonitis* occurred in a 72-year-old patient 2 weeks after beginning treatment with naproxen. Fever and leucocytosis, with eosinophilia, elevated erythrocyte sedimentation rate and abnormal blood gas levels, were present. The drug was discontinued and symptoms disappeared within 3 weeks, but recurred within 24 hours upon rechallenge (112[C]).

CNS *Abnormalities in cognitive capacity* and *altered behavior* have been described in elderly patients taking this drug (101[C]).

Blood A case of Coombs negative hemolytic anemia after a 2-week course of naproxen has been reported. This was the sixth reported case in the UK (113[C]).

Interactions Attenuation of antihypertensive effect of *propranolol* and *methyldopa* has been reported, as is true for other NSAID (114[c]).

Oxaprozin *(SEDA-4, 68; SEDA-7, 113)*

In a 2-week, double-blind controlled study in normal male volunteers, oxaprozin was shown to cause less microbleeding, as measured with ^{51}Cr technique, than aspirin, but more than placebo (115).

Pirprofen *(SED-9, 152; SEDA-4, 68; SEDA-7, 113)*

Short-term comparative studies suggest that pirprofen is as well tolerated as either ketoprofen or indomethacin, but better tolerated than aspirin. Adverse reactions necessitated interrupting treatment in 4–21% of patients and the most frequent side effects involved the gastrointestinal system (116[c]–122[c]). They included *gastric ulceration* (3.7% of 160 rheumatoid patients treated for 12 months) (123[c]) and significant *decreases in hemoglobin* and *hematocrit values* (5[C]).

Concern has been expressed regarding the possible hepatotoxicity of this drug (SEDA-7, 106) but a survey of 994 patients treated in the USA found only 6 (0.6%) subjects with *laboratory signs of hepatic dysfunction* (123[c]).

More data on the long-term tolerability of this drug are needed.

Sutoprofen

This appears to have a similar spectrum of side effects to other propionic acid derivatives. Gastrointestinal effects are the most common; headache, sedation, dizziness, fluid retention, rashes, liver dysfunction, elevation of BUN are also reported.

Tiaprofenic acid *(SEDA-5, 106; SEDA-7, 113)*

When this drug was administered to 57 patients in an open study for an average of 13 days, only minor *gastric lesions* were found in 20% of patients at gastroscopy (124[C]). The gastric lesions were more frequent with higher doses and prolonged therapy and this agrees with reports on the higher incidence of gastrointestinal side effects with raised doses documented during clinical trials (125[c]). Rectally administered tiaprofenic acid can provoke *abdominal pain, rectal burning* and *rectal bleeding* (126[c]).

℞ Zomepirac

In March 1983, due to the USA reporting 5 deaths from anaphylactoid reactions in patients taking this drug (127), the manufacturers decided to withdraw zomepirac temporarily from the world market. Several national drug monitoring centers and the manufacturers themselves had, in fact, already received numerous cases of anaphylactic or anaphylactic-like reactions.

According to the FDA's adverse reaction file on zomepirac, a total of 802 reactions were reported to the agency between November 1980, when the product was launched in the US, and December 1982. The most frequently reported adverse reaction was hypotension, with 47 reports, followed by 45 reports of urticaria, 32 of unspecified rash, 23 of pruritus, 19 of asthma, 6 of maculopapular rash and 3 of angioedema. There were 13 reports of 'allergic' reactions including 11 specified as anaphylactoid, and a total of 42 reports of edema, including 23 of facial edema and 3 of laryngeal edema.

According to the manufacturers a total of 1100 reports of allergic reactions have reached the company from around the world, while according to the company's estimates the drug has been taken by 20 million patients throughout the world (128).

The BGA in Germany claims to have received 36 reports on adverse reactions, 17 of an allergic nature, but no case of death associated with the use of the product (128).

512 reports of adverse effects associated with the drug have been received by the CSM in England, 5 were fatal but not necessarily causally related to the drug. 22 reported severe allergic reactions similar to those described in the USA, but none was fatal (129).

The first report of an allergic reaction appeared in the literature in April 1981 and only another 5 can be traced since then (SEDA-7, 114; 130[C], 131[C]). The information on the characteristics of these potentially life-threatening reactions is therefore scanty. Most of them are characterized by hypotension, bronchospasm and serious respiratory distress, with or without oropharyngeal edema, tracheal stridor and cyanosis. Syncopal episodes, anaphylactic shock with acute renal failure and disseminated intravascular coagulation have also been described. Moreover 2 patients exhibited, after 2–3 months of treatment with the drug, signs and symptoms of a multisystem disease process, consistent with a type-3 allergic reaction. The clinical findings were represented by an acute toxic eruption, fever, lymphadenopathy, arthralgias, angioedema of hands and feet and eosinophilia (132[C]).

It is interesting to note that such 'allergic' reactions were not detected during early clinical experience with the drug but were first observed in post-marketing surveillance studies in early 1982. Thereafter the prescribing information for zomepirac has been amended in some countries to draw attention to the possibility of anaphylactoid reactions (128). It should, however, be remembered that a comparative analysis of anaphylactoid reactions associated with NSAID registered in DDE files of the FDA up to May 1981 revealed that about 11% of the 131 recorded cases indicated zomepirac as the causative agent, a frequency only second to that documented for tolmetin, a structurally very similar compound, and approximately the same as that registered for the two widely used drugs ibuprofen and indomethacin (SEDA-7, 114). Both reports from DDE and published data make it quite clear that many of these reactions were severe, i.e. they required prompt hospitalization and emergency treatment. The fact that most, but not all, of the patients had been exposed to the same drug, aspirin or other NSAID, with, or more often, without any reaction, suggests that a sensitizing mechanism could have been involved. It is not possible to predict when sensitivity will be established, as no information is yet available on the timing of hypersensitivity reactions reported to be due to zomepirac.

A number of immunologically and non-immunologically mediated mechanisms could well be involved in these reactions, but, except for allergy to other NSAID and asthma there are no conditions that allow these serious reactions to be forecast.

New cases reported in the literature suggest that nephrotoxicity may be an additional problem. While some cases manifest clinical findings consistent with acute interstitial nephritis, with (134[C]) or without nephrotic syndrome (135[C]), others, particularly predisposed patients, had intrinsic (ischemic) renal failure (136[C], 137[C], 138[C]) or non-oliguric acute renal insufficiency, possibly due to a direct nephrotoxic effect (139[C], 140[C]) (idiosyncratic reaction). Urinary symptoms not usually associated with other NSAID have also been reported with zomepirac (SEDA-7, 114), but the causal link is not clear.

The decision to withdraw zomepirac from the world market was made voluntarily by the manufacturers who are said to be planning to relaunch the drug after further amendment to the prescribing recommendations (133). Whether or not this will be the case, it remains to be seen whether the benefits of zomepirac, which do not appear to be very specific to this drug, outweigh the risk of prescribing it as an analgesic.

Although the reported problems may reflect the drug's very intensive marketing and also the characteristics of some of the patients, most NSAID have not shown a comparable frequency of serious anaphylactoid reactions. Therefore, unless the analgesic properties of zomepirac are clearly proved to be superior to those of the other NSAID, on the basis of currently available evidence, there is no reason to continue prescribing it for this indication.

ANTHRANYLIC ACID DERIVATIVES

Antrafenine *(SEDA-4, 69; SEDA-5, 93; SEDA-7, 116)*

Acute thrombocytopenic purpura with eosinophilia and complicated by severe hematuria has been reported in a patient who had previously used the drug without problems (141[C]).

Floctafenine *(SED-9, 154; SEDA-5, 107; SEDA-7, 116)*

Acute renal failure has also been attributed to this glafenine derivative (142[C]).

Flufenamic acid

A case of fluoride osteosis has been attributed to prolonged treatment with flufenamic acid (143[C]). The patient was a 75-year-old woman who had taken 600–1000 mg/day of flufenamic acid for 6 years. She developed osteosis similar to that seen after environmental exposure to fluorine, and serum, urine and bone fluoride levels were all above normal. Flufenamic acid contains 20.3% fluorine by weight and the patient had received the equivalent of 300 g fluorine. Fluoride osteosis has also been described after prolonged use of niflumic acid.

Glafenine *(SED-9, 153; SEDA-4, 69; SEDA-5, 106; SEDA-6, 98; SEDA-7, 116)*

Coronary spasm, which affected more than one segment and branch of the right coronary artery, that led to *myocardial infarction* developed during a typical Quincke's edema due to a therapeutic dose of glafenine. The patient did not have any known risk factor for coronary artery disease. There was no evidence of increased myocardial oxygen demand prior to the onset of myocardial ischemia and coronary perfusion pressure was not decreased (144[C]). Coronary vasoconstriction has been attributed to some NSAID (SEDA-7, 108; 145) but the sequence of events supports the allergic reaction as a concomitant or additive cause of coronary spasm.

Meclofenamate

Meclofenamate produced an exacerbation of psoriasis on three occasions in a man given the drug for psoriatic arthritis (146[C]).

Mefenamic acid

A case of psychotic behavior has been reported in the Kuwait University Drug Adverse Reaction's Series. A 65-year-old man showed irritability, and psychotic and irrational behavior on the 2nd day of treatment with mefenamic acid, which resolved on stopping treatment.

A 20-year-old girl developed extrapyramidal symptoms – cervical spasm, rigidity and torticollis, which might have been due to mefenamic acid given for dysmenorrhea. The symptoms were felt to be probably psychogenic but one previous case has been reported (147[C]).

Niflumic acid *(SED-9, 153; SEDA-4, 68; SEDA-5, 107; SEDA-6, 99)*

The 361 cases of niflumic acid *acute intoxication* referred to the Centre Antipoison de Paris, between 1974 and 1981, were reviewed. Most of the 143 patients who ingested excessive amounts (generally less than 7.5 g) of this drug alone were asymptomatic; the others presented mild and transient symptoms such as epigastric pain, somnolence and malaise. More serious side effects may be expected from larger ingested doses (148[C]).

Talniflumate

This new derivative seems to be well tolerated in short-term studies. Gastrointestinal disturbances are the side effects most often reported (149[R]).

MISCELLANEOUS DRUGS

Etodolac

This compound was found to produce no greater fecal blood loss than placebo and was well tolerated in a phase I study. The reported side effects were mild and transient and included *sweating, nausea, vomiting, heartburn, dysuria, weight gain, bitter taste and tiredness* (150[c]).

Isoxepac *(SEDA-7, 106)*

Gastrointestinal bleeding, as measured by ^{51}Cr-labelled red blood cell loss in the stools, was found to be increased compared with pre-treatment levels in 10 patients between the 1st and 4th treatment week (151[c]).

Lefetamine

Clinical experience with this drug is very limited. The side effects detected in short-term or single dose studies included *sedation, tiredness, nausea, vomiting, anorexia, headache, sweating and flushing* (152[R]).

Nabumetone

This new non-acidic compound is a poor inhibitor of prostaglandin synthesis that proved to be almost free of gastrointestinal toxicity in animal experiments (153). However, *dyspepsia, severe heartburn* and *epigastric pain* are quoted as the most common side effects in the few short-term clinical studies that have been carried out (154[c]–156[c]).

Piroxicam *(SED-9, 154; SEDA-4, 69; SEDA-5, 107; SEDA-6, 100; SEDA-7, 117; 157[R])*

Data sheet information on this compound has been the object of minor amendments following an agreement between the UK Committee on Safety of Medicines and the manufacturer regarding a new warning that demands the interruption of treatment should peptic ulceration or gastrointestinal bleeding occur and stresses the possible involvement of the drug in precipitating heart failure in the elderly or patients with compromised cardiac function (158).

Skin Severe adverse skin and/or mucosa reactions after short exposure to this drug may be more common than previously thought (SEDA-6, 100). Four cases of *erythema multiforme* alone (159[C]) or with *localized epidermal necrolysis* (2 patients), and serious diffuse *mucosa erosions* of the lip, oro- and rhino-pharyngeal, ano-genital and conjunctival (3 patients) have been described (160[C], 161[C]). These patients also had fever, general malaise and, in one case, elevated bilirubin and transaminase levels (161[C]). 29 cases of phototoxic reactions were received by the Adverse Drug Reaction Reporting System of the American Academy of Dermatology between May 1982 and July 1983. Skin eruptions occurred within 4 days of starting treatment, and in 19 out of the 29 patients they occurred after their first exposure to the sun. Most cases had vesicles or bullae in sun-exposed areas (163[C]). Phototoxic reactions have also been reported to other adverse reaction monitoring agencies, including the UK and Swedish regulatory authorities (164[C]); and there have been two further case reports (159[C], 165[C]).

Hyperkalemia A 55-year-old man with rheumatoid arthritis, glomerulonephritis and hypertension was found to have a hyperkalemic metabolic acidosis and a BUN of 45 mg/dl. He had been taking piroxicam for 6 months and his hypertension was controlled with propranolol. After stopping piroxicam his electrolytes became normal and his BUN fell to 22 mg/dl. Renal insufficiency and the use of propranolol may have been predisposing factors (166[C]).

Renal failure and hyperkalemia occurred

in an 82-year-old woman who was also taking triamterene (167[C]).

Interactions A patient on lithium developed signs of intoxication and elevated serum lithium concentrations when given piroxicam (168[C]). Other NSAID are also known to increase serum lithium concentrations – indomethacin (SEDA-4, 24), phenylbutazone (SEDA-5, 24), diclofenac (SEDA-7, 112).

Tenoxicam (Tilcotil; Ro-12.0068)

This piroxicam analog, which has a long half-life (75 hr), is just beginning its clinical evaluation. The fecal blood loss, as analyzed by the ^{51}Cr-method, in an open cross-over study on 6 normal volunteers was lower with tenoxicam therapy than after aspirin (169). Side effects developed in 28% of patients during a 2-week comparative study. *Gastrointestinal tract* and *central nervous system* symptoms predominated, but rarely led to discontinuation of treatment. Lower doses seem to be better tolerated (162[c]).

Pyritinol and derivatives *(SEDA-5, 108; SEDA-6, 13, 100; SEDA-7, 117)*

35% of 60 patients with rheumatoid arthritis who had failed to respond, or had shown unfavorable adverse reactions, to gold or d-penicillamine therapy, treated with pyritinol in a long-term open study, discontinued treatment because of undesirable side effects similar to those found with d-penicillamine. The effects included *diarrhea*, sometimes dose-related and the most often seen adverse reaction, *nausea, vomiting, loss of taste*, various types of *pruritic cutaneous reactions, leukopenia, myasthenic-like symptoms, alopecia* and *acute dyspnea*. Cross allergic reactions with penicillamine have been suggested (SEDA-5, 108; SEDA-6, 13), but only one patient manifested the same type of reaction with both drugs in this study (170[C]).

JPC-80 is an analog of pyritinol which is being evaluated as a slow-acting antirheumatoid drug. It was found to have safety advantages over d-penicillamine during preclinical assessment. Three of 12 patients who took part in a 12-week phase I study developed mild reversible side effects (*skin rash, diarrhea* and *elevated liver enzyme levels*), but the long-term safety of this compound needs further evaluation (177[C]).

DRUGS USED IN THE TREATMENT OF GOUT

Allopurinol *(SED-9, 155; SEDA-4, 70; SEDA-5, 108; SEDA-6, 104; SEDA-7, 118)*

Allopurinol has been reported to enhance the myelosuppressive properties of the thiopurine antimetabolites 6-mercaptopurine (6-MP) and azathioprine (SEDA-1, 94; SEDA-3, 96; SEDA-7, 118; 172[C]) but, as intravenous 6-MP combined with allopurinol did not increase the availability of the drug in experimental animals and no toxicity was detected, this reaction probably only occurs with oral 6-MP (173).

Colchicine *(SED-9, 156; SEDA-4, 70; SEDA-5, 109; SEDA-7, 118)*

More experience has been accumulated on the use of this drug in patients affected by familial mediterranean fever (174[C], 175[C]). Prophylactic colchicine was prescribed to 85 patients at doses between 1.2 and 1.8 mg/day and continued for more than 3 years in 73% of them. Virtually all patients had mild transient *diarrhea* and *abdominal discomfort* at the beginning of treatment, but only 2 patients were withdrawn from therapy due to side effects (one for chronic intractable diarrhea and the other for progressive *discrease in libido*) attributed to the drug. No signs of myopathy, hair loss, hematologic changes or malabsorption were observed. The small bowel biopsies taken from a number of patients did not reveal any significant histologic abnormalities (174[C]). *Allergic reactions* are also rare. Only 3 of 1100 patients affected by the disease developed severe enough reactions to warrant the drug being discontinued. The side effects reported were generalized *urticaria, edema, dyspnea* and *severe epistaxis*. All 3 patients were successfully desensitized (175[C]).

Sulfinpyrazone *(SED-9, 157; SEDA-5, 109; SEDA-6, 104; SEDA-7, 118)*

New data cast doubt on the safety of prescribing sulfinpyrazone during the early recovery from acute myocardial infarction

(SEDA-7, 118), as cases of acutely *decreased renal function* have been reported (176[CR], 177[C]–180[C]). The mechanism involved is probably related to the inhibition of renal prostaglandin synthesis. These cases support the proposal that renal function should be carefully monitored in patients with recent myocardial infarction (SEDA-7, 118).

REFERENCES

1. Barron KS, Person DA, Brewer EJ (1982) The toxicity of nonsteroidal antiinflammatory drugs in juvenile rheumatoid arthritis. *J. Rheumatol., 9,* 149.
2. Brewer EJ, Giannini EH, Baum J et al (1982) Aspirin and fenoprofen (Nalfon®) in the treatment of juvenile rheumatoid arthritis. Results of the double-blind trial. A segment II study. *J. Rheumatol., 9,* 123.
3. Brewer EJ, Giannini EH, Baum J et al (1982) Sodium meclofenamate (Meclomen®) in the treatment of juvenile rheumatoid arthritis. A segment I study. *J. Rheumatol., 9,* 129.
4. Brewer EJ, Giannini EH, Baum J et al (1982) Proquazone (Biarson®) in the treatment of juvenile rheumatoid arthritis. A segment I study. *J. Rheumatol., 9,* 135.
5. Bass JC, Giannini EH, Brewer EJ et al (1982) Pirprofen (Rengasil®) in the treatment of juvenile rheumatoid arthritis. A segment I study. *J. Rheumatol., 9,* 140.
6. Brewer EJ, Giannini EH, Baum J et al (1982) Ketoprofen (Orudis®) in the treatment of juvenile rheumatoid arthritis. A segment I study. *J. Rheumatol., 9,* 144.
7. Nicholls A, Hazleman B, Todd RM et al (1982) Long-term evaluation of naproxen suspension in juvenile chronic arthritis. *Curr. Med. Res. Opin., 8,* 204.
8. Levison JE, Brewer EJ, Hanson V (1977) Comparison of tolmetin sodium and aspirin in the treatment of juvenile rheumatoid arthritis. *J. Pediatr., 91,* 799.
9. Haapasaari J, Ylijoki H, Wuolijoki E (1982) Declofenac sodium and acetylsalicylic acid in juvenile rheumatoid arthritis: a placebo controlled double blind study. In: *Voltaren New Findings,* p. 51. Editor: E. Kass. Hans Huber, Bern.
10. Johnson PC, Lidsky M, Amadio P Jr (1975) Evaluation of the endocrine system response to Tolmetin in patients with acute flares of rheumatoid arthritis. In: *Tolmetin: A New Non-Steroidal Antiinflammatory Agent,* p. 184. Editor: J.R. Ward. Excerpta Medica, Amsterdam.
11. Sipilä R, Kuhlbäck B, Skrifvars B et al (1983) Acute renal failure during azapropazone therapy. *Mayo Clin. Proc., 58,* 209.
12. Mitchell H, Muirden KD, Kinkaid-Smith P (1982) Indomethacin-induced renal papillary necrosis in juvenile chronic arthritis. *Lancet, 2,* 558.
13. Jacquot C, Hornych A, D'Auzac de la Martinie C et al (1982) Insuffisance rénale aiguë par la clométacine rechute sous diclofénac, inhibition de la synthèse des prostaglandines. *Rev. Méd. Intern., 3,* 349.
14. Vereerstraeten P, Thoua Y, Goldman M et al (1982) Syndrome néphrotique et azotémie réversibles, associés à l'administration d'alclofénac. *Schweiz. Rundschau Med., 71,* 1222.
15. Anon (1982) Nephrotic syndrome. *Med. J. Aust., 2,* 191.
16. Wachtel A (1982) Nonsteroidal anti-inflammatory agents and acute renal failure. *Mayo Clin. Proc., 57,* 601.
17. Trèves R, Gastine H, Richard A et al (1983) Responsabilité de l'ibuprofen dans une méningite aseptique et une insuffisance rénale aiguë au cours d'un lupus érythémateux disséminé. *Rev. Rhum., 50,* 75.
18. Mourad G, Mimran A, Baldet P et al (1982) Insuffisance rénale aiguë réversible et syndrome néphrotique induits par le fénoprofène. *Néphrologie, 3,* 65.
19. Zech P, Geitner S, Birraux B et al (1982) Insuffisance rénale aiguë et syndrome néphrotique secondaires à la prise de fénoprofène. *Nouv. Presse Méd., 11,* 2227.
20. Thomsen BS, From A, Jacobsen IA et al (1983) Acute renal failure possibly associated with fenoprofen therapy. *Arthritis Rheum., 26,* 234.
21. Guyon B, Ory J-P., Wagschal G et al (1983) Insuffisance rénale aiguë avec syndrome néphrotique due au fénoprofène. *Schweiz. Rundschau Med., 72,* 403.
22. Ducret F, Pointet P, Martin D et al (1982) Insuffisance rénale aiguë réversible induite par le kétoprofène. *Néphrologie, 3,* 105.
23. Wasser WG, Goldstein MH, Barba F et al (1982) Persistent renal failure following administration of naproxen. *Mt Sinai J. Med. N.Y., 49,* 127.
24. McCarthy JT, Schwartz GL, Blair TJ et al (1982) Reversible nonoliguric acute renal failure associated with Zomepirac therapy. *Mayo Clin. Proc., 57,* 351.
25. Levenson DJ, Simmons CE, Brenner BM (1982) Arachidonic acid metabolism, prostaglandins and kidney. *Am. J. Med., 72,* 354.
26. Goodwin JS, Webb DR (1981) Regulation of the immune response by prostaglandins. *Immunol. Ser., 14,* 99.
27. Henrich WL (1983) Nephrotoxicity of nonsteroidal antiinflammatory agents. *Am. J. Kidney Dis., 11,* 478.
28. Calin A (1983) In common clinical usage non-

steroidal anti-inflammatory drugs infrequently produce adverse effects on the kidney. *Am. J. Kidney Dis.*, *11*, 485.
29. Torres VE (1982) Present and future of the non-steroidal anti-inflammatory drugs in nephrology. *Mayo Clin. Proc.*, *57*, 389.
30. Paladini G, Tonazzi C (1982) Indomethacin-induced hyperkalemia and renal failure in multiple myeloma. *Acta Haemat.*, *68*, 256.
31. Boelaert J, Van Eeghem P, Fagard R et al (1982) Renal dysfunction with sulphinpyrazone therapy. *Am. Heart J.*, *104*, 174.
32. James DW, Cleland LG, Robinson CW et al (1982) Reversible renal failure associated with treatment with a beta-adrenergic receptor blocking drug and non-steroidal anti-inflammatory drugs. *Med. J. Aust.*, *1*, 232.
33. Ory JP, Guyon B, Wagschal G et al (1982) Hyperkaliémie et anti-inflammatoires non stéroidiens. *Conv. Méd.*, *1*, 513.
34. Favre L, Glasson P, Vallotton MB (1982) Reversible acute renal failure from combined triamterene and indomethacin. *Ann. Intern. Med.*, *96*, 317.
35. McCarthy JT, Torres VE, Romero JC et al (1982) Acute intrinsic renal failure induced by indomethacin. Role of prostaglandin synthetase inhibition. *Mayo Clin. Proc.*, *57*, 289.
36. Finkelstein A, Fraley DS, Stachura I et al (1982) Fenoprofen nephropathy, lipid nephrosis and interstitial nephritis: a possible T-lymphocyte disorder. *Am. J. Med.*, *72*, 81.
37. Clinton AL, Clark WF, Driedger AA et al (1980) Acute interstitial nephritis due to drugs. *Ann. Intern. Med.*, *93*, 735.
38. Solez K, Beschorner WE, Bender WL et al (1983) The 'unique' lesion of fenoprofen nephropathy – an oversimplification? *Kidney Internat.*, *23*, 198.
39. Bunning RD, Barth WF (1982) Sulindac. A potentially renal-sparing nonsteroidal anti-inflammatory drug. *J. Am. Med. Assoc.*, *248*, 2864.
40. Whelton A, Bender W, Vaghaiwalla F et al (1983) Sulindac and renal impairment. *J. Am. Med. Assoc.*, *249*, 2892.
41. Lomvardias S, Pinn VW, Wadhwas ML et al (1981) Nephrotic syndrome associated with sulindac. *N. Engl. J. Med.*, *305*, 424.
42. Steiness E, Waldorff S (1982) Different interactions of indomethacin and sulindac with thiazides in hypertension. *Br. Med. J.*, *285*, 1702.
43. Cinotti GA (1983) Clinical assessment of renal toxicity of antirheumatic drugs. Presented at the 24th Congress of the Europ. Soc. Toxicology, Rome, 28–30 March 1983.
44. Cinotti GA, Manzi M, Mene P et al (1982) Prostaglandin dependence of renal function in chronic glomerular disease. *Clin. Res.*, *30*, 445A (Abstract).
45. Dunn MJ (1983) The effect of cyclo-oxygenase inhibitors on renal function. Presented at the 24th Congress of the Europ. Soc. Toxicology, Rome, 28–30 March 1983.
46. Templeton JS (1982) Azapropazone or allopurinol in the treatment of chronic gout and/or hyperuricaemia. A preliminary report. *Br. J. Clin. Practice*, *36*, 353.
47. Barkow D (1982) Rheumatherapie mit Mofesal. *Therapiewoche*, *32*, 4526.
48. Müller-Vahl H (1983) Adverse reactions after intramuscular injections. *Lancet*, *1*, 1050.
49. Shafer J (1965) Phenylbutazone-induced pericarditis. *Br. Med. J.*, *2*, 795.
50. Ford MJ, Prescott LF (1982) Phenylbutazone pericarditis. *Scott. Med. J.*, *27*, 252.
51. Speed BR, Spelman DW (1982) Sialadenitis and systemic reaction associated with phenylbutazone. *Aust. N.Z. J. Med.*, *12*, 261.
52. Neoptolemos JP, Locke TJ (1983) Recurrent small bowel obstruction associated with phenylbutazone. *Br. J. Surg.*, *70*, 244.
53. Reshad H et al (1983) Generalised pustular psoriasis precipitated by phenylbutazone and oxyphenbutazone. *Brit. J. Dermatol.*, *108*, 111.
54. Rau R, Konstantinidou D, Braun HD (1982) Wirksamkeit und Verträglichkeit intramuskulär verabreichten Indometacins bei der chronischen Polyarthritis. *Med. Welt*, *33*, 683.
55. Sjödin J-G, Holmlund D (1982) Indomethacin by intravenous infusion in ureteral colic. *Scand. J. Nephrol.*, *16*, 221.
56. Lanza FL, Umbenhauer ER, Nelson RS et al (1982) A double-blind randomized placebo controlled gastroscopic study to compare the effects of indomethacin capsules and indomethacin suppositories on the gastric mucosa of human volunteers. *J. Rheumatol.*, *9*, 415.
57. Vane JR, Whittle BJR (1983) The biochemical basis for the toxicity of non-steroid antirheumatoid drugs. Presented at the 24th Congress of the Europ. Soc. Toxicology, Rome, 28–30 March 1983.
58. Hunt JN, Smith JL, Jiang CL (1983) Gastric bleeding and gastric secretion with sulindac and naproxen. *Dig. Dis. Sci.*, *28*, 169.
59. Marlow N, Chiswick ML (1982) Neonatal Bartter's syndrome, indomethacin and necrotising enterocolitis. *Acta Paediatr. Scand.*, *71*, 1031.
60. Mogilner BM, Ashkenazy A, Borenstein R et al (1982) Hydrops fetalis caused by maternal indomethacin treatment. *Acta Obstet. Gynecol. Scand.*, *61*, 183.
61. Verboom AJ, De Leeuw R (1983) Hydrops foetalis na indometacinegebruik in de zwangerschap. *Ned. Tijdschr. Geneesk.*, *127*, 18.
62. O'Sullivan M, Hanly JG, Molloy M (1983) A case of toxic epidermal necrolysis secondary to indomethacin. *Br. J. Rheumatol.*, *22*, 47.
63. Reasbeck PG, Rice ML, Reasbeck JC (1982) Double-blind controlled trial of indomethacin as an adjunct to narcotic analgesia after major abdominal surgery. *Lancet*, *2*, 115.
64. Young JH, Currie WJC (1983) 'Osmosin' in general practice: preliminary report of a double-

blind study in the treatment of osteoarthritis. *Curr. Med. Res. Opin.*, *8*, 99.

65. Gallacchi G, Strolz F (1983) Clinical evaluation of 'Osmosin' versus piroxicam. *Curr. Med. Res. Opin.*, *8*, 83.

66. Rhymer AR, Sromovsky JA, Dicenta C et al (1983) 'Osmosin': a multi-centre evaluation of a technological advance in the treatment of osteoarthritis. *Curr. Med. Res. Opin.*, *8*, 62.

67. Bobrove AM, Calin A (1983) Efficacy and tolerance of a novel precision-dose formulation of indomethacin: double-blind trials in rheumatoid arthritis and osteoarthritis. *Curr. Med. Res. opin.*, *8*, 55.

68. Anon (1983) 'Osmosin' may not reduce indomethacin's side effects. *Scrip*, *82*, 1.

69. Pasquier P, Desfosses G, Magar Y et al (1982) Insuffisance rénale aiguë réversible à la clométacine. Une observation. *Nouv. Press Méd.*, *11*, 3064.

70. Clerc D et al (1983) Insuffisance rénale aiguë sous kétoprofène et clométacine. *Sem. Hôp. Paris*, *59*, 1613.

71. Parini M, Benevent D, Leroux-Robert C (1982) Insuffisance rénale aiguë et hépatite lors d'un traitement par clométacine. *Nouv. Presse Méd.*, *11*, 2641.

72. Seigneuric C, Oksman F, Tkaczuk J et al (1983) Hépatite et thrombopénie auto-immune au cours d'un traitement par la clométacine. *Nouv. Presse Méd.*, *12*, 106.

73. Bozsoky S, Zahumenszky Z (1982) A 3-month, double-blind study of proglumetacin and naproxen in the treatment of rheumatoid arthritis. *Curr. Med. Res. Opin.*, *8*, 89.

74. Manero Guardiola F, Chillon F, Rodriguez di Guzman F et al (1982) Open evaluation of the efficacy and endoscopic gastric tolerance of proglumetacin in chronic rheumatic in-patients. *Curr. Med. Res. Opin.*, *8*, 14.

75. Giroux Y, Moreau M, Kass TG (1982) Cholestatic jaundice caused by sulindac. *Can. J. Surg.*, *25*, 334.

76. Whittaker SJ, Amar JN, Wanless IR et al (1982) Sulindac hepatotoxicity. *Gut*, *23*, 875.

77. McIndoe GA, Menzies KW, Reddy J (1981) Sulindac (Clinoril) and cholestatic jaundice. *N.Z. Med. J.*, *94*, 430.

78. Health Protection Branch, Drug Adverse Reaction Program (1981) Suspected adverse reactions to sulindac. *Report of Dept. of N.H.W.*, pp. 1–15.

79. Dujovne CA, Pitterman A, Vincek WC et al (1983) Enterohepatic circulation of sulindac and metabolites. *Clin. Pharmacol. Ther.*, *33*, 172.

80. Sprung DJ (1982) Sulindac causing a hypersensitivity reaction with peripheral and mediastinal lymphadenopathy. *Ann. Intern. Med.*, *97*, 564.

81. Anon (1982) Sulindac. *Med. J. Aust.*, *2*, 191.

82. Gross GE (1982) Granulocytosis and a Sulindac overdose. *Ann. Intern. Med.*, *96*, 793.

83. Anon (1982) Benoxaprofen. *Br. Med. J.*, *285*, 459.

84. Anon (1982) Benoxaprofen-benefits and side-effects. *S. Afr. Med. J.*, *62*, 225.

85. Anon (1982) Lessons from the Benoxaprofen affair. *Lancet*, *2*, 529.

86. Anon (1983) 'Opren Scandal'. *Lancet*, *1*, 219.

87. Anon (1982) Lilly refuses UK compensation scheme. *Scrip*, *749*, 9.

88. Wittenborg A, Wilmowsky H (1982) Carprofen in ankylosing spondylitis. *Europ. J. Rheumatol. Inflam.*, *5*, 527.

89. Stein GH, Dickey RA, Cohn PD et al (1983) Controlled comparison of carprofen and aspirin in osteoarthritis of the knee. *Curr. Ther. Res.*, *33*, 415.

90. Merot Y et al (1983) Photosensibilisation au carprofène (Imadyl), un nouvel anti-inflammatoire non stéroïdien. *Dermatologica*, *166*, 301.

91. Tait B (1982) Fenbufen in osteoarthritis of the hip. *Pharmacology*, *25*, 73.

92. Salzman RT, Reid RT (1982) Long-term, double-blind, randomized parallel group studies comparing fenbufen with indometacin in patients with osteoarthritis. *Pharmacology*, *25*, 54.

93. Roth SH, Dryan WS, Harris BK et al (1982) Long-term double-blind comparison of fenbufen with aspirin in the treatment of rheumatoid arthritis. *Pharmacology*, *25*, 63.

94. Siemens P (1982) Fenbufen in the treatment of ankylosing spondylitis. *Pharmacology*, *25*, 51.

95. Salzman RT, Reid RT (1982) Long-term, double-blind randomized parallel group studies comparing fenbufen and indomethacin in patients with osteoarthritis. *Europ. J. Rheumatol. Inflam.*, *5*, 318.

96. Brock PG, Jackson D (1982) UK general practitioners experience of fenbufen in elderly patients. *Europ. J. Rheumatol. Inflam.*, *5*, 326.

97. Teilloe D et al (1983) *Nouv. Presse Méd.*, *12*, 1297.

98. Bunde B, Deckers Y, Dequeker J (1983) Fentiazac in rheumatoid arthritis: comparison with sulindac and long-term tolerance. *Curr. Med. Res. Opin.*, *8*, 310.

99. Kotowski KE, Grayson MF (1982) Side effects of non-steroidal anti-inflammatory drugs. *Br. Med. J.*, *285*, 377.

100. Gall EP, Caperton EM, McComb JE et al (1982) Clinical comparison of ibuprofen, fenoprofen calcium, naproxen and tolmetin sodium in rheumatoid arthritis. *J. Rheumatol.*, *9*, 402.

101. Goodwin JS, Regan M (1982) Cognitive dysfunction associated with naproxen and ibuprofen in the elderly. *Arthritis Rheum.*, *25*, 1013.

102. Griffith JD, Smith CH, Smith RC (1982) Paranoid psychosis in a patient receiving ibuprofen, a prostaglandin synthesis inhibitor: case report. *J. Clin. Psychiat.*, *43*, 499.

103. De Torrenté A (1982) Anti-inflammatoires non stéroidiens et insuffisance rénale aiguë vasomotrice. *Schweiz. Rundschau Med.*, *71*, 944.

104. Sandyk R (1982) Phenytoin toxicity induced by interaction with ibuprofen. *S. Afr. Med. J., 62,* 592.
105. Bruni G, Lavezzari M, Perbellini A et al (1982) Adverse reactions to indoprofen: a survey based on a total of 6764 patients. *J. Int. Med. Res., 10,* 306.
106. Koch H (1982) Lonazolac calcium. *Drugs Today, 18,* 184.
107. Wagenhaüser FJ, Narozna H (1982) Der Einfluss von Lonazolac-Ca (Irritren®) auf aktivierte Arthrosen. *Akt. Rheumatol., 7,* 194.
108. Siegmeth W, Placheta P (1982) Vergleich von Lonazolac-Ca mit Naproxen bei vertebragenen Syndromen und bei Arthrosen der grossen Gelenke: Ergebnisse einer Doppelblindstudie. *Wien. Klin. Wochenschr., 94,* 145.
109. Nobbe-Balogh S, Frenger W (1983) Lonazolac-Ca[1] bei rheumatischen Erkrankungen. *Z. Allg. Med., 59,* 94.
110. Accardo S, Samanta E, Cutolo M et al (1982) Intravenous sodium naproxen: bioavailability on man and relief from pain in rheumatic diseases. *Curr. Ther. Res., 32,* 952.
111. Quigley MR, Richfield M, Krumlovsky FA et al (1982) Concurrent naproxen- and penicillamine-induced renal disease in rheumatoid arthritis. *Arth. Rheum., 25,* 1016.
112. Nader DA, Schillaci RF (1983) Pulmonary infiltrates with eosinophilia due to naproxen. *Chest, 83,* 280.
113. Hughes JA, Sudell W (1983) Haemolytic anaemia associated with naproxen. *Arth. Rheum., 26,* 1054.
114. Adverse Drug Reactions Advisory Committee (1982) An adverse interaction. *Med. J. Aust., 2,* 190.
115. Lussier A, LeBel E, Tétreault L (1982) Gastrointestinal blood loss of oxaprozin and aspirin with placebo control. *J. Clin. Pharmacol., 22* 173.
116. Goebel KM (1982) Essai comparatif en double insu du pirprofène, de l'indométacine et d'un placebo dans la polyarthrite rheumatoide. *Nouv. Presse Méd., 11,* 2484.
117. Ayrolles C, Fournie A (1982) Utilisation du pirprofène dans le traitement de la polyarthrite rhumatoide (P.R.). *Nouv. Presse Méd., 11,* 2487.
118. Jajic I, Nekora A, Chadri HA (1982) Pirprofène, indométacine et placebo dans la spondylarthrite ankylosante. Comparaison en double insu. *Nouv. Presse Méd., 11,* 2491.
119. Renier J-C., Fournier M, Loyau G et al (1982) Spondylarthrite ankylosante. Essai comparatif de deux antiinflammatoires non stéroidiens, le pirprofène et le kétoprofène. *Nouv. Presse Méd., 11,* 2494.
120. Peyron J, Doury P (1982) Etude comparative du pirprofène et du kétoprofène dans le traitement de la cox-arthrose et de la gonarthrose. *Nouv. Presse Méd., 11,* 2497.
121. Dolanc B, Morscher E (1982) Etude comparative en double insu du pirprofène, de l'indométacine et d'un placebo dans le traitement de l'arthrose vertébrale. *Nouv. Presse Méd., 11,* 2500.
122. Crouzet J (1982) Traitement des rhumatismes extra-articulaires par le pirprofène. *Nouv. Presse Méd., 11,* 2503.
123. Roth H, Levasseur Y-J, Ryan R (1982) Activité thérapeutique comparée du pirprofène et de l'acide acétylsalicylique dans le traitement de la polyarthrite rhumatoide. Etude multicentrique contrôlée sur douze mois. *Nouv. Presse Méd., 11,* 2517.
124. Mirelli E (1982) Studio endoscopico sulla tollerabilità gastrica di sostanze antalgico-antireumatiche-antifolgistiche: l'acido tiaprofenico. *Gaz. Med. It., 141,* 427.
125. Berry H, Bloom B, Hamilton EBD (1982) Treatment of osteoarthritis. A dose-ranging study of tiaprofenic acid (Surgam). *Clin. Trials J., 19,* 217.
126. Espirito Santo J, Pereira da Silva J, Teixeira da Costa J et al (1982) Acido tiaprofenico versus indometacina no tratamento da artrite reumatoide. *Arg. Reumatol., 4,* 223.
127. Anon (1983) Zomax withdrawn from market after fatal reactions. *Pharm. J., 230,* 299.
128. Anon (1983) FDA's Zomax ADR reports. *Scrip, 776,* 13.
129. Anon (1983) UK Zomax licence to stay. *Scrip, 780,* 1.
130. Corre KA, Rothstein JR (1982) Anaphylactic reaction to Zomepirac. *Ann. Allergy, 48,* 299.
131. Driver PS, Endo RK, Levin A et al (1982) Anaphylactic-like reactions to zomepirac. *Drug Intell. Clin. Pharm., 16,* 616.
132. Kiani R, Kushner M (1983) Zomepirac induced serum sickness. *J. Am. Med. Assoc., 249,* 2812.
133. Anon (1983) Zomax to be reintroduced. *Scrip, 778,* 8.
134. Mease PJ, Ellsworth AJ, Killen PD et al (1982) Zomepirac, interstitial nephritis, and renal failure. *Ann. Intern. Med., 97,* 454.
135. McCarthy JT, Schwartz GL, Blair TJ et al (1982) Reversible nonoliguric acute renal failure associated with Zomepirac therapy. *Mayo Clin. Proc., 57,* 351.
136. McCarthy JT, Schwartz GL, Pierides AM et al (1982) Drug induced renal failure. *Mayo Clin. Proc., 57,* 671.
137. Boike SC, Rybak MJ, Tintinalli JE et al (1983) Zomepirac-related acute renal failure. *Drug Intell. Clin. Pharm., 17,* 56.
138. Warren SE, Mosley C (1983) Renal failure and tubular dysfunction due to Zomepirac therapy. *J. Am. Med. Assoc., 249,* 396.
139. Ratner SJ (1982) Zomepirac and renal failure. *Ann. Intern. Med., 96,* 793.
140. Lisker WH (1983) Nonoliguric renal failure associated with Zomepirac. *J. Am. Med. Assoc., 249,* 1706.

141. Watrigant Y, Salomez-Granier F, Fournier P et al (1983) Purpura thrombopénique secondaire à la prise d'antrafénine. *Nouv. Presse Méd., 12,* 363.

142. Kessler M, Mertens N, Hurault de Ligny B et al (1982) Insuffisance rénale aiguë associée à la prise de glafénine et dérivés. A propos de 12 observations. *Thérapie, 37,* 455.

143. Leroux JL et al (1983) *Rev. Méd. Thérap., 17,* 785.

144. Weber S, Genevray B, Pasquier G et al (1982) Severe coronary spasm during drug-induced immediate hypersensitivity reaction. *Lancet, 2,* 821.

145. Wennmalm A (1983) Central and peripheral haemodynamic effects of non-steroid anti-inflammatory drugs (NSAI) in man. Presented at the 24th Congress of the Europ. Soc. Toxicology, Rome, 28–30 March 1983.

146. Meyerhoff JO (1983) Exacerbation of psoriasis with meclofenamate. *N. Engl. J. Med., 309,* 496.

147. Cremona-Barbaro A (1983) Extrapyramidal symptoms following mefenamic acid. *J. Roy. Soc. Med., 76,* 435.

148. Garnier R, Riboulet-Delmas G, Rousselin X et al (1982) Intoxication aiguë par l'acide niflumique. Etude rétrospective des observations du Centre Anti-Poisons de Paris 1974–1981. *Sem. Hôp. Paris, 58,* 1443.

149. Torriani H (1983) Talniflumate. *Drugs Today, 19,* 97.

150. Joubert L, Mullane JF, Merlo M et al (1982) Clinical pharmacological profile of Ultradol®, a new non-steroidal anti-inflammatory drug. *Curr. Ther. Res., 32,* 74.

151. Mitchell H, Barraclough D, Muirden KD (1982) Blood-loss studies for new non-steroidal anti-inflammatory drugs. *Med. J. Aust., 1,* 328.

152. De Angelis L (1983) Lefetamine hydrochloride. *Drugs Today, 19,* 82.

153. Boyle EA, Freeman PC, Mangan FR et al (1978) Studies on the anti-inflammatory and gastric irritancy properties of 14-(6-methoxy-2-naphthyl)butan-2-one (BRL 14777). In: *Proc. Intern. Congress of Inflammation, Bologna, Italy 1978,* p. 103.

154. Verbruggen LA, Cytryn E, Pintens H (1982) Double-blind crossover study of nabumetone versus naproxen in the treatment of osteoarthritis. *J. Int. Med. Res., 10,* 214.

155. Ginsberg F, Famaey JP (1982) Double-blind cross-over study of nabumetone versus naproxen in the treatment of osteoarthritis of the knee and hip. *J. Int. Med. Res., 10,* 209.

156. Fostiropoulos G, Croydon EAP (1982) A comparative study of the effectiveness and safety of two non-steroidal anti-inflammatory agents, nabumetone and naproxen in rheumatoid arthritis. *J. Int. Med. Res., 10,* 204.

157. Dahl SL, Ward JR (1982) Pharmacology, clinical efficacy, and adverse effects of piroxicam, a new non-steroidal anti-inflammatory agent. *Pharmacotherapy, 2,* 80.

158. Anon (1982) Feldene side-effects reporting. *Scrip, 748,* 14.

159. Faure M, Goujon C, Perrot H et al (1982) Accidents cutanés provoqués par le piroxicam. A propos de trois observations. *Ann. Dermatol. Vénéréol. (Paris), 109,* 255.

160. Bertail M-A, Cavelier B, Civatte J (1982) Réaction au piroxicam (Feldène®). Un type d'ectodermose érosive pluri-orificielle. *Ann. Dermatol. Vénéréol. (Paris), 109,* 261.

161. Cavaroc Y, Sarrat P, Guillet G et al (1982) Intolérance au piroxicam (Feldène®). *Bordeaux Méd., 15,* 469.

162. Kirchheiner B, Holm P, Jensen EM et al (1982) A new long-acting anti-inflammatory agent, tenoxicam (Tilcotil®): in osteoarthritis of the knee and the hip: a randomized comparison with indomethacin. *Curr. Ther. Res., 32,* 627.

163. Stern RS (1983) Phototoxic reactions to piroxicam and other nonsteroidal anti-inflammatory agents. *N. Engl. J. Med., 309,* 186.

164. Sachs S (1983) Phototoxic reactions to piroxicam and other nonsteroidal anti-inflammatory agents. *N. Engl. J. Med., 309,* 187.

165. Torras H, Marti R (1982) Urticaria aguda por Piroxicam. *Med. Cut. I.L.A., 10,* 351.

166. Grossman LA, Moss S (1983) Piroxicam and hyperkalaemic acidosis. *Ann. Intern. Med., 99,* 282.

167. Frais MA, Burgess ED, Mitchell LB (1983) Piroxicam-induced renal failure and hyperkalaemia. *Ann. Intern. Med., 99,* 129.

168. Kerry RJ, Owen G, Michaelson SOG (1983) Possible toxic interaction between lithium and piroxicam. *Lancet, 1,* 418.

169. Bird HA, Bamford L, Pickup ME et al (1982) A comparison between gastrointestinal blood loss caused by Tilcotil (Ro 12-0068) and aspirin in normal volunteers. *Curr. Med. Res. Opin., 8,* 9.

170. Von Wilmowsky H (1983) Die Behandlung der chronischen Polyarthritis mit Pyrithioxin. Eine offene Studie an 60 Patienten. *Akt. Rheumatol., 8,* 41.

171. Norton WL, Donnelly RJ, Schimmelpfennig W et al (1982): JPC-80, a new slow acting antirheumatoid drug. *J. Rheumatol., 9,* 951.

172. Brooks RJ, Dorr RT, Durie BGM (1982) Interaction of allopurinol with 6-mercaptopurine and azathioprine. *Biomedicine, 36,* 217.

173. Zimm S, Narang PK, Riccardi R et al (1982) The effect of allopurinol on the pharmacokinetics of oral and parenteral (i.v.) 6-mercaptopurine. *Proc. Am. Assoc. Cancer Res., 23,* 210 (Abstract).

174. Peters RS, Lehman TJA, Schwabe AD (1983) Colchicine use for familial mediterranean fever. *West. J. Med., 138,* 43.

175. Cabili S, Shemer Y, Revach M et al (1982) Allergic reactions and desensitization to colchicine in familial Mediterranean fever. *Rhumatologie, 12,* 207.

176. Boelaert J, Daneels R, Schurgers M et al (1982) Sulphinpyrazone-induced decrease in renal function: a review of reports with discussion of pathogenesis. *Acta Clin. Belg.*, *37*, 368.
177. Lijnen P, Boelaert J, Van Eeghem P et al (1983) Decrease in renal function due to sulphinpyrazone treatment early after myocardial infarction. *Clin. Nephrol.*, *19*, 143.
178. Mayrhofer EF, Feilhauer GD, Pilecky I et al (1982) Sulfinpyrazon-assoziierte Niereninsuffizienz. *Dtsch. Med. Wochenschr.*, *107*, 1057.
179. Keidar S, Kohan R, Levy J et al (1982) Non oliguric acute renal failure after treatment with sulfinpyrazone. *Clin. Nephrol.*, *17*, 266.
180. Perez Mijares R, Praga Terente M, Lopez de Novales E (1983) Oliguric acute renal failure after treatment with sulfinpyrazone. *Clin. Nephrol.*, *19*, 54.

J. Descotes and J.Cl. Evreux

11 General anesthetics and therapeutic gases

GENERAL TOPICS

Risk factors

Underlying disease is a factor predisposing surgical patients to an increased rate of anesthesia-related complications. As recently reviewed (1[R]), anesthetic risks are greater in hypertensive patients: closer preoperative patient evaluation and continuous monitoring are therefore warranted. Antihypertensive medications should be continued until the time of surgery and large, rapidly administered doses of short-acting induction agents preferably avoided. Premature ventricular excitation is unlikely to be of particular concern in anesthetic patients, except when specific surgery for premature excitation is needed (2[C]).

Anesthesia may prove hazardous in hypothyroid patients (3[R]). However, most reported complications have occurred in patients with unrecognized hypothyroidism which underlines the need for a preoperative recognition of disease: hypothermia and electrolyte disturbances are relatively common. Surgical patients with cancer are frequently exposed to multiple complications both per- and postoperatively as reviewed by Chung (4[R]), mainly involving decreased cardiac and pulmonary reserve, increased sensitivity to general anesthetics and prolonged neuromuscular blockade.

Peranesthetic respiratory and cardiac complications may be more frequent in patients with muscular dystrophy, especially of the Steinert type, as noted in 3 of their patients by Martin et al (5[C]). Conversely, Recklinghausen's neurofibromatosis, according to Girotti et al (6[C]), is unlikely to involve particular anesthetic problems.

Drug interactions are another important risk factor. Ponten et al (7[C]) conducted a randomized study in 91 patients chronically treated with beta-blocking drugs. In 51, the drug was gradually withdrawn over a period of 4 days preoperatively while treatment was continued in 48. Increased blood pressure or chest pain was noted in hypertensive patients or in those with ischemic heart disease after withdrawal. Surgery was indeed postponed in 4 cases due to the severity of withdrawal. From experimental data obtained in dogs, Foex et al (8) concluded that an adverse interaction is unlikely, between beta-blockade (in casu oxprenolol) and anesthesia with halothane, isoflurane or enflurane. However, enflurane should be avoided in propranolol-treated patients. *Calcium entry blockers* are valuable new drugs in the treatment of many cardiovascular diseases but data concerning their anesthesiological implications are fairly scarce, particularly with respect to preoperative discontinuation of treatment (9).

Lithium salts are known to potentiate anesthetic agents and muscle relaxants, but these interactions have no deleterious consequences in so far as they are fully recognized and compensated for. Furthermore, it is wise to continue lithium until the evening before operation in order to prevent risk of suicide (10[R]).

General anesthesia in the elderly, although usually well tolerated, should take into account the higher frequency of underlying disease and of medication in this population (11[R]). Continuous postoperative monitoring and management of elderly patients are probably of critical importance to avoid side effects (11[R], 12[C]). Postoperative respiratory complications in which surgery-

Side Effects of Drugs Annual 8
M.N.G. Dukes, editor

ISBN 0 444 90339 9
$0.80 per article per page (transactional system)
$0.20 per article per page (licensing system)

induced pulmonary changes play a role (13[R]), may be more frequently encountered in geriatric patients. In that respect, Haljamae et al (14[C]) suggested that locoregional anesthesia is a safer alternative to general anesthesia.

Hemostasis and platelet function

Comparing the effects of general, epidural and spinal anesthesia, Koumblis et al (15[C]) found a larger and significant reduction in fibrinogen during general anesthesia. Platelet number was minimally decreased.

Malignant hyperthermia

Malignant hyperthermia is still a subject of concern as demonstrated by several recent reviews (16[R]–19[R]). Preoperative assessment of susceptibility to malignant hyperthermia is an unsettled issue. Traynor et al (20[C]) showed that the muscle phosphorylase to total phosphorylase ratio is unacceptable owing to a percentage of false-positive responses ranging between 6 and 29%. Fletcher et al (21[C]) provided additional evidence of dantrolene efficacy in an 18-month-old boy with congenital muscular dystrophy who developed malignant hyperthermia after 85 min of halothane/nitrous oxide anesthesia. Kecik et al (22[C]) reported one case of fatal malignant hyperthermia in a scoliotic patient and considered scoliosis a factor of increased risk. Lotstra et al (23[C]) observed a 49-year-old woman with a history of neuroleptic malignant syndrome who underwent general anesthesia without ill effects, thus supporting the theory of distinct pathogenic mechanisms.

General anesthesia and immunocompetence

Three recent reviews can be recommended (24[R]–26[R]).

Neuropsychological complications

57 patients were double-blindly anesthetized with either Althesin, thiopentone or fentanyl combined with diazepam for cystoscopies. The patients of the thiopentone group experienced the highest degree of subjective effects detected with the Beecher's mood scale but the smallest reaction time prolongation, 1.5 hours after anesthesia. Fentanyl-diazepam gave the least subjective effects but the highest reaction time prolongation. Althesin gave intermediate results. About 25% of the patients complained of side effects which had persisted for more than 1 day after anesthesia. These side effects were more frequent and more prolonged in the thiopentone group (27[C]). The psychological alterations related to anesthesia and surgery have recently been reviewed (28[R]).

General anesthesia and endocrine function

The topic has been reviewed by Kehlet (29[R]).

Surgical atmospheric pollution

No new data have been provided but the comprehensive review of Marier (30[R]) can be recommended.

Hypersensitivity reactions

Hypersensitivity reactions in the course of general anesthesia (31[R]) are a matter of frequent reporting and extensive investigation: the frequency of such adverse reactions to Cremophor-containing intravenous anesthetics is about 1 in 1000 cases in the United Kingdom (32[R]). The broadly similar epidemiology of hypersensitivity in anesthesia has recently been reviewed on the basis of German and Dutch (33[R]), French (34[R]) and Australasian (35[R]) experience. General anesthetics were found to be the leading cause of anaphylactic shock in a French multicenter study of 1047 patients; alphadione was involved in 42 cases followed by thiopental in 34 cases and propanidid in 15 cases (115[C]), while Le Cam et al (36[C]) incriminated thiopental more often than alphadione and propanidid in their series of 35 severe peranesthetic anaphylactoid reactions.

It is always hard to distinguish allergenic from pathological mechanisms in a given patient. Based on their own experience (37[R]), Moneret-Vautrin et al (38[R]) have proposed a wide battery of immunological and allergological tests to investigate such patients. Moreover immunological and non-immunological mechanisms may be involved (39[R]): one of these, histamine release, is a matter of controversy despite evidence provided by some investigators (40[R]). A better standardization of assay procedures and closer scrutiny of variations in plasma histamine levels are warranted (41[R]).

General anesthetic drugs may at times not themselves be involved in anaphylactoid reactions to general anesthesia; in one 42-

year-old woman who developed such a reaction, allergological investigation identified sodium benzoate as the causative allergen (42[C]).

INDIVIDUAL COMPOUNDS

Gases

Chloroform

A comprehensive review with 162 references on chloroform toxicity can be recommended (43[R]).

Enflurane

In a preliminary study of 150 patients anesthetized with enflurane, Chan (44[C]) concluded that enflurane is likely to be a safer alternative to halothane. Among 216 patients undergoing plastic surgery, 16 patients developed dysrhythmia after receiving subcutaneous or submucosal infiltration of epinephrine in the course of enflurane general anesthesia. However, no severe accident was noted and the authors considered the combination enflurane-epinephrine safe enough for patients without cardiac disease (45[C]). Chander (46[C]) noted isorhythmic AV dissociation in 15.2% of 105 patients who received 1–1.5% enflurane and reemphasized the potential hazard of this inhalation agent in patients with cardiac disease.

Liver damage In Chan's series, published in Singapore in 1982, one case of moderate cholestatic jaundice was reported in a 61-year-old man following general anesthesia maintained with 1.5% enflurane. Full recovery was rapidly obtained (44[C]). The debate as to the possible toxicity of enflurane has however flared up again with the publication on the one hand of a review of 28 cases of enflurane hepatitis by Lewis et al (116[R]) and on the other of a statement by the U.S. F.D.A.'s Division of Drug Experience in July 1983. The latter refers to more than 35 case reports of patients with mild, moderate or severe hepatic dysfunction following enflurane anesthesia (117[r]). The patients in Lewis's series are largely derived from the F.D.A.'s file. To be brief, Lewis's group found in these patients clinical and biochemical data, very similar to those obtained in cases of halothane or methoxyflurane-induced hepatic injury. They conclude that reasonable evidence exists to suggest that enflurane-induced hepatic dysfunction, though a very rare event, is a real phenomenon. 19 of their 28 cases had jaundice after an average latent period of 8 days (range 3–19 days); eosinophilia was recorded in 7 patients and skin rash in 3. There were 3 cases having associated renal failure. 10 of the patients had previously been exposed to enflurane or halothane and the latent period in these cases was considerably shorter than the mean. 5 cases proved fatal. The clinical symptoms appear to support the belief that enflurane-induced hepatic injury is a hypersensitivity phenomenon, but final judgment on this issue may take as long as has been the case with halothane (see below).

Halothane

Liver damage Despite continuing reporting (48[C]–52[C]), the 15-year-old debate concerning halothane hepatitis has not yet reached its final conclusion (53).

The 'toxic' hypothesis has attracted most recent attention: Plummer et al (54[R]) reviewed extensively the metabolism of volatile anesthetics, reaching the conclusion that halothane biotransformation is likely to play a key role in reported hepatotoxicity, a conclusion similar to that of Van Dyke (55[R]). Experimental data have indeed demonstrated that free radical intermediates of halothane metabolism are involved in the rat (56). Furthermore, this hypothesis is in keeping with evidence supporting a pharmacogenetic predisposition to halothane hepatitis (57).

However, the 'allergic' hypothesis cannot be discarded in so far as specific halothane-related antibodies can be serologically detected in patients with fulminant hepatic failure indicating that these patients were sensitized to halothane-altered liver-cell membrane components (58[C]).

Berendes et al (59[C]) failed to show any evidence of hepatotoxicity in 42 patients receiving repeated halothane anesthesia at short time intervals for treatment of laryngeal stenoses.

Malignant hyperthermia Several additional cases of malignant hyperthermia involving halothane (60[C]–62[C]) or halothane combined with succinylcholine (63[C]–65[C]) have been recently reported.

Cardiovascular Comparing the incidence of cardiac arrhythmias, Sigurdsson et al (66[C]) noted a significantly lower incidence in children receiving enflurane (38.9%) than in those receiving halothane (86.6%). In particular, ventricular arrhythmias were less frequent in the enflurane group.

Miscellaneous Ron et al (67[C]) reported 3 cases of *uterine cornual spasm* which were relieved by halothane.

Herrick and Herrick (68[C]) reported the case of a 43-year-old man who had previously used povidone-solution without adverse effect but who developed contact dermatitis when concurrently exposed to halothane. The meaning of this finding remains unclear.

Chaloche et al (69[C]) described *acute myolysis with myoglobinuria* in an 11-year-old boy following halothane. The outcome was favorable.

Isoflurane

Friesen and Lichtor (70[C]) investigated the *cardiovascular* effects of isoflurane in 60 healthy infants aged 5–26 weeks. Half of them were premedicated with atropine sulfate 0.02 mg/kg intramuscularly. Atropine was found to minimize the decrease of heart rate from 32% to 20% but had no effect on blood pressure which fell by 40% in both cases. A significant increase from baseline in heart rate, cardiac output and plasma epinephrine levels and a significant reduction in systemic vascular resistance index and plasma norepinephrine level was noted in 10 patients undergoing coronary artery bypass surgery after 10 min of isoflurane 1.5–2.0% in oxygen (71[C]).

One case of *malignant hyperthermia* with favorable outcome has been reported in a 17-year-old black man given isoflurane 0.5–2.5% after thiopental induction (72[C]).

Methoxyflurane

Two cases of *hepatitis* have been reported following methoxyflurane obstetric analgesia (73[C]) and Mazzia has reviewed current knowledge concerning methoxyflurane *nephrotoxicity* (74[R]).

Nitrous oxide

Cardiovascular Cardiovascular collapse was described in a 1-year-old infant immediately following supplementation of thiopental and morphine with nitrous oxide. It is likely that nitrous oxide precipitated acute cardiac failure in this infant with partial anomalous pulmonary venous drainage (75[C]).

Hematological Nitrous oxide inactivates vitamin B12 which can result in *megaloblastic anemia* (76[C]), particularly following repeated exposure (77[C]). However, the hemopoietic toxicity of nitrous oxide cannot be reversed by high doses of folinic acid (78[C]).

One case of *hypothromic anemia* has been noted in an anesthetist chronically exposed to nitrous oxide but the causal relationship deserves further investigation (79[C]).

Tympanic membrane rupture Three cases of tympanic membrane rupture have been reported (80[C], 81[C]) in patients undergoing general anesthesia supplemented with nitrous oxide resulting in transient hearing loss. An increase in middle-ear pressure as demonstrated in children (82[C]) is likely to be a critical factor.

Miscellaneous Two cases of *pneumomediastinum* following nitrous oxide abuse have been reported (83[C]).

Oxygen

Hittner et al (84[C]) provided evidence supporting the preventive efficacy of vitamin E 100 mg/kg day in the preterm infant with respect to retrolental fibroplasia.

INTRAVENOUS AGENTS

Inhalation versus intravenous general anesthesia

The comparative effects of inhalation and intravenous general anesthesia have been the subject of recent reviews: owing to their inhibition of the pulmonary vasoconstriction response to hypoxia in man, volatile inhalation agents should be used with caution in patients suffering from airway obstruction (85[R]). Data are otherwise far less conclusive: Prys-Roberts (86[C]) reviewed the cardiovascular effects of most intravenous and inhalation agents, but reached the conclusion that no direct comparison is acceptable at the moment. Andreen (87[R]) has suggested that the consequences of the surgical and anesthetic procedures may be of greater relevance than the effects of various anesthetics inasmuch as the hepatic and splanchnic circulation are concerned, while Steen (88[R]) has proposed that the cerebral effects of various anesthetic agents have no clinical implication for operations other than neurosurgery.

Althesin

Safety for long-term use Although Althesin is frequently used as an induction agent, continuous intravenous infusion for maintenance of general anesthesia is generally considered as safe (89[R], 90[R]), even though long-term sedation of patients in the intensive care unit may prove more hazardous (91[C]). Althesin's solvent, Cremophor El, is again possibly responsible for the suggested hazard: although the observed Cremophor El-related decrease in blood viscosity may have some advantages in critically ill patients (92[C]), Knell et al (91[C]) suspected this polyoxyethylated ricinoleic acid for causing progressive reduction of hemoglobin, plasma albumin and serum sodium values below 130 mmol/l in 4 patients who received prolonged Althesin infusion. These reported effects deserve further investigation to provide more conclusive evidence of any hazard which may exist.

Hypersensitivity Complement activation is likely to play an essential role in Althesin-induced hypersensitivity reactions: Radford et al (93[C]) sequentially investigated 30 patients with clinical signs of hypersensitivity to Althesin in a search for a complement system activation. The alternative complement pathway, but not the classical pathway, was activated in 5 of 13 patients on first exposure to Althesin while the classical complement pathway, but not the alternative pathway, was activated in 5 of 13 patients on first exposure to Althesin; classical complement pathway activation was demonstrated in all 17 patients reacting on repeat exposure. These findings are in keeping with those of Descotes et al (94[C]) who found both complement pathways activated in 8 patients with signs of hypersensitivity. Interestingly, the latter authors suggested that Althesin may be capable of moderately activating complement pathways despite the lack of overt clinical hypersensitivity reaction. Furthermore, such hypersensitivity reactions with complement activation could be noted even though Althesin was very slowly infused (94[C]–96[C]).

Simpson et al (97[C]) suggested that pregnancy is a likely risk factor with respect to Althesin-induced hypersensitivity reactions involving complement activation.

Despite the reported case of a 19-year-old woman who underwent 84 general anesthesias with Althesin between the age of 6 and 15 without ill effects (98[C]), repeated Althesin exposure is generally regarded as a critical risk factor. Recent experimental data provide supportive evidence: Althesin was found to behave as a moderate sensitizer in guinea pigs (99), while Cremophor El proved to be a potent immunological adjuvant in rodents (100).

Barbiturates

Thiopental Three cases of anaphylactoid reactions following administration of thiopental with full recovery have been reported in low-risk patients (101[C], 102[C]). Butler et al (103[C]) have described an unusual fixed drug eruption on 2 consecutive occasions in a 65-year-old man following thiopental.

Comparing thiopental and midazolam for induction of general anesthesia in ASA class I and II patients, Lebowitz et al (104[C]) found no significant difference in cardiovascular effects: there was a moderate decline of mean arterial pressure, stroke volume, cardiac output and heart rate; the mean right atrial pressure increased slightly whereas systemic vascular resistance remained unchanged.

The case of a 17-year-old male patient who was inadvertently injected 15 ml of 2.5% thiopental via the axillary route has been described (105[C]). He experienced mild discomfort and paresthesiae in the fingers which persisted for several hours and subsided without sequelae.

About 1 in 10 patients experienced

local pain or venous complications after injection of thiopental. Similar results were obtained with 1% methohexital and disoprofol while diazepam gave a 40% rate of such side effects (106[C]).

Disoprofol

Disoprofol has been compared to Althesin for maintenance of general anesthesia in 200 surgical patients (107[C]): the main problem encountered with disoprofol was pain at the injection site in 11–12% of patients. Involuntary movements were less frequent however.

Disoprofol contains Cremophor El as a solvent and, as might be expected, hypersensitivity reactions are likely complications following its application: Briggs et al (108[C]) reported one such case with involvement of the complement system in a 42-year-old man.

Ketamine

Cardiovascular Midazolam 0.15 mg/kg proved effective in suppressing the cardiostimulatory action of ketamine but was unable to modify its effects on intracranial pressure (109[C]).

Ketamine infusion was shown to cause only minimal changes in cardiac output and left ventrical performance by contrast to thiopental in ASA class III and IV patients. Both drugs decreased the diastolic pressure time index to systolic time pressure index ratio significantly (110[C]).

Central nervous system Three additional cases of ketamine-induced convulsions have been reported in children (111[C]). Ketamine should be avoided in children with the Kinsbourne syndrome (myoclonic encephalopathy of infants) because it potentiates myoclonus and opsoclonus (112[C]).

Acupuncture may be an effective preventive measure against ketamine-induced hallucinations (113[C]).

Propanidid

Cousin et al (114[C]) reported one case of anaphylactoid reaction with blood clotting problems in a 30-year-old woman following propanidid: fibrinogen levels were decreased by 50%. The patient fully recovered within 24 hours.

REFERENCES

1. Rodriguez PR, Mangano DT (1982) Anesthesia and hypertension. *Semin. Anesth., 1,* 226.
2. Caramella JP, Malbezin S, Valère PE, Desmonts JM (1982) Syndrome de pré-excitation ventriculaire et anesthésie générale. *Ann. Cardiol. Angéiol., 31,* 381.
3. Murkin JM (1982) Anesthesia and hypothyroidism: a review of thyroxine physiology, pharmacology and anesthetic implication. *Anesth. Analg., 61,* 371.
4. Chung F (1982) Cancer, chemotherapy and anesthesia. *Canad. Anaesth. Soc. J., 29,* 364.
5. Martin R, Néron R, Lamarche Y (1982) Dystrophies musculaires et anesthésie. *Union Méd. Canad., 111,* 1.
6. Girotti E, Zanardi R, Dondarini A (1982) Problemi anestesiologici nella neurofibromatosi di von Recklinghausen. *Acta Anaesth. Italica, 33,* 545.
7. Ponten J, Biber B, Bjuro T et al (1982) β-receptor blocker withdrawal: a preoperative problem in general surgery. *Acta Anaesth. Scand., Suppl. 76,* 32.
8. Foex P, Francis CM, Cutfield GR (1982) The interactions between β-blockers and anaesthetics: experimental observations. *Suppl. 76,* 38.
9. Reves JG, Kimin I, Lell WA, Tosone S (1982) Calcium entry blockers: uses and implications for anesthesiologists. *Anesthesiology, 57,* 504.
10. Pottecher T, Galani M, Otteni JC (1982) Lithium et intervention chirurgicale. *J. Méd. Strasbourg, 13,* 363.
11. Cousin MT (1982) Anesthésie du vieillard. *Revue Méd., 23,* 39.
12. Benoît Y, Chadenson O, Descotes J, Bertrix L et al (1983) La pharmacovigilance en anesthésiologie: bilan de l'expérience lyonnaise. *Thérapie, 38,* 437.
13. Spence AA (1982) Pulmonary changes after surgery. *Regional Anesth., 7,* S 119.
14. Haljamae H, Stefansson T, Wickstrom I (1982) Influence of anesthetic technique on postoperative pulmonary complications in geriatric patients. *Regional Anesth., 7,* S 122.
15. Koumblis E, Hondreli E, Skouloudis A (1982) Fibrinolysia and anaesthesia: comparative effects of general, epidural and spinal anaesthesia. *Hellen. Anaesthesiol. Acta, 16,* 67.
16. Rockahr GI (1982) Malignant hyperthermia: Disposition oder abortiver Verlauf? Ein Fallbericht. *Dt. Gesundh. Wesn, 37,* 1066.
17. Schulte-Sasse U, Eberlein HJ (1983) Die maligne Hyperthermie. *Anaesthesist, 32,* 141.
18. Rodgers IR (1983) Malignant hyperthermia:

a review of the literature. *Mount Sinai J. Med.*, *50*, 95.

19. Dodge T, Morris D (1982) Malignant hyperthermia. Identification and confirmation. *Anesthesiol. Rev.*, *9*, 15.
20. Traynor CA, Van Dyke RA, Gronert GA (1983) Phosphorylase ratio and susceptibility to malignant hyperthermia. *Anesth. Analg.*, *62*, 324.
21. Fletcher R, Blennow G, Olsson AK et al (1982) Malignant hyperthermia in a myopathic child. Prolonged postoperative course requiring dantrolene. *Acta Anaesth. Scand.*, *26*, 435.
22. Kecik Y, Tuzuner F, Budayicioglu A, Akkartal B (1982) A case of malignant hyperthermia related to scoliosis. *GATA Bülteni*, *24*, 631.
23. Lotstra F, Linkowski P, Mendlewicz J (1983) General anaesthesia after neuroleptic malignant syndrome. *Biol. Psychiatr.*, *18*, 243.
24. Hole A (1982) Effect of general anesthesia and epidural anaesthesia on some monocyte and lymphocyte function during and after surgery. *Regional Anesth.*, *7*, S 75.
25. Kehlet H, Wandall JH, Hjorts ØNC (1982) Influence of anesthesia and surgery on immunocompetence. *Regional Anesth.*, *7*, S 68.
26. Nalda MA, Garcia MP (1982) A new concept in anesthesiology and reanimation: its immunological interaction. *Rev. Esp. Anest. Rean.*, *29*, 333.
27. Elsass P, Stibolt O, Klauber PV et al (1982) A clinical neuropsychological study of the postoperative course after three types of anaesthesia. *Acta Anaesth. Scand.*, *26*, 151.
28. Hole A (1982) Psychological alterations after anesthesia and surgery. *Regional Anesth.*, 7, S 141.
29. Kehlet H (1982) The modifying effect of general and regional anesthesia on the endocrine-metabolic response to surgery. *Regional Anesth.*, *7*, S 38.
30. Marier JR (1982) Halogenated hydrocarbon environmental pollution: the special case of halogenated anesthetics. *Environ. Res.*, *28*, 212.
31. Stoelting RK (1983) Allergic reactions during anaesthesia. *Anesth. Analg.*, *62*, 341.
32. Clarke RSJ (1982) Epidemiology of adverse reactions in anaesthesia in the United Kingdom. *Klin. Wochenschr.*, *60*, 1003.
33. Langrehr D, Newton D, Agoston S (1982) Epidemiology of adverse reactions in anaesthesia in Germany and the Netherlands. *Klin. Wochenschr.*, *60*, 1010.
34. Laxenaire MC, Moneret-Vautrin DA, Boileau S, Moeller R (1982) Adverse reactions to intravenous agents in anaesthesia in France. *Klin. Wochenschr.*, *60*, 1006.
35. Fisher M (1982) The epidemiology of anaesthetic anaphylactoid reactions in Australasia. *Klin. Wochenschr.*, *60*, 1017.
36. Le Cam B, Tanguy RL, Egreteau JP (1982) Les accidents anaphylactoides graves en anesthésie: a propos de trente cinq cas. *Sem. Hôp. Paris.*, *58*, 2691.
37. Moneret-Vautrin DA, Laxenaire MC et al (1982) Etude allergologique de 28 sujets ayant présenté un choc anaphylactoide à des anesthésiques généraux. *Toxicol. Eur. Res.*, *2*, 95.
38. Moneret-Vautrin DA, Laxenaire MC, Bertrand F (1982) Conduite du bilan immuno-allergologique en cas d'accident anaphylactoide peranesthésique. *Ann. Fr. Anesth. Réanim.*, *1*, 267.
39. Watkins J, Thornton JA (1982) Immunological and non immunological mechanisms involved in adverse reactions to drugs. *Klin. Wochenschr.*, *60*, 958.
40. Lorenz W, Doenicke A, Schöning B et al (1982) Definition and classification of the histamine-release response to drugs in anaesthesia and surgery. *Klin. Wochenschr.*, *60*, 896.
41. Röher HD, Lorenz W, Lennartz H et al (1982) Plasma histamine levels in patients in the course of several standard operations: influence of anaesthesia, surgical trauma and blood transfusion. *Klin. Wochenschr.*, *60*, 926.
42. Moneret-Vautrin DA, Moeller R, Malingrey L, Laxenaire MC (1982) Anaphylactoid reaction to general anaesthesia: a case of intolerance to sodium benzoate. *Anaesth. Intens. Care*, *10*, 156.
43. Davidson IWF, Summer DD, Parker JC (1982) Chloroform: a review of its metabolism, teratogenic, mutagenic and carcinogenic potential. *Drug Chem. Toxicol.*, *5*, 1.
44. Chan CS (1982) Preliminary experience with enflurane. *Singapore Med. J.*, *23*, 26.
45. Gouveia MA, Labrunie GM (1982) Enflurane and epinephrine incidence of cardiac dysrhythmias. *Rev. Bras. Anest.*, *32*, 95.
46. Chander S (1982) Isorhythmic atrioventricular dissociation during enflurane anesthesia. *Southern Med. J.*, *75*, 945.
47. Masone RJ, Goldfarb JP, Manzione NC, Biempica L (1982) Enflurane hepatitis. *J. Clin. Gastroenterol.*, *4*, 541.
48. Lewis RB, Blair M (1982) Halothane hepatitis in a young child. *Br. J. Anaesth.*. *54*. 349.
49. Flores JO, Burlamaque A, Geyer GR (1982) Necrose hepatica maçica apos halotano. Relato de um caso. *Rev. Bras. Anesth.*, *32*, 289.
50. Shiba R, Tsukawaki Y, Ogli K, Miyazaki M (1982) A case report of fulminant hepatitis following exposure to halothane. *Hiroshima J. Anaesth.*, *18*, 56.
51. Kawana S, Namiki A, Shirase M et al (1982) Case reports of postoperative liver dysfunction after halothane anesthesia. *Hiroshima J. Anaesth.*, *18*, 52.
52. Giorgini RJ, Giorgini GL, Lombardo M (1982) Halothane hepatitis: a series of case reports following pediatric surgery. *J. Foot Surg.*, *21*, 270.
53. Pohl LR, Gillette JR (1982) A perspective on halothane induced hepatotoxicity. *Anesth. Analg.*, *61*, 809.
54. Plummer JL, Counsis ML, De la Hall PM

(1982) Volatile anaesthetic metabolism and acute toxicity. *Rev. Drug. Metab. Drug Interact., 4,* 49.

55. Van Dyke RA (1982) Metabolism of anesthetic agents: toxic implications. *Acta Anaesth. Scand., Suppl. 75,* 7.

56. Plummer JL, Beckwith ALJ, Bastin FN et al (1982) Free radical formation in vivo and hepatotoxicity due to anesthesia with halothane. *Anesthesiology, 57,* 160.

57. Cousins MJ, Courlay GK, De la Hall PM, Knights K (1982) Pharmacogenetics and halothane hepatitis. *Anesthesiology, 56,* 484.

58. Neuberger J, Gimson AES, Davis M, Williams R (1983) Specific serological markers in the diagnosis of fulminant hepatic failure associated with halothane anaesthesia. *Br. J. Anaesth., 55,* 15.

59. Berendes S, Bonhoeffer K, Rose KG (1982) Häufig wiederholte Halothannarkosen in der Chirurgie laryngo-trachealer Stenosen. Wie hoch ist das Risiko einer Läberschädigung? *H.N.O., 30,* 307; *Hellen. Anaesthesiol. Acta., 16,* 211.

60. Kocke A, Morimoto M (1982) Reports of two cases with hyperthermia during anesthesia. *Hiroshima J. Anaesth., 18,* 227.

61. Seo K, Inoue S, Kaieda et al (1982) Hyperthermia after halothane anesthesia: a case report. *Hiroshima J. Anesth., 18, Suppl. 1,* 31.

62. Uehara K, Nishida Y, Uno T, Motomatsu K (1982) A case of suspected malignant hyperthermia. *Hiroshima J. Anesth., 18,* 39.

63. Miyamoto K, Sasaki M, Okuda T et al (1982) Four cases of suspected malignant hyperthermia induced by halothane and succinylcholine. *Hiroshima J. Anesth., 18,* 157.

64. Yoshida S, Takahashi N, Yokoyama K (1982) A case of subtype malignant hyperthermia during GOF anesthesia. *Hiroshima J. Anesth., 18,* 44.

65. Nishijima H, Hashimoto K, Aoki A et al (1982) Two cases of postoperative malignant hyperthermia. *Hiroshima J. Anaesth., 18,* 39.

66. Sigurdsson GH, Carlsson C, Lindahl S, Werner O (1983) Cardiac arrhythmias in non-intubated children during adenoidectomy: a comparison between enflurane and halothane anaesthesia. *Acta Anaesth. Scand., 27,* 75.

67. Ron M, Beller U, Hochner-Velnikier, Palti Z (1982) The effect of halothane on uterine cornual spasm during general anaesthesia. *Int. J. Fertil., 27,* 187.

68. Herrick RT, Herrick S (1982) Povidone-iodine-halothane interaction. *Orthopedics, 5,* 1480.

69. Chaloche C, Nordmann Y, Fontaine JL, Lejeune C (1982) Myoglobinurie post-anesthésique. *Arch. Franç. Pediatr., 39,* 169.

70. Friesen RH, Lichtor JL (1983) Cardiovascular effects of inhalation induction with isoflurane in infants. *Anesth. Analg., 62,* 411.

71. Balasarasuwathi K, Glisson SN, El-Etr AA, Mummaneni N (1982) Hemodynamic and catecholamine response to isoflurane anaesthesia in patients undergoing coronary artery surgery. *Canad. Anaesth. Soc. J., 29,* 533.

72. Boheler J, Hamrick JC, MacKnight RL, Eger EI (1982) Isoflurane and malignant hyperthermia. *Anesth. Analg., 61,* 712.

73. Delia JE, Maxson WS, Breen JL (1983) Methoxyflurane hepatitis: two cases following obstetric analgesia. *Int. J. Gynaecol. Obstet., 21,* 89.

74. Mazzia VDB (1982) Kidney failure due to methoxyflurane. *Leg. Med. Annual., 82,* 59.

75. Davidson JR, Chinyanga HM (1982) Cardiovascular collapse associated with nitrous oxide anaesthesia: a case report. *Canad. Anaesth. Soc. J., 29,* 484.

76. Skacel PO, Hewlett AM, Lewis JD et al (1983) Studies on the haemopoietic toxicity of nitrous oxide in man. *Br. J. Haematol., 53,* 189.

77. Nunn JF, Sharer NM, Gorchein A et al (1982) Megaloblastic haemopoiesis after multiple short-term exposure to nitrous oxide. *Lancet, 1,* 1379.

78. Skacel PO, Chanarin I, Hewlett A, Nunn JF (1982) Failure to correct nitrous oxide toxicity with folinic acid. *Anesthesiology, 57,* 557.

79. Novelli GP, Ristori M, Piscitelli P, Festimanni F (1982) Anemia da protossido d'azoto: descrizione di un caso di patologia professionale inconsueta. *Acta Anaesth. Ital., 33,* 161.

80. Perreault L, Normandin, Plamondon L et al (1982) Tympanic membrane rupture after anesthesia with nitrous oxide. *Anesthesiology, 57,* 325.

81. Ravindran RS, Cummins DF (1983) Spontaneous rupture of tympanic membrane following nitrous oxide anesthesia. *Anesthesiol. Rev., 10,* 24.

82. Casey WF, Drake-Lee AB (1982) Nitrous oxide and middle ear pressure. *Anesthesia, 37,* 896.

83. Lipuma JP, Wellman J, Stern HP (1982) Nitrous oxide abuse: a new cause for pneumomediastinum. *Radiology, 145,* 602.

84. Hittner HM, Godio LB, Speer ME et al (1983) Retrolental fibroplasia: further clinical evidence and ultrastructural support for efficacy of vitamin E in the preterm infant. *Pediatrics, 71,* 423.

85. Bjertnaes LJ (1982) Intravenous versus inhalation anaesthesia: pulmonary effects. *Acta Anaesth. Scand., Suppl. 75,* 18.

86. Prys-Roberts C (1982) Cardiovascular effects of continuous intravenous anaesthesia compared with those of inhalational anaesthesia. *Acta Anaesth. Scand., Suppl. 75,* 10.

87. Andreen M (1982) Inhalation versus intravenous anaesthesia: effects on the hepatic and splanchnic circulation. *Acta Anaesth. Scand., Suppl. 75,* 25.

88. Steen PA (1982) Inhalational versus intravenous anaesthesia cerebral effects. *Acta Anaesth. Scand., Suppl. 75,* 32.

89. Towler CM, Garrett RT, Sear JW (1982) Althesin infusion for maintenance of anaesthesia. *Anaesthesia, 37,* 428.
90. Ramsay MAE, Saveze TM, Simpson BRJ, Goodwin R (1974) Controlled sedation with alphadolone-alphaxolone. *Br. J. Anaesth., 2,* 656.
91. Knell AJ, Turner P, Chalmers APD (1983) Potential hazard of steroid anaesthesia for prolonged sedation. *Lancet, 1,* 526.
92. Gramstad L, Stvner J (1979) Plasma viscosity and cremophor-containing anaesthetics. *Br. J. Anaesth., 51,* 1175.
93. Radford SG, Lokyer JA, Simpson PJ (1982) Immunological aspects of adverse reactions to althesin. *Br. J. Anaesth., 54,* 859.
94. Descotes J, Veysseyre CM, Bringuier JP et al (1983) Réactions de type anaphylactoïde sous Alfatésine. Etude préliminaire du rôle du complément. *Thérapie, 38,* 535.
95. Benoit Y, Chadenson O, Ducloux B et al (1983) Hypersensitivity reactions to Althesin infusion: measurement of complement involvement. *Anaesthesia, 38,* 1079.
96. Thompson EEM, Greenhough SG (1982) Adverse response to i.v. anaesthetics. *Br. J. Anaesth., 54,* 1145.
97. Simpson PJ, Radford SG, Lockyer JA, Sear JW (1982) Some factors predisposing to Althesin hypersensitivity. *Br. J. Anaesth., 54,* 1131.
98. Howard DJ, Farag S, Liscombe RM (1982) Multiple general anaesthesia with althesin. *Brit. Med. J., 285,* 99.
99. Tachon P, Descotes J, Laschi-Locquerie et al (1983) Experimental assessment of the allergenic potential of Althesin and its constituents. *Br. J. Anaesth., 55,* 715.
100. Descotes J, Tachon P, Laschi-Locquerie A, Evreux JCl (1983) Adjuvancy of Cremophor El in rodents. *Int. Arch. Allergy Appl. Immunol., 72,* 287.
101. Cabot C, Nailhac N, Pourrut JC et al (1982) A propos de trois cas de réactions anaphylactoides per-anesthésiques. *Rev. Méd. Toulouse, 18,* 423.
102. Guidici JP, Lirzin JD (1983) Choc anaphylactique au penthiobarbital. *Cah. Anesthesiol., 31,* 49.
103. Butler JM, Kazmierowski JA, Brun RD, Hirshman CA (1982) An unusual adverse drug reaction to thiopental. *Anesthesiology, 57,* 51.
104. Lebowitz PW, Cote ME, Daniels AL et al (1982) Comparative cardiovascular effects of midazolam and thiopental in healthy patients. *Anesth. Analg., 61,* 771.
105. Twohy SA, MacEvilly MA (1982) Inadvertent injection of thipentone to the brachial plexus sheath. A case report. *Br. J. Anaesth., 54,* 355.
106. Kawar P, Dundee JW (1982) Frequency of pain on injection and venous sequelae following the iv administration of certain anaesthetics and sedatives. *Br. J. Anaesth., 54,* 935.
107. O'Callaghan AC, Normandale JP, Grundy EM et al (1982) Continuous intravenous infusion of disopropol. *Br. J. Anaesth., 37,* 295.
108. Briggs LP, Clarke RSJ, Watkins J (1982) An adverse reaction to the administration of disoprofol (Diprivan). *Br. J. Anaesth., 37,* 1099.
109. Belopavlovic M, Buchtnal A (1982) Modification of ketamine-induced intracranial hypertension in neurosurgical patients by pretreatment with midazolam. *Acta Anaesth. Scand., 26,* 458.
110. Pedersen T, Engback J, Klausen NO et al (1982) Effects of low-dose ketamine and thiopentone on cardiac performance and myocardial oxygen balance in high-risk patients. *Acta Anaesth. Scand., 26,* 235.
111. De Carvalho AF, De Souza Gouveia JD (1981) Crises convulsivas apos administraças de Quetamina en pacientes pediatrocos. *Rev. Bras. Anest., 31,* 115.
112. Burrows FA, Sceman RG (1982) Ketamine and myoclonic encephalopathy of infants (Kinsbourne syndrome). *Anesth. Analg., 61,* 873.
113. Cechherelli F, Manani G, Ambrosio F, Angel A et al (1981) Influence of acupuncture on the postoperative complications following ketamine anesthesia. *Acupuncture Eletrother. Res. Int., 6,* 255.
114. Cousin MT, Barbe D, Saclier MH, Maneglia R (1982) Anaphylactoid reaction to propanidid. Blood clotting problems. *Ann. Fr. Anésth. Réanim., 1,* 455.
115. Mantz JM, Pauli G, Meyer P et al (1982) Le choc anaphylactique. Résultats d'une enquête nationale portant sur 1047 cas. *Rev. Med. Int., 3,* 331.
116. Lewis JH, Zimmerman HJ, Ishak KG, Mullick FG (1983) Enflurane hepatotoxicity – a clinicopathologic study of 24 cases. *Ann. Int. Med., 98,* 984.
117. Turner WM (1983) Enflurane anesthesia and liver dysfunction. *F.D.R. Highlights, 83–4,* 1–2. (United States Federal Food and Drug Administration, Division of Drug Experience).

J. Descotes and J.Cl. Evreux

12 Local anesthetics

SYSTEMIC TOXICITY

Although generally considered as the main complication of local anesthesia (see SED-10), systemic toxicity is rarely severe. Nevertheless *deaths* have been attributed to local anesthetics and Lalli and Amaranath (1[c]) reported 53 such cases in which no unequivocal evidence implicating allergy could be provided. Inadvertent intravascular injection, overdosage, improper technique and management of patients were the likely causative factors according to these authors.

Drug addiction has been suggested as a *predisposing factor* to local anesthesia-related side effects in dental practice: Scheutz (2[C]) found a significant increase in the rate of anxiety, unrest, sweating, pallor, palpitation, nausea and fainting in drug addicts as compared to controls, while local anesthetic agents proved less effective, in such addicts.

Four local anesthetic drugs (bupivacaine, chloroprocaine, lidocaine and tetracaine were shown to *inhibit platelet aggregation* in vitro at toxic plasma concentrations (3).

HYPERSENSITIVITY

Allergy is an extremely rare complication of local anesthetics of the amide type (4[R], 5) and cases providing conclusive evidence for its involvement certainly do not exceed ten in the literature.

Mc D. Fisher and Pennington (6[C]) have reported one such case involving a severe anaphylactoid reaction in a 35-year-old woman following dental block with 1% lignocaine. Three months later, intradermal testing was found positive at high dilutions of lignocaine, prilocaine and tetracaine. As skin tests were negative with bupivacaine, she underwent episiotomy using 0.25% bupivacaine; there was no adverse response. These authors, like others (7[C]) advocate the use of skin testing to determine the causative drug allergen and thus avoid further hypersensitivity reactions.

Placental transfer of local anesthetics R

Anesthetists are increasingly concerned with analgesia during delivery and anesthesia in the pregnant woman as demonstrated by several recent reviews (8[R]–12[R]). In seeking to achieve safer management of the mother, the newborn and the fetus, placental transfer of local anesthetics is undoubtedly a critical factor to be reckoned with (13[R]–15[R]). Basically, however, placental transfer of local anesthetics is not different from that of unrelated drugs.

The membranes separating fetal capillary blood from maternal blood in the intervillous space resemble cell membranes elsewhere in their general permeability; foreign organic substances readily cross the placenta provided that their molecular size is less than 600 and that they are are unionized and lipid-soluble. Local anesthetics meet all these conditions and arrive in the fetal circulation with astonishing rapidity after maternal injection (16[R]). However, although amide-type agents should theoretically attain comparable maternal and fetal blood levels, this is by no means the case owing to variations in the degree to which these drugs are bound to plasma proteins. Since only unbound drug is capable of crossing the placenta, the proportion of drug gaining access to the fetal circulation will be small if maternal protein binding of the drug is high.

Moreover, several factors leading to variation in the degree of placental transfer deserve careful examination (14[R]): fetal acidosis is one, and of utmost importance.

Side Effects of Drugs Annual 8
M.N.G. Dukes, editor

ISBN 0 444 90339 9
$0.80 per article per page (transactional system)
$0.20 per article per page (licensing system)

Maternal and fetal drug concentrations normally reach a state of equilibrium and fetal drug in excess is returned to the maternal circulation via the placental barrier. However, in the event of fetal acidosis due to hypoxia or local anesthetics (e.g. lignocaine) for instance, the proportion of unionized local anesthetic decreases and higher blood levels are attained in the newborn as compared to the mother with an increased risk of developing overt toxicity. Additional variation-inducing factors comprise decreased maternal protein concentrations, changes in uterine capacity, and addition of epinephrine to an anesthetic solution(14[R]).

The fetal-to-maternal ratio of blood levels is a good indicator of placental transfer. The ratio for bupivacaine is only 0.2 owing to its high degree of plasma protein binding and bupivacaine is generally considered as particularly suited to use in obstetrics because of its long duration of action with a reduced need for subsequent reinjection (17[C], 18[C]). The same holds true for etidocaine with a ratio of 0.2. The ratio for lidocaine lies between 0.5 and 0.7. This ratio is 0.7 for mepivacaine and 1 or more for prilocaine (14[R]). Chloroprocaine readily crosses the placenta, but is so rapidly hydrolized in blood that its half-life is extremely brief and virtually no drug is capable of gaining access to the fetal circulation. Available data concerning narcotic analgesics recently introduced for regional anesthesia are scarce but suggest that potentially toxic concentrations may be attained in the newborn (19[C], 20[C]).

EFFECTS RELATED TO DIFFERENT MODES OF USE

Intraspinal narcotic analgesia

Intraspinal narcotics have been recently introduced for obstetric analgesia (SEDA-7, 134). Despite initial enthusiasm concerning their theoretical safety, side effects are not uncommon, as demonstrated by a Swedish nationwide survey (21[C]): *ventilatory depression* severe enough to necessitate naloxone administration was noted in 0.25–0.40% of patients treated with extradural morphine and in 4–7% given intrathecal morphine. Age over 70, thoracic extradural puncture and reduced ventilatory capacity were likely risk factors.

Epidural and spinal anesthesia *(22[R])*

Among 1417 parturients receiving bupivacaine, followed by 2-chloroprocaine 2 or 3% without epinephrine, only 6 (0.4%) developed temporary neurological complications, i.e *pain* and *numbness* in the lower limbs associated with motor weakness twice (23[C]). One case of *Horner's syndrome* was reported in a 21-year-old woman following 5 ml of 2% mepivacaine and 5 ml of 0.25% bupivacaine epidurally. She fully recovered within 5 days (24[C]). Cakalova et al (25[C]) observed persisting motor and sensitive block 8 days after an epidural puncture. The symptoms, due to an epidural hematoma at the level of the puncture (L3), disappeared completely after 8–9 days.

Peridural anesthesia and obstetric regional anesthesia *(26[R]–28[R])*

Stellate ganglion block

Kozody et al (29[C]) reported 2 cases of *grand mal seizures* following injection into the vertebral artery of 2.5 mg bupivacaine and 1.25 mg bupivacaine + 5 mg lidocaine. The authors reemphasize the need to avoid inadvertent injection into the vertebral artery owing to subsequent central nervous system toxicity.

Olson and Ivy (30[C]) advocated the use of stellate block for trigeminal zoster despite frequent occurrence of *hoarseness, pain* or *paresis of the ipsilateral arm.* One patient out of 27 experienced *Horner's syndrome* and one *mental confusion* probably due to inadvertent intravascular injection.

Paracervical block

Weiss et al (31[C]) compared 2-chloroprocaine for paracervical block in 60 mothers and their child. None of the 60 mothers developed side effects. *Fetal bradycardia* was noted once in the 29 chloroprocaine-treated mothers and twice in the 31 lidocaine-treated mothers.

Neuroleptanesthesia

Respiratory depression is a common complication of neuroleptanesthesia particularly when fentanyl and droperidol are used. The respiratory depressant effects of the latter drug can recur after having dissipated as reported in a 20-year-old healthy male who recovered following use of naloxone (32[C]).

Retzke et al (33[C]), after studying the cardiovascular effects of neuroleptanesthesia with 2.5 mg droperidol and 0.05 mg fentanyl in 10 healthy pregnant women concluded that the observed decrease in mean arterial pressure and elevation of cardiac output does not deserve particular attention except when it subsequently proves necessary to induce general anesthesia.

Regional intravenous anesthesia

Systemic toxic reactions are the commonest complication of this technique, initially proposed by Bier. Choice of the safest agent is critical as shown by a prospective randomized study which demonstrated that prilocaine was significantly less toxic than bupivacaine. Doses of the latter exceeding 1 mg/kg should be avoided because of excessive risk (34[C]). However, intravenous regional anesthesia should be considered a particularly hazardous technique; 5 deaths have been reported to the British health authorities since 1979 (35[C]).

EFFECTS RELATED TO INDIVIDUAL DRUGS

Bupivacaine

In a clinical evaluation of 371 patients undergoing lumbar epidural anesthesia with bupivacaine 0.75%, *nausea* and *vomiting* proved the commonest side effects. Only 2 patients developed *respiratory* and *circulatory complications* probably due to inadequate dural puncture (36[C]).

Cardiotoxicity is an important potential complication of bupivacaine use. Gould and Aldrete (37[C]) have reported one case of severe bradycardia and hypotension in a 52-year-old man with chronic renal failure following injection of bupivacaine (250 mg) for axillary block. Hyperkalemia and acidosis appeared to play a critical role. Hyperbaric bupivacaine, with its mean duration of action of 6.5 hours, proved satisfactory in 61 low-risk patients undergoing spinal anesthesia: only 4 became moderately hypotensive (38[C]). Dysrhythmia is another manifestation of bupivacaine cardiotoxicity as demonstrated in a 77-year-old man who experienced a trial fibrillation following epidural administration of 20 ml of 0.5% bupivacaine. This dysrhythmia persisted until the termination of anesthesia (39[C]). Conklin and Ziadlou-Rad have described a case of ventricular tachycardia requiring cardioversion (54[C]); in their patient excessively rapid administration of a large epidural dose (20 ml) or simultaneous use of succinylcholine (which can raise serum potassium) may have increased the risk.

Respiratory failure is another possible unwanted consequence of bupivacaine: delayed respiratory arrest was described in a 45-year-old healthy man following the use of 40 ml of 0.5% bupivacaine for brachial plexus block (40). Smith (41[R]) stressed the potential risk of respiratory arrest after retrobulbar bupivacaine.

Venous leakage under the tourniquet cuff during a Bier block can result in severe systemic toxicity as exemplified by a 71-year-old man who developed severe bradycardia, hypotension and convulsions 2 minutes after i.v. regional anesthesia with 80 ml of 0.25% bupivacaine (42[C]).

Malignant priapism is a possible, although very rare, complication of bupivacaine infiltration of the dorsal nerves of the penis (43[C]).

Centbucridine

Centbucridine is a new quinoline derivative with local anesthetic action (44). Saxin et al (45[C]) compared 0.5% centbucridine with 2% lidocaine in a double-blind randomized study of 87 patients and concluded that centbucridine may have fewer cardiovascular side effects.

Chloroprocaine

The potential *neurotoxicity* of chloroprocaine is still a matter of controversy (46[R], 47) although basically no really new data has become available.

Abnormality of pseudocholinesterase, the enzyme which rapidly hydrolyses 2-chloroprocaine, is a factor in *prolonged duration of action* and hence of possible toxicity as shown in a 31-year-old woman who experienced prolonged epidural block after 25 ml of 3% chloroprocaine (48[C]).

Cinchocaine

Two children developed severe *neurological* and *cardiovascular disturbance* with the adult respiratory distress syndrome following cinchocaine overdose. Both required intensive care for a period of 6–15 days and fully recovered (49[C]).

Lidocaine

Adult *respiratory distress syndrome* is an extremely rare hypersensitivity reaction to lidocaine: Howard et al (50[C]) reported one such case with rechallenge in a 57-year-old woman who developed the adult respiratory distress syndrome following 5 ml of 4% lidocaine by ultrasonic nebulization, then again days later after inadvertent subcutaneous injection of 0.5 ml of 1% lidocaine. She fully recovered, but another 19-year-old woman died in the course of a similar reaction after 30 ml of 1% lidocaine had been employed for topical anesthesia during fiberoptic bronchoscopy (51[C]). A third (but non-fatal) case has been described by Woelke and Tucker in a woman who received 5 ml of 1% lidocaine without adrenaline for a skin suture (55[C]).

Convulsions are well-known side effects of local anesthetics. Moreover, epinephrine injection into the subarachnoid space in conjunction with lidocaine spinal anesthesia may cause spinal cord ischemia with resultant transient and localized seizures as reported by Nadkarni and Tondare (52[C]).

Prilocaine

One case of *hypersensitivity* to prilocaine has been reported in a 46-year-old woman who complained of nausea, unsteadiness and loss of motor power. Intradermal testing showed a wheal and flare reaction to prilocaine alone (53[C]).

REFERENCES

1. Lalli AF, Amaranath L (1982) A critique on mortality associated with local anesthetics. *Anesthesiol. Rev., 9,* 29.
2. Scheutz F (1982) Drug addicts and local analgesia-efficacy and general side-effects. *Scand. J. Dent. Res., 90,* 299.
3. Gotta AW, Sullivan CA (1982) Local anaesthetics inhibit platelet aggregation. *Canad. Anaesth. Soc. J., 29,* 497.
4. Leynadier F, Pujade-Lauraine MD, Dry J (1983) La place de l'allergie dans les accidents des anesthésiques locaux. *Rev. Méd., 24,* 349.
5. Lampe KF (1982) Allergic hypersensitivity to local anaesthetics. *J. Am. Med. Assoc., 247,* 2155.
6. McD Fisher M, Pennington JC (1982) Allergy to local anaesthesia. *Br. J. Anaesth., 54,* 893.
7. Barrer MR, MacAllen MK (1982) Hypersensitivity to local anaesthetics: a direct challenge test with lignocaine for definitive diagnosis. *Br. Med. J., 284,* 1229.
8. Perriss BW (1981) Analgesia and anaesthesia. *Clin. Obstet. Gynecol., 8,* 475.
9. Schider SM (1981) Choice of anaesthesia for labor and delivery. *Obstet. Gynecol., 58,* 24 S.
10. Redick LF (1982) Epidural analgesia. *Clin. Perinatol., 9,* 63.
11. Abouleish E (1982) Anaesthesia for the high-risk parturient. *Sem. Anesth., 1,* 133.
12. Clark RB, Seifen AB (1982) Complications of obstetrical anaesthesia. *Sem. Anesth., 1,* 155.
13. Garstka G, Stoeckel H (1978) Diaplazentarer Transfer von Lokalanästhetika. *Prakt. Anästh., 13,* 1.
14. Yurth DA (1982) Placenta transfer of local anesthetics. *Clin. Perinatol., 9,* 13.
15. Rietbrok I (1981) Plazentarer Transport von Anästhetika. *Anästhesiol. Intensivmed, 11,* 337.
16. Endler GC (1980) Conduction anaesthesia in obstetrics and its effects upon fetus and newborn. *J. Reprod. Med., 24,* 83.
17. Scebacker J, Chareire F, Galli-Doriant P, Viars P (1978) L'utilisation de la marcaine en analgésie obstétricale. *Ann. Anesth. Fr., 19,* 247.
18. Moore DC, Bridenbaugh LD, Bridenbaugh PO (1971) Bupivacaine hydrochloride: summary of investigational use in 3274 cases. *Anesth. Analg., 50,* 856.
19. Bonnardot JP, Maillet M, Colan JC et al (1982) Maternal and fetal concentration of morphine after intrathecal administration during labour. *Br. J. Anaesth., 54,* 487.
20. Cravey RH, Reed D (1981) Placental transfer of narcotic analgesics in man. *Clin. Toxicol., 18,* 911.
21. Gustafsson LL, Schildt B, Jacobsen K (1982) Adverse effects of extradural and intrathecal opiates: report of a nationwide survey in Sweden. *Br. J. Anaesth., 54,* 479.
22. Redick LF (1982) Epidural analgesia. *Clin. Perinatol., 9,* 63.
23. Abouleish E (1982) Neurologic complications following epidural analgesia in obstetrics. One Centers experience. *Regional Anesth., 7,* 119.
24. Torres Morera LM (1982) Sindrome de Horner tras una anaestesia epidural. *Rev. Esp. Anestesiol. Reanim., 29,* 212.
25. Cakalova E, Smilor I, Minceva-Saeva M (1982) A rare complication of epidural analgesia in gynecologic operations. *Akus Ginekol., 21,* 422.
26. Clark RB, Seifen AB (1982) Complications of

obstetrical anesthesia. *Sem. Anaesth.*, *1*, 155.
27. Abouleish E (1982) Anesthesia for the high-risk parturient. *Sem. Anaesth.*, *1*, 133.
28. Barrier G, Sureau C (1982) Effects of anaesthetic and analgesic drugs on labour, fetus and neonate. *Clin. Gynecol. Obstet.*, *9*, 351.
29. Kozody R, Ready LB, Barsa JE, Murphy TM (1982) Dose requirement of local anesthetic to produce grand mal seizure during stellate ganglion block. *Canad. Anaesth. Soc. J.*, *29*, 489.
30. Olson ER, Ivy EB (1981) Stellate block for trigeminal zoster. *J. Clin. Neuro-Ophthalmol.*, *1*, 53.
31. Weiss RR, Halevy S, Almonte RO et al (1983) Comparison of lidocaine and 2-chlorprocaine in paracervical block: clinical effects and drug concentrations in mother and child. *Anesth. Analg.*, *62*, 168.
32. Rich JM (1982) Biphasic respiratory depression from neurolept anesthesia. *J. Am. Assoc. Nurse Anesth.*, *50*, 472.
33. Retzke U, Schwarz R, Lauckner W (1982) Kardiovaskulare Veränderungen während der kleinen Neuroleptanalgesie in der Geburtshilfe. *Anaesthesiol. Reanim.*, *7*, 327.
34. Tryba M, Hausmann E, Zens M, Wellköner HH (1982) Toxizität von Prilocain und Bupivacain in der intravenösen Regionalanästhesie. *Anästh. Intensivther. Notfallmed.*, *17*, 207.
35. Heath ML (1982) Deaths after intravenous regional anaesthesia. *Br. Med. J.*, *285*, 913.
36. Jörgensen H (1982) Lumbar epidural anaesthesia with bupivacaine 0.75%. *Regional Anaesthesiol.*, *5*, 30.
37. Gould DB, Aldrete JA (1983) Bupivacaine cardiotoxicity in a patient with renal failure. *Acta Anaesthesiol. Scand.*, *27*, 18.
38. Holloway AH, Brock-Utne JG, Dowxing JW (1982) Hyperbaric bupivacaine for spinal analgesia. *S. Afr. Med. J.*, *61*, 314.
39. Pratila MG, Pratilas V (1982) Dysrhythmia occurring during epidural anaesthesia with bupivacaine. *Mount Sinai J. Med.*, *49*, 130.
40. Lauckner ME (1982) Delayed respiratory arrest after bupivacaine. *Anaesthesiology*, *37*, 697.
41. Smith JL (1982) Retrobulbar bupivacaine can cause respiratory arrest. *Ann. Ophthalmol.*, *14*, 1005.
42. Rosenberg PH, Kalso EA, Tuomisien MK, Linden HB (1983) Acute bupivacaine toxicity as a result of venous leakage under the tourniquet cuff during a Bier block. *Anesthesiology*, *58*, 95.
43. Wilson F, Staff WG (1982) Malignant priapism: an unexpected response to local anaesthetic infiltration of the dorsal nerves of the penis. *Br. J. Surg.*, *69*, 469.
44. Gupta PP, Tangri AN, Saxena RC, Dhawan BN (1982) Clinical pharmacology studies on 4-N-butylamino-1,2,3,4-tetrahydroacridine hydrochloride (centbucridine) a new local anaesthetic agent. *Indian J. Exp. Biol.*, *20*, 344.
45. Samsi AB, Bhalerao RA, Shah SC et al (1983) Evaluation of Centbucridine as a local anaesthetic. *Anesth. Analg.*, *62*, 109.
46. Covino BG (1983) Potential neurotoxicity of local anaesthetic agents. *Canad. Anaesth. Soc. J.*, *30*, 111.
47. Riggi SJ (1982) Chlorprocaine: neurotoxicity and formulations in perspective. *Anesth. Analg.*, *61*, 715.
48. Kuhxert BR, Philipson EH, Pimental R, Kuhnert PP (1982) A prolonged chloroprocaine epidural block in a postpartum patient with abnormal pseudocholinesterase. *Anesthesiology*, *56*, 477.
49. Sutter M, Pfenninger J (1982) Adult respiratory Distress Syndrome nach Intoxikation durch Lokalanästhetika. *Schweiz. Med. Wochenschr.*, *112*, 1710.
50. Howard JJ, Mohsenifar Z, Simons SM (1982) Adult respiratory distress syndrome following administration of lidocain. *Chest*, *81*, 644.
51. Promisloff RA, Dupont DC (1983) Death from ARDS and cardiovascular collapse following lidocaine administration. *Chest*, *83*, 585.
52. Nadkarni AV, Tondare AS (1982) Localized clonic convulsions after anesthesia with lidocaine and epinephrine. *Anesth. Analg.*, *61*, 945.
53. Yeoman CM (1982) Hypersensitivity to prilocaine. *Br. Dent. J.*, *153*, 69.
54. Conklin KA, Ziadlou-Rad F (1983) Bupivacaine cardiotoxicity in a pregnant patient with mitral valve prolapse. *Anesthesiology*, *58*, 596.
55. Woelke RJ, Tucker RA (1983) Lignocaine. Adult respiratory distress syndrome. *Chest*, *83*, 933.

F.J. Richardson and S.A. Agoston

13 Muscle relaxants

Immune reactions and histamine release

Immune responses and histamine release are of prime importance in many of the adverse reactions to intravenous drugs and fluids administered during anesthesia. Serious life-threatening anaphylactoid reactions are assessed as occurring in between 1 in 1 000 and 1 in 10,000 anesthesias, but minor reactions probably occur in 1% or more of patients and many of these go unnoticed. The extent to which neuromuscular blocking agents contribute to this incidence is unknown, though almost all have been claimed to have caused "anaphylaxis", and "anaphylactoid" or "allergic" reactions. The difficulties in diagnosis begin with the confusing terminology, and are compounded by the simultaneous use of several drugs and fluids during anesthesia and by the multitude of differential diagnoses which might all account for the modified signs of these reactions under the conditions of anesthesia. Furthermore, confirming or refuting a suspicion that a particular drug has been responsible for an anaphylactoid reaction is hampered by the lack of reliable specific tests. Skin testing is most commonly used, but can be highly misleading, particularly where neuromuscular blocking agents are concerned. d-Tubocurarine, for example, is well known as the muscle relaxant which most often gives rise to reactions mediated by histamine release (SEDA-7, 140), but skin testing yields many false positive histamine-release phenomena with this agent, the majority of "skin reactors" showing no adverse systemic effects when d-tubocurarine is injected intravenously.

In the last 2 years there have been some publications which attempt to put the problems in perspective and to increase the accuracy of diagnosis. A paper by Laxenaire et al (1[Cr]) reviews 18 cases of anaphylaxis produced by suxamethonium in eastern France over a 9-year period, describing the incidence of the various presenting signs and the associated factors in relation to the general population. In addition he discusses a battery of suitable tests and when they should be carried out to confirm the diagnosis. Cardiovascular collapse accompanied by sinus tachycardia was the presenting sign in more than 70% of the patients; bronchospasm was seen in only a third of the cases; cardiac arrest occurred in 5 of the 18 patients. While mucocutaneous manifestations were present in 72% of the cases, these were often only noticed later, after circulatory resuscitation. Of the associated factors, a history of a previous drug reaction was claimed to increase the likelihood of a subsequent reaction 4-fold. 16 patients were women, supporting an increased risk for females. Spasmophilia and skin hyperreactivity to histamine were also significantly increased in comparison to the general population. The best time for performing diagnosic tests was considered to be between 6 weeks and 3 months after the incident. Three tests were chosen as most satisfactory – the intradermal injection of the drug concerned (in this case suxamethonium) and other drugs possibly responsible for the reaction, plus control and histamine injections for hyperreactivity, the Prausnitz-Kustner test, and the human basophil degranulation test. For confirmation of an anaphylactoid reaction 2 of the 3 tests had to be positive, and, if only 1 was, then they were repeated a month later. In the prevention of anaphylactoid reactions Laxenaire et al advocate the taking of careful preoperative case histories in regard to previous reactions, issuing "allergy" cards – a measure already practised in many coun-

Side Effects of Drugs Annual 8
M.N.G. Dukes, editor

ISBN 0 444 90339 9
$0.80 per article per page (transactional system)
$0.20 per article per page (licensing system)

tries – and a reduction in the use of suxamethonium, avoiding its use particularly during 2 consecutive anesthetics. In the case of closely repeated anesthetics it is advisable to vary the drugs used so as to avoid the production of antibodies.

Diagnostic procedures in cases where such reactions are suspected have been summarized in a short report from the same authors (2[r]) which also includes details on the blood samples (one put into EDTA for complement assays and the other into heparin for hematology and serology other than complement) which should be taken as soon as possible and repeated at 1, 6, 24 and 72 hours after the incident.

Further discussions on the topics of the assessment of complement involvement (3) and the study of human basophils (4) in anaphylactoid reactions, together with full suggestions for the immunological and allergological investigation of reactions during anesthesia (5) and the assay of plasma histamine (6) emanated from a workshop on the subject of immuno-allergology and anesthesia held in Nancy in 1982. Another symposium on "histamine and antihistamines in anesthesia and surgery" (7[CR]) has been reported on by Thornton and Lorenz (8).

In clinical studies involving conscious volunteers and orthopedic patients Lorenz et al (9[Cr]) studied the symptoms and signs produced by the intravenous injection of histamine and the response to polygeline(Haemaccel)-induced histamine release and correlated these with plasma histamine levels, determined by means of a fluorometric-fluoroenzymatic assay. Systemic anaphylactoid reactions were associated with plasma histamine levels greater than 1 ng/ml. Levels above 1 ng/ml were defined as pathological. Tachycardia was the most frequent sign of a reaction in both groups, with flushing or wheals being the commonest cutaneous manifestation in the histamine-injection or polygeline group respectively.

According to Moss et al (10[C]) plasma histamine levels correlate in a positive fashion with the dose and rate of administration of d-tubocurarine and some other neuromuscular blocking agents and with the resulting fall in blood pressure and rise in heart rate. The clinical implications are that agents known to give rise to allergoid or anaphylactoid reactions should be injected slowly and in the smallest dosage commensurate with the desired effect – as concluded in SEDA-7, p. 141. Finally, on this subject Stoelting (11[R]) reviews 'allergic reactions during anesthesia', covering the mechanisms, treatment and diagnosis and discussing the drugs, including muscle relaxants, and intravenous fluids associated with allergic reactions in anesthesia in an easily assimilable way, although his opinions, particularly in the treatment section, may not always be the generally accepted ones.

DEPOLARIZING NEUROMUSCULAR BLOCKING AGENTS

Suxamethonium

An unusual presentation of a *possible anaphylactoid reaction* to suxamethonium is described by Cohen et al (14[C]). *Upper airway edema* producing respiratory distress was seen postoperatively in a young patient following detubation after an emergency Caesarean section. Laryngoscopy revealed 'marked edema of palate, pharynx and larynx; moderate swelling of lips and eyelids was also evident'. No cardiovascular effects, skin rash or bronchospasm were present. Skin testing was negative for all the agents used except suxamethonium, which gave a strongly positive reaction. There were predisposing factors present, namely, a history of asthma and previous penicillin allergy. The authors point out that two previously reported cases with upper-airway edema were accompanied by other more usual signs of anaphylactoid reactions; they were also both 'allergic' for penicillin. In the present case the hypervolemia and relative hypoproteinemia of pregnancy may have aggravated the edema.

There are of course some centers which have accumulated much experience with anaphylactic reactions attributed to suxamethonium. Vervloet et al (51[C]) have presented data on reactions in 41 patients, all but 5 of these having had anesthesia on a previous occasion. They found positive skin reactions to suxamethonium in the treated patients but not in controls.

The paper on 18 cases of suxamethonium-induced *anaphylactic shock* by Laxenaire et al (1[Cr]) is reported on in the introduction, in the section on immune responses and histamine release. It is worth commenting here that 15 of the patients received *suxamethonium iodide* and only 3 the *chloride*. Does the use of suxamethonium *iodide* increase the risk of an anaphylactoid reaction developing?

An exceptionally *long-lasting phase-II block* following suxamethonium, in a patient with a probable $E^u_1E^a_1$ genotype, is reported (15[C]). The patient, a middle-aged healthy woman of 59 kg, was operated on for correction of a maxillo-mandibular dysplasia. She was not taking any drugs. Anesthesia was induced with thiopental and intubation facilitated by suxamethonium 150 mg, preceded by d-tubocurarine 3 mg. Small doses of fentanyl and droperidol together with nitrous oxide-oxygen and 0.5% halothane with controlled ventilation were used to maintain anesthesia. Cardiovascular parameters were adequate throughout. No spontaneous respiratory efforts could be elicited at the end of the operation, even after 0.4 mg naloxone and 40 mg doxapram. A phase-II block "in the non-depolarizing stage" was demonstrated by ulnar nerve stimulation. Extubation was only possible about 9.5 h after the administration of suxamethonium. Plasma cholinesterase was 17 Warburg units (normal (44–90 units) and the dibucaine number was 67 (normal 80). The patient had been given suxamethonium (100 mg) during a previous operation which lasted about 2 hours, but showed no muscle weakness on that occasion. Barring the accidental administration of additional relaxants, the explanation for this unusually prolonged phase-II block remains obscure.

Hyperkalemia following the injection of suxamethonium is a well-known side effect which can be life-threatening in certain circumstances (SED-10, Ch 13; SEDA-4, 89; SEDA-5, 134; SEDA-6, 128). Its association with *severe intra-abdominal infection* was described by Kohlschütter (16[C]) and is now confirmed by Popović (17[Cr]) and Khan (18[C]). Popović describes 18 cases with *severe and prolonged intra-abdominal infection* in whom the serum potassium rose from a mean of 5.23 ± 0.18 to 7.14 ± 0.22 mmol/l in 3–6 min following the injection of suxamethonium 1 mg/kg. Kahn, measuring potassium after 1.5 mg/kg suxamethonium in 21 control patients and 21 patients with infections of varying severity (acute or chronic osteomyelitis, gangrene of a limb, and one case of amebic liver abscess), found that there was a significant rise in the infected patients but not in the controls. 7 of the infected patients had increases of 1 meq/l or more and one patient exhibited a rise of 2.3 meq/l. In the control patients the maximum increase was 0.4 meq/l. Furthermore, he reports that the increase was proportional to the severity of the infection and was greater in those with infections of 8–21 days' duration. The circumstances in this report are somewhat different from the others in that almost all of these patients had *infections other than intra-abdominal.*

Rhabdomyolysis and myoglobinuria, particularly in children and in combination with the use of halothane, are featuring increasingly in reports on adverse reactions to suxamethonium (see also SEDA-3, 114). McKishnie et al (19[Cr]) describe a case involving a previously healthy 3-year-old boy, who developed *myoglobinuria and renal failure* after an otherwise uneventful anesthesia (suxamethonium 1 mg/kg, with nitrous oxide/oxygen/halothane) for orchidopexy. No temperature elevation was noted at any time. Features often commonly associated with rhabdomyolysis, as the authors found from their survey of 12 similar reports, were also present. There was a history of myopathy in the family (two maternal uncles had muscular dystrophy of the Duchenne type), the child had a massively-elevated serum CPK, 1000 times normal, later falling to levels of 12–60 times normal), was male, and received suxamethonium and halothane. No muscle biopsy was done, but while recovering from renal failure, the boy was observed to display muscle *weakness characteristic of Duchenne muscular dystrophy.* The authors postulate that patients with underlying myopathies may be more susceptible to muscle injury caused by depolarizing agents.

The suggestion that *rhabdomyolysis and malignant hyperthermia (MH)* may represent different degrees of severity of a syndrome involving muscle damage resulting from the use of certain triggering agents in susceptible patients is still further supported by three other reports. One (20[C]) is entitled 'Four cases suspected of *malignant hyperthermia* induced by halothane and succinylcholine' and describes 4 infants who developed *myoglobinuria*, together with *raised CPK* and other enzymes, all 'without high fever' and the operations were completed without remarkable problems. Although muscular rigidity was seen in 3 of the cases and (electron) microscopic abnormalities are described, this sounds more like rhabdomyolysis than MH.

Lewandowski (21[Cr]) presents a case in which an apparently healthy 6-year-old boy was anesthetized for correction of strabismus.

Halothane and suxamethonium (1.5 mg/kg) were both used. Intubation was difficult due to *stiffness of the jaw.* Tachycardia occurred and later ventricular and supraventricular extrasystoles developed. Cyanosis was not present. An hour postoperatively the child was still not awake, the *tachycardia persisted,* and *stiffness of the extended limbs was present.* Rectal temperature at this stage was 37.8°C and there was a slight metabolic acidosis; serum potassium and sodium were normal. He was treated with surface cooling and bicarbonate. Serum CPK, aldolase and LDH were elevated: oliguria was treated with furosemide and fluids; *large amounts of myoglobin* were found in the urine. *On recovery, muscle weakness,* initially with inability to walk, lasted 2 days. An EMG was normal. The strabismus in the patient himself, together with strabismus and minimal scoliosis in his brothers, and Duchenne dystrophy in a distant relative led to the conclusion that the patient (and his family) were affected by *subclinical myopathy*, and thus 'prone to MH and/or rhabdomyolysis'.

Incomplete relaxation after suxamethonium, rigidity, or unexplained tachycardia are emphasized as possible warning signs of rhabdomyolysis or MH.

Linter et al (22[C]) describe a case with a more serious outcome.

Again, a young boy for squint correction, given both halothane (plus nitrous oxide/cyclopropane) and suxamethonium, and who immediately developed *hypertonicity.* On this occasion *inability to ventilate* the patient led to cyanosis and *asystole.* Resuscitation was successful. Serum potassium was almost normal and the temperature was at no time raised. Although he was alert and talking 6 hours later, *tachycardia* persisted, together with acidosis and, due to diminishing spontaneous ventilatory ability, he required artificial ventilation for 4 days. Despite bicarbonate infusions acidosis persisted for two days. *CPK was greatly increased,* and was still raised (10,000 I.U.) on the 10th day. Striking features were that physiotherapy was required for *progressive foot drop* and his *calves became hypertrophic* during his early recovery period, and that later he could only rise from the floor by climbing up his legs and had a *typical Duchenne walk.* The diagnosis of *pseudohypertrophic muscular dystrophy* was subsequently confirmed by muscle biopsy and EMG.

Many of the features in this case, as in the others, could be attributed to MH or rhabdomyolysis – although myoglobinuria was not apparently looked for here. The apparent 'precipitation' of muscular dystrophy is unsettling. Consideration should be carefully given to avoiding the use of suxamethonium, particularly in combination with halothane, in (male) children – as in adults – if there are any signs or symptoms in the patient or his family, distant relatives included, of possible (sub)clinical myopathy. The potential dangers of using non-depolarizing agents, such as the shorter-acting vecuronium or atracurium, in place of suxamethonium need to be re-assessed.

Various *methods for prevention of the unwanted side effects of suxamethonium* have been tried (SED-10, Ch 13; SEDA-2, 117; SEDA-4, 89; SEDA-5, 135, 136; SEDA-6, 129, 130; SEDA-7, 147). None of them is always successful. Recently, Cozanitis et al (23[C]) have reported on a trial in 60 patients aged 6–56 years with *strabismus*, comparing four previously described methods with respect to the *severity of fasciculations, and rises in serum potassium and CPK.* The four methods were (1) suxamethonium 1 mg/kg i.v. over 3 sec, (2) suxamethonium 0.14 mg/kg injected 45–60 sec before suxamethonium 1 mg/kg given over 5 sec (the 'self-taming' method), (3) suxamethonium 0.6 mg/kg given over 30 sec into a fast-running glucose solution, and (4) d-tubocurarine 0.05 mg/kg, followed by thiopentone and then immediately (3 min after the d-tubocurarine) suxamethonium 1.5 mg/kg given over 3 sec. The last method was by far the best, producing the lowest incidence (still 13.3%) of adverse grades of fasciculations. CPK rose in all groups, the mean increase being lowest (though not significantly so) in the last group where the range was also smallest. The 'self-taming' method produced cardiac slowing in two-thirds of the patients, but the extent is not reported. A surprising finding, contrasting with previous studies using similar methods, was the *very small rise in serum potassium* found in all groups. In the first group, for example, the serum potassium rose from 4.11 ± 0.35 mmol/l (mean ± SD) to a maximum of 4.22 ± 0.23 10 min after injection of the suxamethonium. It is suggested in the paper that this may correlate with some biochemical muscle abnormality in patients with strabismus (24[C]). More detailed studies on this aspect of suxamethonium and (possible) muscle disease are needed before it can be concluded if there is any foundation in this hypothesis or not.

Another method is described (25[C]) for the *prevention of post-suxamethonium myalgia* which seems to be effective. 10 ml of *calcium gluconate* 10% were injected intravenously immediately before thiopentone and suxamethonium 100 mg in 40 healthy adult patients. The incidence of myalgia (5%) was significantly less than that (45%) in a control group of patients given only thiopentone and suxamethonium. Significant rises in serum potassium at 2 min, seen in the control patients who subsequently developed muscle pains, were not observed in any of the calcium-treated patients, whether they complained of myalgia or not. A membrane-stabilizing effect of calcium is postulated as a possible explanation of these findings.

An interesting case report (26[C]), illustrative of *organophosphorus poisoning*, comes from Bloemfontein in South Africa, where they have a local experience of about 30 cases every year.

The patient was 34–35 weeks *pregnant. Plasma cholinesterase and (red cell) acetylcholinesterase activities 'were essentially zero'.* Caesarean section was performed 11 hours after admission because optimal atropine therapy for the mother produced unacceptable tachycardia in the fetus. Suxamethonium (30 mg) was given and 11 min later a *floppy baby* was delivered with an Apgar score of 3 at 1 min. His cholinesterase activities were less than 2% of normal. Subsequently, the mother failed to breathe spontaneously and both she and the baby required artificial ventilation, the mother for 8 days, the baby for 2 days. Atropine therapy for the effects of organophosphorus poisoning was given to the mother for 11 days and to the neonate for 8 days. The contribution of the maternal suxamethonium to the durations of ventilatory insufficiency in mother and baby cannot be assessed since, unfortunately, neuromuscular transmission was not monitored.

In their discussion the authors suggest that the virtual absence of plasmacholinesterase activity in the mother might have led to higher than usual amounts of suxamethonium being available for transfer to the fetus, who also had an extreme deficiency of the normal enzyme necessary for its hydrolysis. Organophosphorus compounds, they also point out, are highly lipid soluble and can easily cross the placenta to affect the fetus. However, it is possible that high amounts of acetylcholinesterase and plasmacholinesterase in the placenta may have reduced the amounts of the cholinesterase inhibitor transferred to the fetus. Cholinesterase activities recovered more quickly in the neonate than in the mother, though they were still below normal when both were discharged. No geno-typing was done, so the possibility that the mother or baby might also have an atypical cholinesterase is not excluded.

The varied *interactions between depolarizing and non-depolarizing neuromuscular blocking agents* are well known (SED-10, Ch 13). The potentiation of a subsequently administered non-depolarizer by an intubation dose of suxamethonium is seen daily by most anesthetists. It is often believed, however, that this potentiation occurs only if the non-depolarizing agent is given within a short time of the suxamethonium. A paper by D'Hollander et al (27[C]) clearly shows this belief to be erroneous. Following suxamethonium 1 mg/kg i.v. the isometric twitch tension of the indirectly stimulated adductor pollicis muscle was allowed to recover fully and 0.04 mg/kg vecuronium was given 5, 15 or 30 min later. *Even 30 min after apparent full recovery from the suxamethonium the block produced by vecuronium was significantly potentiated and recovery was prolonged* (the effects being approximately doubled); the onset was also significantly faster. These effects almost certainly apply to all non-depolarizing neuromuscular blocking agents and imply that their doses can be reduced when they are given up to half-an-hour – and, possibly, much longer – after suxamethonium. Dose-response studies of relaxants performed 'after full recovery from suxamethonium' may well overestimate the response (degree of blockade) produced by a given dose of a non-depolarizing relaxant.

NON-DEPOLARIZING NEUROMUSCULAR BLOCKING AGENTS

Increased dosage requirements in patients with burns have already been shown for *d-tubocurarine* (28[C]). Plasma concentrations 5 times greater than normal were required to achieve a given twitch height depression. The cause of this resistance does not appear to be altered pharmacokinetics (29[C]). Martyn et al (30[C]) further report on *metocurine requirements in burned pediatric patients.* They found that, in comparison with non-burned children, *2–3 times greater doses were required* for a given degree of neuromuscular blockade and that a given degree of recovery occurred at plasma levels twice as great. Recovery times (5–25% of control twitch heights) were not different from those in the non-burned children. Increased plasma protein binding (31) was insufficient to account for the increased dosage requirements. Various possible mechanisms are discussed, an increased number of acetylcholine receptors being one possible explanation.

In another paper Martyn et al (32[C]) present a case of a child who was anesthetized on several occasions spread over a 15-month period after he suffered 35% body surface area burns. He was always anesthetized in a similar fashion and received *metocurine* for muscle relaxation. Dose-response (paralysis) and plasma concentration-effect relationships were obtained on each occasion. His dose requirements (for 95% twitch height depression) decreased over this period from 12 to 2 times those of a control group of non-burned children. Plasma concentrations for given degrees of block were also initially much higher than normal and subsequently fell to normal during the observation period, rising again, inconsistently, on the last admission. This case shows that *increased dose requirements for non-depolarizing relaxants may persist more than a year after complete burn coverage.* It also raised the *suggestion* that, if a common underlying mechanism exists, *the danger of a hyperkalemic response to depolarizing agents may also last 15 months or more after burns.*

Sarubin (33[C]) reports that the dosage requirements of *alcuronium* are also increased in burned patients. The increase (about 70%) was not as striking as in the cases for d-tubocurarine or metocurine. However, the skin area involved here was rather small (17.5% mean). His 12 patients were operated on 7–21 days after the injury for the excision of necrotic skin and skin-grafting. It is not clear if necrosis/infection could have contributed to the results obtained.

2 cases are reported by Yamashita et al (34[C]) who suggest that *resistance to pancuronium* also occurs in burned patients. The requirements for pancuronium were based on clinical observations and were not, considering the apparently light anesthesia levels, exceedingly high. One patient required 25 mg during an operation lasting more than 6 hours, the other 13 mg over 8⅓ hours. Nevertheless, it seems likely that burned patients require higher doses of non-depolarizing agents in general.

There have been few other recent papers of note on side effects or interactions of non-depolarizing relaxants that have not been previously reported. Atracurium, being a new agent has, however, received considerable attention.

Atracurium *(SED-10, Ch 13; SEDA-5, 134; SEDA-7, 146).*

Histamine release with atracurium is, according to animal experiments, highly unlikely in the clinical dose-range (35), although there are occasional references in several studies to signs which could be attributable to this. Basta et al (36[C]) confirmed the expected cardiovascular stability under thiopentone/fentanyl/nitrous oxide anesthesia, reporting atracurium to be more favorable than metocurine. However, at higher doses (0.5 and 0.6 mg/kg) *arterial pressure decreased* 13% and 20% *and heart rate increased* 5% and 8% respectively. These effects were maximal 1–1.5 min after the injection of atracurium and lasted less than 5 min. They 'were (often) associated with *slight facial flushing'*, suggesting that they may have resulted from histamine release. Hunter et al (37[c]), using doses of 0.5 mg/kg for intubation, observed *minimal cardiovascular changes* and no adverse reactions, but also noted that in 3 (out of 25) patients a *transient flush* was seen over the face and shoulders which cleared within 2–3 min – unaccompanied by any change in arterial pressure.

Comparing skin induration and redness resulting from *intradermal injections of vecuronium, atracurium and d-tubocurarine* in 6 awake male volunteers, Robertson et al (38[C]) found that atracurium and d-tubocurarine were almost indistinguishable in their reactions and vecuronium caused a significantly smaller response. Basta et al (39[C]) measured *plasma histamine levels* in 40 patients given a 5-sec bolus of atracurium and in 28 given metocurine; twitch height depression, heart rate and blood pressure were also measured. The maximal cardiovascular changes occurred at 1–2 min and returned to normal by 5 min. The lowest doses which produced *significant cardiovascular effects* were *0.6 mg/kg for atracurium* and 0.5 mg/kg for metocurine (and 0.5 mg/kg for d-tubocurarine, from an earlier study). At this dose level for atracurium the mean arterial pressure was 79.5% and the heart rate 108.3% of the control values (in 10 patients); the plasma histamine was 192% of control. They conclude that the ability of atracurium to release histamine, relative to its neuromuscular blocking potency, is approximately one-half that of metocurine and less than one-third that of d-tubocurarine.

One case of *possible atracurium-induced bronchospasm* has been reported (40[C]). The patient was on chronic phenytoin therapy for epilepsy. He received thiopentone 7 mg/kg and atracurium 0.5 mg/kg and bronchospasm was first noticed some 2–3 min later, after intubation. It resolved quickly with halothane. A local weal-and-flare reaction at the injection site was present and skin tests during the operation (using rather high concentrations of various agents) were (strongly) positive for atracurium alone. Atracurium is perhaps not the agent of choice for patients with asthma or a tendency to allergic responses.

According to an in vitro study in the guinea pig (41) atracurium is most *unlikely to produce effects from ganglion blockade.* In comparison with d-tubocurarine, its ganglion blocking potency is 5 times less.

As regards its effects upon the heart rate Carter has reported on 4 cases of severe bradycardia during surgery in patients receiving atracurium in doses somewhat higher than those usually employed. In all cases sinus rhythm was restored by giving intravenous atropine. The author could find no clear explanation for this phenomenon, but he made two suggestions. One was that atracurium's lack of cardiovascular effects might mean that the cholinergic actions of other agents used during anesthesia were unattenuated; the other possibility would be that a metabolite was capable of producing bradycardia, especially since laudanosine (the main metabolite) has a structure similar to that of apomorphine. At the time of the present review, no similar cases appear to have been reported, either in the journals or to the British Committee on Safety of Medicines (52[Cr]). Carter's report has in the meantime produced a spate of reactions (to be found in the British Medical Journal of September 10th, 1983) from anesthetists who consider the bradhcardia which he observed to have been due to the operation itself or the other agents given (fentanyl, morphine or halothane).

Some of the *breakdown products of atracurium* produce dose-dependent neuromuscular blockade, hypotension and autonomic effects in cats (42), but these are not expected to be seen in man, considering their low potencies and the quantities likely to be formed. *Prior suxamethonium* (about 35 min beforehand) is reported to *potentiate* the block produced by atracurium in man but not to prolong its duration (43[C]). These authors also confirm the earlier reported *potentiation and prolongation* of atracurium blockade by *halothane* (44[C]). Sokoll et al (45[C]) demonstrate that *isoflurane* also *potentiates atracurium* in man, the ED95 (under balanced anesthesia) being reduced from 0.27 mg/kg to 0.13 mg/kg (after more than 15 min of isoflurane 0.6 – 0.65% end-tidal, together with nitrous oxide).

Chapple et al (46) report on a series of experiments assessing the *interaction in cats between atracurium and numerous drugs used in anesthesia.* In general the results are as expected from the interactions reported for other non-depolarizing neuromuscular blocking drugs (SED-10, Ch 13), but the numbers are small for assessing significance. Neostigmine reversed the enhanced blocks produced by neomycin and polymyxin B.

Atracurium appears to be a very acceptable relaxant, perhaps the agent of first choice, for *use in patients with no renal function* (47[C]). Initial doses of 0.5 mg/kg followed by increments of 0.2 mg/kg at 10% return of twitch response (to a mean total dose of 2.3 mg/kg over 2.5 h) resulted in no prolongation of its action in comparison with normal patients.

Interactions of relaxants

Verapamil, an antidysrhythmic drug whose action is thought to be through calcium, or slow-channel, blockade, has been reported to produce significant dose-related depression of twitch height in vivo in cats and dogs (12, 13). Spontaneous recovery was slow. After intravenous doses of 0.1 mg/kg (not much greater than the usual therapeutic dose in humans) indirectly stimulated twitch height of the flexor carpi radialis muscle was reduced by 25% approximately and took 60–90 min to recover fully. Larger doses produced greater effects which also lasted much longer. The authors draw the tentative conclusion that verapamil is neither a specific nor a selective slow-channel blocker and make the suggestion that potent inhalational agents, relaxants, or antibiotics and other drugs reducing neuromuscular function may interact with verapamil in therapeutic dosage to promote muscle weakness. Their findings, however, are controversial and require confirmation before definite conclusions can be reached, particularly with regard to man.

SKELETAL MUSCLE RELAXANTS

There are almost no recent reports on adverse reactions to this group of drugs, which have not previously been described.

Dantrolene

Among usual side effects, such as drowsiness, dizziness, nausea and diarrhea, 3 patients are described (in a short-term double-blind cross-over trial with 17 patients) who developed *numbness in hands and feet* (48[c]). The maximum dose of dantrolene was 400 mg daily. Dantrolene is a hydantoin derivative and long-term use of diphenylhydantoin has been incriminated in the causation of polyneuropathy in 7–30% of patients. However, it is not possible from the article to ascertain the extent to which the numbness may have been due to the underlying neurological disease or injury, and 'concurrent medication' was not defined, although most patients were receiving treatment for urinary infection. (This lack of detail is a constant problem in assessing the significance of side effects mentioned 'en passant' in papers on this group of relaxants.) 'Bright yellow coloration of the urine of most patients' is also reported here. No conclusions can be reached as to whether dantrolene was the causative, or a contributory, agent in these cases. If nitrofurantoin was used for treating the urinary infections this hydantoin derivative could just as easily have produced the effects described. Vitamin B preparations may also give yellow coloration of urine. More details are required.

Baclofen

A case of *mania* is described by Wolf et al (49[C]) in a schizophrenic patient, whose condition was, however, stabilized by lithium therapy. It is known that baclofen may produce *euphoria or depression*, and auditory, visual and paranoid *hallucinations* SEDA-2, 118; SEDA-6, 132) have all been described on (sudden) withdrawal of the drug. *Cumulation* in patients with *renal dysfunction* SEDA-7, 148) has also led to the development of a *psychotic syndrome and myoclonia*. Baclofen should be avoided in psychotic, schizophrenic or mentally disturbed patients, as well as in those with renal dysfunction. If used, such patients should be exceptionally carefully observed for changes in their psychic state. *The drug should always be withdrawn gradually.*

An interesting paper by Wimmer (50[C]) describes 4 cases of *absolute or relative overdose* of baclofen which illustrate several of the points above, such as *renal insufficiency leading to toxic accumulation*, and *hallucinations and psychoses on sudden withdrawal* (by forced diuresis). The *muscle weakness* produced was demonstrated by the need to *ventilate one patient artificially* (after 1.250 mg) and by *swallowing difficulties* in another. Hypotonia and mental confusion have been reported earlier when daily doses of more than 60 mg have been used. One of the patients, who became disorientated and paranoid on 37.5 mg/day, was later restarted on 10 mg/day and, even on this small dose, showed psychomotor disturbances and became very confused at night. The patient was 66 years old. *Elderly patients* often tolerate baclofen badly.

REFERENCES

1. Laxenaire M-C, Moneret-Vautrin DA, Boileau S (1982) Choc anaphylactique au suxaméthonium à propos de 18 cas. *Ann. Franç. Anesth. Réanim.*, *1*, 29.
2. Laxenaire M-C, Moneret-Vautrin DA, Watkins J (1983) Diagnosis of the causes of anaphylactoid

anaesthetic reactions, a report of the recommendation of the joint Anaesthetic and Immuno-allergological Workshop, Nancy. *Anaesthesia, 38*, 147.

3. Watkins J (1982) Evaluation pratique de l'implication du complément au cours des réactions anaphylactoïdes. *Ann. Franç. Anesth. Réanim., 1*, 279.
4. Theobald-Segalen C, Sainte-Laudy J, Pons A et al (1982) Intérêt de l'exploration des basophiles humains dans le diagnostic de l'allergie médicamenteuse. *Ann. Franç. Anesth. Réanim., 1*, 285.
5. Moneret-Vautrin DA, Laxenaire M-C, Bertrand F (1982) Conduite du bilan immuno-allergologique en cas d'accident anaphylactoïde peranesthésique. *Ann. Franç. Anesth. Réanim., 1*, 267.
6. Lorenz W, Neugebauer E, Schmal A (1982) Le dosage de l'histamine plasmatique lors de réactions anaphylactoïdes chez le sujet anesthésié. *Ann. Franç. Anesth. Réanim., 1*, 271.
7. Ahnefeld FW, Doenicke A, Lorenz W (1982) Symposium on histamine and antihistamines in anaesthesia and surgery, Munich 3–5 June 1982. *Klin. Wochenschr., 60*, 871.
8. Thornton JA, Lorenz W (1983) Histamine and antihistamine in anaesthesia and surgery, report of a symposium. *Anaesthesia, 38*, 373.
9. Lorenz W, Doenicke A, Schöning B et al (1982) Definition and classification of the histamine-release response to drugs in anaesthesia and surgery: studies in the conscious human subject. *Klin. Wochenschr., 60*, 896.
10. Moss J, Philbin DM, Rosow CE et al (1982) Histamine release by neuromuscular blocking agents in man. *Klin. Wochenschr., 60*, 891.
11. Stoelting RK (1983) Allergic reaction during anesthesia. *Anesth. Analg., 62*, 341.
12. Kraynack BJ, Lawson NW, Gintautas J (1983) Neuromuscular blocking action of verapamil in cats. *Canad. Anaesth. Soc. J., 30*, 242.
13. Lawson NW, Kraynack BJ, Gintautas J (1983) Neuromuscular and electrocardiographic responses to verapamil in dogs. *Anesth. Analg., 62*, 50.
14. Cohen S, Liu KH, Marx GF (1982) Upper airway edema – an anaphylactoid reaction to succinylcholine? *Anesthesiology, 56*, 467.
15. O'Ryan F, Epker BN (1981) Prolonged apnea after orthognathic surgery due to atypical cholinesterase. *Int. J. Oral Surg., 10*, 338.
16. Kohlschütter B, Baur H, Roth F (1976) Suxamethonium-induced hyperkalaemia in patients with severe intra-abdominal infections. *Br. J. Anaesth., 48*, 557.
17. Popović BM (1981) Succinylcholine-induced hyperkalaemia in patients with intra-abdominal infections. SRPSKI ARHIV (Serbian Archive) 109, 1003 (in Serbian).
18. Kahn TZ, Khan RM (1983) Changes in serum potassium following succinylcholine in patients with infections. *Anesth. Analg., 62*, 327.
19. McKishnie JD, Muir JM, Girvan DP (1983) Anaesthesia induced rhabdomyolysis – a case report. *Canad. Anaesth. Soc. J., 30*, 295.
20. Miyamoto K, Sasaki M, Okudo T et al (1983) Four cases suspected of malignant hyperthermia induced by halothane and succinylcholine. *Hiroshima J. Anesth., 18*, 157.
21. Lewandowski KB (1982) Strabismus as possible sign of subclinical muscular dystrophy predisposing to rhabdomyolysis and myoglobinuria: a study of an affected family. *Canad. Anaesth. Soc. J., 29*, 372.
22. Linter SPK, Thomas PR, Withington PS et al (1982) Suxamethonium associated hypertonicity and cardiac arrest in unsuspected pseudohypertrophic muscular dystrophy. *Br. J. Anaesth., 54*, 1331.
23. Cozanitis DA, Karhunen U, Brander P et al (1982) A matched comparison of four suxamethonium administration techniques in patients with strabismus. *Br. J. Anaesth., 54*, 1283.
24. Tammisto T, Brander P, Airaksinen MM et al (1970) Strabismus as a possible sign of latent muscular disease predisposing to suxamethonium-induced muscular injury. *Ann. Clin. Res., 2*, 126.
25. Shrivastava OP, Chatterji S, Kachhwa S et al (1983) Calcium gluconate pretreatment for prevention of Succinylcholine-induced myalgia. *Anesth. Analg., 62*, 59.
26. Weis OF, Müller FO, Lyell H et al (1983) Materno-fetal cholinesterase inhibitor poisoning. *Anesth. Analg., 62*, 233.
27. D'Hollander AA, Agoston S, De Ville A et al (1983) Clinical and pharmacological actions of a bolus injection of suxamethonium: two phenomena of distinct duration. *Br. J. Anaesth., 55*, 131.
28. Martyn JAJ, Szyfelbein SK, Ali HH et al (1980) Increased d-tubocurarine requirement following major thermal injury. *Anesthesiology, 52*, 352.
29. Martyn JAJ, Matteo RS, Greenblatt DJ et al (1982) Pharmacokinetics of d-tubocurarine in patients with thermal injury. *Anesth. Analg., 61*, 241.
30. Martyn JAJ, Goudsouzian NG, Matteo RS et al (1983) Metocurine requirements and plasma concentrations in burned paediatric patients. *Br. J. Anaesth., 55*, 263.
31. Leibel WS, Martyn JAJ, Szyfelbein SK et al (1981) Elevated plasma binding cannot account for the burn related d-tubocurarine hyposensitivity. *Anesthesiology, 54*, 378.
32. Martyn JAJ, Matteo RS, Szyfelbein SK et al (1982) Unprecedented resistance to neuromuscular blocking effects of metocurine with persistence after complete recovery in a burned patient. *Anesth. Analg., 61*, 614.
33. Sarubin J (1982) Erhöhter Bedarf an Alloferin bei Verbrennungspatienten. *Anaesthesist, 31*, 392.
34. Yamashita M, Shiga T, Matsuki A et al (1982) Unusual resistance to pancuronium in severely burned patients: case reports. *Canad. Anaesth.*

Soc. J., *29*, 630.

35. Hughes R, Chapple DJ (1981) The pharmacology of atracurium: a new competitive neuromuscular blocking agent. *Br. J. Anaesth.*, *53*, 31.
36. Basta SJ, Ali HH, Savarese JJ et al (1982) Clinical pharmacology of atracurium besylate (BW 33A): a new non-depolarizing muscle relaxant. *Anesth. Analg.*, *61*, 723.
37. Hunter JM, Jones RS, Utting JE (1982) Use of atracurium during general surgery monitored by the train-of-four stimuli. *Br. J. Anaesth.*, *54*, 1243.
38. Robertson EN, Booij LHDJ, Fragen RJ et al (1983) Intradermal histamine release by 3 muscle relaxants. *Acta Anaesth. Scand.*, *27*, 203.
39. Basta SJ, Savarese JJ, Ali HH et al (1983) Histamine-releasing potencies of atracurium, dimethyl tubocurarine and tubocurarine. *Br. J. Anaesth.*, *55*, *Suppl. 1*, 105S.
40. Sale JP (1982) Bronchospasm following the use of atracurium. *Anaesthesia*, *38*, 511.
41. Healy TEJ, Palmer JP (1982) In vitro comparison between the neuromuscular and ganglion blocking potency ratios of atracurium and tubocurarine. *Br. J. Anaesth.*, *54*, 1307.
42. Chapple DJ, Clark JS (1983) Pharmacological action of breakdown products of atracurium and related substances. *Br. J. Anaesth.*, *55*, *Suppl. 1*, 11S.
43. Stirt JA, Katz RL, Murray AL et al (1983) Modification of atracurium blockade by halothane and by suxamethonium: a review of clinical experience. *Br. J. Anaesth.*, *55*, *Suppl. 1*, 71S.
44. Payne JP, Hughes R (1981) Evaluation of atracurium in anaesthetized man. *Br. J. Anaesth.*, *53*, 45.
45. Sokoll MD, Gergis SD, Mehta M et al (1983) Safety and efficacy of atracurium (BW33A) in surgical patients receiving balanced or isoflurane anesthesia. *Anesthesiology*, *58*, 450.
46. Chapple DJ, Clark JS, Hughes R (1983) Interaction between atracurium and drugs used in anesthesia. *Br. J. Anaesth.*, *55*, *Suppl. 1*, 17S.
47. Hunter JM, Jones RS, Utting JE (1982) Use of atracurium in patients with no renal function. *Br. J. Anaesth.*, *54*, 1251.
48. Luisto M, Möller K, Nuutila A et al (1982) Dantrolene sodium in chronic spasticity of varying etiology. *Acta Neurol. Scand.*, *65*, 355.
49. Wolf ME, Almy G, Toll M et al (1982) Mania associated with the use of baclofen. *Biol. Psychiatr.*, *17*, 757.
50. Wimmer C (1982) Über Lioresal[R]-(Baclofen)-Intoxikationen – ein kasuistischer Beitrag. *Dtsch. Gesundheitsw.*, *37*, 1500.
51. Vervloet D, Nizankowska E, Arnaud A et al (1983) Adverse reactions to suxamethonium and other muscle relaxants under general anaesthesia. *J. Allergy Clin. Immunol.*, *71*, 552.
52. Carter ML (1983) Bradycardia after the use of atracurium. *Brit. Med. J.*, *287*, 247.

Z. Fastner

14 Drugs affecting autonomic functions or the extrapyramidal system

SYMPATHICOMIMETIC DRUGS

Drugs predominantly stimulating β-receptors.

Isoproterenol

The risks of use (and abuse) of β-sympathicomimetics are well known but it is very unusual to encounter a report on a follow-up of a case of myocardial necrosis due to isoproterenol abuse (1[C]).

A female patient, suffering from asthma since childhood, had always been a heavy smoker. By the age of 32 she was steroid-dependent (prednisone 30–100 mg daily) and used aminophylline suppositories and tablets (total 1700 mg daily), as well as isoproterenol by nebulization and inhaler (totalling up to 500 μg daily). At the age of 43, she had a severe asthma attack and used the whole content of an isoproterenol inhaler within 12 hours prior to developing signs of angina pectoris. Electrocardiogram and enzymes were positive, but she recovered after 3 weeks of uneventful hospitalization. She remained reasonably well 2 years later.

This case, although not isolated, is interesting because of the gross overdose of isoproterenol; it also illustrates the fact that asthmatics in distress do not count their inhalations. Naturally, one must wonder about the role of her excessive smoking in the development of coronary insufficiency, as well as the part played by prednisone.

Side Effects of Drugs Annual 8
M.N.G. Dukes, editor

ISBN 0 444 90339 9
$0.80 per article per page (transactional system)
$0.20 per article per page (licensing system)

DRUGS PREDOMINANTLY STIMULATING β_1-RECEPTORS

Dopamine and dobutamine

Dopamine is considered as a safe drug for the treatment of reduced cardiac output in patients with pulmonary hypertension. However, recently a patient was described in whom during treatment for acute respiratory distress syndrome with dopamine the pulmonary vascular resistance and pulmonary arterial pressure rose with the fall of cardial index. Dopamine was replaced by isoproterenol, producing gradual improvement (2[Cr]). It may be concluded that if dopamine aggravates pulmonary hypertension and right ventricular failure, isoproterenol must be considered as an alternative inotropic drug.

When used for the treatment of low-output congestive heart failure, dopamine was shown to inhibit platelet aggregation in vivo and in vitro. This is in contrast to the platelet-aggregating properties of many catecholamines. Three of six patients investigated developed slight *petechial bleeding* when their dobutamine infusion was continued for more than 3 days (3[C]). As aggravation of myocardial ischemia can follow circulating platelet aggregation, dobutamine inhibition of platelet aggregation can however be desirable, preventing further coronary occlusion.

Dopamine was considered to have produced *myoclonic encephalopathy* in a 55-year-old patient suffering from endocarditis. As dopamine does not pass the blood–brain barrier, it was postulated that cerebral vasculitis, secondary to endocarditis, had produced permeability of that barrier to dopamine. Although the onset of seizures appeared 2 weeks after the start of the treatment, the disappearance of the symptoms soon after cessation of dopamine treatment was striking (4[c]).

Levodopa

Diurnal cortisol rhythm disruption was found in 62% of patients (n = 73) receiving levodopa. In these patients sleep disturbance and psychic side effects of levodopa were more frequent than usual. A normal cortisol rhythm reappeared and psychiatric symptoms disappeared when levodopa was discontinued. It was suggested that neuroendocrine changes must underlie these side effects (5[c]).

A curious side effect was observed in Parkinson patients taking levodopa, namely *asterixis,* a jerky relaxation of tonically contracted postural muscles. It is more usually seen in patients with structural lesions of the brain or metabolic encephalopathy, but not in Parkinson patients. Fourteen patients have been described, out of 60 treated with levodopa who displayed asterixis. If the picture is not recognized it may be wrongly labelled as chorea or tremor. The condition alleviates when the dose is reduced. It was characteristic of this group of patients that asterixis occurred mainly in those with mental disorders and myoclonus. Moreover, the patients with asterixis tended to be demented (6[C]).

OTHER DRUGS INCREASING DOPAMINE ACTIVITY

Amantadine and rimantadine

Rimantadine is an amantadine analog (α-methyl-1-adamantanemethylamine hydrochloride) and has been found to be more active than amantadine against influenza A viruses in vitro and in laboratory animals.

In a 6-week field experiment during an influenza outbreak 450 volunteers received amadantine, rimantadine or placebo (7[C]). Influenza occurred in 41% of placebo users, but for amantadine and rimantadine users these figures were 9% and 14% respectively. While the prophylactic value of the two drugs, used in a dose of 200 mg per day during 6 weeks, seemed to be equal, side effects were much less common with rimantadine. CNS adverse effects (insomnia, jitteriness and concentration difficulties) were twice as frequent with amantadine as with rimantadine. With other side effects the difference was not statistically significant.

The validity of the findings is limited by the composition of the trial group (young healthy individuals), and they should be confirmed by trials on elderly and other high risk individuals. The findings have indeed been challenged (8[r]) but no detailed criticism of them has been offered.

DRUGS STIMULATING DOPAMINERGIC RECEPTORS

Bromocriptine

Side effects limiting the use of bromocriptine in Parkinson patients are quite common, but are certainly dose related. This view was confirmed in a recent study (9[C]).

29 Parkinson patients were treated with bromocriptine, in addition to levo-dopa or amantadine; the initial dose of bromocriptine was 1 mg daily, augmented by 1 mg daily at weekly intervals to a 15 mg/day maximum. The improvement of Parkinson symptoms was as great as in patients using dosages of 50–150 mg/day, but the optimum response was delayed, sometimes by weeks, and this may have led others to increase dosage too soon and too radically. Hallucinations and postural hypotension occurred in the same frequency as with higher doses, but were always milder and were readily reversible with slight dose reduction.

Bromocriptine-induced *psychosis* is well known and it seems that particular caution is warranted in patients having a family history of mental disorders (10[C]).

A 32-year-old man with acromegalia, but without a personal history of psychiatric disorders, was treated with 30 mg bromocriptine per day for 3 months. His mental condition started to deteriorate as little as 2 weeks after bromocriptine was started, when the daily dosage was only 10 mg. He developed a full paranoic state leading to his admission to a psychiatric unit. As the mother of the patient had a history of paranoic schizophrenic episode at the age of 60, genetic vulnerability must be considered a possibility in this patient.

Another case, involving a 22-year-old woman, has been reported by Einarson (48[C]).

An interesting but highly unusual sequel of bromocriptine administration may be *CSF rhinorrhea* (11[Cr]).

A 28-year-old woman with prolactinemia was treated with 5 mg bromocriptine daily; after a week she noticed left sided rhinorrhea, the discharge comprising cerebrospinal fluid. The leakage was repaired by a transsphenoid operation.

One cannot say with certainty that bromocriptine produced rhinorrhea, but an empty sella, resulting probably from pituitary adenoma suppression, was filled with CSF. Pulsations of CSF have erosive effects, and leakage of the CSF is a known, albeit rare, complication of pituitary tumors.

Interaction bromocriptine–tamoxifen Of a group of 12 women, treated with bromocriptine for their prolactin producing hypophyseal adenomata, 3 withstood the treatment poorly, suffering from vomiting, headache and dizziness. When tamoxifen in a dose of 10–20 mg/day was added to bromocriptine (2.5–7.5 mg/day), side effects at once disappeared. This experience is interesting, offering perhaps a possibility of bromocriptine treatment to patients who cannot otherwise tolerate it (12[C]).

Pergolide

A 31-year-old woman with schizophrenia well controlled on depot flupenthixol, also had a prolactinoma for which she was taking pergolide to suppress lactation. During the first 2 weeks of pergolide therapy, she suffered a relapse of her schizophrenia with depressive and suicidal psychosis. The psychosis was resolving within 2 days of discontinuing pergolide.

Ergoline

8-α-Ergoline (CU 32-085) was compared in an open study with bromocriptine. It appeared to be more effective and to have less side effects. However, these results are not entirely reliable, not only because of the open character of the investigation, but because the author compared two dissimilar groups of patients (13[c]).

DRUGS PREDOMINANTLY STIMULATING BETA-RECEPTORS

Drugs in use in asthma and respiratory distress. Abnormalities in serum immunoglobin levels in asthmatic patients have been reported earlier, but the possibility of a relation with the treatment (steroid or otherwise) has not previously been examined.

In a recent study 65 adult asthmatic patients receiving steroid treatment were compared with patients receiving β-adrenergic agents. It was found that the patients receiving β-adrenergic agents had significantly lower serum IgG levels. This effect was seen both in subjects never receiving steroids but also in steroid users; in the group receiving combined treatment, this depressive effect was indeed even more pronounced. The mechanism of the effect is not clear and has yet to be elucidated (14[C]).

Terbutaline

Terbutaline tolerance Continuous oral terbutaline use during 2 weeks in a dose of 5 mg t.i.d. has led to a reduced β-adrenergic response in various in vitro parameters and a decrease in the number of β-adrenergic receptors. A reduced response in vivo was also seen. Basal lung function in asthmatic subjects remained clinically improved. It is suggested that desensitization occurred, but the therapy remained beneficial. Desensitization is interpreted as a form of cellular protection against overstimulation and exhaustion. It is concluded that monotherapy should be avoided, in order to prevent domination of constrictive mechanisms in asthmatics. Combination of β-adrenergic drugs with theophylline and/or anticholinergics is advocated, especially when prophylactic treatment with cromoglycate or corticosteroids are insufficient (15[C]).

Terbutaline, like other adrenergic agents, can produce irritability and muscular tremor. However, a greater degree of CNS stimulation, leading to *convulsions* can apparently occur in some circumstances.

An asthmatic girl, 7.5 years old, was treated with terbutaline and tolerated high doses (7.5 mg every 8 hr) but treatment was discontinued for 4 days because of intercurrent febrile disease. When terbutaline, along with theophylline and beclomethasone, was restarted, she developed seizures, necessitating phenobarbital and phentoin treatment. It is speculated, that the patient developed tolerance to high doses of terbutaline, but that this tolerance was lost during the short withdrawal. Most probably theophylline also reduced the patient's seizure threshold (16[Cr]).

Bronchospasm due to terbutaline Bronchospasm must be added to the list of side effects due to terbutaline.

A 53-year-old female patient with 8 years of asthma, was given oral terbutaline sulfate b.i.d. Severe bronchospasm appeared and persisted for 12 hours. The patient suspected a causal relationship and skipped treatment the next day. However, when reassured by her physician that such an effect was impossible, she took a second dose 48 hours after the first one, only to develop after 4 hours the worst dyspnea she ever experienced. She was admitted with coma and respiratory depression. As oxygen inhalation together with 240 mg i.v. theophylline and 500 mg prednisolone did not bring relief, i.v. treatment with orciprenaline sulfate was started (5 mg in 500 ml isotonic saline). After 100 ml during the first 20 min, then 100 ml/hr for 2 hours and 50 mg/hr for the next 4 hours, she improved rapidly.

Although an isolated instance, this case is quite instructive. The physician should take into consideration an unexpected side effect if the patient suspects a relation between his or her treatment and an adverse effect, even if this is not warned against in the package insert.

The long lag between intake and onset (4–6 hr) is worthy of note, suggesting that bronchospasm was elicited by some metabolite rather than by the drug itself (17[c]).

Terbutaline and blood pressure drop In patients with quadriplegia, a deep and life threatening hypotensive reaction was registered after terbutaline administration. It seems that an absence of autonomic spinal functions produces deeper hypotension than otherwise described during terbutaline treatment. As these patients had received theophylline as well, an interaction is not excluded. In view of this observation, it seems warranted to warn against indiscriminate use of β-adrenergic agents in patients with quadriplegia (18[C]).

Risks of inhalation therapy Risks of inhalation therapy of asthma by inhalation of β-agonists have been discussed in SEDA-7 (p. 151). To these risks, that of overt abuse must be added. When inhalers are used, careful monitoring and advice are needed, especially in young people, although the elderly are certainly not immune for abuse. It could be advisable to prescribe salbutamol in a rotacap inhaler, as fluorocarbon use is thereby avoided and the dosage is better controlled (19[Cr]).

When *salbutamol* is used in a nebulizer, a marked increase in dosage often occurs. The dose from a pressurized aerosol dispenser amounts to 200 to 400 μg, while a nebulizer yields much more, up to 10 mg. Such a dose produces tachycardia and palpitations. As tachycardia shortens diastole, the time for coronary perfusion is shortened, and in cases of existing coronary disease this may result in an anginal attack or even a myocardial infarct. Three such cases have been recently published, but it is suspected that many other cases remain unrecognized. Caution is therefore recommended when salbutamol is used in a nebulized form in older patients or in individuals with known coronary disease. The dose must be kept low, initially not more than 1 mg, increasing it only until adequate bronchodilatation is achieved (20[c]).

Terbutaline and migraine In 2 pregnant migraine patients, use of terbutaline was followed by evidence of *cerebral ischemia.*

One of these women was treated for asthma at 25 weeks' gestation. She had a history of migraine, increasing during pregnancy. After having received 0.25 mg terbutaline s.c. at 6-hour intervals, she developed signs of focal cerebral ischemia. A computed tomographic scan was positive for a small lesion of the right parietal lobe. She recovered and delivered a normal baby at term. Cerebral angiography performed post partum was within normal limits.

Another patient with a history of migraine was seen at the 28th week of pregnancy for premature uterine contractions. After a second dose of 0.25 mg s.c. of terbutaline, she complained of severe throbbing headache, nausea and vomiting, right hemianospia and spotty scotomas. The right arm showed motor and sensory disturbances accompanied by mild aphasia. She recovered spontaneously within 60 min.

The mechanism of these 2 cases of focal neurological signs is unclear, but they provide sufficient warning to refrain from use of terbutaline (and its congeners) in pregnant patients with a history of migraine or vascular headache. This seems to apply both to asthmatic patients and to use of the drug for tocolysis (23c).

Ritodrine

Not only tachycardia can result from the use of β-sympathicomimetics, but bradycardia also, as illustrated in a recent case report.

A 33-year-old woman was admitted at the 33rd week of pregnancy for preterm uterine contractions. After initial treatment with ritodrine i.m. 60 mg/day, she was given 50 mg/day orally. At the 38th week she was delivered by cesarean section. Twelve days later she developed a syncopal episode and on admission she showed sinus bradycardia of 40 beats/min. After 1 mg atropine i.v. the pulse rate rose to 60/min.

This retarded bradycardia was regarded by the authors concerned as an expression of reduced sensitivity to endogenous catecholamines, since β-adrenoreceptor sensitivity decreases after β-adrenoreceptor stimulation (24[c]).

A curious finding is that of Desir et al (45[C]) to the effect that brief infusions of ritodrine (150 μg/min for 4 hours) rapidly raise plasma melatonin levels in healthy women. This is believed to be the first demonstration of a pharmacological stimulation of melatonin release in normal humans.

To the known side effects of tocolytic treatment with ritodrine, hypertensive crisis should now be added.

A woman, aged 32, in the 27th week of gestation, was admitted because of premature labor. She was treated with 300 mg ritodrine orally the first day, followed by 60 mg/day i.v. during the next 2 days and 40 mg/day for the 4 following days. Due to renewed uterine contractions, 400, 300 and 120 mg i.v. were given together with 10 mg orally on the 8th, 9th and 10th day. She also had 12 mg of dexamethasone on the 1st and 8th day.

After having had 120 mg during the 10th day, the patient became restless, dyspneic and tremolous. The pulse rate rose to 110/min, but the arterial pressure rose to 300/120, with no ECG changes. Administration of ritodrine was stopped, and 5 mg of diazepam was given parenterally. The blood pressure dropped to 150/100 within 15 min and normalized completely within 1 hour. Follow-up showed complete normalization.

The pathophysiology of this episode remains obscure, but it is obvious that during i.v. use of ritodrine a patient must be under close hemodynamic monitoring (25[c]).

One other recent case developed a curious complex of side effects to the use of ritodrine as a tocolytic agent.

A 21-year-old primipara was admitted for the treatment of preterm labor. She received ritodrine, 10 mg every 2 hours during 36 hours. Despite the treatment, she was delivered of a baby the same day. Next day the white blood cell count rose to 531,000/mm^3, falling gradually in the subsequent days, but at the same time hemolytic anemia and altered liver tests of the hepatitis type were found. Beside this, hypokalemia and acidosis were transiently noted. All these signs cleared spontaneously within a week (26[C]).

Synergism atropine-ritodrine When ritodrine is used to alleviate fetal distress, atropine premedication prior to cesarean section must be avoided. The vagolytic action of atropine is synergistic to the action of ritodrine, resulting in severe maternal tachycardia and systolic hypertension (27[c]).

Isoetharine

In several patients described by Hooper (46[c]), administration of isoetharine resulted in pink coloration of the sputum, due to the presence of a reddish metabolite; in such cases, hemoptysis may be suspected.

Hexoprenaline

When used as a tocolytic agent, hexoprenaline has been described as producing atrial fibrillation, which disappeared 8 hours after withdrawal. It is possible that this complication appears more frequently than reported, as ECG monitoring is not always permanent, and only tachycardia and palpitations are registered (28[c]).

Tulobuterol

Tulobuterol is a relatively new Japanese β_2-sympathicomimetic agent. When used in a dose of 2 mg, its effect seemed to be comparable to 4 mg salbutamol. However, the frequency of typical side effects was high (6 of 10 patients). When a higher dose, 4 mg, was used, side effects were noted in 9 of 10 patients (21[c]).

New compounds

In the hope of avoiding muscular tremor due to the use of adrenergic β-stimulants, many new compounds have been synthetized (22[c]). Two of these, D-2343 and

QH-25, have in some animal experiments shown dissociation of bronchial and skeletal muscle effects. When tested in asthmatic patients, however, no such dissociation could be observed.

SYMPATHICOLYTIC AGENTS

Drugs blocking α-receptors

Tolazoline

Tolazoline has a pulmonary vasodilator action, and is therefore used to improve arterial oxygenation in infants. However, it also has a histamine-like action, increasing gastric juice secretion. This property apparently led to *duodenal perforation* in a 31-hour-old infant treated with tolazoline for 6 hours because of meconium aspiration. At the age of 5 days, operation was performed, and the duodenal defect repaired (29[c]).

THE ERGOT ALKALOIDS AND RELATED AGENTS

Ergotamine

When ergotamine tartrate, as used in Cafergot suppositories for migraine treatment, is taken during pregnancy, caution is indicated as the consequences for the fetus cannot be foreseen, and ergotamine is not free of effects on the myometrium. In 2 cases recently described, a single suppository, containing 2 mg of ergotamine tartrate, was administered late in pregnancy. In both cases signs of peripheral vasoconstriction appeared and intrauterine death of the fetus was established (30[Cr]).

A similar report concerns a pregnant patient suffering from orthostatic hypotension. At the 29th week, she received dihydroergotamine in a dose of 1 mg t.i.d. Ten days afterwards, she developed uterine contractions, which disappeared only after withdrawal of the drug. Despite tocolytic treatment with fenoterol, delivery followed in the 36th week, happily without damage to the infant (31[cr]). It is obvious that the contraindications to ergot alkaloids are sometimes disregarded. Both the above preparations are contraindicated in pregnancy, as clearly stated in the manufacturer's package insert leaflet.

Combination ergotamine–heparine

The combination of heparine with dihydroergotamine is frequently used for the prevention of thromboembolic complications. It is claimed that these two components act synergistically, allowing a lower dosage of heparine to be used. However, the lower risk of hemorrhagic complications is certainly not counterbalanced by a lowered risk of ergotism, despite the claims of manufacturers (31a[C], 32[C], 33[C], 34[r], 35[r], 36[R]).

Dihydroergotamine is a potent vasoconstrictor and its risks should not be underestimated. This view is supported by recent clinical reports on 9 patients receiving heparine-dihydroergotamine prophylaxis for thromboembolic complications. It is to be deplored that the manufacturers have deemed fit to claim that this combination only rarely produces arterial vasospasms, when enough clinical evidence exists that this complication may occur. Moreover, as monitoring of dihydroergotamine levels in the blood is not routinely possible, its dosage remains a delicate problem and careful observation is needed to detect early signs of arterial spasms and to withdraw the drug. Even after withdrawal the regression of clinical symptoms is not as rapid as could be desired.

Methysergide has long been known to produce retroperitoneal fibrosis, but the incidence of this complication after the use of ergotamine was described only once before. It is therefore interesting to cite a newer case report on a patient, a 37-year-old woman using Cafergot, taking in this way 3–4 mg ergotamine per day, probably for more than a year before admission. On admission, *retroperitoneal fibrosis* was found. The diagnosis was confirmed by laparoscopy. As ergotamine was thought to be the cause of the fibrosis, it was discontinued. After withdrawal, the fibrosis did not reappear. As methysergide and ergotamine are chemically closely related, the appearance of the same side effect is hardly surprising; this complication, although rare, must therefore be borne in mind (37[cr]).

AGENTS WITH CHOLINERGIC EFFECTS

Carbachol

In 3 patients receiving carbachol for problems with their micturition, extreme bradycardia, combined with severe arterial hypotension, developed. Dosage had been normal, not exceeding 2 mg (2–4 tablets per day). Usually, only transitory and mild bradycardia is seen, but these 3 patients reacted with extremely severe symptoms. They recovered upon receiving atropine intravenously. As carbachol is not destroyed by choline esterase, a cumulative effect is possible in patients receiving regular doses at shorter intervals, but one patient developed hypotension on the 3rd treatment day. There were no signs of organic heart damage in any of the patients (38[C]).

CHOLINESTERASE INHIBITORS

Neostigmine and physostigmine

Neostigmine or other anticholinesterase preparations are regularly used in anesthesiology to reverse neuromuscular block. However, in patients, suffering from neuromuscular disorders, this reversal may present unforeseen difficulties. Two patients recently described, one with dystrophia myotonica and the other with progressive muscle dystrophy, presented with respiratory difficulties, necessitating prolonged mechanical ventilation. As these difficulties are as good as impossible to predict, short acting neuromuscular blockers should preferably be used, thus avoiding the need for reversal agents (39[C]).

Although *diazepam* does not have anticholinergic properties, it is possible to reverse diazepam-induced delirium by the use of cholinesterase inhibitors such as physostigmine. The latter can however on occasion induce severe *arterial hypertension.*

An 86-year-old man admitted for minor ophthalmic surgery was sedated with 15 mg diazepam i.v. (after having received 5 mg per os). He became agitated and it was decided to administer physostigmine to reverse his agitation. The dose administered was 5 mg i.v. over the next 15 min. Agitation ceased by the patient's arterial blood pressure rose to 260/120 (from 140/90 prior to surgery). To reverse this sudden hypertension, hydralazine was given i.v., 5 mg every 5 min, until after 20 min the pressure was under control. No further sequelae were observed (40[Cr]).

Although physostigmine hypertension is known in animal experiments, it seems that clinicians are not sufficiently aware of this possibility. It is recommended to limit physostigmine dosage to 2 mg i.v. to avoid this complication and its risks.

AGENTS WITH ANTICHOLINERGIC EFFECTS

Atropine

That atropine can produce bradycardia is well known but recently a case was described in which it proceeded to *asystole.* The patient, who was being prepared for dental surgery, developed bradycardia after having received 0.5 mg atropine i.v. The bradycardia became rapidly more severe until asystole was registered on the ECG. The exact duration of asystole was not registered, but after 10 min recovery was complete, with a pulse rate of 60/min. Whether this accident was due to atropine alone, or whether cardial syncope also played a role, is not clear (41[c]).

Atropine was considered to have produced *hypothermia* in a boy aged 14, who was being treated with paracetamol and cooling blankets for hyperthermia. When 0.4 mg atropine i.v. was added because of present bradycardia, his temperature dropped to 34°C within 2 hours. After rechallenge, 10 hours later, the same effect was produced. It can be argued that the patient was under a heavy acetaminophen load, and the exclusive role of atropine cannot be proven. However, as in the animal experiment atropine can produce hypothermia, a causal relationship cannot be excluded, even if concomitant action with acetaminophen is taken for granted (42[C]). Loss of temperature control is naturally a well-known effect of various drugs with anticholinergic properties, notably the neuroleptics.

Hyoscine butylbromide

One isolated case of *angioneurotic edema* has been described during the use of hyoscine butylbromide (Buscopan). Buscopan was used in the usual dose of 10 mg t.i.d., but the total dose was not registered. The symptoms subsided 18 hours after withdrawal and administration of 100 mg hydrocortisone i.v. (43[c]).

Orphenadrine

Orphenadrine overdosage has already been warned against (SEDA-3, 124; SED-9,

231). Although usually well tolerated in therapeutic doses, overdosage, even slight, can lead to atropine-like symptomatology, and overt overdosage of 2–3 g must be considered lethal. In patients with orphenadrine intoxication, mortality is very high and exceeds 10% of all cases described. As deterioration of vital functions progresses very quickly, early recognition and rapid help are of crucial importance (44[R]).

REFERENCES

1. Jacobs RL, Koppes GM (1982) Myocardial necrosis associated with isiproterenol abuse; a ten-year follow-up. *Tex. Med., 78,* 58.
2. Klausen NO, Qvist J, Brynjolf I et al (1982) Pulmonary hypertension in a patient with ARDS – a possible side-effect of dopamine treatment. *Intensive Care Med., 8,* 155.
3. Smith RE, Briggs B, Unverferth DV, Leier CV (1982) Dobutamine-induced inhibition of platelet function. *Int. J. Clin. Pharmacol. Res., 2,* 89.
4. Boudouresques G, Tafani B, Benichou M, Sarlon B (1982) Encéphalopathie myoclonique à la dopamine. *Sem. Hôp. Paris, 58,* 2729.
5. Nausieda PA, Baum RA, Weiner WJ (1982) Cortisol rhythm disruption as a side effect of chronic levodopa therapy. *Neurology, 32,* A180.
6. Glantz R, Weiner WJ, Goetz CG et al (1982) Drug-induced asterixis in Parkinson disease. *Neurology, 32,* 553.
7. Dolin R, Reichman RC, Madore HP et al (1982) A controlled trial of amantadine in the prophylaxis of influenza A infection. *N. Engl. J. Med., 307,* 580.
8. Douglas Jr RG (1982) Amantadine as an antiviral agent in influenza. *N. Engl. J. Med., 307,* 617.
9. Teychenne PF, Bergsrud D, Anis Racy PA-C et al (1982) Bromocriptine: low-dose therapy in Parkinson disease. *Neurology, 32,* 577.
10. Le Feuvre CM, Isaacs AJ, Frank OS (1982) Bromocriptine-induced psychosis in acromegaly. *Br. Med. J., 285,* 1315.
11. Afshar F, Thomas A (1982) Bromocriptine-induced cerebrospinal fluid rhinorrhea. *Surg. Neurol., 18,* 61.
12. Völker W, Gehring WG, von zur Mühlen A, Schneider J (1982) Bromocriptin plus Tamoxifen. Ein neuer therapeutischer Ansatz bei nicht supprimierbaren prolaktinbildenden Adenomen. *Geburtshilfe Frauenheilkd., 42,* 790.
13. Jellinger K (1982) Adjuvant treatment of Parkinson's disease with dopamine agonists: open trial with bromocriptine and CU 32-085. *J. Neurology, 227,* 75.
14. Mansfield LE, Nelson HS (1982) Effect of beta-adrenergic agents on immunoglobin G levels in asthmatic subjects. *Int. Arch. Allergy Appl. Immunol., 68,* 13.
15. Van den Berg W, Leferink JG, Fokkens JK et al (1982) Clinical implications of drug-induced desensitization of the beta receptor after continuous oral use of terbutaline. *J. Allergy Clin. Immunol., 69,* 410.
16. Friedman R, Zitelli B, Jardine D, Fireman P (1982) Seizures in a patient receiving terbutaline. *Am. J. Dis. Child., 136,* 1091.
17. Drexel H, Regele M, Längle U (1982) Successful treatment of terbutaline-induced bronchospasm with orciprenaline sulphate. *Lancet, 2,* 446.
18. Pingleton SK, Schwartz O, Szymanski D, Epstein M (1982) Hypotension associated with terbutaline therapy in acute quadriplegia. *Am. Rev. Respir. Dis., 126,* 723.
19. Pratt HF (1982) Abuse of salbutamol inhalers in young people. *Clin. Allergy, 12,* 203.
20. Neville E, Corris PA, Vivian J et al (1982) Nebulized salbutamol and angina. *Br. Med. J., 285,* 796.
21. Maesen F, Smeets J, Polderman J (1983) Tulobuterol, a new beta-2-sympathomimetic agent. *J. Drug Res., 8,* 1635.
22. Löfdahl CG, Bengtsson B, Svedmyr K, Svedmyr N (1982) Two new beta-2 adrenoceptor agonists, D-2343 and QH 25, studied in asthmatic patients. *Allergy, 37,* 351.
23. Rosene KA, Featherstone HJ, Benedetti TJ (1982) Cerebral ischemia associated with parenteral terbutaline use in pregnant migraine patients. *Am. J. Obstet. Gynecol., 143,* 405.
24. Dean H, Berliner S, Garfinkel D et al (1982) Sinus bradicardia following ritodrine withdrawal. *J. Am. Med. Assoc., 247,* 1810.
25. Gonen R, Samberg I, Sharf M (1982) Hypertensive crisis associated with ritodrine infusion and betamethasone administration in premature labor. *Europ. J. Obstet. Gynecol. Reprod. Biol., 13,* 129.
26. Alcena V (1982) Severe hemolytic anemia, leukemoid reaction, acidosis, hypokalemia, and transient hepatitis associated with the administration of ritodrine hydrochloride (Yutopar). *Am. J. Obstet. Gynecol., 144,* 852.
27. Sheybany S, Evans D, Newcombe RG, Pearson JF (1982) Ritodrine in the management of fetal distress. *Br. J. Obstet. Gynecol., 89,* 723.
28. Frederiksen MC, Toig RM, Depp III R (1982) Atrial fibrillation during hexoprenaline therapy for premature labor. *Am. J. Obstet. Gynecol., 145,* 108.
29. Matsuo M, Yamada T, Takemine H et al (1982) Duodenal perforation with tolazoline therapy. *J. Pediatr., 100,* 1005.
30. Van Aken B, Knipscheer RJJL, Lameijr W (1982) Acuut ergotisme in de zwangerschap. *Ned. Tijdschr. Geneeskd., 126,* 1620.

31. Lippert TH, Böhm HR (1982) Über das Risiko einer Dihydroergotamin-Behandlung in der Schwangerschaft. *Geburtsh. Frauenheilkd., 42,* 866.

31a. Van den Berg E, Rumpf KD, Fröhlich H et al (1982) Vascular spasm during thromboembolism prophylaxis with heparin-dihydroergotamine. *Lancet, 2,* 268.

32. Van den Berg E, Walterbusch G, Gotzen L et al (1982) Ergotism leading to threatened limb amputation or to death in two patients given heparin-dihydroergotamine prophylaxis. *Lancet, 1,* 955.

33. Van den Berg E, Walterbusch G, Gotzen L et al (1982) Ergotismus – eine ernste Komplikation der medikamentosen Thromboemboliephrophylaxe. *Dtsch. Med. Wochenschr., 107,* 716.

34. Krupp P, Majer M (1982) Vasospasmen nach Heparin-Dihydroergotamin. *Dtsch. Med. Wochenschr., 107,* 995.

35. Urbanyi B (1982) Erfahrungen bei der Thromboembolieprophylaxe in der Gefässchirurgie. *Dtsch. Med. Wochenschr., 107,* 996.

36. Woodcock BG, Rietbrock N (1982) Ergotismus unter Thromboembolieprophylaxe mit Heparin-Dihydroergotamin. *Dtsch. Med. Wochenschr., 107,* 996.

37. Lepage-Savary D, Vallières A (1982) Ergotamine as a possible cause of retroperitoneal fibrosis. *Clin. Pharm., 1,* 179.

38. Van der Meer FJM, Van der Vijver JCM (1982) Bradicardie en cardiogene shock veroorzaakt door carbachol. *Ned. Tijdschr. Geneeskd., 126,* 1010.

39. Buzello W, Krieg N, Schlickewei A (1982) Hazards of neostigmine in patients with neuromuscular disorders. *Br. J. Anaesth., 54,* 529.

40. Wood DG, Weng J-T, Youngberg JA (1982) Severe hypertension following physostigmine reversal of diazepam-induced delirium. *Anesth. Rev., 9,* 29.

41. Weinstein IR (1982) Atropine... Bradicardia ... Asystole...? Arrest. *Anesth. Prog., 29, 112.*

42. Lacouture PG, Lovejoy Jr FH, Mitchell AA (1983) Acute hypothermia associated with atropine. *Am. J. Dis. Child., 137,* 291.

43. Robinson ACR, Teeling M (1982) Angioneurotic oedema and urticaria induced by hyoscine butylbromide. *Postgrad. Med. J., 58,* 316.

44. Sangster B (1982) Intoxicatie door orfenadrine. *Geneesmiddelenbull., 16,* 53.

45. Desir D, Kirkpatrick C, Fevre-Montange M et al (1983) Ritodrine increases plasma melatonin in women. *Lancet, 1,* 184.

46. Hooper PL, Harrelson LK, Johnson GE (1983) Pseudohemoptysis from isoetharine. *N. Engl. J. Med., 1,* 1602.

47. Beeley L (1983) Personal Communication to the Editor of the Side Effects of Drugs Annual.

48. Einarson TR (1983) Psychotic reaction to low-dose bromocriptine. *Clin. Pharm., 2,* 273.

J.P. Nater and A.C. de Groot

15 Dermatologicals and cosmetics

Benzoyl peroxide in acne: risk of sensitization? *(SEDA-7, 168)*

Benzoyl peroxide is widely used as a topical agent for the treatment of acne vulgaris because of its antimicrobial and keratolytic properties; in addition, chronic leg ulcers have successfully been treated with this compound (85).

In experimental situations benzoyl peroxide has a high potential for contact sensitization (90[C], 93[C]) and indeed it is well-documented that when used for leg ulcers, benzoyl peroxide readily induces contact allergy (86[C], 87[C]). However, data on the sensitizing potential of benzoyl peroxide when used for the topical treatment of acne are conflicting, estimations of the incidence of contact allergic reactions ranging from 1–2% (88[C]) to 25% of patients treated (89[R]).

Some authors (90[C]) have suggested that the estimate of 1–2% sensitization in acne patients is too low due to: (1) mild allergy with erythema and pruritus being interpreted as irritancy; (2) allergy manifesting on the face as edema only; (3) allergy manifesting as worsening of acne.

Recently, two new studies on this subject have been published (91[r], 92[C]). Rietschel and Duncan (91[r]) patch tested 60 patients with benzoyl peroxide 1% and 0.1% (vehicle: commercial gel basis 2–20% in petrolatum), after a 12-week acne study comparing 4 treatments: benzoyl peroxide, benzoyl peroxide combined with salicylic acid, salicylic acid alone, and a vehicle control group. Of 28 patients treated with benzoyl peroxide 7 (25%) gave a 1^+ or 2^+ reaction to benzoyl peroxide 1%, one of whom also reacted to 0.1%; these patients were considered to be allergic to benzoyl peroxide. However, none of these patients had clinical manifestations of contact allergy, and only 3 of them had erythema of the face equal to that seen in the vehicle control group. There was thus a striking discrepancy between clinical findings and patch test results. In 6 of 32 patients (19%) treated with the vehicle or salicylic acid only, a 1^+ reaction (considered to be relevant) was noted to benzoyl peroxide 1%; this was explained by past usage of topical benzoyl peroxide, mostly within the last year, but these reactions may have been false-positive patch test reactions since none reacted to 0.1% benzoyl peroxide.

In another study (92[C]) 445 patients using benzoyl peroxide were observed regularly over a 12-month period. Many of these displayed mild 'irritant' dermatitis, usually in the first few weeks of treatment, and settling with continued use. Six patients had severe redness and scaling; 5 of them were patch tested with benzoyl peroxide 1% and 0.1% (commercial gel basis). One patient had a strong reaction to both concentrations, 4 had mild erythema at 1%; in these 4, treatment could later be reintroduced without ill effects. The authors thus concluded that benzoyl peroxide as acne therapy has a low incidence of allergic reactions; however, to establish the true incidence all patients should have been patch tested, especially in view of the results of the study of Rietschel and Duncan (91[r]).

From these data it would seem that no definite conclusions can yet be drawn concerning the sensitizing potential of benzoyl peroxide used for acne treatment. For future studies and observations an adequate non-irritant test concentration of benzoyl peroxide for patch testing should be established; it may well be that 1% causes irritant patch test reactions in 'susceptible' individuals, while 0.1% is too low a concentration for detecting allergy in some cases. Preferably both concentrations should be tested, and in addition a use test may be needed for correct interpretation (91[r]).

Side Effects of Drugs Annual 8
M.N.G. Dukes, editor

ISBN 0 444 90339 9
$0.80 per article per page (transactional system)
$0.20 per article per page (licensing system)

In spite of the uncertainty about the frequency of sensitization of benzoyl peroxide for acne it would seem clear that a clear-cut case of contact allergic dermatitis only occasionally develops, forcing the withdrawal of topical benzoyl peroxide; the frequently observed 'irritant' reactions (or are they sometimes allergic?) usually decrease with time, rendering interruption of treatment unnecessary.

ORAL PHOTOCHEMOTHERAPY

Cataractogenesis One of the major concerns of long-term photochemotherapy is the possible development of cataracts, which has been demonstrated in experimental animals. In human subjects, cataracts thought to be due to PUVA have been reported previously (SEDA-6, 146; 73[C]).

Lerman et al (74[C]) examined the lenses of 2 patients on PUVA who required cataract surgery. The lens homogenates showed phosphorescence peaks identical in shape and lifetime with the previously reported 8-methoxypsoralen lens protein photoproduct seen in PUVA-treated cataractous rat lenses. This evidence seems to substantiate the previous clinical reports of presumptive PUVA cataracts.

Nail pigmentation Of 10 psoriatic patients taking *8-methoxypsoralen* followed by sunlight exposure, 3 developed pigmentation of the nails. All patients involved in this study from India were heavily pigmented (52[C]). This effect has been observed previously in the same center in vitiligo patients undergoing photochemotherapy (SEDA-4, 105).

Bullous eruptions Several authors have reported on bullous eruptions due to oral photochemotherapy, some of which were designated as bullous pemphigoid (59[CR]). However, it has been shown that bullous eruptions mimicking bullous pemphigoid both clinically and histologically may lack the typical immunofluorescence findings (60[Cr]) necessary for ascertaining the diagnosis.

Maculae and freckles A 40-year-old man with a long history of psoriasis who was treated with PUVA noted within 2 years of starting therapy the development of ashen-grey maculae on the trunk; after 2 further years of treatment the maculae had spread to most parts of the trunk and the proximal segments of the limbs. Marked dysplastic changes were found in the keratinocytes and melanocytes in the affected areas (100[C]).

ORAL RETINOIDS

Nail changes Nail changes due to oral *etretinate* were studied by Baran (55[C]): fragility with onychorrhexis and onychoschizia was the commonest finding. Other changes included onychomadesis, nail shedding, paronychia, and onycholysis (rare).

Bone changes Yoder (56[c]) treated 7 patients with keratinizing disorders with *isotretinoin* 3 mg/kg for 3 years: symptoms and/or radiological evidence of skeletal hyperostosis developed in 5. Although admitting that the recommended dosage for treating cystic acne is lower and of shorter duration, the author warns that the potential toxicity of this drug, which has recently been approved by the Food and Drug Administration for marketing for the treatment of severe recalcitrant cystic acne, may have been seriously underemphasized.

Flare of cystic acne Of 8 patients with cystic acne treated with *isotretinoin* 1 mg/kg/day, 3 developed explosive cystic flares within 1 week, requiring hospitalization in 1 patient (57[c]).

Effects on the eye Seven patients with acne conglobata were treated with *13-cis-retinoic acid* 0.5–1 mg/kg/day. They were examined ophthalmologically 3 months after starting and again 3 months after stopping the use of this retinoid. One patient complained of dry eyes and slight visual blurring during therapy, and another was unable to continue to wear his contact lenses. The basal tear secretion as assessed by the Schirmer test appeared unchanged during and after therapy, but the tearfilm breakup time (BUT) was significantly reduced during therapy with 13-cis-retinoic acid. This drug is known to cause a decrease in sebum excretion rate, and it is therefore suggested that this effect is due to a reduction of lipid content of the tearfilm, thereby increasing evaporation (94[c]).

CONTACT ALLERGY

Newly described contact allergies and updated information concerning contact sensitivity to (ingredients of) topical drugs are summarized in Table 1. Included are occupational and/or accidental contact with drugs causing contact allergic reactions. Table 2 deals with contact allergy to cosmetic ingredients.

PHOTOCONTACT DERMATITIS

Photocontact allergy to 2-hydroxy-4-methoxybenzophenone in one patient has been described (23[C]). In another report (24[C]) an acute photosensitivity was reported to 2-ethoxyethyl-p-methoxycinnamate in a sunscreen used by two patients. Patch tests and photopatch tests were negative, but it was shown that the sunscreen produced concentration-related decrease in the MEDs in the patients *and* controls, thus suggesting a 'toxic' photosensitivity rather than photocontact allergy.

Kroon (36[Cr]) photopatch tested 495 patients with Musk Ambrette 5% in petrolatum, and found 4 positive reactions; 2 of these were related to typical perfume dermatitis, in the other 2 patients the relevance was uncertain. The same author also performed routine photopatch tests with Waxtar (5% coal tar), p-aminobenzoic acid, potassium bichromate and balsam of Peru (37[Cr]); the results are shown in Table 3.

Photocontact urticaria to Waxtar was noted in a few patients. Two more patients with photoallergic dermatitis to Musk Ambrette have been described from Germany (49[CR]); one of them also had a positive photopatch test to Musk Xylol.

Five patients with photocontact allergy to sunscreens were reported from Finland (97[C]). In 3 PABA produced a positive photopatch test, in the 4th the responsible ingredients were 6-ethoxy-2,4-dimethyl-m-dioxane (dimethoxane, a preservative) and 2-phenylbenzimidazole-5-sulfonate, and the last patient had positive reactions to photopatch tests with p-methoxyisoamylcinnamate, 2-ethoxyethyl-p-methoxycinnamate and cinnamic aldehyde.

CONTACT URTICARIA

A laboratory worker employed in a pathology department had daily outbreaks of urticaria on the face, neck, forearms and dorsa of the hands while at work. The symptoms were ascribed to exposition to formaldehyde vapor: open tests with formaldehyde 1% and 2% were positive, whereas 20 controls tested with formaldehyde 10% were negative. Although this would suggest this case of the contact urticaria syndrome to be of immunological origin, a passive transfer test was negative (41[C]).

A 1-year-old child with atopic dermatitis developed contact urticaria when being bathed in a wheat bran bath. Skin prick tests showed strong reactions to both the bran bath and the wheat extract; in addition, the Prausnitz-Küstner test was positive. When the child was given a gluten-free diet, its atopic dermatitis was essentially improved, and when wheat products were introduced, an exacerbation was registered (42[C]).

Angioedema of the lips and face, followed by faintness due to eating an ice cream cone in a 38-year-old female patient suffering from chronic urticaria, has recently been reported (43[C]). The etiologic agent was Cremodan SE 40, used as a food consolidater; its components are mono-, di- and triglycerides of fatty acids, sodium alginate, polysorbate 80, guar gum and carrageenan. The ingredients could not be tested separately, but polysorbate was suggested as the cause of the contact urticarial response.

Generalized erythema, whealing and pruritus developed in an atopic child after the application of a diethyltoluamide containing insect repellent. An open test and prick test were positive, and remained positive 6 years later. The Prausnitz-Küstner test was positive, thus suggesting an immunological mechanism (69[C]).

SYSTEMIC SIDE EFFECTS OF TOPICAL DRUGS

Camphor

Gossweiler (53[R]) has reported the experience of the Swiss Toxicological Information Center with camphor poisoning from 1966 to 1981. It was noted that both (unintentional) oral administration and topical administration may lead to serious intoxication: breathing difficulties, convulsions, and coma have been reported after repeated topical application of camphor-containing externa. The author con-

Table 1. *Contact allergy to topical drugs*

Drug	Use	Patch testing (4^R)	No. pat.	Cross-reactions	Comment	Ref.
benzyl alcohol	vehicle ingredient	5% pet.	1		the patient was also allergic to isopropyl palmitate and triamcinolone acetonide	44[C]
benzyl benzoate	scabicide, ingredient of cosmetics	5–10% pet.	1	*not* to balsam of Peru		9[C]
bufexamac	nonsteroidal antiinflammatory agent	5% pet.	3		it is suggested that photocontact allergy to bufexamac may occur	15[C]
certrimonium bromide	antiseptic	0.1% aqua	1		patch tests not performed. the diagnosis of non-accidental injury was suspected. irritant dermatitis not excluded	17[C]
chloridazon-(5-amino-4-chloro-2-phenyl-pyridazine-3-one)	herbicide in agriculture	0.1–1% aqua	1		accidental contact in a farmer	6[C]
clindamycin HCl	antibiotic	1% aqua	1			11[C]
dodecyl maleamic acid	in adhesive bandages	5% pet.	2	N-octadecyl maleamic acid (1% aqua/alc.), undecyl polyethylene oxymaleic acid ester (1% aqua/alc.), octyl maleic acid ester (1% pet.)		50[C]
econazole nitrate	antifungal drug	1% pet.	1	*not* to miconazole nitrate	the contact allergic reaction mimicked erythema exsudativum multiforme	7[C]
enilconazole	veterinary antifungal drug	2% pet.	1	econazole, isoconazole, miconazole	all antifungals mentioned are β-substituted 1-phenethyl imidazoles	64[C]
erythromycin sulfate	antibiotic	2–10% pet.	1		the authors used 25% pet. for patch testing	8[C]

Table 1. *(continued)*

Drug	Use	Patch testing (4[R])	No. pat	Cross-reactions	Comment	Ref.
fluocortolonhydrat mikro 20	topical cortico-steroid in Ultralanum ointment	1% and 10% pet.	1	see comment	the patient was apparently (diagnosis made *per exclusi-onem*) also allergic to hydro-cortisone-17-butyrate. from the case report it is not evident which steroid was the primary sensitizer	16[C]
gelatin	constituent of paste bandage	pure	1		*see also under* paste bandages	18[C]
gentian violet	antiseptic	0.25% aqua	1		*see under* white soft paraffin	3[C]
glutaraldehyde	disinfectant	1% aqua	2	patch tests with formalde-hyde not mentioned	occupational allergy	34[C]
idoxuridine	antiviral drug	1% pet.	2			45[CR]
imidazoline chlor-hydrate	sympathicomi-metic agent in a nasal spray	0.1% pet.	1			14[C]
isoconazole	antifungal drug	2% pet.	1	*not* to other imidazoles		1[C] 31[C]
isopropyl palmitate	vehicle ingredient	2% pet.	1		*see under* benzyl alcohol	44[C]
ketoprofen	topical anti-inflammatory drug	1% pet	1			67[C]
mesulfen	scabicide and antifungal drug	5% pet.	4		also has irritant properties	9[C]
miconazole nitrate	antifungal drug	2% pet.	1	*not* to other imidazoles		1[C]
miconazole nitrate	antifungal drug	2% pet.	1	*not* to other imidazoles	the diagnosis of contact allergy to the active ingredient miconazole nitrate was made *per exclusionem*; it is con-cluded that testing with micon-azole nitrate 2% may give false negative results	2[C]

Table 1. *(continued)*

Drug	Use	Patch testing (4^R)	No. pat.	Cross-reactions	Comment	Ref.
nifuratel	antimycotic and antitrichomonas agent	1% acet.	1			68^C
octyl dodecanol	vehicle ingredient	13.5% aqua	1		the patient was sensitized to octyl dodecanol in an antimycotic cream, and had a rash later due to dodecanol in a moisturizing lotion	35^C
2-n-octyl-4-isothiazolin-3-one	antifungal drug (paint mildewcide)	1% o.o.	2		occupational allergy	12^C
paste bandages		as is, and the ingredients separately	9		allergic reactions to the ingredients parabens (9) coal tar (3) lanolin (2) gum acacia (1) gelatin (1) cetostearyl alcohol (1) and emulsifying wax (1)	18^C
piperazine	anti-inflammatory drug (combined with phenylbutazone)	5% aqua	2		occupational contact dermatitis in one patient	13^C
preservatives (n = 29)			465			72^C
propolis	folk medicine	1–5% pet.	22	'pseudo-cross-reactions' to balsam of Peru and several essential oils	both propolis and balsam of Peru contained cinnamyl cinnamate, benzyl cinnamate, benzyl benzoate, cinnamic alcohol and vanillin	38^{Cr}
resorcinol	ingredient of carbolfuchsin paint	2% pet.	1			19^r
sodium fusidate	antibiotic	1% pet.	1			10^C
sorbitan monolaurate (Span 20)	emulsifyer	5% aqua	1		*see under* white soft paraffin	3^C
sorbitan monooleate	emulsifyer	5% aqua	1			5^c

Table 1. *(continued)*

Drug	Use	Patch testing (4[R])	No. pat.	Cross-reactions	Comment	Ref.
sulconazole nitrate cream	antifungal drug	cream 1% pet.	1	other imidazoles *not* tested	the causative ingredient was not looked for	61[c]
tetramisole HCl	anthelmintic drug for cattle	0.01–3% aqua (?)	1	levamisole (0.01–1% aqua?)	occupational allergy	21[C]
triamcinolone acetonide	corticosteroid	1% pet.	3		concomitant sensitization to hydrocortisone and prednisolone (in 1 case)	40[CR] 44[C]
tromantadine HCl	antiviral drug	1% pet.	21		the commercial preparation was tested, as the active ingredient is nearly always the sensitizer	62[CR]
vitamin K3 sodium bisulfite	vitamin	0.1% pet./aqua	1		occupational allergy. nausea, dizziness, giddiness, vomiting and diffuse pigmentation were noted	20[C]
white soft paraffin	vehicle constituent	pure	1		the patient described had multiple contact allergies to medicaments ('ampliative medicament allergy')	3[C]
yellow soft paraffin	vehicle constituent	pure	1		*see under* white soft paraffin	3[C]

Table 2. *Contact allergy to cosmetic ingredients*

Ingredient	Cosmetic	Patch testing (4[R])	No. pat.	Cross-reactions	Comment	Ref.
α-amyl cinnamic alcohol	perfume ingredient	2% pet.	11	α-amyl cinnamic aldehyde		51[CR]
α-amyl cinnamic aldehyde	perfume ingredient	2% pet.	13	α-amyl cinnamic alcohol		51[CR]
benzoin	cream	10% alc.	1		the primary sensitizer was probably balsam of Peru	25[C]
castor oil	lipstick	pure	1		the patient reacted to many lipsticks and lipcreams; they all proved to contain castor oil	32[C]
cocobetaine	amphoteric detergent in shampoo	2% aqua	2	Tegobetaine (1 patient)		68[C]
colophony	various	20% pet.	–		valuable review of colophony allergy	22[R]
D & C Yellow 11	soap	soap 5% aqua (open test)	1		the patient had previously been sensitized by a modified Draize test; 9/149 subjects were sensitized to D & C Yellow 11 in this test!	26[C]
cis-3-hexenyl salicylate	perfume ingredient in a toilet lotion	3% pet.	1	*not* to hexyl, methyl, phenyl, or benzyl salicylate		65[C]
hinokitiol (β-thujaplicin=4-isopropyl-2-hydroxy-2,4,6-triene-1-one	hair liquid	0.1% alc.	1		the patient had a concomitant sensitization to pyridoxine 3,4-dioctanoate (*see under* pyridoxine)	39[C]
2-hydroxy-4-methoxy benzophenone	1) sunscreen 2) lipstick	2% pet. 2% pet.	1		the authors have tested the ingredient 10% aqua. caused *photo*contact allergy	23[C]
lead acetate	hair dye	0.5% pet., 1% aqua	1		the positive patch test reaction may have been due to patch test sensitization	28[c]

Table 2. *(continued)*

Ingredient	Cosmetic	Patch testing (4^R)	No. pat.	Cross-reactions	Comment	Ref.
lilial (p-tert-butyl-α-methylhydrocinnamic aldehyde)	perfume ingredient in antiperspirant	1% pet.	1		lilial is a synthetic fragrance ingredient	66[C]
mercury	toilet soap	0.5% pet. (report)	1		the patient also reacted to colophony, benzalkonium chloride, and an eau de Cologne	33[C]
oakmoss	various, mostly after-shaves	2% pet.	7		positive reactions were noted to the aromatic compounds atranorin (4), usnic acid (5), evernic acid (4), physodic/physodalic acid (3) and diffractaic acid (1), tested 1% in petrolatum	30[C]
propantheline bromide	antiperspirant	1–5% aqua	1			26[c]
pyridoxine 3,4-dioctanoate	hair liquid	0.001% alc., 1% pet.	1	pyridoxine hydrochloride	the patient had a concomitant sensitization to hinokitiol (*see under* hinokitiol)	39[C]
tertiary butyl alcohol	sunscreen	70% aqua	1			29[c]
triethanolamine stearate	sunscreen	5% pet.	1		the patient was also sensitive to methyl paraben	70[C]

Table 3. *Standard photopatch tests with Waxtar, PABA, potassium bichromate and balsam of Peru*

	Waxtar (as is)	PABA (5% alc.)	Potassium bichromate (0.5% pet.)	Balsam of Peru (as is)
No. of patients tested	194	161	161	161
Negative reactions	154	160	161	159
Positive reactions	40	1	0	2
Phototoxic	40	0	0	2
Photoallergic	0	0	0	0

cludes that camphor-containing ointments for colds and coughs should not be used in the newborn and in small infants.

Clindamycin

In 13 patients treated with 1% clindamycin hydrochloride topically for acne vulgaris, the serum level and urinary excretion of clindamycin were measured on the 3rd and 27th day of therapy. There was no detectable antibiotic in the serum of any subject (<0.4 μg/ml) but in 10 clindamycin was found in the urine. It was calculated that after topical application of 1% clindamycin hydrochloride, an average of 4% to 5% of clindamycin was absorbed (46[C]).

Dinitrochlorobenzene

Generalized urticaria, pruritus and dyspepsia developed in a previously healthy individual treated with dinitrochlorobenzene (DNCB) for alopecia totalis; after the therapy was stopped all symptoms disappeared within 10 days. As the symptomatology returned after re-institution of the DNCB applications, the authors suggest a causal relationship (47[c]).

Glycopyrrolate

Twenty-two patients suffering from the Frey syndrome (localized facial gustatory sweating and flushing) were treated with topical glycopyrrolate, a quaternary ammonium compound, 0.5–2% in a solution, cream or roll-on lotion (99[C]). A total of 1012 applications was recorded, and 7 episodes of side effects were noted: blurred vision (1), minor eye infections (2), itchy or dry eyes (1) and dry mouth (3). It should be appreciated that in the control group blurred vision and dry mouth were also recorded as side effects.

Mafenide acetate

A patient with less than 30% body surface area burn was placed on topical therapy with mafenide acetate cream during the 14th post-burn day. Within 15 hours, his course was complicated by *pulmonary insufficiency*. The authors assume that the respiratory failure might be the result of a hypersensitivity reaction to the mafenide acetate, the lung being the shock organ, or the result of high doses of carbonic anhydrase inhibitors formed from the mafenide acetate and its metabolic products. It should be mentioned that the patient received several other drugs, and that he had complained of progressive shortness of breath prior to the first application of the mafenide acetate cream (71[C]).

Monobenzylether of hydroquinone

Although brown discoloration of the conjunctiva and cornea is a well-known adverse effect of hydroquinone in industrial workers, no ocular adverse reactions to monobenzylether of hydroquinone (monobenzone), which is used topically by patients with extensive vitiligo to depigment their remaining normally pigmented skin, have been reported.

However Hedges et al (98[Cr]) have examined a patient who had been applying this drug for one year: an anterior linear deposition of pigment in both corneas was noted. Subsequently, 15 additional patients with vitiligo were screened, 11 of whom were using monobenzone; in 2 acquired conjunctival melanosis, and pingueculae in 3 patients were discovered, which according to the authors may have been related to monobenzone use. The findings, which appeared to have no clinical significance, resembled those known to occur after hydroquinone exposure, and in their report the possible mechanisms are discussed by the authors.

Monosulfiram

A 26-year-old patient treated himself with a monosulfiram and benzyl benzoate containing alcoholic solution for topical use on 10 consecutive days. The 3rd and 7th applications were made just before a meal, during which the patient drank two glasses of wine; after 10 min generalized flushing with malaise and rhinorrhea ensued, lasting for 20 min on the first and 30 min on the second occasion. The authors compare this reaction to an Antabus (disulfiram) effect, and ascribe this adverse event to the monosulfiram content of the topical medication used (95[c]).

Scopolamine hydrobromide

Scopolamine hydrobromide 1–3% as cream or lotion was used to treat patients suffering from the Frey syndrome (localized facial gustatory sweating and flushing). Side effects included blurred vision, itching or dry eyes, dry mouth, and one rash. It should be noted, however, that blurred vision and dry mouth were also recorded as side effects in the placebo group (99[C]).

Sulfadiazine-silver

Transient leukopenia due to sulfadiazine-silver in burn patients has been well-documented (SED-9). Of 9 patients with thermal burns greater than 25% t.b.s., 5 developed leukopenia, defined as white blood count of less than 5,000 (63[CR]).

The clinical significance of leukopenia due to topical sulfadiazine-silver therapy, which thus seems to be a frequent event, is unclear. It always resolves spontaneously and apparently does *not* induce an increase in mortality.

MISCELLANEOUS

Henna

Occupational asthma due to exposure to henna dust, used for hair dyeing, was noted in 2 beauticians (54[C]). Scratch and prick tests with a glycerated preparation of henna powder revealed 3^+ reactions in both patients, and IgE antibodies were demonstrated in the serum.

Topical corticosteroids

Björnberg (58[C]) has shown that when normal skin on the forearms of healthy individuals is exposed to corticosteroids under occlusion for several weeks, a severe skin reaction, notably *erythema craquelé*, may be provoked in some persons in the test area after finishing the course of application. The reactions, which become visible 0.5–2 days after finishing the continuous treatment, reach their maximum after about 3 days, but occasionally remain visible for up to 6 weeks.

Mechlorethamine HCl

Previous studies have led to the suspicion that mechlorethamine HCl (nitrogen mustard), which is used topically for mycosis fungoides, may act as a (co)carcinogen (SEDA-4, 106).

In another study (48[CR]) *skin cancers* developed in 4 patients treated with daily topical applications of nitrogen mustard (for a period of 12 to 38 months). As there was a reversal of the ratio of basal cell to squamous cell carcinomas, as all of the cancers were on normally covered skin, and as other significant risk factors were absent in 2 patients, the authors also suggest a role for topical nitrogen mustard as a carcinogen or tumor promoter.

Hydroquinone ethers

Creams containing hydroquinone and hydroquinone ethers (usually monobenzylether of hydroquinone = monobenzone) are widely used for bleaching of hyperpigmented lesions.

Sometimes disfiguring leukoderma is the result of monobenzone treatment. In a recent report (96[CR]) it is shown that the mono*methyl* ether of hydroquinone may also cause long-lasting *depigmentation*, both locally and at a distance from the treated areas.

Mutagenic and tumor promoting properties of dithranol ℞

Several publications (75, 76) indicate mutagenicity of dithranol, in particular the induction of a high frequency of 'petite mutants' in haploid strains of saccharomyces cerevisal (77). Using the Ames adapted test frameshift mutagenicity on strains of Salmonella typhimurium could be noted (75). In other investigations (79, 80) only marginal effects were found.

A tumor-provoking activity of dithranol on mice pretreated with 7,12-dimethylbenz(a)anthracene (DMBA) has been reported (81). Furthermore malignant lymphomas appeared in mice treated with daily paintings of dithranol (77, 82); the incidence increased after prior intraperitoneal injections of urethan. A tumor-provoking activity of dithranol in mice was also reported by Boch and Burns (81). Dithranol is thus not only active as a promoter but also capable of tumor production by itself. A tumor promoter effectively elicits tumors only in a tissue, usually mouse skin, that has previously been exposed to a small noncarcinogenic dose of a carcinogen. On the other hand, although dithranol is capable of promoting tumor formation in mice previously treated with a subcarcinogenic dose of DMBA, dithranol administered in conjunction with the potent tumor promoter tetradecanoyl-phobol-13-acetate (TPA) inhibits tumor formation (84).

It has been stated that although dithranol is a potent tumor promoting agent on mouse skin, the available clinical evidence suggests that it does not have any deleterious effects in humans at the dosages used (83). However, reliable clinical reports on the long-term effects of dithranol therapy are not available.

REFERENCES

1. Jelen G (1982) Allergie gegen imidazolhaltige Antimykotika: Kreuzallergie? *Dermatosen, 30,* 53.
2. Foged EK, Hammershøy O (1982) Contact dermatitis due to miconazole nitrate. *Contact Dermatitis, 8,* 284.
3. Lawrence CM, Smith AG (1982) Ampliative medicament allergy: concomitant sensitivity to multiple medicaments including yellow soft paraffin, white soft paraffin, gentian violet and Span 20. *Contact Dermatitis, 8,* 240.
4. Nater JP, De Groot AC (1983) *Unwanted Effects of Cosmetics and Drugs Used in Dermatology.* Excerpta Medica, Amsterdam.
5. Austad J (1982) Allergic contact dermatitis to sorbitan monooleate (Span 80). *Contact Dermatitis, 8,* 426.
6. Bruze M, Fregert S (1982) Allergic contact dermatitis to chloridazon. *Contact Dermatitis, 8,* 427.
7. Valsecchi R, Tornaghi A, Tribbia G, Cainelli T (1982) Contact dermatitis from econazole. *Contact Dermatitis, 8,* 422.
8. Lombardi P, Campolmo P, Spallanzani P, Sertoli A (1982) Delayed hypersensitivity to erythromycin. *Contact Dermatitis, 8,* 416.
9. Meneghini CL, Vena GA, Angelini G (1982) Contact dermatitis to scabicides. *Contact Dermatitis, 8,* 285.
10. De Groot AC (1982) Contact allergy to sodium fusidate. *Contact Dermatitis, 8,* 429.
11. De Groot AC (1982) Contact allergy to clindamycin. *Contact Dermatitis, 8,* 428.
12. Thormann J (1982) Contact dermatitis to a new fungicide, 2-n-octyl-isothiazolin-3-one. *Contact Dermatitis, 8,* 204.
13. Menezes Brandão F, Foussereau J (1982) Contact dermatitis to phenylbutazone-piperazine suppositories (Carudol®) and piperazine gel (Carudol®). *Contact Dermatitis, 8,* 264.
14. Romaguera C, Grimalt F (1982) Contact dermatitis from nasal sprays and amyl nitrite. *Contact Dermatitis, 8,* 266.
15. Reiffers J (1982) Contact dermatitis to bufexamac. *Dermatologica, 164,* 354.
16. Brown R (1982) Simultaneous hypersensitivity to 3 topical corticosteroids. *Contact Dermatitis, 8,* 339.
17. Inman JK (1982) Cetrimide allergy presenting as suspected non-accidental injury. *Br. Med. J., 284,* 385.
18. Hardie RA, Benton EC, Hunter JAA (1982) Adverse reactions to paste bandages. *Clin. Exp. Dermatol., 7* 135.
19. Fisher AA (1982) Resorcinol – a rare sensitizer. *Cutis, 29,* 331.
20. Camarasa JG, Barnadas M (1982) Occupational dermatosis by vitamin K3 sodium bisulphite. *Contact Dermatitis, 8,* 268.
21. Pambor M, Hein K (1982) Tetramisolhaltiges Anthelminthikum (Nilverm®) als berufliches Ekzematogen in der Viehwirtschaft. *Dermatol. Monatsschr., 168,* 314.
22. Hausen BM, Kuhlwein A, Schulz KH (1982) Kolophonium-Allergie. *Dermatosen, 30,* 145.
23. Hölzle E, Plewig G (1982) Photoallergische Kontaktdermatitis durch benzophenonhaltige Sonnenschutzpräparate. *Hautarzt, 33,* 391.
24. Davies MG, Hawk JLM, Rycroft RJG (1982) Acute photosensitivity from the sunscreen 2-ethoxyethyl-p-methoxycinnamate. *Contact Dermatitis, 8,* 190.
25. Mann RJ (1982) Benzoin sensitivity. *Contact Dermatitis, 8,* 263.
26. Gall H, Kempf E (1982) Kontaktallergie auf das lokale Antiperspirant Propanthelinbromid. *Dermatosen, 30,* 55.
27. Jordan WP Jr (1981) Contact dermatitis from

D & C Yellow 11 dye in a toilet bar soap (letter). *J. Am. Acad. Dermatol.*, *4*, 613.
28. Edwards EK Jr, Edwards EK (1982) Allergic contact dermatitis to lead acetate in a hair dye. *Cutis*, *30*, 629.
29. Edwards EK Jr, Edwards EK (1982) Allergic reaction to tertiary butyl alcohol in a sunscreen. *Cutis*, *29*, 476.
30. Thune P, Solberg Y, McFadden N et al (1982) Perfume allergy due to oak moss and other lichens. *Contact Dermatitis*, *8*, 396.
31. Frenzel UA, Gutekunst A (1983) Contact dermatitis to isoconazole nitrate. *Contact Dermatitis*, *9*, 74.
32. Sai S (1983) Lipstick dermatitis caused by castor oil. *Contact Dermatitis*, *9*, 75.
33. Alomar A, Camarasa JG, Barnadas M (1983) Addison's disease and contact dermatitis from mercury in a soap. *Contact Dermatitis*, *9*, 76.
34. Hansen KS (1983) Glutaraldehyde occupational dermatitis. *Contact Dermatitis*, *9*, 81.
35. Tucker WFG (1983) Contact dermatitis to Eutanol G. *Contact Dermatitis*, *9*, 88.
36. Kroon S (1983) Standard photopatch testing with Musk Ambrette. *Contact Dermatitis*, *9*, 1.
37. Kroon S (1983) Standard photopatch testing with Waxtar®, para-aminobenzoic acid, potassium dichromate and balsam of Peru. *Contact Dermatitis*, *9*, 5.
38. Rudzki E, Grzywa Z (1983) Dermatitis from propolis. *Contact Dermatitis*, *9*, 40.
39. Fujita M, Aoki T (1983) Allergic contact dermatitis to pyridoxine ester and hinokitiol. *Contact Dermatitis*, 9, 61.
40. Esser B (1982) Beitrag zur Kortison-Allergie. *Z. Hautkr.*, *58*, 29.
41. Lindskov R (1982) Contact urticaria to formaldehyde. *Contact Dermatitis*, *8*, 333.
42. Langeland T, Nyrud M (1982) Contact urticaria to wheat bran bath: a case report. *Acta Derm. Venereol. (Stockh.)*, *62*, 82.
43. Camarasa JMG (1982) Acute contact urticaria. *Contact Dermatitis*, *8*, 347.
44. Lazzarini S (1982) Contact allergy to benzyl alcohol and isopropyl palmitate, ingredients of topical corticosteroid. *Contact Dermatitis*, *8*, 349.
45. Lombardi P, Spallanzani P, Giorgini S, Seroli A (1982) Allergic contact dermatitis from idoxuridine. *Contact Dermatitis*, *8*, 350.
46. Barza M, Goldstein JA, Kane A et al (1982) Systemic absorption of clindamycin hydrochloride after topical application. *J. Am. Acad. Dermatol.*, *7*, 208.
47. McDaniel DH, Blatchley DM, Welton WA (1982) Adverse systemic reaction to dinitrochlorobenzene (letter to the Editor). *Arch. Dermatol.*, *118*, 371.
48. Lee LA, Fritz KA, Golitz L et al (1982) Second cutaneous malignancies in patients with mycosis fungoides treated with topical nitrogen mustard. *J. Am. Acad. Dermatol.*, *7*, 590.
49. Galosi A, Plewig G (1982) Photoallergisches Ekzem durch Ambrette Moschus. *Hautarzt*, *33*, 589.
50. Heskel NS, Samour CM, Storrs FJ (1982) Allergic contact dermatitis from dodecyl maleamic acid in Curad adhesive plastic bandages. *J. Am. Acad. Dermatol.*, *7*, 747.
51. Guin JD, Haffley P (1983) Sensitivity to α-amylcinnamic aldehyde and α-amylcinnamic alcohol. *J. Am. Acad. Dermatol.*, *8*, 76.
52. Naik RPC, Parameswara YR (1982) 8-Methoxypsoralen-induced nail pigmentation. *Int. J. Dermatol.*, *21*, 275.
53. Gossweiler B (1982) Kampfervergiftungen heute. *Schweiz. Rundschau. Med. (Praxis)*, *71*, 1.
54. Starr JC, Yunginger J, Brahser GW (1982) Immediate Type I asthmatic response to henna following occupational exposure in hairdressers. *Ann. Allergy*, *48*, 98.
55. Baran R (1982) Action thérapeutique et complications du rétinoïde aromatique sur l'appareil unguéal. *Ann. Dermatol. Vénéreol. (Paris)*, *109*, 367.
56. Yoder FW (1983) Isotretinoin: a word of caution (letter). *J. Am. Med. Assoc.*, *249*, 350.
57. Katz RA, Jorgensen H, Nigra TP (1983) Flare of cystic acne from oral isotretinoin (letter). *J. Am. Acad. Dermatol.*, *8*, 132.
58. Björnberg A (1982) Erythema craquelé provoked by corticosteroids on normal skin. *Acta Derm. Venereol. (Stockholm)*, *62*, 147.
59. Brun P, Baran R (1982) Pemphigoïde bulleuse induite par la photochimiothérapie du psoriasis. *Ann. Dermatol. Vénéreol. (Paris)*, *109*, 461.
60. Pullmann H, Trost T, Witte U (1982) Akrale Blasenbildung unter PUVA-Therapie. *Z. Hautkr.*, *57*, 288.
61. Lassus A, Forström S, Salo O (1983) A double-blind comparison of sulconazole nitrate 1% cream with clotrimazole 1% cream in the treatment of dermatophytoses. *Br. J. Dermatol.*, *108*, 195.
62. Schneider KW (1982) Tromantadin-Kontaktallergien. *Therapiewoche*, *32*, 5691.
63. Hollis Caffee H, Bingham HG (1982) Leukopenia and Silver sulfadiazine. *J. Trauma*, *22*, 586.
64. Van Hecke E, De Vos L (1983) Contact sensitivity to enilconazole. *Contact Dermatitis*, *9*, 144.
65. Van Ketel WG (1983) Sensitization to cis-3-hexenyl salicylate. *Contact Dermatitis*, *9*, 154.
66. Larsen WG (1983) Allergic contact dermatitis to the fragrance material lilial. *Contact Dermatitis*, *9*, 158.
67. Valsecchi R, Falgheri G, Cainelli T (1983) Contact dermatitis from ketoprofen. *Contact Dermatitis*, *9*, 163.
68. Bedella PG, Goitre M, Cane D, Fogliano MR (1983) Contact dermatitis from Nifuratel. *Contact Dermatitis*, *9*, 166.
69. Von Mayenburg J, Rakoski J (1983) Contact

urticaria to diethyltoluamide. *Contact Dermatitis, 9,* 171.
70. Edwards EK Jr, Edwards EK (1983) Allergic reaction to triethanolamine stearate in a sunscreen. *Cutis, 31,* 195.
71. Albert LT, Lewis NS, Warpeha RL (1982) Late pulmonary complications with use of mafenide acetate. *J. Burn Care Rehabilit., 3,* 375.
72. Meynadier J-M, Meynadier J, Colmas A et al (1982) Allergie aux conservateurs. *Ann. Dermatol. Vénéreol. (Paris), 109,* 1017.
73. Lerman S (1982) Ocular phototoxicity and PUVA therapy: an experimental and clinical evaluation. Proceedings of the 7th FDA-symposium. *J.N.C.I., 69,* 287.
74. Lerman S, Megaw J, Gardner K (1982) Psoralen-long-wave ultraviolet therapy and human cataractogenesis. *Invest. Ophthalmol. Vis. Sci., 23,* 801.
75. Brown JP, Dietrich PS, Brown RJ (1972) Frameshift mutagenicity of certain naturally occurring phenolic compounds in the 'Salmonella/Microsome' test: activation of anthraquinone and flavonol glycosides by gut bacterial enzymes. *Biochem. Soc. Transact., 5,* II.
76. Gillberg BO, Zetterberg G, Swanbeck G (1967) Petite mutants induced in yeast by dithranol (1,8,9-trihydroxyanthracene), an important therapeutic agent against psoriasis. *Nature, 214,* 415.
77. Yasuhira K (1968) Induction of malignant lymphoma and other tumors during experiments with Anthralin painting of mice. *Gann, 59,* 195.
78. Ames BN, McCann J, Yamasaki E (1975) Methods for detecting carcinogens and mutagens with Salmonella/mammalian microsome mutagenicity test. *Mutat. Res., 31,* 347.
79. Brown JP, Brown RJ (1976) Mutagenesis by 9,10-Anthraquinone derivatives and related compounds in Salmonella typhimurium. *Mutat. Res., 40,* 203.
80. Clark JM, Hanawalt PC (1981) Inhibition of DNA replication and repair in cultured human cells by anthralin or danthron. *Br. J. Dermatol., 105, Suppl. 20,* 49.
81. Bock FG, Burns R (1963) Tumor promoting properties of anthralin (1,8,9-anthratriol). *J. Nat. Canc. Inst., 30,* 393.
82. Yasuhira K (1968) Skin papilloma production by Anthralin painting after urethan initiation in mice. *Gann, 59,* 184.
83. Segal A, Katz C, Van Duuren BL (1971) Structure and tumor-promoting activity of anthralin (1,8-dihydroxy-9-anthrone) and related compounds. *J. Med. Chem., 21,* 26.
84. Boutwell RK, Hoel MJ, Digiovanni J (1981) The role of anthralin in mouse skin tumour promotion. *Br. J. Dermatol., 105, Suppl. 20,* 68.
85. Colman GJ, Roenigk HH (1978) Topical therapy of leg ulcers with 20% benzoyl peroxide lotion. *Cutis, 21,* 491.
86. Vena GA, Angelini G, Meneghini CL (1982) Contact dermatitis to benzoyl peroxide. *Contact Dermatitis, 8,* 338.
87. Jensen O, Petersen SH, Vesterager L (1980) Contact sensitization to benzoyl peroxide following topical treatment of chronic leg ulcers. *Contact Dermatitis, 6,* 179.
88. Pace WE (1965) A benzoyl peroxide-sulfur cream for acne vulgaris. *Canad. Med. Assoc. J., 93,* 252.
89. Plewig G, Kligman AM (1975) *Acne: Morphogenesis and Treatment,* pp. 290–291. Springer Verlag, Berlin–Heidelberg.
90. Leyden JJ, Kligman AM (1977) Contact sensitization to benzoyl peroxide. *Contact Dermatitis, 3,* 273.
91. Rietschel RL, Duncan SH (1982) Benzoyl peroxide reactions in an acne study group. *Contact Dermatitis, 8,* 323.
92. Cunliffe WJ, Burke B (1982) Benzoyl peroxide: lack of sensitization. *Acta Derm. Venereol. (Stockholm), 62,* 458.
93. Poole RL, Griffith JF, McMillan FSK (1970) Experimental contact sensitization with benzoyl peroxide. *Arch. Dermatol., 102,* 635.
94. Ensink BW, Van Voorst Vader PC (1983) Ophthalmological side-effects of 13-cis-retinoid therapy (Letter). *Br. J. Dermatol., 108,* 627.
95. Plouvier B, Lemoine X, De Coninck P et al (1982) Effet antabuse lors de l'application d'un topique à base de monosulfirame. *Nouv. Presse Méd., 11,* 3209.
96. Grojean M-F, Thivolet J, Perrot H (1982) Leucomélanodermies accidentelles provoquées par les topiques dépigmentants. *Ann. Dermatol. Venéréol. (Paris), 109,* 641.
97. Fagerlund V-L, Kalimo K, Jansén C (1983) Valonsuoja-aineet fotokontaktiallergian aiheuttajina. *Duodecim., 99,* 146.
98. Hedges TR, Kenyon KR, Hanninen LA, Mosher DB (1983) Corneal and conjunctival effects of monobenzone in patients with vitiligo. *Arch. Ophthalmol., 101,* 64.
99. Hays LL, Novack AJ, Worsham JC (1982) The Frey Syndrome: A simple, effective treatment. *Otolaryngol. Head Neck Surg., 90,* 419.
100. Kanerva L et al (1983) Psoralen + UVA. Ashen-gray maculae and freckles. *Dermatologica, 166,* 281.

C.B.M. Tester-Dalderup

16 Antihistamines

H1 RECEPTOR ANTAGONISTS
(SEDA-4, 117; SEDA-5, 156; SEDA-6, 157; SEDA-7, 171)

Sedative effects of antihistamines
(27[R])

The treatment of asthmatic and allergic conditions with antihistamines has always been hampered by the sedative effects of the antihistamines and the resulting daytime drowsiness, lack of concentration and diminished mental acuity, resulting in an impaired ability to handle machinery and drive vehicles. For many years researchers have tried to find antihistamines lacking this marked sedative effect and every so often it is proclaimed that this has now been achieved; nearly as often clinical experience has shown that such claims were too hasty; only where an antihistamine has little penetration to the CNS, as is the case with terfenadine, may some real improvement be anticipated.

A division of the antihistamines into those with marked and those with moderate sedative effect is possible. The division lines are not sharp and classification often depends on which studies and how many studies are taken into account. Reported figures may vary wildly. Pharmacokinetic data, penetration of the drug and/or its active metabolites into the CNS and speed of elimination are important, but, especially with the older preparations, not always well known. Dosage per administration and total daily dosage do play a role as does the age of the patient, the sedative effect often being more pronounced in the older patient.

The sedative effect is marked and common, with an incidence of 25–60% or even higher with substances like brompheniramine, chlorpheniramine, cyproheptadine, d-chlorpheniramine, diphenhydramine, hydroxyzine and pizotifen. Methapyrilene is indeed more often used as a sedative than as an antihistamine (SED-9, 268), promethazine being used mainly if a sedative effect is desired to supplement the desired therapeutic action (1[cr], 2[R]).

For other antihistamines it has been more difficult to find figures. Azatadine was reported to cause sedation in 30% of cases in one study and none in another (2[rc]). Astemizole, a new long-acting antihistamine, is stated to have little or no sedative effect, but in a report relating to the treatment of seasonal allergic rhinitis, a sedative effect was observed in 2 out of 16 cases (3[rc]).

Clemastine fumarate was reported to have an incidence of drowsiness/sedation of 9% (SED-7, 253), of 50% in a sample of 108 cases (1[r]) and of 22.4% in a group of 259 patients on a dose of 1 mg b.d.; in this study in which sedation-related side effects were reported in 11.4% of the 729 cases treated with placebo (2[rc]).

For ketotifen an incidence of 10% and 12.6% was noted in SEDA-5 (p. 157). Barlow et al (2[rc]) remark that in 6 reports the incidence varied from 10–82%, but the dosages used are recorded. Lebeau et al (4[C]) state somnolence to be the most common side effect during treatment with ketotifen with an incidence of 13% seen in 1791 cases treated, usually with doses of 2 mg daily. In a ketotifen versus d-chlorpheniramine comparison using daily doses of 2–3 mg in the treatment of allergic rhinitis the incidence of sedation was 11% with ketotifen and 15% with d-chlorpheniramine (5[c]).

Mequitazine, another of the newer products with a fairly prolonged action, was said to have no influence on concentration and reaction tests in a group of 32 children with asthma (6[rc]). However, in earlier reports, drowsiness or somnolence was noted. In a mequitazine versus placebo comparison somnolence was seen in 10/23

Side Effects of Drugs Annual 8
M.N.G. Dukes, editor

ISBN 0 444 90339 9
$0.80 per article per page (transactional system)
$0.20 per article per page (licensing system)

cases on mequitazine and 10/25 treated with placebo (SEDA-6, 157); a figure of 10% was reported in a publication reviewed in SEDA-7 (p. 173). Barlow (2[rc]) quotes 8 and 26% as having been observed in two more studies.

Oxatomide caused drowsiness in 37% of cases in one study (2[rc]), while in an oxatomide versus placebo comparison drowsiness was reported in 56% of the 43 cases given oxatomide and in 20% of the 44 cases given placebo (7[c]).

Terfenadine, another of the newly developed antihistamines is said not to pass the blood-brain barrier and supposedly has no sedative effect in full antihistamine doses (8[r]). Backhouse et al. as reported in SEDA-7 (p. 173) found an incidence for sedation of 2.2% and with placebo 4.4%. Barlow et al (2[rc]) using doses varying from 120–400 mg daily reported an incidence of 12.6% in 965 persons while in the 729 patients treated with placebo an incidence of 11.4% was recorded. In a comparison of dexachlorpheniramine 2 mg t.d.s., terfenadine 60 mg b.d. and placebo in 312 patients, drowsiness occurred in 24% of cases in the dexachlorpheniramine-treated group, in 13% in the placebo-treated and in 11% in the terfenadine-treated group (9[cr]). Similar results were reported by Brandon et al (10[c]) in two studies comparing terfenadine with chlorpheniramine maleate. CNS depression was seen in 18% of cases on chlorpheniramine, 11% on terfenadine and in 7.5% of cases treated with placebo. Terfenadine was found as effective as the older antihistamines in seasonal allergic rhinitis; it has to be mentioned however that in the first of the two studies no statistically significant difference could be found between the efficacy of placebo, chlorpheniramine and terfenadine, which raises the classic question as to whether therapeutically adequate doses had been compared.

Tripolidine 2.5 mg in a comparison with placebo and with cyclizine 50 and 100 mg caused no sedation according to the authors while the cyclizine 100 mg did have a marked influence upon the CNS as shown with performance tests (11[C]). In prior publications drowsiness was reported to be a major side effect with tripolidine.

Nicholson (27[R]) has recently provided an overview of the entire topic of antihistamines and sedation. Of the newer drugs claimed to be largely free of sedative effects, astemizole is in his view likely to be free of sedative effects in doses up to 20 mg, i.e. twice the currently advised adult dose. Mequitazine does not impair performance at the recommended dose level of 5 mg twice daily, but a 10 mg dose does have central effects; there seems to be a useful therapeutic window around the 5 mg dose level. Terfenadine in a 60 mg dose (recommended for twice daily use) does not sedate and may even have some alerting effect. Its lack of central activity is due mainly to its difficulty in crossing the blood-brain barrier, though its specificity of action may be a contributory factor. For these three drugs as a group, Nicholson nevertheless concludes that sedative effects in the individual can never be entirely excluded in advance; to avoid them, a trial and error approach may be advisable, and perhaps also a regimen based on chronopharmacological principles, which is currently under investigation.

Sudden cot death and antihistamines

Care should be exercised in the administration of antihistamines, especially those with a marked sedative effect, to children and infants. In 1982 Kahn and Blum (12[C]) published a study into the circumstances surrounding cases of sudden infant cot death, the so-called near misses and sleep apnoe. Among 52 cases of sudden death and 36 cases of near misses the use of phenothiazines including alimemazine and promethazine was significantly higher than in the 175 control cases. Medications had been used in 23% of the sudden death cases, in 22% of the near misses and in 2% of the control group. Possibly in these infants sensitivity is excessive, or the metabolic rate of the drug is decreased; there may be other reasons. It will be interesting to learn whether similar findings are forthcoming in other groups of cases of sudden infant death.

Interactions

The combined administration of H1 receptor antagonists and *H2 receptor antagonists* has been discussed by Sewing (13[R]); the advantages of such a combination in trying to antagonize the effects of endogenously released histamine is considered a zero-option, there being more effective ways. According to this writer the minor side effects of the H1-receptor antagonists (sedation, GI disturbances, atropine-like effects, allergy and rarely leucopenia or agranulocytosis) are sufficiently different from those of the H2 receptor antagonists (rare renal disorders, endocrine disorders, mental disorders including confusion, cardiovascular problems and interactions with other drugs) not to lead to major problems when the two are given together. This statement by Sewing however underestimates the effect of the H2 receptor antagonist on the CNS and the possible interference with metabolism and elimination of the H1 receptor antagonist, especially if cimetidine is used in the combination.

The possibility of interaction of antihistamines (and also oral antibiotics) with the effectiveness of *oral contraceptives* was raised in an American study (14[C]). 15 out of 16 patients who had become pregnant while using birth control pills had claimed to have been totally compliant with the schedule were found to have used antimicrobial agents and/or 'cold tablets' during the suspected time of conception, a not unexpected finding which however is far from proving an interaction.

INDIVIDUAL ANTIHISTAMINES

Astemizole

Astemizole (R-43512) is a new long-acting antihistamine intended for use in atopic patients. In an astemizole versus placebo double-blind study using 16 patients with hayfever in each group, side effects were mild. Besides sedation, which was seen in 2 (1) cases, the following complaints were listed; dry mouth in 1 (1); nausea 2 (2); headache 2 (1); weight gain 2 (0) (3[C]). (The figures between brackets represent the number of cases in the placebo group having the symptom in question).

Azatadine

This antihistamine was given in combination with pseudoephedrine to 132 patients with symptoms of upper respiratory allergy or common cold; doses were 1–2 mg azatadine maleate and 30–60 mg pseudoephedrine depending on age. The tolerance was stated to be good. Somnolence was seen in 18% of cases, asthenia in 2%. In a group of patients treated with placebo somnolence was noted in 5% of cases and headache in 1 case (2%).

Dexchlorpheniramine

Dexchlorpheniramine 6 mg used for common cold symptoms in combination with pseudoephedrine 120 mg caused an overall incidence of side effects in 56% in the treated group (25 of 44 cases) as compared with 40% in the placebo group, 19 of 48 in a double blind comparison. The main difference in incidence was for the side effects drowsiness (23% against 13%) and dry mouth (11% against 4%). Nausea, vertigo and palpitations were mentioned in one case each in the group on dexchlorpheniramine with pseudoephedrine (16[c]).

Diphenhydramine

Intoxications with diphenhydramine continue to be reported. Two cases reported in Germany both presented with restlessness, hallucinations, disorientation and confusion. Symptoms abated after about 16 hours and recovery seemed complete with amnesia for the period of delirium (17[C]). The third case, a 14-year-old girl, ingested a large dose of about 7.5 g. She was found with tonic-clonic convulsions, shallow respiration and in coma. Circulatory failure preceded death (18[C]). Again attention was drawn to the different reactions seen in different age groups. Children and young adults commonly present with symptoms of CNS stimulation; hyperactivity, tremors, dilated pupils and tonic-clonic seizures. The older adult more readily develops sedation and coma but rarely seizures.

Interactions The diphenhydramine-methaqualone interaction was studied in 12 healthy volunteers. Clinically the sedative effect of methaqualone is enhanced. There were no differences in serum levels of methaqualone and metabolite or for the area under the curve. There was no evidence for a pharmacokinetic interaction which of course does not rule out a pharmacological interaction (19[C]).

Hydroxyzine

Tardive dyskinesia has been described after the use (especially long-term use) of many of the major tranquilizers, but only rarely with the use of antihistamines. A case of tardive dyskinesia was described in a 74-year-old woman after 7.5 months of therapy with hydroxyzine 50 mg twice daily. There is mention of the concomitant use of doxepin 100 mg at night, but doxepin had been used earlier without problems. The woman had also been treated with phenothiazine preparations in the past. Discontinuation of the hydroxyzine therapy was followed by some improvement but not by disappearance of the symptoms which could be controlled by chlorazepate 15 mg at bedtime (20[c]).

Ketotifen

This antihistamine, one of the group of the benzocycloheptatiophenes, has been marketed for the treatment of asthma. It is dealt with in Chapter 17 in this volume.

Mebhydrolin

In SEDA-7 (p. 173) the occurrence of agranulocytosis connected with the use of mebhydrolin was reported. Recently the Australian Adverse Drug Reactions Advisory Committee reported that during the period from June 1973 till November 1981, 11 cases of reversible agranulocytosis or leukopenia associated with the use of mebhydrolin napadisylate were recorded. In 7 of the cases no other drug was recorded as having had a causative role, either by the original reporter or by the Committee. In the other cases one or more other drugs had been used that could have been causative (21[R]). From the Sydney Hospital, again in Australia, comes a report of two more cases. In one, a 55-year-old woman, a multitude of drugs had been used including co-trimoxazole, but a recurrence occurred at a time when she was using only mebhydrolin. In the other case, a 45-year-old woman, the drug exposure consisted of iron and vitamin supplements and about 10 doses of mebhydrolin. In an addendum to the article the occurrence of a third case is mentioned but no details are given (22[C]). These cases do not seem to appear in the list issued by the Australian Drug Committee.

A possible sedative effect of mebhydrolin was investigated with the help of performance tests by 17 volunteers. In the cross-over study the combination with placebo and ethanol was also investigated. A single therapeutic dose of mebhydrolin did not cause a significant impairment of any of the tests (standing steadiness, auditory and visual reaction time, complex reaction time, finger dexterity, numerical reasoning, hand-arm coordination and perceptual speed). In the combination of mebhydrolin with ethanol an enhancement of the ethanol induced performance deficits was found. Pre-treatment with mebhydrolin did not have a significant effect on ethanol blood concentration (23[C]).

Pyrimethamine

Harpey et al (28[c]) have drawn attention to a possible case of teratogenicity attributable to pyrimethamine. The male infant in question was born with a severe defect of the abdominal and thoracic wall and a missing left arm. The mother had taken both chloroquine and maloprim (i.e. pyrimethamine with dapsone). They consider the possible causal link with pyrimethamine because the two other drugs are not thought to be teratogenic, whereas pyrimethamine is a teratogen in animals. The drug is an inhibitor of dihydrofolate reductase, and might be a risk factor in women with a pre-existing low folate store.

Terfenadine *(see also general section above)*

In the few reports available concerning this new antihistamine (SEDA-7, 174) tolerance seems to be quite good (2[rc], 8[r], 10[c]). Sedation was noted in about the same frequency as with placebo treatment. There were few other side effects. Headache, sweating and mild gastrointestinal disturbances were reported infrequently, according to one article (6[r]). One will be anxious to see whether this favorable picture persists as more experience is gained and the drug becomes more widely used.

Tripolidine HCl

The use of tripolidine alone and in combination with pseudoephedrine was commented upon in two articles. A report in Spanish of a study carried out in England concerns the use of this medication for the treatment of the symptoms of the common cold. In this group of 466 otherwise healthy adults side effects seem to have been absent

(24[c]). In the other article the case is described of a 33-year-old woman who after one day of treatment with the combination complained of ocular pain and was found to have some punctate staining of the epithelium of the cornea inferiorly. Discontinuation of the medication quickly solved the problem, which the patient had never experienced during the use of other antihistamine preparations (25[c]).

The combination of tripolidine HCl, pseudoephedrine and paracetamol caused the appearance of abnormal movements (myoclonia) in a 58-year-old woman some hours after the ingestion of the medication. Symptoms disappeared spontaneously within 24 hours. The causative relation could not be confirmed (26[c]).

REFERENCES

1. Kriz RJ (1981) Patient evaluation of clemastine fumarate and comparison with other anti-histamines. *Wisc. Med. J., 80,* 31.
2. Barlow JLR, Beitman RE, Tsai TH (1982) Terfenadine, safety and tolerance in controlled clinical trials. *Arzneim.-Forsch./Drug Res., 32,* 1215.
3. Wilson JD, Hillas JL (1982) Astemizole: a new long-acting antihistamine in the treatment of seasonal allergic rhinitis. *Clin. Allergy, 12,* 131.
4. Lebeau B, Gence B, Bourdain M, Loria Y (1982) Le kétotifène dans le traitement préventif de l'asthme: Analyse synthétique de 1791 observations de médicine praticienne. *Poumon-Coeur, 38,* 125.
5. Langrick AF, Wallace MG (1982) A new approach to the treatment of seasonal allergic rhinitis. *Br. J. Clin. Pract., 36,* 312.
6. Baran D (1982) Biologische en klinische tolerantie van een nieuw synthetisch antihistaminicum. *Ars. Med., 2,* 485.
7. Brompton Hospital Medical Research Council Collaborative Trial (1981) A controlled trial of oxatomide in the treatment of asthma with or without perennial rhinitis. *Clin. Allergy, 2,* 483.
8. Weiner M (1982) Sedation and antihistaminics. *Arzneim.-Forsch./Drug Res., 32,* 1193.
9. Owen RT (1982) Terfenadine. *Drugs Today, 18,* 444.
10. Brandon ML, Weiner M (1982) Clinical studies of terfenadane in seasonal allergic rhinitis. *Arzneim.-Forsch./Drug Res., 32,* 1204.
11. Hamilton M, Bush M, Bye C, Peck AW (1982) A comparison of triprolidine and cyclizine on Histamine (H_1) antagonism, subjective effects and performance tests in man. *Br. J. Clin. Pharmacol., 13,* 441.
12. Kahn A, Blum D (1982) Phenothiazines and sudden infant death syndrome. *Pediatrics, 70,* 75.
13. Sewing K-Fr (1982) Comment: Effects and side effects of H_1 and H_2-receptor antagonists in clinical situations. *Klin. Wochenschr, 60,* 1046.
14. DeSano EA, Hurley SC (1982) Possible interactions of antihistamines and antibiotics with oral contraceptive effectiveness. *Fertil. Steril., 37,* 853.
15. Kaminszczik I, Barbon L (1983) Relieving symptoms of upper respiratory allergies and the common cold: Azatadine Maleate/Pseudoephedrine sulphate syrup versus placebo. *J. Intern. Med. Res., 11,* 101.
16. Virtanen H (1983) A slow release combined preparation (dexchlorpheniramine + pseudoephedrine) for symptomatic treatment of the common cold. *J. Laryngol. Otol., 97,* 159.
17. Hladny J (1982) Akute Psychosen durch Intoxikation mit Diphenhydramin. *Münch. Med. Wochenschr., 124,* 977.
18. Krenzelok EP, Anderson GM, Mirick M (1982) Massive diphenhydramine overdose resulting in death. *Ann. Emerg. Med., 11,* 212.
19. Hindmarsh KW, Wallace SM, Schneider CB, Korchinski ED (1983) Methaqualone-Diphenhydramine interaction study in humans. *J. Pharm. Sci., 72,* 176.
20. Clark BG, Araki M, Brown HW (1982) Hydroxyzine associated tardive dyskinesia. *Ann. Neurol., 2,* 435.
21. McEwen J, Strickland W (1982) Mebhydrolin napadisylate. *Med. J. Aust., 2,* 523.
22. Young GAR, Forrest P, Deveridge SF et al (1982) Mebhydrolin induced agranulocytosis. *Aust. NZ J. Med., 12,* 173.
23. Franks HM, Lawrie M, Schabinsky VV et al (1981) Interaction between ethanol and antihistamines: 3. mebhydrolin. *Med. J. Aust., 2,* 477.
24. Bye CE, Cooper J, Empey DW et al (1981) Efectos terapéuticos de la pseudoephedrine y de la triprolidine, solas y en combinación, sobre la sintomatología del resfriado común. *Compendium, 1,* 9.
25. Farber AS (1982) Ocular side effects of antihistamine-decongestant combinations. *Am. J. Ophthalmol., 94,* 565.
26. Jacquesson M, Saudeau D, Pantin B et al (1982) Myoclonies imputables a une association de tri-prolidine, de pseudo-éphédrine et de paracétamol. *Nouv. Presse Méd., 2,* 2298.
27. Nicholson AN (1983) Antihistamines and sedation. *Lancet, 2,* 211.
28. Harpey JP, Darbois Y, Lefèbre G (1983) Teratogenicity of pyrimethamine. *Lancet, 2,* 399.

F.A. Nelemans

17 Antiallergic and antitussive drugs

ASTHMA

Editorial note *Several of the drugs used in bronchial asthma and cough are dealt with primarily in other chapters. They include xanthine compounds (Ch. 1), the opiates (Ch. 8), sympathomimetic and parasympatholytic agents (Ch. 14), the antihistamines (Ch. 16), and the corticosteroids (Ch. 41).*

Cromolyn sodium (disodium cromoglycate)
(SED 9, 275; SEDA-5, 169; SEDA-6, 171; SEDA-7, 189)

Hypersensitivity reactions to cromolyn sodium are uncommon, but well documented. They may occur after many months of use of this drug. Regular taking of prednisolone (10–40 mg daily) does not give protection as has been shown by the case of a 41-year-old man with severe asthma. After 11 months' use of cromolyn sodium by oral inhalation 4 times per day he complained of burning sensations in the eyes. On the next day, he developed an itchy erythematous facial rash and periorbital edema. Cromolyn sodium inhalation was stopped and the symptoms disappeared within 3 days (1[c]).

Kallós and Kallós in 1982 reviewed in extenso the available evidence on *pseudo-allergic reactions* due to cromolyn (16[R]). Surveying the world literature on the drug up to that moment they detected 13 cases of facial rash, urticaria and/or generalized dermatitis, 1 of nasal congestion, 19 of severe bronchospasm and/or pulmonary edema, eventually culminating in shock, 4 of eosinophilic or granulomatous pulmonary infiltration, 5 of gastrointestinal disturbances, 2 of dysuria and urinary frequency, 1 of liver disease and vasculitis, 1 of pericarditis, and 3 of polymyositis. They do however remind the reader that there must be much unpublished material, e.g. 4 cases of anaphylactic shock known to them personally but not described in print. They consider that at present there is no proof that the adverse reactions to cromolyn which mimic allergic processes of the immediate or delayed type are mediated by IgE and/or specifically reactive lymphocytes; consequently these reactions fulfil the criteria which characterize pseudoallergic reactions. Kallós and Kallós also note the much higher incidence of adverse reactions when cromolyn is used orally (50–100 mg q.i.d.) to prevent food allergic reactions, a matter discussed earlier in these volumes. All in all, they conclude that inhaled cromolyn produces major adverse reactions, most probably of pseudo-allergic origin, in at least 2% of cases, whilst oral use produces minor reactions in about 29% of patients.

A striking negative finding with respect to adverse effects relates to the absence in man of serious effects upon the kidney circulation, despite the fact that such effects had been detected around 1970 when the drug was investigated toxicologically in monkeys (17); such instances point to the risks of allowing animal toxicity studies to determine the fate of a new drug.

Ostler reported earlier on 2 cases of an acute chemotic reaction of the conjunctiva (SEDA-7, 189). He later reported that uninterrupted use of cromolyn sodium relieved the symptoms and signs in one of the patients, suggesting that when he used medication after being without it for a period of time, the drug acted as an allergen and induced degranulation of the mast cells, whereas continuous use of the drug stabilized the mast cells, resulting in relief of the symptoms. The alpha-1 AT levels in both patients were found to be normal (150–240 as compared with a normal range of 111–270 in the laboratory). The alpha-1 AT level in the tears was not determined in the crucial period but was previously found

Side Effects of Drugs Annual 8
M.N.G. Dukes, editor

ISBN 0 444 90339 9
$0.80 per article per page (transactional system)
$0.20 per article per page (licensing system)

in the presence of normal serum levels (2[c]). These data suggest that a deficiency of alpha-1 AT played no role in the reaction.

Ketotifen (Zaditen) *(SEDA-5, 157; SEDA-7, 189)*

Ketotifen is an orally active antihistamine with antiallergic properties. Side effects are rarely a problem. In a double-blind study with 40 skin-test-positive perennial asthma patients (20 ketotifen, 20 placebo) (1 mg twice a day for 12 weeks) the only side effect was drowsiness. The drowsiness occurred in 8 patients on ketotifen and in 3 patients on placebo ($p = 0.078$). Sedation in the ketotifen group appeared suddenly and was rated as mild in 4 patients (duration 3–8 days), moderate in 3 (duration 7–12 days) and severe in 1 (duration 18 days). Even in the latter case it was not necessary to interrupt the treatment nor to reduce the dosage (3).

In an open trial of 433 outpatients with bronchial asthma (219 men and 214 women, and 20% under 12 years, recruited from 74 hospitals) the dosage was 0.5–1 mg twice a day for children and 1 mg twice a day for adults during 3 months. The most common side effect was once again drowsiness (22% of the adults and 11.5% of the children). In 4% the drowsiness was rated as severe. 10 patients dropped out because of adverse reactions. Other side effects were weight gain (3 adults, 2 children), vertigo (3 adults) and dyspepsia (3 adults) (4).

Recently a patient was described in whom oral ketotifen was associated with erythema multiforme bullosum (5[c]). The ketotifen treatment (1 mg twice daily) had started 1 month beforehand. The diagnosis was confirmed by biopsy and a challenge test. The family and personal history pointed to various types of hypersensitivity reaction.

Desensitization *(SEDA-7, 190)*

In 242 patients treated with 3500 injections of polymerized ragweed for immunotherapy two very mild systemic reactions were observed as the only side effects. The patients developed high levels of blocking antibody (6[c]).

In a 3-year double-blind study 40 typical grass pollen allergic patients were allocated to specific immunotherapy (hyposensitization) with whole pollen allergens and purified pollen allergens (2 isolated timothy major allergens, Ag 19 and Ag 25). The systemic side effects set in after 1.5–5 hours and lasted without further treatment for 30 min to 10 hours. Treatment with the 2-component extract showed a preponderance of minor systemic side effects (arthralgia, rhinitis, tiredness, headache, conjunctivitis, nausea, flu-like symptoms) but major systemic side effects (urticaria, angioedema, asthma) were equally distributed between treatments with the two extracts. Major systemic side effects complicated the treatment before the first grass pollen season in 33% of the patients versus only 3% during the subsequent perennial therapy. Systemic and local (side) effects were delayed when using aluminium-absorbed extracts. Major systemic side effects were predicted by means of high nasal sensitivity but not by immediate local skin reactions (7).

Tiaramide *(SEDA-7, 189)*

29 patients with moderate to severe bronchial asthma cooperated in a double-blind cross-over study using placebo, salbutamol and tiaramide (800 mg/d). No difference in therapeutic effect was found between tiaramide and salbutamol; both were better than placebo. Few patients experienced side effects with tiaramide; these comprised headache, diarrhea and nausea (8).

Mucolytic agents *(SED 9, 277; SEDA-4, 121; SEDA-5, 170; SEDA-6, 171; SEDA-7, 189)*

Although the clinical usefulness of mucolytic agents is still under discussion, all authors agree that side effects are no problem. In a balanced article on *bromhexine* Jørgensen pointed out that few side effects have been detected with this agent. Reactivation of intestinal ulcers is the most important, but has only been described in a few patients. As far as the author knows no hematemesis, melena or other complications have been found (9[r]). Milder gastrointestinal symptoms have been referred to in earlier volumes in this series.

In a group of 27 patients (16 males and 11 females) the tolerance of *ambroxol* was excellent in 15, good in 10, moderate in 1; in 1 patient with duodenal ulcer there were complaints about pyrosis and dyspepsia (10[c]).

In a double-blind study 224 pregnant women received ambroxol or placebo daily over a period of 5 days (500 ml infusion of 5% glucose with 1000 mg ambroxol or placebo within 2 hours). All these women were already in premature labor or had premature rupture of the membranes between the 28th and 36th week. Side effects such as nausea were described in 3 women on placebo and in 5 on ambroxol. All 8 had received betamimetic drugs (11[C]).

Acetylcysteine (NAC) is used not only as a mucolytic but also systemically as an antidote in paracetamol poisoning. Side effects are rare.

A 49-year-old woman had ingested about 50 tablets of paracetamol and a bottle of sherry. She had for many years taken phenytoin and phenobarbitone for the control of epilepsy. The plasma paracetamol on admission (at least 8 hr post ingestion) was 146 mg/l. Intravenous NAC 150 mg/kg over 15 min was started. Within 5–10 min a patchy erythematous rash appeared over the patients face and arms and she complained of wheeziness and difficulty in breathing. The infusion was discontinued and the symptoms subsided within 10 min (12[c]).

Using the De Vilbiss inhaler various concentrations of *Mesna* (usually 1:1 diluted solution) have been used in 29 patients without severe complications. There were 2 cases of bronchospasm and 1 case produced blood-tinged sputum (13).

Cough remedies

Mofoxine (Arphosal) is an antitussive substance possibly having antiphlogistic and sedative properties. When it was administered to 41 children (1–12 years) in an amount of 4 mg/kg per day, no side effects, either clinical or biochemical, were observed (14).

A 21-year-old female had 2 epileptic attacks after swallowing 25 mg of *tipepidine hibenzate* (3-di(2-thienyl)methylene-1-methylpiperidinium 4-hydroxybenzophenone-2-carboxylate). Under EEG control she took again a therapeutic dose and epileptiform changes in the EEG were detected. The piperidine ring can be considered as convulsant, its convulsant action being antagonized by GABA. It is therefore not entirely surprising that, after having given the patient 300 mg vitamin B6 per day intramuscularly for 8 consecutive days and then rechallenging here with the drug, the EEG remained normal (15[c]).

REFERENCES

1. Adverse Drug Reactions Advisory Committee (1982) Seven case studies. *Med. J. Aust., 1,* 524.
2. Ostler HB (1982) Alpha-1-Antitrypsin and ocular sensitivity to cromoglycate. *Lancet, 2,* 1287.
3. Baronti A, Vibelli C (1983) Ketotifen in skin-test-positive perennial asthma. *Curr. Ther. Res., 33,* 401.
4. Vibelli C, Rudelli G (1982) Multicentre study for the evaluation of ketotifen in the prophylaxis of bronchial asthma: an interim report. *Curr. Ther. Res., 32,* 686.
5. Goihman-Yahr M, Rothemberg A, Essenfeld-Yahr E (1983) Erythema multiforme and ketotifen. *J. Am. Acad. Derm., 8,* 429.
6. Grammer LC, Zeiss CR, Suszko IM et al (1982) A double-blind placebo-controlled trial of polymerized whole ragweed for immunotherapy of ragweed allergy. *Am. Acad. All. Immunol., 69,* 494.
7. Østerballe O (1982) Side effects during immunotherapy with purified grass pollen extracts. *Allergy 37,* 553.
8. Bonifazi F, Sanguinetti CM, Vennarucci LS, Gasparini S (1982) La tiaramide, un nuovo farmaco per via orale, nel trattamento dell'asma. *Riv. Pat. Clin. Tubercol. Pneumol., 53,* 69.
9. Jørgensen PH (1982) Bromhexin, en genvurdering ud fra litteraturen. *Ugeskr. Laeg., 144,* 1327.
10. Piantedosi FV, Cordedda M (1982) Efficacia terapeutica e tollerabilita dell'ambroxol in uno studio su 27 pazienti broncopneumopatici. *Osp. Ital. Pediatr., 17,* 812.
11. Wauer RR, Schmalisch G, Menzel K et al (1982) The antenatal use of ambroxol (bromhexine metabolite VIII) to prevent hyaline membrane disease: a controlled double-blind study. *Biol. Res. Pregn., 3,* 84.
12. Vale JA, Wheeler DC (1982) Anaphylactoid reactions to acetylcysteine. *Lancet, 2,* 988.
13. Choi KH, Kim KR, Kim JM et al (1982) Clinical effects of mercaptoethane sylphonate (MESNA) in various respiratory diseases. *Tuber. Resp. Dis., 29,* 157.
14. Romagny G, Karman JF (1982) Intérêt d'une molécule tussiplégique nouvelle en pédiatrie. La mofoxine. *Prog. Méd. (Paris), 5,* 87.
15. Cuomo RM (1982) On the possible convulsive activity of an antitussive piperidinic

derivative ('tipepidina ibenzato') in man. *Acta Neurol., 37,* 110.
16. Kallós P, Kallós L (1982) Pseudo-allergic reactions due to disodium cromoglycate. In: *Pseudo-Allergic Reactions. Involvement of Drugs and Chemicals, Vol. 3,* pp. 122–132. Karger, Basel.
17. Parker JM (1983) Paper delivered to the Drug Information Association, Washington DC, July 1983 (Personal communication to the Editor).

Jeffrey K. Aronson

18 Cardiac glycosides and drugs used in dysrhythmias

DIGITALIS GLYCOSIDES *(SED-9, 180; SEDA-4, 123; SEDA-5, 172; SEDA-6, 173; SEDA-7, 193)*

Monitoring therapy

It is known from a combination of theoretical considerations, anecdotes, and a few prospective studies that the risk of digitalis toxicity is increased by hypokalemia and probably by hypercalcemia (SED-10). It has now been shown that the combination of mild hypokalemia with mild hypercalcemia (expressed as an increase in the ratio of serum ionized calcium to serum potassium concentrations) increases the risk of digoxin toxicity manifesting as ectopic dysrhythmias (1^C). By contrast patients with digoxin toxicity manifesting as either gastrointestinal symptoms or evidence of atrioventricular nodal block did not have an increased Ca:K ratio but had high serum digoxin concentrations. In addition, the patients with ectopic dysrhythmias had an increased arterial pH (7.498), while in the other patients the pH was not raised. The authors suggest that when toxicity occurs in association with serum digoxin concentrations in the recognised 'therapeutic' range (0.8–2.0 ng/ml; 1.0–2.6 nmol/l) it may be due to alterations in the Ca:K ratio and arterial pH, and when that happens increased automaticity may result in ectopic dysrhythmias. The other manifestations of digitalis toxicity are more likely to occur at high serum digoxin concentrations without marked changes in Ca:K ratio or arterial pH. However, in the patients with AV nodal block, more than half had serum digoxin concentrations in the 'therapeutic' range and although there may be further subgroups within this group of patients, they were not identifiable on the basis of the Ca:K ratio or arterial pH.

Side Effects of Drugs Annual 8
M.N.G. Dukes, editor

ISBN 0 444 90339 9
$0.80 per article per page (transactional system)
$0.20 per article per page (licensing system)

Toxic effects

Children There has been a report of the dangers of even low dosages of digoxin in seriously ill, low-birth-weight (<1500 g) children (2^C). Of 18 sick children given digoxin for the treatment of circulatory congestion secondary to patent ductus arteriosus, 9 developed one or more signs of clinical deterioration attributed to digoxin toxicity and resolving on discontinuation of digoxin. Digoxin maintenance dosages were between 3 and 5 μg/kg and while it is known that the dose:serum concentration ratio is lower in neonates than in older children (3^C), these dosages would be expected to result in serum digoxin concentrations of between 1.0 and 1.5 ng/ml (1.3 and 1.9 nmol/l). However, in these 9 low-birth-weight neonates, serum digoxin concentrations were between 3.5 and 4.1 ng/ml, presumably because of markedly reduced renal clearance. Even so, these serum concentrations are not necessarily high enough to have been associated with digitalis toxicity in children under one month of age (SEDA-3, 151) and other factors may also have played a part. For example, all the children had respiratory distress syndrome and acidosis may have potentiated the effects of digoxin. Whatever the causes of toxicity in these low-birth-weight children it is clear that great care must be taken if digoxin is to be used.

Cardioversion The increased risk of serious dysrhythmias following electrical cardioversion in patients taking digitalis is well known and if cardioversion is necessary in such patients, it is recommended that initial attempts should be with low energies (e.g. 10 Joules). In a study (4[C]) of 50 patients with plasma digoxin concentrations at 0.7–2.4 ng/ml, 6 of whom had clinical and symptomatic evidence of digoxin toxicity, successful cardioversion was carried out using energies of between 10 and 200 Joules, using a procedure in which electrical shocks were administered in increasing energies, starting at 10 Joules. The distribution of successful cardioversions was as follows: 10–20 J in 16 patients (2 toxic); 30–40 J in 14 patients (1 toxic); 50–75 J in 5 patients (2 toxic); 100–150 J in 5 patients (2 toxic); 200 J in 5 patients (1 toxic).

Following cardioversion 21 patients had premature atrial beats, 12 had occasional premature ventricular beats, and one had ventricular tachycardia. The ventricular tachycardia resolved following a single i.v. injection of lignocaine and no other treatment of dysrhythmias, all of which resolved within 24 hours, was needed. The authors concluded that cardioversion in patients taking digitalis was safe and that initially low energies should be used, confirming the views of others. However, they stressed the importance of correcting potassium depletion before attempting cardioversion, and one could perhaps add to that the suggestion that other electrolyte abnormalities and acidosis should also be remedied before cardioversion.

Endocrine In Annual 7 the effects of digitalis on sex hormones and gonadotrophins were reviewed and it was concluded that in *patients* on digitalis there was an increase in serum FSH and estrogen concentrations, and a reduction in LH and testosterone concentrations (SEDA-7, 194). However, it has recently been reported (5[C]) that in *healthy male volunteers*, 25–39 years of age, β-acetyldigoxin caused no changes in plasma concentrations of androstenedione, dehydroepiandrosterone, estrone, estradiol, progesterone, 17-hydroxyprogesterone, cortisol, and aldosterone. There was no change in the plasma steroid response to ACTH or HCG and LH concentrations rose normally after LHRH (GnRH or gonadorelin). Plasma digoxin concentrations were 1.5 ± 0.6 ng/ml (1.9 ± 0.8 nmol/l) and β-acetyldigoxin was given for 43 days. The reasons for the discrepancies in results between patients and healthy volunteers are not clear but since plasma steroid hormone concentrations are known to be altered by, for example, age, obesity, liver disease, and some forms of cardiovascular disease, the results in patients may be attributable to a drug-disease interaction rather than to a simple drug effect. The duration of treatment may also be important, since the effect of digitoxin in causing stratification of vaginal epithelium in post-menopausal women was noted only after 2 years of therapy (SEDA-7, 194). The results in healthy volunteers do not, as the authors suggest, necessarily exonerate digoxin, as opposed to digitoxin, as a direct cause of feminizing effects in patients.

Treatment of toxicity There continue to appear reports of the successful use of Fab fragments of anti-digoxin antibodies in the treatment of digitalis toxicity and self-poisoning, in the case not only of digoxin but also of digitoxin and lanatoside C. We have mentioned some of these reports in previous editions of SEDA (SEDA-5, 173; SEDA-6, 178) and there has recently appeared a review of the experience of one group in 26 cases of life-threatening digitalis intoxication, including 4 cases which have been published before (6[C]). Of the 26 patients, 23 had taken digoxin, 20 of whom were taking it for known heart disease, and 13 of whom took overdoses accidentally or with suicidal intent. Of those 23, 19 had serum digoxin concentrations over 5 ng/ml (6.4 nmol/l). Of the 3 patients who took digitoxin, all had plasma digitoxin concentrations over 100 ng/ml (131 nmol/l). The manifestations of digitalis toxicity were: severe nausea and vomiting (20 patients); hyperkalemia (>5.6 mmol/l) (11 patients); advanced cardiac rhythm disturbances (all patients: accelerated atrioventricular functional rhythm < 100/min or tachycardia > 100/min (13 patients), ventricular dysrhythmias (VT or VF) (20 patients), high-grade atrioventricular block (19 patients).

Treatment with Fab fragments was initiated before irreversible myocardial or brain damage had occurred in 22 of the patients; 21 recovered completely and 1 died with recurrence of dysrhythmias (attributed to inadequate dosage of antibody). The other 4 patients died, albeit after an apparently initial favorable response.

In no case was there any adverse reaction attributable to the use of antibody, and in particular, there was no evidence of hypersensitivity reactions.

Risk factors The risks presented by the presence both of mild hypokalemia and mild hypercalcemia are discussed under 'monitoring therapy' (above).

Interactions

Nifedipine Nifedipine in a dose of 10 mg t.d.s. has been reported to increase plasma digoxin concentrations in healthy subjects by about 45% (7[c], 8[C]). However, in a formal study of the effect of nifedipine on the pharmacokinetics of digoxin in healthy subjects, no effect whatsoever was found apart from a slight *increase* in non-renal clearance (9[C]). The reason for this discrepancy is not clear, and it is not known what the clinical significance of this interaction might be, even if it exists.

Amiodarone There are now 4 reports that amiodarone increases plasma digoxin concentrations (10[c], 11[c], 12[C], 13[C]). Three of these reports are anecdotal, and in the other (12[C]) the evidence was indirect, consisting of a weak but significant correlation between plasma amiodarone and plasma digoxin concentrations in patients taking digoxin or β-methyldigoxin. In one other study no such effect was found (despite the title of the paper!) (14[c]). This interaction awaits formal elucidation and assessment of its clinical significance.

Cytotoxic drugs It has been reported that certain combinations of cytotoxic drugs may reduce plasma digoxin concentrations by approximately 50% during treatment with β-acetyldigoxin (15[C]). The cytotoxic drug combinations studied were cyclophosphamide, vincristine, and prednisone, with and without procarbazine. The suggested mechanism was impairment of absorption of β-acetyldigoxin. In another similar study no such effect was described for digitoxin (16[C]).

Lidocaine (lignocaine)

The adverse effects resulting from two different infusion regimens of lidocaine have been compared (17[C]). In both regimens an initial dose of 75 mg was given i.v. over 2 min and was followed 2 min later by administration of 150 mg over 18 min. In one regimen the 150 mg was infused continuously over the whole 18 min; in the other three 50 mg injections were given at 6 min intervals. In both cases treatment was continued with a continuous infusion at a rate of 2 mg/min. Mean plasma lidocaine concentrations were the same in the two groups although some patients in the multiple dose group had higher concentrations at around 20 min after the initial dose. Of the 18 patients studied, 13 had either drowsiness or tinnitus following the initial 75 mg dose. During the subsequent administration of 150 mg, all 6 of the patients given 50 mg three times had symptoms of mild to moderate toxicity (drowsiness, tinnitus, dysarthria, or paresthesiae). In comparison, only 1 of the 12 patients given the continuous infusion of 150 mg experienced symptoms of toxicity (drowsiness). Adverse effects were not closely related to plasma lidocaine concentrations.

These data stress the need for relatively slow infusion of lidocaine during the period of loading.

As to the duration of infusion of lidocaine, it is known that because of its conversion to toxic metabolites with longer half-times than the parent drug, lidocaine should not be given for more than 36–48 hours. An additional complication appears to be that with prolonged infusion (24 hours or more), the total body clearance rate of lidocaine is reduced by about 30% and its half-time proportionately prolonged (18[C]). This effect may be due to lidocaine-induced alterations in liver blood flow.

Disopyramide

Liver In addition to the rather sketchy information published by the Japanese Ministry of Health and Welfare (albeit from a large number of patients) suggesting that disopyramide may cause liver damage (19[cr]), there are other anecdotal reports.

Intrahepatic *cholestasis* has been reported in at least 2 cases (20[c], 21[c]) and *hepatocellular damage* in conjunction with disseminated intravascular coagulation in 1 case (22[c]). However, disopyramide may also cause heart failure and has been reported to have twice caused *secondary hepatic impairment* without direct hepatotoxicity

(23[c]). Thus, reports of hepatic damage must be viewed critically. On the basis of the Japanese experience the incidence of hepatic damage is 0.35% and since this may represent an overestimate, the incidence is clearly very low.

Endocrine Anecdotal reports of disopyramide-induced *hypoglycemia* continue to appear (24[c], 25[c], 26[cr]). In 2 cases (26[cr]) hypoglycemia was associated with lactic acidosis of uncertain cause. This appears to be a very uncommon reaction and its pathogenesis has not been worked out.

Skin There has been a single report of cutaneous *blisters* attributed to disopyramide and occurring in conjunction with intravascular coagulation (27[c]).

Breast milk Disopyramide and its N-monodesalkyl metabolite are excreted in breast milk, but an anecdotal report suggests that the amounts so excreted are probably too small to affect a suckling infant (28[c]).

Overdosage Experience of 20 cases of acute overdosage with disopyramide has been reported with a review of 23 other cases in the literature (29[CR]). The clinical manifestations include cardiac and non-cardiac effects. The *cardiac effects* include a variety of dysrhythmias (sinus tachycardia, sinus bradycardia, ventricular extrasystoles, tachycardia, and fibrillation, torsade de pointes, atrial fibrillation), different forms of heart block (AV nodal block, bundle branch block, intraventricular conduction defects), cardiogenic shock, and cardiac arrest. The non-cardiac effects include those of *anticholinergic poisoning* (e.g. urinary retention, dry mouth, constipation, tachycardia, blurred vision), neurological abnormalities (drowsiness and coma, convulsions), respiratory failure, and hypothermia.

The main principles of suggested treatment were reviewed in SEDA-4 (p. 128).

Interaction There has been a single anecdotal report that disopyramide might potentiate the effects of *warfarin* (SEDA-3, 156). A study of 3 patients on disopyramide and warfarin has failed to confirm such an interaction (30[c]). However, the same authors also reported no interaction of quinidine with warfarin in 2 cases and the question of whether disopyramide interacts with warfarin must still be considered open, since quinidine is known to interact with warfarin.

Amiodarone

A comprehensive review of the clinical pharmacology, uses and adverse effects of amiodarone has recently appeared (31[CR]).

With continuing use of this highly effective drug, more experience is accumulating of its long-term adverse effects.

In one series of 140 patients (32[C]) who had been taking amiodarone for up to 5 years (mean 2 years) in dosages of 100–1200 mg/day, the following adverse effects were recorded.

Lung One patient in this series developed pulmonary *interstitial* changes with a restrictive defect on lung function testing.

Nervous system In 8 patients *proximal muscle weakness,* involving the thighs in particular, occurred during the first few weeks and was dose-dependent, occurring at dosages over 800 mg/day, and resolving on reduction of dosage. Two other patients taking high dosages had delayed nerve conduction, but normal electromyograms.

Although a peripheral neuropathy is a well-described risk of amiodarone therapy, none of the patients in this series developed it.

Thyroid In 10 patients systematically studied serum thyroxine (T4) and reverse triiodothyronine (rT3) rose in all. In 85 other patients the mean serum T4 was increased 20% above the control mean; in 5 serum T4 was reduced and TSH increased. Two of those were clinically hypothyroid; 4 patients had increased serum T4 concentrations > 25% above the control mean and 2 were clinically hyperthyroid (both with raised T3 concentrations).

Liver In 15 of 100 patients studied there was a 1.5- to 4-fold increase in serum aspartate aminotransferase activity. This effect correlated well with the plasma concentrations of both amiodarone and its main metabolite desethyl amiodarone. The serum alanine aminotransferase was similarly increased and there was a minimal rise in γ-glutamyl transpeptidase. Bilirubin and alkaline phosphatase were unaffected. In 2 subjects liver biopsies showed no abnormalities. At present, changes in 'liver' enzymes need not dictate withdrawal of amiodarone.

Skin Photosensitivity occurred in 57% of the patients studied. This photosensitivity was not related to plasma concentrations of drug or metabolite but could be alleviated by a reduction in dosage. In contrast, only 2 patients developed the well-known slate-grey/purple *pigmentation*, affecting the face. In those cases biopsy revealed deposition of lipofuscin, a decrease in melanin content, and intense elastic degeneration. This effect was thought to be dose/duration-dependent. In 6 patients a transient, pruritic, erythematous, maculopapular *rash* was seen during the first few days of treatment.

Eyes All patients developed *corneal microdeposits* by 1 month and some as early as 10 days after starting therapy. In only 2 cases were the deposits close enough to the centre of the cornea to cause visual symptoms.

In a different series of 80 patients (33[C]) who had been taking amiodarone for up to 4.5 years (mean 14.8 months) in dosages of 100–1200 mg/day, adverse effects occurred in an overall 82% (requiring withdrawal in 18%) as follows.

Cardiovascular Sinus node arrest occurred in 3 patients and required cardiac pacing. All 3 were also taking digoxin, which may have contributed to the adverse effects.

In 4 patients with recurrent ventricular tachycardia, treatment resulted in incessant *ventricular tachycardia* after 7–35 days of treatment. Resolution followed withdrawal and although 3 of these patients were also taking digoxin, it was felt that that had not contributed in at least 2 of the cases.

Lung Interstitial *pneumonitis* occurred in 4 patients (5%), with restrictive defects on lung function testing. Withdrawal led to resolution in all cases, but one patient was also given prednisone. None of the patients had a history or symptoms of lung disease before starting amiodarone.

Nervous system 19 patients (24%) had *central neurological disorders,* including ataxia, dizziness, tremor, headaches, and nightmares. *Neuromuscular* complaints occurred in 11 (14%), including generalized weakness, proximal muscle weakness, and muscle tenderness. In 2 cases withdrawal of therapy was required because of muscle weakness.

Thyroid The mean free thyroxine index of the population rose, and there were also increases in the mean values of the T3 resin uptake and rT3 concentrations, with a great deal of variability among individual changes. Only 1 patient developed clinical evidence of thyroid disease (hypothyroidism).

Liver In 14 patients (40% of those studied) there were increases in serum alanine aminotransferase and lactic dehydrogenase of more than 50%. One patient presented with malaise, fever, abdominal tenderness, and an enlarged tender liver. Resolution followed withdrawal and reintroduction at a lower dosage caused smaller increases in liver enzymes without clinical effects.

Gastrointestinal 27 patients (34%) had gastrointestinal disturbances, mostly nausea and anorexia, requiring withdrawal in 3 cases.

Skin Photosensitivity occurred in only 7 patients (9%), blue-grey discoloration in 3 and transient urticaria in 1.

Eyes All patients developed *corneal microdeposits* by 6 months but in only 2 cases did visual symptoms result.

Other Hair loss and *hyperhidrosis* were reported, each in 2 patients. *Hypercalcemia* occurred in 1 patient and necessitated withdrawal.

Frequency and severity of adverse effects The general incidence of adverse reactions to amiodarone in children was discussed in SEDA-6 (p. 181), and an accumulation of recent evidence makes it possible to draw conclusions as to adults. From the data of the two large studies outlined above, and one previous study (SEDA-9, 204), it appears that the incidence of interstitial *pneumonitis* may be as high as 5% and anecdotal reports continue to appear (34–38[c]). In 1 case there was accompanying *bone-marrow suppression* with an anemia, but normal white cell and platelet counts (34[c]). The pneumonitis appears to be dose/duration-related, most of the cases having occurred in patients taking at least 400 mg/day for at least 1 month, although there have been two reports in patients taking 200 mg/day, both for at least 2–3 months (35[c], 37[c]). Most of the affected patients have had no recorded evidence of preexisting lung disease and in the majority of cases recovery has occurred following the withdrawal of amiodarone with or without the addition of corticosteroids. In 2 patients who died, however, corticosteroids had not been used (36[c]), and it is suggested that corticosteroids be given to such patients routinely, since there is experience of their efficacy in drug-induced pulmonary disease (39[R]).

The difficulty in treating amiodarone-induced *hyperthyroidism* because of fully iodinated thyroglobulin stores has been pointed out in the context of 2 cases in which prednisone treatment appears to have been effective (40[c]). In 1 case there had been failure of response to carbimazole 60 mg/day for 3 weeks.

A case of generalized pustular *psoriasis* in a patient with psoriasis previously confined to the fingernails has been reported and attributed to amiodarone (41[c]). However, the patient was also taking prednisone, which is more likely to have been to blame. *Photosensitivity* is much more frequent (up to 57%) but its incidence is very variable; *discoloration* seems to involve a constant but small minority.

There has been a case report of the use of amiodarone, 400 mg/day, during *pregnancy* from the 16th week on. The child was healthy, apart from a sinus bradycardia, and at 9 weeks postpartum had plasma amiodarone concentrations of only 25% of those of its mother (42[c]). The concentrations of amiodarone and desethyl amiodarone were measured in breast milk and the daily intake of amiodarone calculated to be at the lower end of the adult therapeutic range (1.5 mg/kg/day). The potential clinical relevance of this dosage in a neonate is not known.

Interactions

Digoxin See above under Cardiac glycosides.

Warfarin That amiodarone potentiates the effects of warfarin is well described (SEDA-6, 181). A series of 10 further cases of such potentiation has been reported (42[C]). In 1 case blood was assayed for concentrations of factors V, VII, IX and X. The last 3 were markedly reduced and it was suggested that amiodarone acts by further reducing the circulating concentration of clotting factors. Normal plasma returned the prothrombin activity to normal, suggesting that amiodarone was in some way affecting the activity via an alteration in vitamin K activity, rather than by changing the activity of circulating clotting factors. The data provided did not, however, yield any information as to the possible mechanism of such an effect. The time-course of the interaction appears to rule out protein-binding displacement of warfarin as a mechanism.

Class I antidysrhythmics In 3 cases amiodarone has been reported to have interacted with Class I antidysrhythmic drugs (43–45[c]).

In 2 cases the combination of amiodarone with quinidine reportedly caused torsade de pointes secondary to prolongation of the QT interval (43[c]), a well-known effect of both amiodarone and quinidine. In a healthy volunteer it was shown that quinidine prolonged the QT interval by 20% and that the QT interval was further prolonged, to a total of 40%, on the addition of amiodarone. The plasma quinidine concentration in the volunteer rose slightly following the addition of amiodarone but there is insufficient information to say whether the interaction was pharmacokinetic (involving an increase in quinidine concentrations) or pharmacodynamic (involving an additive or synergistic effect of the two drugs). The authors reported dysrhythmias and prolongation of the QT interval in 4 other patients in whom amiodarone was combined with disopyramide, propafenon, and mexiletine, and that suggests that the interaction is more likely to be predominantly pharmacodynamic.

In another case sinus arrest was reported in a patient with sick sinus syndrome following the i.v. injection of 300 mg lidocaine in a patient taking amiodarone, 600 mg/day. Both drugs may suppress sinus node function and this too may have been a pharmacodynamic interaction.

Finally, amiodarone has been reported to have increased steady-state plasma aprindine concentrations and thereby to cause slow ventricular tachycardia in one case and ataxia and light-headedness in the other (45[c]). The mechanism of this apparent interaction is not clear.

REFERENCES

1. Sonnenblick M, Abraham AS, Meshulam Z, Eylath U (1983) Correlation between manifestations of digoxin toxicity and serum digoxin, calcium, potassium and magnesium concentrations and arterial pH. *Br. Med. J., 286,* 1089.
2. Johnson GL, Desai NS, Pauly TH, Cunningham MD (1982) Complications associated with digoxin therapy in low-birth-weight infants. *Pediatrics, 69,* 463.
3. Iisalo E, Dahl M, Sundqvist H (1973) Serum digoxin in adults and children. *Int. J. Clin. Pharmacol., 7,* 213.
4. Ali N, Dais K, Banks T, Sheikh M (1982) Fibrated electrical cardioversion in patients on digoxin. *Clin. Cardiol., 5,* 417.
5. Kley HK, Müller A, Peerenboom H, Krüskemper HL (1982) Digoxin does not alter plasma steroid levels in healthy men. *Clin. Pharmacol. Ther., 32,* 12.
6. Smith TW, Butler VP, Haber E et al (1982) Treatment of life-threatening digitalis intoxication with digoxin-specific Fab antibody fragments. *N. Engl. J. Med., 307,* 1357.
7. Belz GG, Aust PE, Munkes R (1981) Digoxin plasma concentrations and nifedipine. (Letter). *Lancet, 1,* 844.
8. Belz GG, Doering W, Munkes R, Matthews J (1983) Interaction between digoxin and calcium antagonists and antiarrhythmic drugs. *Clin. Pharmacol. Ther., 33,* 410.
9. Pedersen KE, Dorph-Pedersen A, Hvidt S et al (1982) Effect of nifedipine on digoxin kinetics in healthy subjects. *Clin. Pharmacol. Ther., 32,* 562.
10. Moysey JO, Jaggarao NJV, Grundy EN, Chamberlain DA (1981) Amiodarone increases plasma digoxin concentrations. *Br. Med. J., 282,* 272.
11. Berdeaux A, Valette H, Auzepy P et al (1981) Influence de l'amiodarone et la digoxinémie. *Nouv. Presse Méd., 10,* 3650.
12. Furlanello F, Inama G, Ferrari M et al (1981) Un altro tipo di interazione fra livelli ematici della digitale e di farmaci antiaritmici: digoxina ed amiodarone. *G. Ital. Cardiol., 11,* 1725.
13. McGovern B, Garan H, Kelly E, Ruskin JN (1983) Adverse reactions during treatment with amiodarone hydrochloride. *Br. Med. J., 287,* 175.
14. Achilli A, Serra N (1981) Amiodarone increases plasma digoxin concentrations. (Letter) *Br. Med. J., 282,* 1630.
15. Kuhlmann J, Zilly W, Wilke J (1981) Effects of cytostatic drugs on plasma level and renal excretion of β-acetyldigoxin. *Clin. Pharmacol. Ther., 30,* 518.
16. Kuhlmann J. Wilke J, Rietbrock N (1982) Cytostatic drugs are without significant effect on digitoxin plasma level and renal excretion. *Clin. Pharmacol. Ther., 32,* 646.
17. Stargel WW, Shand DG, Routledge PA et al (1981) Clinical comparison of rapid infusion and multiple injection methods for lidocaine loading. *Am. Heart J., 102,* 872.
18. Bauer LA, Brown T, Gibaldi M et al (1982) Influence of long-term infusion on lidocaine kinetics. *Clin. Pharmacol. Ther., 31,* 433.
19. Anon (1981) Hepatic damage due to disopyramide. *Jpn. Med. Gaz., June 20th, 11.*
20. Meinertz T, Langer KH, Kasper W, Just H (1977) Disopyramide-induced intrahepatic cholestasis. (Letter). *Lancet, 2,* 828.
21. Riccioni N, Bozzi L, Susini N, Roni P (1977) Disopyramide-induced intrahepatic cholestasis. (Letter) *Lancet, 2,* 1362.
22. Doody PT (1982) Disopyramide hepatotoxicity and disseminated intravascular coagulation. *South Med. J., 75,* 496.
23. Scheinman SJ, Poll DS, Wolfson S (1980) Acute cardiac failure and hepatic ischemia induced by disopyramide phosphate. *Yale J. Biol. Med., 53,* 361.
24. Koizumi J, Kawasaki S, Ueno H et al (1981) A diabetic woman showing a hypoglycemic effect induced by disopyramide (Rythmodan). *J. Jpn Diab. Soc., 24,* 861.
25. Chaussade S, Beucler A, Lafaix C (1982) Hypoglycémie induite par le disopyramide. Une observation. *Nouv. Presse Méd., 11,* 1951.
26. Nappi JM, Dhanani S, Lovejoy JR, van der Ark C (1983) Severe hypoglycemia associated with disopyramide. *West. J. Med., 138,* 95.
27. Handa SP (1982) Disopyramide-induced toxic cutaneous blisters and coagulopathy. *Dialysis Transpl., 11,* 706.
28. Barnett DB, Hudson SA, McBurney A (1982) Disopyramide and its N-monodesalkyl metabolite in breast milk. *Br. J. Clin. Pharmacol., 14,* 310.
29. Larcan A, Lambert H, Laprévote-Heully MC et al (1981) Les intoxications aiguës volontaires au disopyramide. A propos de 20 observations. *Ann. Méd. Nancy, 20,* 901.
30. Sylvén C, Anderson P (1983) Evidence that disopyramide does not interact with warfarin. *Br. Med. J., 286,* 1181.
31. Krikler DM, McKenna WJ, Chamberlain DA (Ed) (1983) Amiodarone and arrhythmias. Pergamon Press, Oxford.
32. Harris L, McKenna WJ, Rowland E et al (1982) Side effects of long-term amiodarone therapy. *Circulation, 67,* 45.
33. McGovern B, Garan H, Kelly E, Ruskin JN (1983) Adverse reactions during treatment with amiodarone hydrochloride. *Br. med. J., 287,* 175.
34. Wright AJ, Brackenbridge RG (1982) Pulmonary infiltration and bone marrow depression complicating treatment with amiodarone. *Br. Med. J., 284,* 1303.
35. Schlaeffer F, Gold B, Hirsch M, Keynan A (1982) A case of interstitial pneumonitis during amiodarone therapy. *Isr. J. Med. Sci., 18,* 809.

36. Sobol SM, Rakita L (1982) Pneumonitis and pulmonary fibrosis associated with amiodarone treatment: a possible complication of a new antiarrhythmic drug. *Circulation, 65,* 819.
37. Chebat J, Caubarrère I (1983) Pneumopathie grave et amiodarone. *Thérapie, 38,* 107.
38. Suárez LD, Poderoso JJ, Elsner B et al (1983) Subacute pneumopathy during amiodarone therapy. *Chest, 83,* 566.
39. Rohfling BM, Hanffer JL (1980) Drug-induced pulmonary disease. In: Prager L (Ed) *Induced Disease,* p. 45, Grune & Stratton, New York.
40. Wimpfheimer C, Stäubli M, Schädelin J, Studer H (1982) Prednisone in amiodarone-induced thyrotoxicosis. *Br. Med. J., 284,* 1835.
41. Muir AD, Wilson M (1982) Amiodarone and psoriasis. (Letter) *NZ Med. J., 95,* 711.
42. Hamer A, Peter T, Mandel WJ et al (1982) The potentiation of warfarin anticoagulation by amiodarone. *Circulation, 65,* 1025.
43. Tartini R, Kappenberger L, Steinbrunn W, Meyer UA (1982) Dangerous interaction between amiodarone and quinidine. *Lancet, 1,* 1327.
44. Keidar S, Grenadier E, Palant A (1982) Sinoatrial arrest due to lidocaine injection in sick sinus syndrome during amiodarone administration. *Am. Heart J., 104,* 1384.
45. Southworth W, Friday KJ, Ruffy R (1982) Possible amiodarone-aprindine interaction. (Letter) *Am. Heart J., 104,* 323.

J.R. Lawrence

19 Anti-anginal and beta-adrenoceptor blocking drugs

BETA BLOCKERS *(SED-9, 295; SEDA-4, 131, 144; SEDA-5, 184; SEDA-6, 185; SEDA-7, 210)*

Central nervous system

Significant psychiatric morbidity during beta-blocker therapy; how common are depression and 'tiredness'? While insomnia and hallucinations are recognized side effects of beta-blocker therapy, a high incidence of depression was noted in one early trial (1[C]) and more recently Petrie et al (2[C]) documented 3 cases of apparent psychotic depression soon after the start of propranolol therapy. In a further 2 patients (3[C]) a cause-effect relationship between beta-blocker therapy and depressive reactions appeared validated by rechallenge experience. Both of these patients developed symptoms while taking propranolol but in 1 case it was the subsequent introduction of metoprolol, another relatively lipophilic agent, which precipitated relapse. However, a very similar case of severe depression occurred during treatment with nadolol (4[C]), a compound of very low lipophilicity (5[R]).

Acute toxic confusional states due to propranolol therapy have been reported in the past (SED-9, 297; SEDA-4, 134; SEDA-5, 185; SEDA-7, 210) and further severe reactions of this type, again attributed to propranolol as confirmed by rechallenge, have recently been documented (6[C], 7[C]).

Significant but less severe degrees of depression and tiredness (which symptoms may also result from the effect of beta-blockers on exercise tolerance – vide infra) have been reported in several large prospective placebo controlled studies designed to examine the efficacy of therapy following myocardial infarction (8[c]–10[c]).

Lipophilicity will control central nervous system penetration of a particular compound and hence may affect its potential to produce some side effects such as vivid dreams and nightmares (5[R], 11[R]). Even atenolol, an extremely hydrophilic compound, has however been associated with severe nightmares and insomnia in the occasional patient (12[c]).

Complicated migraine and cerebrovascular disease Propranolol has long been used as prophylactic therapy by migraine sufferers and nadolol was recently shown to be efficacious in this regard. In an occasional patient, however, the vasospastic features of migraine may actually be provoked by beta-blocker therapy and in one patient a migraine attack during propranolol therapy was complicated by cerebral infarction (13[C]). This resulted in a permanent left hemiparesis whose onset, at an unspecified time after a typical prodrome of left-sided scintillating scotomata, followed right-sided headache and occurred when the patient was erect. Postural hypotension was postulated as a contributory factor in this case and certainly an adverse vasomotor reaction may well have contributed to worsening of hemiparesis and aphasia in a previously described case of propranolol-associated complicated migraine (14[C]). Of interest in this regard is the lack of adverse neurological effect to acebutolol or oxprenolol in circa 30 patients with established cerebrovascular disease, one of whom, however, had recurrence of stroke at the end of a placebo wash-out period (15[c]).

Reduced exercise tolerance and impaired exercise and conditioning It has long been recognized that beta-blockers reduce left ventricular work capacity and exercise

Side Effects of Drugs Annual 8
M.N.G. Dukes, editor

ISBN 0 444 90339 9
$0.80 per article per page (transactional system)
$0.20 per article per page (licensing system)

tolerance in normal subjects (SEDA-6, 186; 16[R]). A variety of possible mechanisms – such as reduced cardiac output, impaired muscle blood supply, effects on intermediary metabolism and a direct effect on muscle contraction – have been proposed as of relevance to this side effect (17[R]).

Most studies have concerned healthy volunteers given single doses of beta-blockers and studied under laboratory conditions. Reduced running performance and an increase in subjectively assessed fatigue have also been documented in healthy regular joggers (18[C]).

In theory, $beta_1$-selective agents might produce less impairment in performance but this was not always substantiated in some earlier single-dose volunteer studies (19[C], 20[C]). The cardioselectivity of atenolol did, however, appear to produce less impairment of exercise performance, compared with propranolol in apparently comparable doses, in two other volunteer studies (18[C], 21[C]). Both these studies claimed that subjects with a high proportion of slow-twitch fibres had a greater relative impairment of performance than subjects whose muscle biopsy specimens showed a high percentage of fast-twitch fibres. How cardioselectivity relates to this finding is unclear in view of the similarities of adrenoreceptor innervation of fast- and slow-twitch fibres (22[R]). At present cardioselective agents may be preferable in physically active patients, particularly in view of the superiority of atenolol over propranolol in terms of subjective fatigue in joggers (18[C]). Partial agonist activity appeared to explain the previously described (23[C]) superiority of oxprenolol over propranolol in terms of exercise duration. Further work is, however, required before this and the other ancillary properties of beta-blockers can be definitely graded in terms of effect on exercise.

Finally, in relation to the difficulty in extrapolating the results of single-dose studies to effects during long-term treatment a double-blind volunteer study comparing propranolol and placebo showed clear attenuation of exercise conditioning with propranolol (24[C]). At the end of a 5-week treatment period significantly increased exercise duration, maximal oxygen uptake and decreased diastolic blood pressure at maximal exercise were seen in subjects on placebo but to a lesser extent or not at all in those on active therapy.

Local anesthetic activity Labetalol has been shown to produce effective analgesia when administered by peridural injection to patients with chronic pain from pelvic organ carcinoma (25[c]). Mild burning discomfort at the site of infiltration was attributed to the low pH of the preparation used and was readily controlled by prior steroid or local anesthetic injection.

Sexual dysfunction Beta-blockers have been reported to cause male impotence (SEDA-5, 187; 26[C], 27[C]) and substantiation of this relationship came from the preliminary report of the UK Medical Research Council prospective study of mild hypertension (28[c]) where men given beta-blockers were significantly more impotent than those given placebo. In another large-scale prospective placebo-controlled study reduced sexual activity was a significant side effect of sufficient severity to lead to withdrawal from the trial (29[c]). These two latter reports do, of course, suggest that the effect is separate from or at least superimposed upon any influence of either hypertension or ischemic heart disease. This claim could not be made for a retrospective questionnaire-based study which examined the sexual dysfunction in some detail (30[C]). In this assessment of patients receiving a variety of treatments for hypertension, angina or migraine (where male diabetic patients were excluded) perceived sexual dysfunction was greater in patients receiving beta-blockers, either alone or in combination. Perceived changes in libido were noted by 65% of 112 subjects, being related to disease category but noted 4 times as commonly by males as females. Indeed no pattern of female orgasmic change was noted while in males decrease in ability to maintain an erection was significantly related to drug category and was particularly marked in subjects receiving beta-blockers in combination with other agents.

This rather characteristic finding of erectile dysfunction in men was noted in previous studies (31[c], 32[c]) but has not been documented in single-dose studies of propranolol (33[C]) or labetalol (34[C]). This last study, which used penile plethysmography, did, however, document dose-related delayed ejaculation and detumescence.

Cardiovascular effects

Reduced peripheral circulation *(SEDA-4, 132; SEDA-5, 192; SEDA-6, 188)* It is considered well established that beta-blockers worsen intermittent claudication and the view that this reaction is common has recently been reiterated (11[R]). There is difficulty in establishing the causality of beta-blocker therapy in this regard, however, because of the common occurrence of intermittent claudication in patients with ischemic heart disease and the variable progress of peripheral vascular disease (SED-9, 297). Moreover a previously reported prospective study of patients already suffering from intermittent claudication was unable to demonstrate any relationship between deterioration of claudication and propranolol use (35[C]).

Two brief reviews (36[R], 37[R]) have recently challenged the view that production or exacerbation of intermittent claudication by beta-blocker therapy is at all common. This view seems entirely justified when one considers the results of large placebo controlled prospective trials. In one such study (28[c]), in patients with mild hypertension, intermittent claudication was not mentioned as a side effect, nor did the myocardial infarction secondary prevention trials in which claudication was not a specific contraindication to inclusion (9[c], 10[c], 38[c], 39[c]) report on claudication as a significant side effect – an omission unlikely to be caused by oversight. Thus the conclusion of Diehm (36[R]) and Cameron and Ramsay (37[R]) that patients with intermittent claudication should not be denied possible benefit from beta-blocker therapy seems entirely justifiable. Such patients should, of course, be carefully observed for any possible deterioration in claudication.

Worsening of vasospastic (Prinzmetal's) angina It is recognized that blockade of vasodilatory $beta_2$-receptors in the coronary arteries might result in reduction of myocardial blood flow and this possibility assumes increased importance in light of the recognition of the probable pathophysiological significance of coronary artery spasm in angina (SEDA-5, 184; SEDA-7, 212). A recent reviewer (40[R]) cited evidence that the use of beta-blockers in patients with arteriographic evidence of coronary artery spasm had not consistently induced worsening of the disorder, but concluded that the evidence for occasional provocation of symptomatic coronary artery spasm by beta-blockers indicated the need for caution when initiating therapy.

Withdrawal syndrome The provocation of severe angina or production of myocardial infarction by abrupt beta-blocker withdrawal in patients on treatment for longer than 1–2 weeks is widely accepted (SED-9, 299; SEDA-5, 193; SEDA-6, 190; SEDA-7, 214). While the prevalence of morbidity attributable to beta-blocker withdrawal is unknown, a retrospective survey (41[C]) of 195 patients with myocardial infarction revealed 13 patients (6.7%) with an average duration of 63 hours between beta-blocker withdrawal (for various reasons) and the occurrence of acute myocardial infarction.

Some previous prospective studies (SEDA-6, 190; SEDA-7, 214) have failed to document the phenomenon, so a simple study of short-term propranolol, atenolol, acebutolol and oxprenolol therapy in normal volunteers and patients with ischemic heart disease or hyperthyroidism is of particular interest (42[C]). These authors observed little change in resting heart rate but increased sympathetic drive – provoked by assumption of the erect posture with or without glyceryltrinitrate vasodilatation or during a Valsalva maneuvre – consistently led to rebound tachycardia after at least a week's treatment with all the agents studied.

Recent work has clearly shown that pindolol withdrawal, after a treatment period of at least one month, was not associated with any significant rebound in isoprenaline sensitivity (43[C]–45[C]). This lack of withdrawal phenomena after pindolol therapy has been attributed to the intrinsic sympathomimetic activity of the compound.

The beta-blocker withdrawal syndrome is generally attributed to enhanced beta-receptor sensitivity, perhaps due to an increased beta-receptor population; other factors of potential importance include reversal of the reduced free triiodothyronine levels, the rightward shift of the oxyhemoglobin dissociation curve or of reduced platelet aggregation – when drug is withdrawn – and finally unmasked progression of the disease process may play a role (46[R]).

Finally, while there is some evidence that continued low-dose beta-blocker therapy might protect against the consequence of receptor hypersensitivity (47[C]), prolonged low-dose metoprolol before complete withdrawal of the drug lessened, but did not prevent, the rebound observed on cessation of therapy (48[C]). There appears to be a real need for further study of the theoretically rather complex dose/response characteristics which pertain during gradual drug withdrawal.

Arrhythmias induced by beta-blockers Beta-blockers are widely applied as antiarrhythmic agents, but one recent study demonstrated a rather convincing provocation or increased frequency of paroxysmal atrial arrhythmias (particularly atrial fibrillation) following the intravenous administration of 25 mg atenolol (49[C]). This was however a highly selected patient group prone to a variety of supraventricular dysrhythmias: nonetheless, an apparent arrhythmogenic effect of this low dose atenolol was seen in 6 of 12 patients.

There have been two further reports (SEDA-7, 211) of Q-Tc prolongation with ventricular tachycardia (torsade de pointes) following sotalol (50[C], 51[C]). In one of these instances (51[C]) the arrhythmia occurred in the setting of self-poisoning.

Use of beta-blockers in portal hypertension While it is accepted that propranolol may have a role in the medical management of some cirrhotic patients with portal hypertension and gastrointestinal bleeding, caution has been advised on the grounds that such treatment will be associated with decreased hepatic blood flow (52[C]). Certainly propranolol therapy seems to be increasingly and perhaps ill-advisedly (53[r]) applied in this setting but few reports of adverse reactions have appeared. One group (54[C]) have however reported increased arterial ammonia levels in 5 of 6 patients with cirrhosis, but not in 3 with fatty liver, treated with 80 mg propranolol per day for 6 days. The mechanism of this effect is necessarily speculative but may involve increased portosystemic shunting.

Pulmonary function

Beta-blockers and asthma

Beta-blockade has the potential for upsetting the balance of smooth muscle tone and thus causing or aggravating bronchospasm; other possible mechanisms contributing to a reduction in respiratory function are promotion of mast cell degranulation and depression of central responsiveness to carbon dioxide (SED-9, 297; SEDA-5, 188; SEDA-6, 189; SEDA-7, 216). The general trend in clinical practice has been to avoid the use of beta-blockers altogether in patients with obvious asthma and, while it has been suggested that the risk is relatively less in cases of 'fixed' airways obstruction, to limit such therapy in patients with chronic obstructive airways disease to cardioselective agents. It is recognized however that bronchospasm can, on occasion, be provoked in patients with no relevant past history (SEDA-5, 188; SEDA-6, 189; SEDA-7, 216).

Recently the emphasis appears to have changed and several pieces of experimental work have shown that at least a number of asthmatic subjects will tolerate certain agents; this argues against the suggestion of Gauld et al (55[C]) that beta-blockers should never *be used in subjects with a history of asthma. The evidence suggests that the cardioselective agents in general, and perhaps labetalol, can be reasonably well tolerated in patients with a history of asthma who either continue regular bronchodilator therapy with inhaled beta$_2$-stimulants or who at least have ready access to such agents. Lawrence et al (56[C]) compared against placebo the effects of atenolol or metoprolol following acute or chronic administration in 14 hypertensive patients with a history of asthma. This randomized blind crossover study in patients was preceded by a dose-ranging study in volunteers to ascertain the equivalent metoprolol/atenolol doses for 24 hr blood pressure control (100 mg twice daily and 100 mg per day respectively were the doses ultimately used). In an initial single-dose dynamic study in the patients metoprolol produced a more marked fall in several indices of airways resistance; active agents were significantly different from placebo, but not from each other, in measurements performed at 2 and 5 hr after dosing. Salbutamol inhalation improved the measures of airways resistance under all conditions. During subsequent 3-week treatment periods however only metoprolol produced significant airway obstruction compared with placebo and this apparent superiority of atenolol was supported by diary records of* *asthmatic attacks and bronchodilator therapy. The authors pointed out, however, that these differences were of clinical significance in only 3 patients and it must be reiterated that dosage equivalence had been determined by prior study in healthy volunteers. Their justifiable conclusion was that if it were decided to prescribe a beta-blocker in patients of this type a cardioselective agent was preferable in order to retain sensitivity to beta$_2$-stimulants and that atenolol might be preferable to metoprolol. A separate large study of the tolerability of metoprolol in hypertension identified 81 asthmatic patients all but 3 of whom tolerated metoprolol therapy and it was not clear whether any attempt had been made to increase the dose of bronchodilators in these subjects (57[c]). With regard to whether labetalol, with its alpha-blocker activity, confers any protection from bronchospasm as a result of reciprocal shift from beta- to alpha-adrenoreceptors in experimental asthma (58[c]), two recent pieces of experimental work disagree, though perhaps this discrepancy is quantitative rather than qualitative. Larsson (59[C]) showed pronounced bronchoconstriction after intravenous labetalol (but not after practolol or placebo) in 14 asthmatic subjects and documented significantly increased airways resistance, compared with placebo, during a subsequent 2-week treatment period with labetalol although sensitivity to isoprenaline was retained. Jackson and Beevers (60[C]) on the other hand showed no significant difference in the small fall of FEV$_1$, induced by single doses of atenolol or labetalol in 11 asthmatic subjects with hypertension, although a greater mean fall followed labetalol. Here too, however, salbutamol inhalation did restore mean FEV$_1$, at least to baseline, which would appear to justify the conclusion that labetalol, like atenolol, may lessen the risk of precipitating an asthmatic attack 'should beta-adrenoreceptor blocking drugs be inadvertently given to patients with airways obstruction'.*

It should be stressed however that, no doubt because of the relative and dose-dependent selectivity of beta-blockers, worsening of bronchospasm can occur even if a beta$_1$-selective drug is used combined with a beta$_2$-receptor agonist (SEDA-5, 188). Recent reports of severe acute asthma occurring in a subject with no significant past history after conventional doses of atenolol (61[C]) and comparability of increased airways resistance in chronic bronchitics after single doses of propranolol and atenolol (62[C]) support the need for caution.

No-one is advocating the wholesale usage of beta-blockers in patients with any history of bronchospasm but if no readily available therapeutic alternative exists a cautious trial of a beta$_1$-selective agent, or perhaps labetalol, would seem justified.

Deterioration of sleep apnea Experimental work showing reduced ventilatory responses to carbon dioxide in animals and man (SEDA-5, 188; SEDA-7, 216) may be relevant to the observation of well-documented increased severity of sleep apnea in 2 subjects (63[C]).

Pneumonitis, pulmonary fibrosis/granulomata and pleurisy Pulmonary fibrosis occurs with sclerosing peritonitis as part of the practolol syndrome (SEDA-9, 297) but has also been described in association with pindolol therapy (SEDA-4, 134). Two separate reports have recently documented superficially similar and unusual lung reactions to acebutolol. One patient experienced recurrent pleurisy associated with a high ESR which resolved on withdrawal of the drug (64[C]). Lung biopsy in this case showed pulmonary granulomata associated with fibrosis as well as patchy fibrosis of the visceral pleura. Another patient experienced a pneumonitic reaction to acebutolol (65[C]) and this report evoked the memory of a patient who appeared to respond similarly to propranolol (66[C]).

Endocrinological and metabolic effects

Hyperthyroxinemia The efficacy of beta-blocker therapy in controlling most features of hyperthyroidism assures their place in routine endocrinological practice. Part, at least, of this effect stems from altered thyroid hormone metabolism with enhanced inactive reverse T3 formation (SED-9, 298; 67[R]) and inhibition of the peripheral deiodination of thyroxine to triiodothyronine (68[C]). It seems all the more surprising, therefore, that a recent report should document hyperthyroxinemia associated with high-dose (mean 480 mg/day) propranolol therapy (69[C]). The authors concluded that the principal mechanism involved was reduction in the rate of thyroxine deiodination and noted that the phenomenon had been alluded to previously (70[C], 71[C]). One of the 6 recently described patients may truly have been hyperthyroid but the remainder, in spite of high thyroxine levels and elevated free thyroxine index, were clearly euthyroid by triiodothyronine levels and TSH response to TRH.

Hypoglycemia Beta-blocker therapy can cause hypoglycemia coma in non-diabetic subjects, particularly in children and in adults after prolonged fasting, severe exertion or in association with hemodialysis (SED-9, 298; SEDA-6, 188; SEDA-7, 215). A recently described case is noteworthy because of its occurrence in a patient with unstable angina treated with modest doses of propranolol (72[C]). The authors noted that this clinical condition may simulate cardiogenic shock, an observation which has been made previously in relation to propranolol induced hypoglycemia in the setting of myocardial infarction (73[C]).

Blood lipids Increased plasma VLDL triglyceride levels result from therapy with both $beta_1/beta_2$-unselective and $beta_1$-selective blockers (SEDA-4, 134; SEDA-6, 188; SEDA-7, 215). In a recent crossover study of short-term (8 weeks) propranolol or prazosin therapy for hypertension this effect was clearly restricted to beta-blocker therapy (74[C]). Of interest are the brief details that have been published purporting to show a correlation between the blood pressure lowering and plasma lipid imbalance effects of propranolol and sotalol therapy (75[c]). Finally, in an unusual case of severe hypertriglyceridemia and pancreatitis associated with beta-blocker therapy marked impairment of triglyceride clearance occurred in rechallenge with atenolol and metoprolol (76[C]).

Reduced plasma immunoreactive parathyroid hormone This effect has been noted in uremic patients receiving propranolol (SEDA-6, 189) and 6 weeks of pindolol therapy for hypertension has now been shown to reduce parathyroid hormone levels by about two-thirds (77[C]). The authors argue that this result is unlikely to be attributable to altered hemodynamics.

Beta-blockers in pregnancy Controversy persists about the safety of beta-blocker therapy during pregnancy. The matter has been extensively discussed in earlier editions of this series (SED-9, 299; SEDA-4, 131; SEDA-5, 194; SEDA-6, 190 and SEDA-7, 215). Certainly opinion seems to have been moving towards according beta-blocker therapy an accepted place in treatment of pregnancy hypertension although the last conclusion expressed on these pages (SEDA-7, 215) was that more data were needed.

Further clinical observations have appeared which may be relevant to this controversy. Apparent neonatal beta-blockade attributed to atenolol was associated with bradycardia, hypoglycemia and extended atenolol excretion (78[C]). The inevitably anecdotal nature of this report has however been criticized and in a recently reported placebo-controlled study of atenolol in 120 women with pregnancy-associated hypertension there was no increased incidence of common neonatal complications (79[C]). Also pertinent to this question are a brief account of a prospective study of labetalol in pregnancy (80[c]) and a full account of parallel treatment (non-randomized) metoprolol/hydralazine versus hydralazine/thiazide therapy (81[C]) where beta-blocker therapy was not associated with any increased neonatal morbidity. Nonetheless a case of intrapartum fetal death associated with propranolol, taken for paroxysmal tachycardia, has also been reported recently (82[C]).

Allergic and fibrosing disorders: skin reactions *(SED-9, 295; SEDA-4, 134; SEDA-5, 190; SEDA-6, 187; SEDA-7, 217)*

Drug-induced lupus A lupus erythematosus like syndrome was a well-recognized reaction to practolol therapy (SEDA-5, 190) but stimulation of antinuclear antibody formation and/or production of a lupus-like syndrome has also been reported with acebutolol, labetalol, pindolol and propranolol (SEDA-4, 134; SEDA-5, 190; 83[C], 84[C]). While many previous accounts linked antinuclear antibodies and the practolol oculomucocutaneous syndrome, the dissociation of the fibrosing practolol syndrome and antinuclear antibody positivity has been stressed more recently (85[R]). This reviewer concluded that the weight of evidence did *not* favor a link between the drug-induced lupus syndrome and the practolol oculomucocutaneous syndrome. Of interest with regard to drug-induced lupus in general is the finding of an association between hydralazine-induced arthritis and HLA type DR4 (86[C]).

Retroperitoneal fibrosis Retroperitoneal fibrosis has long been recognized as an adverse reaction to drug (methysergide) treatment, but an increasing number of cases have been described in association with beta-blocker therapy (SEDA-4, 134; SEDA-5, 191; SEDA-6, 187). Taking recently reported cases into account (87[C]–89[C]), the list of beta-blockers so implicated comprises acebutolol, atenolol, metoprolol, oxprenolol, pindolol, propranolol, sotalol and timolol. Although beta-blockers may not have been incriminated with certainty as causing retroperitoneal fibrosis, the idiopathic variety is rare so that, in spite of the wide nature of beta-blocker usage, the association may well be causal and should be considered when balancing the benefits and risks of long term beta-blocker therapy. Finally it is asserted that this reaction generally occurs in isolation, without other features of the practolol syndrome (89[C]); while sclerosing peritonitis is recorded after non-practolol beta-blockers (SEDA-5, 191; SEDA-6, 187; 90[C]), a causal association is unproven.

Skin and mucous membrane lesions Lichenoid, psoriasiform, eczematous or other cutaneous reactions have all been reported previously in patients on beta-blocker therapy (SEDA-4, 134; SEDA-5, 191; SEDA-6, 187; SEDA-7, 214). Recent additions to this list of rare reactions include single cases of erythematous papules on the legs after acebutolol (91[C]), poikiloderma with premycotic features with tolamolol (92[C]), Lyell's syndrome in association with timolol (93[C]) and a lichen bullous-like eruption during labetalol therapy (94[C]). Finally labetalol has also been implicated in causing a case of aphthoid stomatitis (95[C]).

Miscellaneous reports in relation to allergic disorders Another case of thrombocytopenia (SEDA-4, 135), confirmed by rechallenge and associated with platelet antibodies, has been observed following oxprenolol therapy (96[C]).

Another individual case of exacerbation of the features of anaphylaxis by beta-blocker therapy (SEDA-7, 216) has recently been described (97[C]).

The role of altered immunological mechanisms as a basis for side effects not obviously attributable to beta-blockade

The basis of the group of side effects discussed above, which have been considered to represent formes frustes of the full-blown practolol mucocutaneous syndrome, remains obscure. An attractive hypothesis on how these apparently immunologically mediated phenomena may depend upon the principal pharmacological effect of beta-blockers invokes upset in the T lymphocyte biochemical control mechanisms originally described by Allison et al (98[R]). Thus it has been proposed that practolol, by interacting with suppressor T lymphocyte beta-receptors, might in turn lead to emergence of self-directed B lymphocyte populations (99[r]–102[r]). These suggestions have been reviewed and extended by Duggan and Court (103[R]) who have proposed a unifying hypothesis linking the pharmacological action of beta-blockers and the side effects whose pharmacological basis is far from immediately obvious. The crux of this hypothesis (which they extend to the murine lymphosarcomata induced by pronethalol) is that a rise in cAMP, which would initiate cell division, could be produced by interaction of T-lymphocyte adrenoreceptors and beta-blockers, particularly those with significant partial agonist activity.

There are major difficulties in accepting this argument however, not least of which is the apparent dissociation between the practolol mucocutaneous syndrome and autoantibody formation referred to above. Furthermore the widespread use of pindolol, an agent with a high level of partial agonist activity, has not been associated with any significant number of side effects in this class (104[R]). Finally an in vitro study has shown that the immunomodulatory effect (not shared by metoprolol and atenolol) of propranolol on peripheral blood lymphocytes may be ascribed to the membrane stabilizing effect of the drug rather than its beta-blocker effect (105[C]).

Beta-blockers in renal disease *(SED-9, 294; SEDA-4, 143; SEDA-6, 189; SEDA-7, 214)*

The influence of renal failure on beta-blocker pharmacokinetics and the implications of these findings for clinical practice have been discussed previously (SEDA-4, 132; SEDA-6, 189; SEDA-7, 214) and in a recent review (106[R]).

Decreased renal plasma flow (RPF) and glomerular filtration (GF) are recognized features of beta-blocker therapy and have been considered in two detailed review articles (106[R], 107[R]). These reviewers agree that the theoretically lesser degree of renal vasoconstriction, which is a property of cardioselective agents, might favor the use of these agents, particularly atenolol, where renal function is of concern. Wilkinson (106R) concluded however that during chronic treatment these renal hemodynamic changes were of limited clinical significance and noted comparable small falls in GFR during a crossover study of propranolol, metoprolol and atenolol in 10 patients with renal disease. Both Wilkinson (106[R]) and Epstein and Oster (107[R]) single out nadolol for particular mention as far as its beneficial acute effects (after intravenous administration) on renal hemodynamics are concerned: Wilkinson also notes the desirable properties of tolamolol in this regard. With regard to long-term nadolol therapy the weight of evidence appears to support lack of depression of RPF and GFR (106[R], 107[R]).

While clinically important reduced renal function attributable to beta-blocker therapy alone may be uncommon, that these agents may well enhance the effects of other compounds is suggested by a report of 2 cases of reversible renal failure attributed to combined beta-blocker and nonsteroidal antiinflammatory drug therapy (108[C]). Moreover, in certain circumstances reduced cardiac output may have disastrous consequences on renal function as shown by a case of fatal renal failure due to renal artery thrombosis in an elderly patient with Leriche's syndrome who had received atenolol (109[C]).

High-dose intoxication

The treatment of beta-blocker poisoning was reviewed in SEDA-5 (p. 193) where the principles of treatment with high-dose isoprenaline and glucagon by infusion were stressed. An interesting brief report (110[C]) recorded a dramatic response to intravenous calcium chloride in a case of metoprolol overdose where 'vasopressors and chronotropins were universally to no avail'.

A serious degree of cardiovascular collapse seems, thankfully, to be relatively uncommon in this setting – occurring in only 4 of 40 cases seen in one center over 4 years (111[C]). In this series 90% of the patients showed sinus bradycardia and/or moderate hypotension; atrioventricular block – commonly first degree – occurred in only 20%. A rather low incidence of serious clinical manifestations was also observed in a German series of 77 cases of beta-blocker poisoning in children and adolescents, only 10 of whom showed cardiovascular signs (112[C]). Of interest was the predominance (12 cases) of neurological signs (SEDA-5, 194) in this series and the high incidence (6 cases) of hypoglycemia or symptoms based on hypoglycemia.

Interactions

Interactions between beta-blockers and Class I antiarrhythmic agents such as lidocaine or tocainide may result in depressed myocardial contractility and asystole (SEDA-6, 191), while increased liability to lidocaine intoxication has also been described (SEDA-7, 218). In a recently reported case severe paranoia followed the co-administration of tocainide and propranolol (113[CR]); the true causality of this interaction and its basis remain unclear but the proposed pharmacokinetic interaction of lidocaine and propranolol (SEDA-7, 218) may be relevant to this case.

In view of reports of inhibition of the hypotensive effects of diuretics (SEDA-7, 248) and captopril (SEDA-6, 202) by the non-steroidal, antiinflammatory agent indomethacin, it is of interest that a reduced hypotensive effect may also follow combined indomethacin/beta-blocker therapy (114[r]). Although the effect is small, aspirin has also been shown to negate the hypotensive effect (but not the negative inotropic or chronotropic effect) of intravenous pindolol or propranolol (115[C]). Further work would seem to be required to confirm these effects and determine their clinical relevance.

Maintenance of high- or intermediate-dose beta-blockade during nitrous oxide anesthesia with fentanyl induction was well tolerated by 13 patients with severe renovascular hypertension (116[C]) while thoracic epidural analgesia in patients on beta-blockers receiving neuroleptanesthesia was shown to afford certain cardioprotective effects (117[C]).

Cimetidine has been shown previously to double the plasma concentrations of oral doses of propranolol and labetalol (118[C], 119[C]), this effect being mediated by reduction in liver blood flow. The single dose kinetics and dynamic effect of metoprolol were not altered by prior cimetidine therapy and although the half-life of atenolol was unexpectedly (for a hydrophilic compound eliminated by renal excretion) marginally prolonged, this effect is unlikely to be of practical importance (120[C]).

Debrisoquine oxidation status and beta-blockers

It has been suggested that individuals who experience marked bradycardia while taking conventional doses of alprenolol, timolol or metoprolol may have impaired drug hydroxylation. Alvan et al (121[C]) reported results in 4 subjects who showed excessively high plasma levels after single doses of these drugs and were subsequently shown to be poor hydroxylators of debrisoquine. Two other groups have reported results which appear to confirm this finding, at least as far as metoprolol is concerned (122[C], 123[C]). The implication of these results is that typing of debrisoquine hydroxylator status may predict susceptibility to beta-blockade by agents subject to oxidative metabolism, but more data are required.

NITRATE DERIVATIVES *(SED-9, 301; SEDA-4, 88; SEDA-5, 195; SEDA-6, 191; SEDA-7, 218)*

Hypotension, particularly upon the introduction of oral or sublingual nitrate therapy, is a common reaction which is sometimes associated with bradycardia (SEDA-5, 196; SEDA-6, 192; SEDA-7, 218). The severity of the reaction in 2 recently reported cases may have been attributable to concomitant clonidine (124[C]) and propranolol (125[C]) therapy, the latter in the setting of ethanol intoxication. Treatment of this complication occurring in the course of intravenous nitroglycerin administration has been discussed in a recent, practically oriented, review article (126[R]).

That review of intravenous nitroglycerin usage (126[R]) also mentions the occurrence of hypoxemia (SEDA-6, 191; SEDA-7, 218) and methemoglobinemia (SEDA-5, 196; SEDA-6, 191) with this method of drug delivery. That the latter complication of nitroglycerin infusion is unlikely to be of general importance is suggested by a methemoglobin fraction of only 0.037 following a 24 hr infusion at the rather high rate of 8 μg/kg/min (127[C]). Two G6PD deficient subjects have been reported however, who developed marked hemolytic anemia following oral isosorbide dinitrate (128[C]), so in this subgroup of patients there would seem to be a need for caution.

An unusual case of hemicrania with oculosympathetic paresis occurring during isosorbide dinitrate therapy, which resolved on withdrawal of the drug, has been reported (129[C]). Although the authors propose this as a case of drug-induced 'pericarotid syndrome', rechallenge resulted in generalized, rather than unilateral, headache without any focal features.

The appearance of AIDS and the increased incidence of Kaposi's sarcomata in homosexual men has led to a suggestion that N-nitrosamine formation following the abuse of amyl nitrite inhalation might be an important mutagenic/carcinogenic factor here (130[r]). More convincing in terms of evidence in man is the hypothesis, also implicating amylnitrite abuse, that the drug may have an immunosuppressive effect on T lymphocyte function (131[C]). This latter work did not however speculate on the biochemical mechanisms involved. These suggestions are of course highly speculative but the possible implication of amyl nitrite may be relevant to Kaposi's sarcoma whether regarded as a neoplasm or a multicentric proliferative lesion secondary to opportunistic viral infection.

Attention has recently been drawn to potential for a possible 'adverse effect', essentially physical in nature, relating to a novel formulation of nitroglycerin. Following the use of nitroglycerin ointment applied to the anterior chest there have been reports of current arcing during attempted defibrillation and an animal experiment confirmed this effect, attributable to increased electrical resistance of the skin-defibrillation paddle interface (132[C]).

CALCIUM ANTAGONISTS *(SED-9, 302; SEDA-4, 136; SEDA-5, 196; SEDA-6, 193; SEDA-7, 219)*

Verapamil, nifedipine and diltiazem

Exacerbation of angina on initiation and withdrawal of therapy

A number of calcium antagonists have been shown to be valuable in the treatment of angina that occurs predominantly at rest and beneficial responses have also been found in patients with stable exercise angina. It is increasingly recognized however that the initiation of nifedipine therapy may actually be associated with the provocation of ischemic cardiac pain (SED-9, 302; SEDA-4, 136; SEDA-5, 198; SEDA-7, 219). A further two examples of this reaction have been described recently (133[C]) and in one of these patients single doses of dipyridamole or hydralazine also appeared to provoke anginal pain and ECG changes associated, in each case, with an increased heart rate but no significant change in blood pressure. The relevance of this apparent first-dose effect to the results of a study showing the importance of dose titration when using the drug in patients with stable angina pectoris (134[Cr]) is unclear. Of the 10 patients participating only 3 showed a consistent improvement in work load on all drug doses (ranging from 30–120 mg nifedipine per day), 5 patients improved with 30 mg/day but deteriorated with higher doses and 2 subjects showed no response to any drug dose. So while nifedipine is undoubtedly an effective drug in both unstable (135[C]) and stable (136[C]) angina pectoris caution is certainly required when initiating therapy with this agent. The mechanisms whereby angina may be provoked by nifedipine are unclear but fall in blood pressure or increased heart rate resulting in diminished regional myocardial perfusion or a coronary steal phenomenon may be implicated (134[Cr]).

That a calcium antagonist withdrawal phenomenon may be important clinically is suggested by the reported individual cases of worsening angina or occurrence of myocardial infarction soon after delayed/reduced dosing or of cessation of verapamil (SEDA-5, 198; 137[C]–140[C]), nifedipine (141[C]–145[C]) or diltiazem (146[C]) therapy. This last quoted reference describes 5 patients (2 on verapamil, 3 on diltiazem) where exacerbation of ST segment changes and angina after interruption of therapy was particularly well documented. These cases were encountered during routine ambulatory monitoring of 143 patients on calcium antagonist trials, which would lead to an incidence of withdrawal effects of about 3.5% which the authors note comparable to a reported incidence of 5% during beta-blocker treatment. While Balasubramanian et al tentatively proposed a biochemical mechanism, based on an increased transmembrane calcium gradient, for withdrawal effects following cessation of calcium antagonist therapy this hypothesis is necessarily speculative. Indeed compared with the weight of evidence that exists for a beta-blocker withdrawal syndrome the evidence to date for a calcium antagonist withdrawal 'syndrome' may point to no more than withdrawal of a useful therapeutic effect or unmasking of progressive disease rather than any true rebound (with overshoot) phenomenon.

Other cardiovascular effects

Inherent in the pharmacological action of verapamil and diltiazem in particular is the potential to produce disordered atrioventricular conduction (SEDA-5, 198; SEDA-6, 194; SEDA-7, 219). Adverse reactions of this type would be expected to be more common in the presence of other drugs with negative chronotropic activity; sinus arrest following diltiazem and amiodarone (147[C]), varying degrees of heart block with diltiazem and beta-blockers (148[C]) and nodal bradycardia in the setting of combined verapamil/oxprenolol usage (149[C]) can be readily understood on these grounds. Therapy with verapamil (SEDA-6, 194; SEDA-7, 219) or diltiazem (148[C], 150[C]) alone can however be associated with similar adverse reactions.

It is well known that prenylamine, an agent with calcium blocking activity, can cause ventricular tachycardia (torsade de pointes) in association with QT prolongation but the causality of this dysrhythmia occurring during nifedipine usage (151[C]) has been questioned (152[r]).

The low potential of calcium antagonist therapy for producing congestive cardiac failure or severe hypotension has been discussed in previous editions of this series

(SEDA-5, 197; SEDA-6, 194). Relatively fixed impedance to left ventricular ejection probably explains decompensation apparently produced by those agents on their own (SEDA-5, 197), and may be relevant to deterioration in cases of hypertrophic obstructive cardiomyopathy treated with nifedipine (153[C]) or verapamil (SEDA-7, 219). Another patient with hypertrophic cardiomyopathy (secondary to amyloid) who deteriorated after nifedipine appeared to show no evidence of left ventricular outflow tract obstruction (154[C]): both verapamil and nifedipine have, however, been used successfully in the treatment of non-obstructive cardiac failure (SEDA-6, 194; 155[C]). While caution must still be advised when co-prescribing calcium antagonists, particularly verapamil, and beta-blocking drugs, recent pieces of work have again shown (SEDA-7, 220) that verapamil and propranolol (156[C], 157[C]) or nifedipine and beta-blocker (158[C]) co-administration can be efficacious and well tolerated. The need for caution when initiating such combined therapy is shown by another (SEDA-6, 194) reported case of cardiac failure during treatment with nifedipine and atenolol (159[C]). This whole subject of combined calcium antagonist/beta-blocker use has been discussed in detail in two recent review articles (160[R], 161[R]).

Miscellaneous adverse reactions/interactions

There is evidence that both verapamil and nifedipine can upset *hepatic function* (SEDA-6, 193; SEDA-7, 220), the reaction generally being a mild asymptomatic hepatitis. Two recent reviews of diltiazem usage note rare reactions of this type – amounting to increased transminase levels and/or jaundice – after this more recently introduded agent (162[R], 163[R]).

A case of respiratory failure, which occurred during intravenous verapamil therapy for supraventricular tachycardia, has been described in a patient with Duchenne-type muscular dystrophy (164[C]). It was postulated that this might result from interference with excitation/contraction coupling in skeletal muscle but this, as well as the true causality of the reaction, must remain speculative.

Edema and erythema of the legs after nifedipine (SEDA-5, 198) is a well-recognized reaction. A recently described case of unusual severity involved all 4 limbs and was associated with an erysipeloid reaction (165[C]).

Severe *muscle cramps* in the legs and hands followed nifedipine treatment of angina in 3 patients (166[C]). Rechallenge experience made a cause-effect relationship seem likely.

Whether or not calcium antagonists affect *carbohydrate tolerance* consistently would still seem to be sub judice (SEDA-6, 194; SEDA-7, 220). Diltiazem certainly reduced hypoglycemic symptoms in a case of insulinoma (167[C]), but there is some doubt that this was achieved by influencing glucose levels. A recently published piece of experimental work seems to confirm that chronic verapamil therapy does not impair carbohydrate tolerance (168[C]), at least in non-diabetic subjects. No fresh evidence seems to have come to hand as far as nifedipine is concerned but I have personal knowledge of a previously stable maturity onset diabetic who developed marked hyperglycemia soon after starting nifedipine treatment for hypertension.

There seems little in the way of published observations on calcium antagonist usage and renal function, so it is of interest to note that nifedipine infusion increased renal blood flow (RBF) and glomerular filtration rate in one sub-group of 47 subjects with/without hypertension and/or glomerulonephritis (169[C]). It is intriguing that this increase in RBF was maximal and significant only in individuals with essential hypertension.

One report briefly describes 2 women in whom nifedipine appeared to provoke menorrhagia, possibly as a result of vasodilatation (181[c]).

With regard to the recognised pharmacokinetic interaction between digoxin and verapamil (SEDA-6, 195), this has been shown to be a complex phenomenon involving reduced renal and extrarenal clearance of digoxin, the former effect apparently being due to inhibition of digoxin's tubular secretion by verapamil (170[C]).

High-dose intoxication

Only a small number of cases of calcium antagonist poisoning have been reported (SEDA-6, 195), so the recently described treatment of a severely affected patient is of particular interest. This was a previously healthy young woman who showed marked bradycardia and hypotension, both responding poorly to intravenous calcium and dobutamine infusion. Infused isoprenaline did however produce a dramatic improvement in heart rate and blood pressure (171[C]). The authors note that hyperglycemia and metabolic acidosis reported as 'features' of this overdose would seem to be related to the general clinical condition and treatment (glucagon/isoprenaline) more than to verapamil per se. Combined isoprenaline and calcium infusion combined with AV sequential pacing improved the blood pressure in another reported case (172[C]) in whom unresponsive asystole ultimately ensued while only adrenaline infusion (173[C]) raised blood pressure at all satisfactorily in a third.

Bepridil

Like prenylamine, this more recently introduced agent appears to be associated with typical torsade de pointes; 16 cases have been reported, usually occurring some time after initiation of therapy and commonly in association with hypokalemia (174[C]).

Perhexiline

Peripheral neuropathy and hepatocellular damage are extremely well recognized adverse reactions to the use of this now third-line antianginal agent (SEDA-6, 195; SEDA-7, 220). A few recent observations on these side effects are of interest.

It has been suggested that HLA B8 may predispose to perhexiline, as nitrofurantoin and possibly ethanol, liver damage. This was the tissue type of one recently reported case of perhexiline hepatitis (175[C]). The histological similarity of perhexiline- and ethanol-induced liver damage (176[C]) may be relevant to this observation. Recently one case of cirrhosis was attributed to 4 years of perhexiline therapy (177[C]) but there were unusual features in the absence of Mallory bodies histologically and the presence of circulating immune complexes.

While peripheral neuropathy is well recognized as a side effect of perhexiline, an electrophysiological study has suggested that many asymptomatic patients show changes in nerve conduction which suggest latent neuropathy (178[C]). The biochemical mechanisms involved are unknown but increased ganglioside levels were seen in nerve biopsy specimens (179[C]) from 18 patients. As to the possible relationship of neuropathy to high circulating perhexiline levels it has been suggested that impaired drug oxidation ability – as identified by debrisoquine hydroxylator status – may predispose to this side effect (180[C]).

REFERENCES

1. Waal HJ (1967) Propranolol-induced depression. *Br. Med. J., 2,* 50.
2. Petrie WM, Maffuci RJ, Woosley RL (1982) Propranolol and depression. *Am. J. Psychiatry, 139,* 92.
3. Cremona-Barbaro A (1983) Propranolol and depression. *Lancet, 1,* 185.
4. Russell JW, Schuckit MA (1982) Anxiety and depression in patient on Nadolol. *Lancet, 2,* 1286.
5. Woods PB, Robinson ML (1981) An investigation of the comparative liposolubilities of beta adrenoreceptor blocking agents. *J. Pharm. Pharmacol., 33,* 172.
6. Judd F, Mass A (1982) Propranolol psychosis. *Med. J. Aust., 1,* 370.
7. Horn JR, Rylander ML, Hicks HM (1982) Propranolol-induced hallucinosis. *Clin. Pharmacol., 1,* 464.
8. Norwegian Multicentre Study Group (1981) Timolol-induced reduction in mortality and reinfarction in patients surviving acute myocardial infarction. *N. Engl. J. Med., 301,* 801.
9. Hansteen V, Møinichen E, Lorentsen E et al (1982) One year's treatment with propranolol after myocardial infarction; preliminary report of Norwegian multicentre study. *Br. Med. J., 284,* 155.
10. Julian DG, Prescott RJ, Jackson FS et al (1982) A controlled trial of sotalol for one year after myocardial infarction. *Lancet, 1,* 1142.
11. Breckenridge A (1983) Which beta-blocker. *Br. Med. J., 286,* 1085.
12. Trafford JAP, McGonigle R, Bowles J et al (1982) A two-year clinical evaluation of atenolol and metoprolol in the treatment of hypertension. *Br. J. Clin. Pract., 36,* 351.
13. Gilbert GJ (1982) An occurrence of complicated migraine during propranolol therapy. *Headache, 22,* 81.
14. Prendes JL (1980) Considerations on the use of propranolol in complicated migraine. *Headache, 20,* 93.
15. Ranakusuma TAS, Samino, Tobing SML et al (1981) Comparative study of acebutolol and

oxprenolol in the management of hypertensive cerebrovascular diseased (CVD) patients. *Ann. Acad. Med., 10, Suppl.*, 15.
16. Editorial (1980) Fatigue as an unwanted effect of drugs. *Lancet, 1,* 1285.
17. Breckenridge A (1982) Joggers blockade. *Br. Med. J., 284,* 532.
18. Kaiser P (1982) Running performance as a function of the dose-response relationship to beta-adrenoreceptor blockade. *Int. J. Sports Med., 3,* 29.
19. Pearson SB, Banks DC, Patrick JM (1979) The effect of beta-adrenoreceptor blockade on factors affecting exercise tolerance in normal man. *Br. J. Clin. Pharmacol., 8,* 143.
20. Anderson SD, Bye PTP, Perry CP et al (1979) Limitation of work performance in normal adult males in the presence of beta-adrenergic blockade. *Aust. N.Z. J. Med., 9,* 515.
21. Kaijser L, Kaiser P, Karlsson J et al (1980) Beta-blockers and running. *Am. Heart J., 98,* 542.
22. Bowman WC (1980) Effect of adrenergic activators and inhibitors on the skeletal muscles. In: Szekeres, L (Ed) *Adrenergic Activators and Inhibitors.* Springer-Verlag, Berlin.
23. Franciosa JA, Johnson SM, Tobian LJ (1980) Exercise performance in mildly hypertensive patients. *Chest, 78,* 291.
24. Sable DL, Brammell HL, Sheenan MW et al (1982) Attenuation of exercise conditioning by beta-adrenergic blockade. *Circulation, 65,* 679.
25. Margaria E, Gagliardi L, Palieri S et al (1983) Analgesic effect of peridural labetalol in the treatment of cancer pain. *Int. J. Clin. Pharmacol. Ther. Toxicol., 21,* 47.
26. Knarr JW (1976) Impotence from propranolol. *Ann. Intern. Med., 85,* 259.
27. Miller RA (1976) Propranolol and impotence. *Ann. Intern. Med., 85,* 682.
28. Report of M.R.C. Working Party on mild to moderate hypertension (1981) Adverse reactions to bendrofluazide and propranolol for the treatment of mild hypertension. *Lancet, 2,* 539.
29. Beta-blocker Heart Attack Trial Research Group (1982) A randomised trial of propranolol in patients with acute myocardial infarction. *J. Am. Med. Ass., 247,* 1707.
30. Mann KV, Abbott EC, Gray JD et al (1982) Sexual dysfunction with beta-blocker therapy: more common than we think. *Sexuality Disability, 5,* 67.
31. Rosenthal J, Kaiser H, Raschig A et al (1979) Treatment of hypertension with a beta-adrenoreceptor blocker. *Br. J. Clin. Pract., 33,* 165.
32. Veterans Administration Co-operative Study Group in anti-hypertensive agents (1977) Propranolol in the treatment of essential hypertension. *J. Am. Med. Ass., 237,* 2303.
33. Wagner G, Brindley G (1980) The effect of atropine, alpha- and beta-blockers on human penile erection – a controlled pilot study. In: Zorgniotti A (Ed) *First International Conference on Vascular Impotence,* pp. 77–81. Thomas Publishing, New York.
34. Riley AJ, Riley EJ, Davies HJ (1982) A method for monitoring drug effects on male sexual response: the effect of single dose labetalol. *Br. J. Clin. Pharmacol., 14,* 695.
35. Reichert N, Shibolet S, Ador R et al (1975) Controlled trial of propranolol in intermittent claudication. *Clin. Pharmacol. Ther., 17,* 612.
36. Diehm C (1983) Beta-blocker und periphere Durchblutung. *Münch. Med. Wochenschr., 125,* 27.
37. Cameron HA, Ramsay LE (1983) Which beta-blocker – correspondence. *Br. Med. J., 286,* 1439.
38. Baber MS, Wainwright ED, Evans D et al (1980) Multicentre post-infarction trial of propranolol in 49 hospitals in the United Kingdom, Italy and Yugoslavia. *Br. Heart J., 44,* 96.
39. Hjalmarson A, Elmfeldt D, Herlitz J et al (1981) Effect on mortality of metoprolol in acute myocardial infarction. *Lancet, 2,* 823.
40. McMahon MTV, McPherson MA, Talbert RL et al (1982) Diagnosis and treatment of Prinzmetal's variant angina. *Clin. Pharmacol., 1,* 34.
41. Brandes JW, Körst HA, Sen C et al (1982) Herzinfarkte nach Absetzen von Betarezeptorenblockern. *Med. Klin. (Munich), 77,* 770.
42. Ross PJ, Lewis MJ, Sheridan DJ et al (1981) Adrenergic hypersensitivity after beta-blocker withdrawal. *Br. Heart J., 45,* 637.
43. Szécsi E, Kohlschülter S, Schiess W et al (1982) Abrupt withdrawal of pindolol or metoprolol after chronic therapy. *Br. J. Clin. Pharmacol., 13,* 353S.
44. Walden RJ, Bhattacharjee P, Tomlinson B et al (1982) The effect of intrinsic sympathomimetic activity on beta-receptor responsiveness after beta-adrenoreceptor blockade withdrawal. *Br. J. Clin. Pharmacol., 13,* 359S.
45. Rango RE, Langlois S (1982) Comparison of withdrawal phenomena after propranolol, metoprolol and pindolol. *Am. Heart J., 104,* 473.
46. Prichard BNC, Tomlinson B, Walden RJ et al (1983) The β-adrenergic blockade withdrawal phenomenon. *J. Cardiovasc. Pharmacol., 5,* S56.
47. Dollery CT, Maling TJB (1979) Beta-blocker withdrawal syndrome. *Br. Med. J., 2,* 1074.
48. Rango RE, Langlois S, Lutterodt A (1981) Metoprolol withdrawal phenomena: mechanism and prevention. *Clin. Pharmacol. Ther., 31,* 8.
49. Rasmussen K, Andersen K, Wang H (1982) Atrial fibrillation induced by atenolol. *Eur. Heart J., 3,* 276.
50. Desoutter P, Medioni J, Lerasle S et al (1982) Bloc auriculo-ventriculaire et torsades de pointe après surdosage par le sotalol. *Nouv. Presse Méd., 11,* 3855.
51. Belton P, Sheridan J, Mulcahy R (1982) A case of sotalol poisoning. *Ir. J. Med. Sci., 151,* 126.

52. Sherlock S (1981) In: *Disease of the Liver and Biliary System, 6th Ed.*, p. 163. Blackwell Scientific Publications, Oxford.
53. Conn HO (1982) Propranolol in the treatment of portal hypertension: a caution. *Hepatology, 2,* 641.
54. Van Buuren HR, Van der Velden PC, Koorevaar G et al (1982) Propranolol increases arterial ammonia in liver cirrhosis. *Lancet, 2,* 951.
55. Gauld DR, Pain MCF, Rubinfeld AR (1979) Beta-blocking drugs and airways obstruction. *Med. J. Aust., 66,* 88.
56. Lawrence DS, Sahay JN, Chatterjee SS et al (1982) Asthma and beta-blockers. *Eur. J. Clin. Pharmacol., 22,* 501.
57. Assaykeen TA, Michell G (1982) Metoprolol in hypertension – an open evaluation. *Med. J. Aust., 1,* 73.
58. Barnes PJ, Dollery CT, MacDermot J (1980) Increased pulmonary alpha-adrenergic and reduced beta-adrenergic receptors in experimental asthma. *Nature, 285,* 569.
59. Larsson K (1982) Influence of labetalol, propranolol and practolol in patients with asthma. *Eur. J. Respir. Dis., 63,* 221.
60. Jackson SHD, Beevers DG (1983) Comparison of the effects of single doses of atenolol and labetalol on airways obstruction in patients with hypertension and asthma. *Br. J. Clin. Pharmacol., 15,* 553.
61. Mignot P, Brun J (1982) Tolérance respiratoire des beta bloqueurs chez l'asthmatique. *J. Méd. Caen, 17,* 39.
62. Ranchod A, Keeton GR, Benatar SR (1982) The effect of beta-blockers on ventilatory function in chronic bronchitics. *S. Afr. Med. J., 61,* 423.
63. Boudoulas H, Schmidt H, Geleris P et al (1983) Case reports on deterioration of sleep apnoea during therapy with propranolol – preliminary studies. *Res. Commun. Chem. Pathol. Pharmacol., 39,* 3.
64. Wood GM, Bolton RP, Muers MF et al (1982) Pleurisy and pulmonary granulomata after treatment with acebutolol. *Br. Med. J., 285,* 936.
65. Akoun GM, Herman DP, Mayaud CM (1983) Acebutolol-induced hypersensitivity pneumonitis. *Br. Med. J., 286,* 266.
66. Thompson RM, Grennan DM (1983) Acebutolol-induced hypersensitivity pneumonitis – correspondence. *Br. Med. J., 286,* 894.
67. Anonymous editorial (1980) Beta-blockers in thyrotoxicosis. *Lancet, 1,* 184.
68. Lumholtz IB, Siersbaek-Nielsen K, Faber J et al (1978) Effect of propranolol on extrathyroidal metabolism of thyroxine and 3 3'5'-triiodothyronine-evaluation by non-compartmental kinetics. *J. Clin. Endocrinol. Metab., 47,* 587.
69. Cooper DS, Daniels GH, Ladenson PW et al (1982) Hyperthyroxinaemia in patients treated with high dose propranolol. *Am. J. Med., 73,* 867.
70. Wiersinga WM, Touber JL (1977) The influence of beta-adrenoreceptor blocking agents on plasma thyroxine and triiodothyronine. *J. Clin. Endocrinol. Metab., 45,* 293.
71. Kristensen BO, Weeke J (1977) Propranolol-induced increments in total and free serum thyroxine in patients with essential hypertension. *Clin. Pharmacol. Ther., 22,* 864.
72. Weiner P, Pelled B, Alster R et al (1982) Propranolol-induced hypoglycaemia in a non-diabetic patient during acute coronary insufficiency. *Isr. J. Med. Sci., 18,* 725.
73. Wray R, Sutcliffe SBJ (1972) Propranolol-induced hypoglycaemia and myocardial infarction. *Br. Med. J., 2,* 592.
74. Gemma G, Montanari G, Suppa G et al (1882) Plasma lipid and lipoprotein changes in hypertensive patients treated with propranolol and prazosin. *J. Cardiovasc. Pharmacol., 4,* 233S.
75. Ames R, Hill P (1982) Disturbance in serum total cholesterol and lipoprotein cholesterol ratios during control of hypertension with beta-adrenoreceptor blocking drugs. *Clin. Res., 30,* 630A.
76. Durrington PN, Cairns SA (1982) Acute pancreatitis: a complication of beta-blockade. *Br. Med. J., 284,* 1016.
77. Shasha SM, Shiller M, Aryeh HB et al (1981) Effect of pindolol on blood parathyroid hormone concentration. *Isr. J. Med. Sci., 17,* 1189.
78. Woods DL, Morrell DF (1982) Atenolol: side effects in a newborn infant. *Br. Med. J., 285,* 691.
79. Rubin PC, Butters L, Clark DM et al (1983) Placebo controlled trial of atenolol in treatment of pregnancy associated hypertension. *Lancet, 1,* 431.
80. Smith AM (1982) Atenolol: side effects in a newborn infant – correspondence. *Br. Med. J., 285,* 972.
81. Sandström B (1982) Adrenergic beta-receptor blockers in hypertension of pregnancy. *Clin. Exp. Hyper., 1,* 127.
82. Buechler AA, Palmer SK (1982) Intrapartum fetal death associated with propranolol: case report and review of physiology. *Wis. Med. J., 81,* 23.
83. Griffiths ID, Richardson J (1979) Lupus-type illness associated with labetalol. *Br. Med. J., 2,* 496.
84. Harrison T, Sisca TS, Wood WH (1976) Propranolol-induced lupus erythematosus syndrome? *Postgrad. Med., 59,* 24.
85. Hughes GRV (1982) Hypotensive agents, beta-blockers, and drug-induced lupus. *Br. Med. J., 284,* 1358.
86. Batchelor JR, Welsh KI, Tinoco RM et al (1980) Hydralazine-induced systemic lupus erythematosus: influence of HLA-DR and sex upon susceptibility. *Lancet, 1,* 1107.
87. Laakso M, Arvala I, Tervonen S et al (1982) Retroperitoneal fibrosis associated with sotalol. *Br. Med. J., 285,* 1085.

88. Rimmer E, Richens A, Forster ME et al (1983) Retroperitoneal fibrosis associated with timolol. *Lancet, 1,* 300.
89. Thompson J, Julian DG (1982) Retroperitoneal fibrosis associated with metoprolol. *Br. Med. J., 284,* 83.
90. Clark CV, Terris R (1983) Sclerosing peritonitis associated with metoprolol. *Lancet, 1,* 937.
91. Perrot H, Faure M, Dupouy M (1982) Accidents cutanes des beta-bloquants. A propos d'un cas de toxidermie sous acebutolol. *Lyon Med., 247,* 585.
92. Fierens F, Bowland P, Clerens A et al (1982) Etat poikilodermique et tolamolol. *Dermatologica, 164,* 109.
93. Gérard A, Roche G, Presles O et al (1982) Syndromes de Lyell medicamenteux. *Therapie, 37,* 475.
94. Bertani E, Sala F, Crosti C et al (1982) Eruzione cutanea lichenoide de labetalolo. *G. It. Derm. Vener., 117,* 229.
95. Pradalier A, Ory J, Baron J-F (1982) Stomatite aphtoide induite par le labétolol. *Therapie, 37,* 689.
96. Patrassi GM, Fabris F (1982) Thrombocytopenia secondary to oxprenolol, a beta-blocking agent. *Acta Haematol., 68,* 75.
97. Cathala B (1982) Choc anaphylactique aggravé par béta-bloquant. *Rev. Méd. Toulouse, 18/Suppl.,* 416.
98. Allison AC, Denman AM, Barnes RD (1971) Co-operating and control functions of thymus-derived lymphocytes in relation to autoimmunity. *Lancet, 2,* 135.
99. Felix RH, Ive FA, Dahl MGC (1974) Cutaneous and ocular reactions to practolol. *Br. Med. J., 4,* 321.
100. Raftery ED, Denman AM (1973) Systemic lupus erythematosus syndrome induced by practolol. *Br. Med. J., 2,* 452.
101. Madsen SM, Sondergaard J (1977) Cyclic nucleotides, practolol and the peritoneum. *Lancet, 1,* 1055.
102. Behan PO, Behan WM, Zacharias FJ et al (1976) Immunological abnormalities in patients who had the oculomucocutaneous syndrome associated with practolol therapy. *Lancet, 2,* 984.
103. Duggan MAK, Court JB (1981) A proposed mechanism of production of the autoimmune and lymphoproliferative side effects of beta-adrenergic site blocking drugs and hydantoin anticonvulsants. *Ann. Clin. Res., 13,* 406.
104. Krupp P, Fanchamps A (1982) Pindolol: experience gained in 10 years of safety monitoring. *Am. Heart J., 104,* 486.
105. Hallengren B, Forsgren A, Melander A (1982) Influence of beta-adrenoreceptor blocking agents on lymphocyte function in vitro. *Br. J. Clin. Pharmacol., 13,* 543.
106. Wilkinson R (1982) Beta-blockers and renal function. *Curr. Ther., 23,* 65.
107. Epstein M, Oster JR (1982) Beta-blockers and the kidney. *Miner. Electrolyte Metab., 8,* 237.
108. James DW, Cleland LG, Robinson CW et al (1982) Reversible renal failure associated with treatment with a beta-adrenergic receptor blocking drug and non-steroidal anti-inflammatory drugs. *Med. J. Aust., 1,* 232.
109. Shaw AB, Opalka SK (1982) Renal artery thrombosis caused by antihypertensive treatment. *Br. Med. J., 285,* 1617.
110. Jones JL (1982) Metoprolol overdose. *Ann. Emerg. Med., 11,* 114.
111. El Rharrat D, Bismuth C (1982) Acute intoxication by beta-blocking agents: no mortality in 40 cases. *Int. J. Clin. Pharmacol. Res., 2,* 207.
112. Eibs HG, Oberdisse U, Brambach U (1982) Vergiftungen mit Beta-rezeptoren Blockern bei Kindern und Jungendlichen. *Monatsschr. Kinderheilkd., 130,* 292.
113. Rubino M, Jackson E (1982) Severe paranoia with concomitant tocainide and propranolol therapy. *Clin. Pharmacol., 1,* 177.
114. Hansten PD (1981) Propranolol drug interactions. *Drug Interact. Newsletter, 1,* 8.
115. Sziegoleit W, Rausch J, Polak G et al (1982) Influence of acetylsalicylic acid on acute circulatory effects of the beta-blocking agents pindolol and propranolol in humans. *Int. J. Clin. Pharmacol. Ther. Toxicol., 20,* 423.
116. Prys-Roberts C (1982) Interactions of anaesthesia and high pre-operative doses of beta-receptor antagonists. *Acta Anaesthesiol. Scand., Suppl., 76,* 47.
117. Reiz S, Häggmark S, Rydvall A et al (1982) Beta-blockers and thoracic epidural analgesia. Cardioprotective and synergistic effects. *Acta Anaesthesiol. Scand., Suppl., 76,* 54.
118. Feely J, Wilkinson GR, Wood JJ (1981) Reduction of liver blood flow and propranolol metabolism by cimetidine. *N. Engl. J. Med., 304,* 692.
119. Daneshmed TK, Roberts CJC (1981) Cimetidine and bioavailability of labetalol. *Lancet, 1,* 565.
120. Houtzagers JJR, Streurman O, Regardh CG (1982) The effect of pre-treatment with cimetidine on the bio-availability and disposition of atenolol and metoprolol. *Br. J. Clin. Pharmacol., 14,* 67.
121. Alvan G, Van Bahr C, Seideman P et al (1982) High plasma concentrations of beta-receptor blocking drugs and deficient debrisoquine hydroxylation. *Lancet, 1,* 333.
122. Shah RR, Oates NS, Idle JR et al (1982) Beta-blockers and drug oxidation status. *Lancet, 1,* 508.
123. Lennard MS, Silas JH, Freestone S et al (1982) Defective metabolism of metoprolol in poor hydroxylators of debrisoquine. *Br. J. Clin. Pharmacol., 14,* 301.
124. Pradalier P, Canny M, Pailleret JJ et al

(1982) Bradycardie et hypotension sévéres induites par la prise de clonidine et de dinitrate d'isosorbide. *Thérapie, 37,* 213.
125. Baillie GR, Nelson MV, Krenzelok EP (1983) Profound hypotension following sublingual nitroglycerin. *Vet. Hum. Toxicol., 25,* 11.
126. Jaffe AS, Roberts R (1982) The use of intravenous nitroglycerin in cardiovascular disease. *Pharmacother., 2,* 273.
127. Husum B, Lindeburg T, Jacobsen E (1982) Methaemoglobin formation after nitroglycerin infusion. *Br. J. Anaesth., 54,* 571.
128. Aderka D, Garfinkel D, Bograd H et al (1983) Isosorbide dinitrate-induced haemolysis in G6PD-deficient subjects. *Acta Haematol., 69,* 63.
129. Mueller RA, Meienberg O (1983) Hemicrania with oculosympathetic paresis from isosorbide dinitrate. *N. Engl. J. Med., 308,* 458.
130. Jørgensen KA, Lawesson S-O (1982) Nitroseringsreagenser (f. eks. amylnitrit) som mulig årsag til Kaposisarkom hor homoseksuelle maend. *Ugeskr. Laeg., 144,* 3727.
131. Goedert JG, Wallen WC, Mann DL et al (1982) Amylnitrite may alter T lymphocytes in homosexuals. *Lancet, 1,* 412.
132. Parke JD, Higgins SE (1982) Hazards associated with chest application of nitroglycerin ointments. *J. Am. Med. Ass., 248,* 427.
133. Yokoyama M, Koizumi T, Fujitani K (1982) Adverse response to nifedipine in unstable angina pectoris. *Chest, 81,* 646.
134. Deanfield J, Wright C, Fox K (1983) Treatment of angina pectoris with nifedipine: importance of dose titration. *Br. Med. J., 286,* 1467.
135. Gerstenblith G, Duyang P, Achuff SC et al (1982) Nifedipine in unstable angina: a double-blind randomized trial. *N. Engl. J. Med., 306,* 885.
136. Maskowitz RM, Piccini PA, Nacarelli GV et al (1979) Nifedipine therapy for stable angina pectoris: preliminary results of effects on anginal frequency and treadmill exercise response. *Am. J. Cardiol., 44,* 811.
137. Balasubramanian V, Bowles MJ, Penalver H et al (1981) Verapamil in ischaemic heart disease – an objective study of 100 patients. In: Zanchetti and Krikler (Eds) *Calcium Antagonism in Cardiovascular Therapy: Experience with Verapamil,* pp. 118–139. Excerpta Medica, Amsterdam.
138. Raftos J (1980) Verapamil in the long-term treatment of angina pectoris. *Med. J. Aust., 2,* 78.
139. Solberg LE, Nissen RG, Vlietstra RE et al (1978) Prinzmetal's variant angina response to verapamil. *Mayo Clin. Proc., 53,* 256.
140. Freedman B, Richmond DR, Kelly DT (1980) Coronary spasm management with verapamil (Isoptin). *Med. J. Aust., 2,* 22.
141. Heupler Jr EA, Proudfit WL (1979) Nifedipine therapy for refractory coronary artery spasm. *Am. J. Cardiol., 44,* 798.
142. Bertrand ME, Lablanche JM, Tilmant PY (1981) Treatment of Prinzmetal's variant angina. *Am. J. Cardiol., 47,* 174.
143. Müller JE, Gunther SJ (1978) Nifedipine therapy for Prinzmetal's angina. *Circulation, 57,* 137.
144. Moses JW, Wertheimer JH, Bodenheimer MM et al (1981) Efficacy of nifedipine in rest angina refractory to propranolol and nitrates in patients with obstructive coronary disease. *Ann. Intern. Med., 94,* 425.
145. Schick EC, Liang C-S, Heupler FA et al (1982) Randomized withdrawal from nifedipine: placebo-controlled study in patients with coronary artery spasm. *Am. Heart J., 104,* 690.
146. Balasubramanian V, Bowles MJ, Khurmi NS et al (1983) Calcium antagonist withdrawal syndrome: objective demonstration with frequency-modulated ambulatory ST-segment monitoring. *Br. Med. J., 286,* 520.
147. Briand H, Peltier B (1982) Complications cardiaques du diltiazem. *Ouest Med., 35,* 1171.
148. Hossack KF (1982) Conduction abnormalities due to diltiazem. *N. Engl. J. Med., 307,* 953.
149. Voga G, Skrabl-Mocnik F (1982) A case of the simultaneous action of verapamil and oxprenolol. *Zdrav. Vestn., 51,* 31.
150. Schroeder JS, Feldman RL, Giles TD et al (1982) Multiclinic-controlled trial of diltiazem for Prinzmetal's angina. *Am. J. Med., 72,* 227.
151. Grayson HA, Kennedy JD (1982) Torsades de pointes and nifedipine. *Ann. Intern. Med., 97,* 144.
152. Krikler DM, Rowland E (1982) Torsade de pointes and nifedipine. *Ann. Intern. Med., 97,* 618.
153. Fedor JM, Stack RS, Pryor DB et al (1983) Adverse effects of nifedipine therapy on hypertrophic obstructive cardiomyopathy. *Chest, 83,* 704.
154. Griffiths BE, Hughes P, Dowdle R et al (1982) Cardiac amyloidosis with asymmetrical septal hypertrophy and deterioration after nifedipine. *Thorax, 37,* 711.
155. Bellocci F, Ansalone G, Santarelli P et al (1982) Oral nifedipine in the long-term management of severe chronic heart failure. *J. Cardiovasc. Pharmacol., 4,* 847.
156. Balasubramanian V, Bowles MJ, Davies AB et al (1982) Combined therapy with verapamil and propranolol in chronic stable angina. *Am. J. Cardiol., 49,* 125.
157. Bassan M, Weiler-Ravell D, Shalev O (1982) Additive antianginal effect of verapamil in patients receiving propranolol. *Br. Med. J., 284,* 1067.
158. Terry RW (1982) Nifedipine therapy in angina pectoris: evaluation of safety and side effects. *Am. Heart J., 104,* 681.
159. Robson RH, Vishwanath MC (1982) Nifedipine and beta-blockade as a cause of cardiac failure. *Br. Med. J., 284,* 113.

160. Oesterle SN, Schroeder JS (1982) Calcium entry blockade, beta-adrenergic blockade and the reflex control of circulation. *Circulation, 65,* 669.
161. Packer M, Leon MB, Bonow RO et al (1982) Haemodynamic and clinical effects of combined verapamil and propranolol therapy in angina pectoris. *Am. J. Cardiol., 50,* 903.
162. Tartaglione TA, Pepine CJ, Pieper JA (1982) Diltiazem: a review of its clinical efficacy and use. *Drug Intell. Clin. Pharm., 16,* 371.
163. McGraw BF, Walker SD, Hemberger JA (1982) Clinical experience with diltiazem in Japan. *Pharmacother., 2,* 156.
164. Zalman F, Perloff JK, Durant NN et al (1983) Acute respiratory failure following intravenous verapamil in Duchenne's muscular dystrophy. *Am. Heart J., 105,* 510.
165. Grunwald Z (1982) Painful oedema, erythematous rash and burning sensation due to nifedipine. *Drug Intell. Clin. Pharm., 16,* 492.
166. Keidar S, Binenboim C, Palant A (1982) Muscle cramps during treatment with nifedipine. *Br. Med. J., 285,* 1241.
167. Taniguchi H, Murakami K, Morita S et al (1977) Calcium antagonist (diltiazem) for reversal of hypoglycaemic symptoms in insulinoma. *Lancet, 2,* 501.
168. Semple CG, Thomson JA, Beastall GH et al (1983) Oral verapamil does not affect glucose tolerance in non-diabetics. *Br. J. Clin. Pharmacol., 15,* 570.
169. Yokoyama S, Kaburagi T (1983) Clinical effects of intravenous nifedipine on renal function. *J. Cardiovasc. Pharmacol., 5,* 67.
170. Pedersen KE, Dorph-Pedersen A, Hvidt S et al (1981) Digoxin-verapamil interaction. *Clin. Pharmacol. Ther., 30,* 311.
171. Crump BJ, Holt DW, Vale JA (1982) Lack of response to intravenous calcium in severe verapamil poisoning. *Lancet, 2,* 939.
172. Orr GM, Bodansky HJ, Dymond DS et al (1982) Fatal verapamil overdose. *Lancet, 2,* 1218.
173. Jain SC, Bharadwaj RPS, Shukla RK et al (1982) Severe hypotension and bradycardia after suicidal consumption of 100 tablets of verapamil: a case report. *Indian Heart J., 34,* 175.
174. Leclerq JF, Kural S, Valère PE (1983) Bepridil and torsade de pointes. *Arch. Mal. Coeur Vaiss., 76,* 341.
175. Dawes P, Moulder C (1982) Perhexiline hepatitis HLA B8. *Lancet, 2,* 109.
176. Paliard P, Evreux JC, Bonvoisin S et al (1982) Manifestations hépatiques liées à l'emploi du maléate de perhexiline (Pexid). *Ann. Gastroenterol. Hepatol., 18,* 209.
177. Hamchi L, Pirotte J, Borlee G et al (1982) Cirrhose induite par le maléate de perhexiline. *Acta Gastro-Enterol. Belg., 45,* 210.
178. Mabin D, Penther PL, Perrot J et al (1982) Neuropathies périphériques latentes induites par le maléate de perhexiline. *Bordeaux Med., 15,* 891.
179. Hauw JT, Mussini JM, Boutry JM et al (1981) Perhexiline maleate induced lipidosis in human peripheral nerve and tissue culture: ultrastructural and biochemical changes. *Clin. Toxicol., 18,* 1405.
180. Shah RR, Oates NS, Idle JR et al (1983) Prediction of subclinical perhexiline neuropathy in a patient with inborn error of debrisoquine hydroxylation. *Am. Heart J., 105,* 159.
181. Rodger JC, Torrance TC (1983) Can nifedipine provoke menorrhagia? *Lancet, 2,* 460.

M. Verstraete

20 Drugs acting on the peripheral circulation

Focus on serotonin and its inhibition

Serotonin (5-hydroxytryptamine, 5-HT) has direct vasoconstrictive properties and is, in addition, a potent vasoactive agent which appears to amplify the vasoconstrictor effect of noradrenaline and angiotensine II. Serotonin stimulates or inhibits a variety of smooth muscles and nerves but its effect is heterogeneous as it can differ between species and even between animals of the same species. In the brain, 5-HT is a more potent vasoconstrictor agent, often with greater intrinsic activity than noradrenaline. Outside the brain, serotonin mainly affects the cardiovascular, respiratory and gastrointestinal systems.

The lack of specific antagonists to serotonin has hampered the precise delineation of serotonin in a number of diseases in which a role of serotonin has been suspected. It was recently discovered that there are at least two distinct 5-HT receptors. The 5-HT_1 receptor (S_1-receptor) is labeled selectively by (^3H)-serotonin and the 5-HT_2 receptor (S_2-receptor) by (^3H)-spiperone in the rat frontal cortex (1,2). The 5-HT_1 receptor cannot be correlated with any physiological or pharmacological effect of serotonin. The physiological importance of the 5-HT_2 receptors is better understood as they were shown to mediate the antagonism of various serotonergic effects measured in vivo, e.g. tryptamine-induced clonic seizures and serotonin-induced contractions in isolated rat caudal arteries (3). 5-HT_2 receptors are present in the smooth muscle of the vessel wall, in bronchial tissue, and in blood platelets.

These serotonin receptors are different from the serotonin receptors which can be blocked by morphine (M-receptors) and those blocked by phenoxybenzamine (D-receptors) (4). Morphine is inactive in both 5-HT_1 and 5-HT_2 receptor binding assays while phenoxybenzamine has a weak activity (3).

A selective antagonist to 5-HT_2 receptors, ketanserin, has been developed, which blocks at low doses the effects of serotonin on the 5-HT_2 receptors present in the smooth muscle of the vessel wall, in bronchial tissue, and in platelets; 5-HT_1 receptors are not affected (3). Its specificity is high although it has slight $alpha_1$-adrenoreceptor and H_1-histamine receptor blocking properties (5). It could thus be that by virtue of its greater specificity for certain receptors it will be largely free of some effects (e.g. sedative, antihistamine-like) of the older antiserotonin compounds, such as the appetite stimulator cyproheptadine and the antidepressant mianserin. Ketanserin does not appear to mimick the pharmacological effects of serotonin and seems therefore to be devoid of agonistic properties.

The effects of ketanserin in animals are multiple and one of the best studied is the hypotensive effect in spontaneous hypertensive rats and dogs with (at lower doses) virtually no reduction of blood pressure in normotensive animals. High doses of ketanserin induce a dose-depending blood pressure reduction. The substance acts on the microcirculation and can largely reverse the cardiovascular alterations observed after experimental pulmonary embolism, endotoxic shock, exercise-induced muscular degeneration and malignant hyperthermia, probably by restoring the impaired microcirculation. Ketanserin inhibits serotonin induced vasoconstriction, bronchoconstriction and platelet aggregation and also the amplifying effect of serotonin on

---

Side Effects of Drugs Annual 8
M.N.G. Dukes, editor

ISBN 0 444 90339 9
$0.80 per article per page (transactional system)
$0.20 per article per page (licensing system)

vasoconstriction or platelet aggregation induced by other vasoactive agents. It has no effect on serotonin-induced vasodilation.

The clinical effects of ketanserin are being evaluated in patients with hypertension, in patients with partial obstruction or spasm in limb arteries and in patients with low-output conditions. Most data seem to suggest that ketanserin causes an improvement of nutritive flow in the microcirculation.

Adverse reactions during parenteral treatment *Only a limited number of clinical reports have been published (6–19) but there are numerous abstracts at meetings and unpublished reports to the manufacturers of ketanserin. Most often ketanserin is well tolerated when administered as a bolus in arteries or veins or as a continuous intravenous infusion. Clinical investigators have mainly administered 2.5 mg ketanserin per minute in doses up to 30 mg under monitoring of blood pressure and heart rate; the intravenous maintenance dose varied between 2 to 6 mg/hr. A transient hypotensive reaction is observed occasionally, particularly in hypovolemic patients, and reverses spontaneously by fluid administration or with a vasopressor (e.g. norepinephrine, dopamine). A few patients experienced transient light-headedness or sleepiness immediately after injection, and some reported slight flushing or a dry mouth. It is estimated that over 1,000 patients have received parenteral treatment with ketanserin.*

High doses of ketanserin (100 mg boluses and infusions at a rate up to 50 mg/hr) have been given in anesthesia; even these very high doses are apparently well tolerated, at least in the particular circumstances of anesthesia.

The longest duration of intravenous continuous infusion (2 mg/hr) was 19 days. A rise in SGOT, SGPT and alkaline phosphatase was observed but may be due to concomitant treatment with amino acids and lipids.

Adverse reactions during oral treatment *Oral treatment with ketanserin has been reported in approximately 1,500 patients of whom 326 in placebo-controlled studies. The daily dose ranged from 20 to 160 mg, divided over 1 to 4 intakes. The usual doses were 20 mg t.i.d. and 40 mg b.i.d. or t.i.d. The maximal dose per intake was 160 mg, given once daily for 8 weeks.*

Some patients experience subjective symptoms such as drowsiness, dizziness, fatigue, light-headedness, which may occur 1 or 2 hours after oral intake of 40 mg, particularly the first few days of treatment. These and other reactions are rare with 20 mg per intake but become more frequent as the dose per intake increases. Controlled studies in over 500 patients with essential hypertension treated with 20 to 40 mg ketanserin during 1 month or more showed that the frequency and intensity of adverse reactions are directly related to the dose per intake and not to the total daily dose. With 20 mg per intake the incidence of adverse reactions in the first weeks is 23.6% (40/169 patients), with 40 mg taken the following weeks 26.4% (9/34 patients), while 17% of the placebo patients (35/206) had side effects in these placebo-controlled studies lasting more than 1 month. There is no difference in the dropout rate in the ketanserin-treated (6/326) and in the placebo-treated (3/286) patients. Most adverse reactions are transient and can be prevented by starting treatment with a low dose (e.g. 20 mg b.i.d. or t.i.d.) and increasing the dose 1 or 2 weeks later.

Allergic reactions have been reported in 4 patients only; they consist of skin rash, facial edema, anxiety-hyperventilation syndrome or bronchospasm.

Three patients had a prolongation of the QT-interval with rhythm disturbances. A systematic analysis of the QT-interval corrected for heart rate in 35 patients treated with a single intravenous injection of 10 mg ketanserin, prolonged the QT_c-intervals by 4% (from a mean of 0.43 ± 0.005 to 0.45 ± 0.005), without clinical signs. The QT/QS_2 ratio remained virtually unchanged.

Interactions *In 8 of 100 diabetic patients well under control with insulin or oral antidiabetic agents, an asymptomatic hypoglycemia was noted which normalized after reduction of the antidiabetic agent.*

Ketanserin is additive to beta-blockers and diuretics in hypertensive patients whose blood pressure is not well controlled with either drug alone; it partially counteracts the bradycardic effect of beta-blockers.

Safety *A transient rise in transaminase has been observed during the first days of treatment with ketanserin. This effect is transient and is often observed with drugs that are* *metabolized in the liver. Numerous hematological and other biochemical data have been collected in 259 patients involved in 10 controlled trials with ketanserin. Except for the very occasional transient increase in SGOT or SGPT early in the treatment and a decrease observed once in triglycerides after 38 weeks of treatment, no consistent changes in laboratory results have been observed.*

OTHER DRUGS

Pentifylline and nicotinic acid

Among the older generation of drugs used in the hope of improving cerebral or peripheral circulation are the xanthines and the nicotinic acid derivatives. They have often been employed in combination, sometimes indeed in a chemical combination (xanthinol nicotinate). As pointed out earlier in this series the adverse effects of the two types of compound are additive (SED-9, 735). An instance of this is to be found in a recent report from Kuwait of a 60-year-old man with suspected cerebral atheroma who was given Cosaldon Retard tablets, each containing 200 mg pentifylline and 50 mg nicotinic acid, in a dose of 2 tablets daily. The patient was also receiving propranolol and was suffering from hepatosplenomegaly. Shortly after the first dose of Cosaldon the patient experienced severe headache, flushing and dizziness which receded when the drug was withdrawn (20^c).

REFERENCES

1. Leysen JE, Niemegeers CJE, Tollenaere JP, Laduron PM (1978) Serotonergic component of neuroleptic receptors. *Nature (London), 272,* 168.
2. Peroutka SJ, Snyder SH (1979) Multiple serotonin receptors: differential binding of (^{3}H)-5-hydroxytryptamine, (^{3}H)lysergic acid diethylamide and (^{3}H)spiroperidol. *Mol. Pharmacol., 16,* 687.
3. Leysen JE, Awouters F, Kenis L et al (1981) Receptor binding profile of R 41 468, a novel antagonist at 5-HT$_2$ receptors. *Life Sci., 28,* 1015.
4. Gaddum JH, Picarelli ZP (1957) Two kinds of tryptamine receptors. *Br. J. Pharmacol., 12,* 322.
5. Kalkman HO, Timmermans PBMWM, Van Zwieten PA (1982) Characterization of the antihypertensive properties of ketanserin (R 41468) in rats. *J. Pharmacol. Exp. Ther., 222,* 227.
6. De Cree J, Leempoels J, De Cock W et al (1981) The antihypertensive effects of a pure and selective serotonin-receptor blocking agent (R 41468) in elderly patients. *Angiology, 32,* 137.
7. De Cree J, Leempoels J, Geukens H et al (1981) The antihypertensive effects of ketanserin (R 41468), a novel 5-hydroxytryptamine-blocking agent, in patients with essential hypertension. *Clin. Sci., 61,* 473.
8. Demoulin JC, Bertholet M, Soumagne D et al (1981) 5-HT$_2$ receptor blockade in the treatment of heart failure. *Lancet, 1,* 1186.
9. De Cree J, Verhaegen H, Symoens J (1981) Acute blood pressure lowering effect of ketanserin. *Lancet, 1,* 1161.
10. Kalenda Z, Hoelzenspies AJ (1981) Restoration of pulmonary perfusion by a serotonin antagonist. *Angiology, 32,* 463.
11. Wenting G, Man in 't Veld AJ, Woittiez AJ et al (1982) Treatment of hypertension with ketanserin, a new selective 5-HT$_2$ receptor antagonist. *Br. Med. J., 284,* 537.
12. De Roose J, Symoens J (1982) Ketanserin (R41468) in superficial thrombophlebitis. *Lancet, 2,* 440.
13. Van den Broeke JJW, Karliczek GF, Brenken U et al (1982) Is prevention of hypertension after open heart surgery possible by blocking 5HT$_2$-receptors with ketanserin? *Acta Anaesthesiol. Belg., 33 (2),* 115.
14. Wenting GJ, Man in 'tVeld AJ, Woittiez AJ et al (1982) Haemodynamic effects of ketanserin, a new selective 5-hydroxytryptamine (serotonin) receptor antagonist in essential hypertension. *Clin. Sci.,* in press.
15. Andrén L, Svensson A, Dahlof B, Eggertsen R, Hansson L (1983) Ketanserin in hypertension. Early clinical evaluation and dose-finding study of a new 5-HT$_2$ receptor antagonist. *Acta Med. Scand., 214,* 125.
16. Van der Starre PJA, Scheijgrond HW, Reneman RS, Bach Kolling J (1983) The use of ketanserin, a 5-hydroxytryptamine receptor antagonist, for treatment of postoperative hypertension following coronary artery bypass surgery. *Anesth. Analg. (Cleveland), 62,* 63.
17. Seibold JR, Jageneau AHM (1983) Treatment of Raynaud's phenomenon with ketanserin, a selective antagonist of the 5-HT$_2$ receptor. *Arthritis Rheum.,* in press.
18. Gerritsen HA, Perquin JWA, De Smet HL et al (1983) Continuous imaging of regional blood flow in peripheral vascular disease using Krypton-81M: effect of ketanserin, a new selective sero-

tonin antagonist. *Diagnostic Imaging, 52,* 85.
19. Hedner T, Persson B, Berglund G (1983) Ketanserin, a novel 5-hydroxytryptamine antagonist: monotherapy in essential hypertension. *Br. J. Clin. Pharmacol., 16,* 121.
20. Kuwait University Drug Adverse Reaction Series (1983) Pentifylline and nicotinic acid. *2,* 29.

J.A. Steiner

21 Antihypertensive drugs

The literature surrounding antihypertensive medications has, this year, followed the pattern set over the previous 1–2 years. Major newcomer to the scene, captopril, has taken a large proportion of the publications, especially since two large symposia have been published. General favorites like methyldopa and minoxidil also continue to receive considerable attention.

A new and interesting observation is the effect of antihypertensive agents on serum lipid concentrations. This arises from a number of large cardiac risk factor studies (1[C]–4[C]) noting the relationship between high low-density lipoprotein (LDL) and low high-density lipoprotein (HDL) cholesterol fractions and increased coronary risk. Beta adrenoceptor antagonists and diuretics have both been associated with lipid abnormalities including changes in LDL/HDL cholesterol ratios and increases in serum triglyceride concentrations (5[CR], 6[CR]). Both these drug groups are more appropriately discussed elsewhere (Chapters 19 and 22). Their relevance to hypertension is that it has been suggested that the induced lipid abnormalities may account for the known failure of control of hypertension to decrease the incidence of coronary artery events. It goes without saying that this is a hypothesis which needs to be proved and that the proof may require many years' work. Within this context, prazosin has been shown in a small group of patients (6[CR]) to lower serum LDL cholesterol and triglyceride levels and to maintain HDL cholesterol levels, but the clinical significance of this is not established.

Another excellent review of *withdrawal syndromes* has appeared in the literature (7[R]). The treatment of hypertension in pregnancy is also reviewed (8[CR]). It seems that both methyldopa and labetalol are safe enough although labetalol may cause tremulousness or shakiness in the mother, a symptom apparently not frequently reported in non-gravid individuals. It should be pointed out that the study cited in this reference which compares labetalol and methyldopa was, it seems, not blind and therefore subject to certain restrictions of interpretation.

Further reviews have appeared concerning the *sexual side effects* of antihypertensive agents. Clearly quite marked differences of opinion are current with Paykel et al (9[R]) virtually discounting all the evidence that such adverse reactions may occur. At the end of the day, faced with sexual problems in patients taking antihypertensives, the physician is still probably best advised to stop the drugs and at least see what happens.

Captopril

Several major reviews of captopril as a therapeutic agent have appeared in the last year (10[R]). None says anything especially new, although the problem of initial hypotension is well highlighted. It is suggested that patients taking diuretics or on salt restricted diets are most vulnerable to such effects and such therapy should therefore be suspended for a few days prior to commencement of captopril. This view is disputed by Ram (11[r]) who points out that many patients cannot tolerate a separation from their therapy and the best approach is to start with low doses of captopril with patients under close supervision. Fortunately the postural hypotension generally wears off with continued use. From Denmark 2 cases of severe initial hypotension are described in cases of renovascular hypertension with high plasma renin (12[C]).

Captopril has now been extensively used in both hypertension and heart failure and a number of large studies have been reported. The Veterans' Administration Cooperative Study Group on Antihypertensive Agents reports its results from 475 patients, black

Side Effects of Drugs Annual 8
M.N.G. Dukes, editor

ISBN 0 444 90339 9
$0.80 per article per pate (transactional system)
$0.20 per article per page (licensing system)

and white, treated double blind with either placebo or captopril initially, and hydrochlorothiazide, captopril or a combination of the two after 7 weeks (13[C]). Whites responded to the captopril better than blacks, but blacks responded well to the combination of captopril and hydrochlorothiazide. Doses of captopril used were 37.5 mg, 75 mg or 150 mg daily. Eighteen patients were withdrawn for drug intolerance which included urticaria, maculopapular rash, dysgeusia, nausea, vomiting, proteinuria, headaches and hypotension. These adverse reactions were not dose-related. There were two withdrawals in the placebo group for drug intolerance.

Weinberger (14[C]) reports a placebo-controlled randomized double blind comparison of captopril 75 mg daily, hydrochlorothiazide 15 mg 3 times daily or a combination of the two in hypertensives. The incidence of side effects was higher in those patients taking combination therapy (22%) than in those taking captopril (16%) or hydrochlorothiazide (14%) alone. The most common side effects were rashes and dizziness. No serious perturbations of renal or hematological function were encountered. The authors do not report uncommon side effects (i.e. reported by 1 or 2 patients only).

Havelka et al (15[C]) report on 76 severely hypertensive patients given captopril in open fashion. The dose was titrated against blood pressure response and the mean daily dose was between 240 and 340 mg/day. Ranges are not given. Patients with renovascular hypertension required marginally less drug than patients with essential hypertension. The study continued for 30 months. Most side effects occurred in patients with impaired renal function. 26 patients experienced side effects, mostly in the first 12 months of therapy. These included taste disturbances, rash, dry cough, reversible leukopenia, nephrotic syndrome, fluid retention, sinus tachycardia, Raynaud's phenomenon and dizziness.

Raine and Ledingham (16[C]) report on 33 patients with severe hypertension. Drug was administered in open fashion and adjusted against arterial pressure response up to a maximum of 450 mg weekly. Four patients were withdrawn because of side effects. Reported side effects were rash, fever, anorexia, nausea, diarrhea, impotence and dysgeusia. Similar patterns of adverse reactions continue to be described in other recent studies (17[C]–19[C]).

Chatterjee et al (20[cR]) review their experience of using captopril in congestive heart failure. The major problem was that of hypotension. Clearly much smaller doses (less than 25 mg) may be required than in hypertension. Skin rash was the only significant problem and this may reflect the small doses used.

Higher doses were used in some other studies in congestive heart failure. Dahlstrom and Karlberg (21[C]) report on 20 patients given up to 75 mg captopril daily in association with digitalis and diuretics. Six patients developed hypotension which necessitated withdrawal of therapy in 2, the doses at the time are not given. One patient developed a rash which reappeared on rechallenge. Doses up to 150 mg daily were used by Awan and Mason (22[C]), one of whose patients developed a persistent eczematoid reaction while another developed proteinuria. Finally, Steingo et al (23[C]) gave captopril 75–450 mg daily to 25 patients with severe chronic congestive heart failure. Although the authors felt that captopril was highly effective, side effects were also frequent. Five patients developed erythematous rashes, associated in one with temporary alopecia and in the other with angioedema of the hands and periorbital tissues. Taste abnormalities, aphthous ulcers, dizziness, nausea, pleural rub, pericardial rub and acute tenosynovitis were reported. No patient developed positive tests for antinuclear factor or clinically significant blood or urine abnormalities.

There were further reports of unusual skin reactions. Aurell et al (24[C]) report on 17 patients receiving hemodialysis. Three developed rashes, one urticaria, one a *bullous exanthema* and one pruritus. All these resolved on stopping the drug. The patients were not rechallenged. Wizemann (25[R]) reports a patient developing *necrotizing blepharitis* as part of agranulocytosis presumably related to captopril. Christeler et al (26[C]) report a case of *pemphigus* appearing in a woman who had taken captopril for 16 months; the eruption persisted for 17 months after cessation of treatment and its relation to treatment may reasonably be queried. Reinhardt et al (27[C]) report *pityriasis rosea* developing into a lichenoid eruption occurring in a patient with hypertension, diabetes mellitus and renal insufficiency, who was taking a number of other medications. The eruption settled despite continuation of captopril therapy. Solinger (28[C]) reports a man with diagnosed polyarteritis nodosa who developed an *exfoliative dermatitis* while taking captopril. The patient responded to steroid therapy and suspension of captopril. Rechallenge was not performed.

Luderer (29[C]) reports on 7 of 23 hypertensive patients who developed skin eruptions while taking captopril. All these eruptions were generalized macropapular rashes and some were associated with systemic symptoms and signs. In 6 of the 7 patients, the eruptions were self-limiting despite continued therapy.

The etiology of these rashes remains to be elucidated. Some have suggested that they may be the result of binding by captopril of zinc or other metallic ions in the skin. If that is the case, it is hard to see why such rashes resolve despite continued therapy. On the other hand, searches for increased antibody titres have not been successful to date.

Further *renal side effects* relating to captopril have been reported. The difficulties of interpreting renal abnormalities in hypertensives have previously been reviewed (SEDA-6, 201; SEDA-7, 232). Palla et al (30[C]) report on 10 patients whose renal function and selective urinary protein content was monitored while taking captopril 400 mg daily for 4 weeks. No consistent or clinically significant changes occurred but, of course, the number of patients is very small and the duration of treatment rather short. Textor et al (31[C]) report on 2 cases of biopsy proven membranous glomerulonephritis occurring in patients taking 600 mg captopril daily. Neither patient previously had signs of nephrotic syndrome nor did either suffer from any concomitant disease likely to cause membranous glomerulonephritis. Despite suspension of therapy, proteinuria and renal biopsy changes were present 12 months later. The authors make the point that, although glomerulonephritis as a side effect of captopril may be rare, it may persist once therapy has ceased.

Hymes and Warshaw (32[C]) report on 6 children including a preterm neonate treated for severe hypertension with captopril. The preterm infant and one older child developed decreases in renal function. In the infant, the renal insufficiency was transient and in the child the effect of captopril could not be differentiated from the underlying disease process. Aurell et al (33[C]) reporting on a group of hypertensive patients mention increased proteinuria in 2 cases. This resolved despite continuation of captopril therapy.

Hooke et al (34[C]) report a 7-year-old girl transplanted for renal failure secondary to cystinosis. Following an episode of transplant rejection she developed intractable hypertension. She was treated with captopril on 3 occasions and each time renal function deteriorated. The renal biopsy showed interstitial nephritis but it is not clear whether this or drug-induced falls in arterial pressure accounted for the changes in renal function.

Patients with renal artery stenosis seem to be particularly at risk. Chrysant et al (35[C]) report on 3 patients, all with this condition, who developed decreasing renal function while taking captopril and other drugs. Two also had a fever and skin rash. The abnormalities resolved when captopril was stopped. Hricik et al (36[C]) describe 11 similar patients and suggest that captopril may be acting via changes in regional blood flow in the kidney. Creager et al (57[C]) reported a case in which captopril caused acute renal failure in a patient with bilateral renal artery stenoses. This was related to a precipitous fall in blood pressure and was reversible.

Further reports of *leukopenia* have appeared (38[c], 39[c]). Cooper, in two separate statements (40[r], 41[r]) concludes that leukopenia is much more common in patients with renal failure, especially if this is due to systemic lupus erythematosus (SLE) or scleroderma. In 3028 patients studied carefully without such complications, the incidence of leukopenia was 0.03%. In patients with renal failure alone, the incidence was 0.5%. In patients with SLE or scleroderma, the incidence was 7.0%. Leukopenia generally occurs within the first 90 days of starting therapy, resolves within 3 weeks of stopping therapy in 90% of patients and does not necessarily recur on rechallenge with lower doses of the drug.

Infections, in Cooper's report, were associated with the leukopenia. These were trivial in patients with normal renal function but very serious and sometimes fatal in patients with compromised renal function with or without associated collagen disease. For this reason, it seems wise to withhold or at least be extremely wary of captopril in patients with these disorders. In patients with normal renal function, the incidence of leukopenia is so infrequent that it is not worthwhile to monitor white cell count. Patients should however be instructed to report all infections including oral ulceration promptly.

Two further cases of hepatitis have been reported. The first (42[C]) occurred in a man requiring peritoneal dialysis in the past who had impaired renal function at the time of treatment with 375 mg daily. In the other case (43[C]) the dose of captopril was 200 mg daily. This patient was also in renal failure.

Antinuclear antibodies have been found in 13 out of 78 patients taking captopril over a period of months (44[C]). These were transient and without clinical sequelae apart from one patient who developed a serum sickness-like illness. The cause of these antibodies is not clear.

Silberbauer et al (45[C]) report a study carried out in volunteers and hypertensives. They show quite convincingly that the hypotensive and hormonal effects of single doses of captopril may be blocked by indomethacin. Whether this can necessarily be interpreted as proving that captopril exerts its effects via prostaglandin release is open to query. However, it seems likely that the possibility of chronic interaction between captopril and indomethacin and/or other prostaglandin synthetase inhibitors should be investigated.

Enalapril maleate

There is a single case report (46[c]) of a man with uncomplicated mild hypertension developing azotemia and glycosuria while taking enalapril maleate (MK-421) 20 mg twice daily. This was reversible on withdrawal of the drug. A letter from Barnes et al (47[c]) relates to a man of 66 with chronic renal failure secondary to polyarteritis nodosa, who developed a maculopapular rash, eosinophilia and hyperkalemia 10 days after being started on enalapril 2.5 mg/day. The authors suggest that the polyarteritis nodosa may have predisposed the patient to these complications and that the drug may have to be given at reduced dosage in impaired renal function.

VASODILATING AGENTS

Hydralazine and dihydralazine

Two further cases have been reported of deterioration in primary pulmonary hypertension treated with hydralazine (SEDA-7, 236; 48[C]) and more cases of *hepatotoxicity* have been presented (49[C], 50[C]).

A case of reversible *monoclonal gammopathy* associated with SLE is reported in a 66-year-old woman also taking hydralazine, atenolol, methyldopa and cyclopenthiazide (51[C]). She was a slow acetylator.

In another patient, *cardiac tamponade* associated with positive ANF titres and DNA binding occurred while he was taking hydralazine, clonidine, propranolol and chlorthalidone (52[C]). This was tapped, hydralazine was ceased and labetalol substituted. The effusion eventually required high-dose steroids and surgical drainage before resolving 9 months later. At this time ANF titre and DNA binding had returned to normal.

The nature of the anti-DNA antibodies has again been assessed in more detail (53[C]). In this study, the authors compared antibodies related to procainamide and to hydralazine therapy. On both immunofluorescence and radioimmunoassay the antibodies are distinctly different, although in both cases the antibodies are to histones rather than to DNA as such, nuclear ribonucleoprotein or other non-histone nuclear antigens.

The cardiovascular complications of hydralazine have been investigated in some more detail. In one study in 5 hypertensives (54[C]) plasma norepinephrine was shown to rise acutely in direct relationship to the rise in heart rate and fall in arterial pressure. This rise persisted for some 4 hours after hydralazine was given. In another study of hydralazine given to patients with congestive heart failure (55[C]), 12 out of 52 patients developed ischemic events. There were 12 episodes of angina and 4 myocardial infarctions. Interestingly, these occurred in the absence of tachycardia and hypotension. The investigators went on to give nitroprusside to 35 of their patients, including 8 who had had ischemic events associated with hydralazine. They make the point that, although greater falls in arterial pressure occurred with nitroprusside than with hydralazine, only one ischemic episode occurred with nitroprusside. They attribute this to the observation that nitroprusside decreased left ventricular filling pressure more than hydralazine although cardiac output was similar for the two drugs. They postulate that subendocardial blood flow and oxygen supply would therefore be greater with nitroprusside than with hydralazine.

A pharmacokinetic interaction has been demonstrated between timolol and dihydralazine (56[C]). Dihydralazine increased timolol C_{max} although this did not reach statistical significance. It is unlikely to be of any clinical importance.

Endralazine

This analogue of hydralazine has recently been reviewed (57[r]). The main side effects mentioned were palpitations, headache, flushing and gastrointestinal intolerance. A small trial of 23 hypertensives compared endralazine 10–20 mg 3 times daily with dihydralazine 25–50 mg 3 times daily in a double-blind crossover design. All patients also received pindolol. The most common side effects were sleep disturbances, headache, dizziness and flushing (58[C]).

Endralazine has also been reported to cause sexual arousal in 7 out of 10 normal male volunteers (59[c]). The dose used was 0.05 mg/kg given intravenously by open label.

Prazosin

Prazosin has been reported to cause recurrent *urticaria, facial edema* and *asthma* in a 70-year-old woman (60[C]). This stopped when prazosin was removed from her treatment. Subcutaneous rechallenge with prazosin was followed by a full blown *anaphylactic attack.*

Three papers have appeared addressing the effect of prazosin on serum lipid profiles (61[C]–63[C]). This is a topic of current interest because of the relationship of HDL and LDL cholesterol content to ischemic heart disease. In all three papers, prazosin was shown to elevate HDL cholesterol content relative to LDL content. Unfortunately all the studies are small and open and patients' diets were not previously stabilized. A very real need exists for well designed large scale prospective studies in this area.

Minoxidil

A number of open label long term studies have appeared in a symposium in the German literature (64[C]–69[C]). These cover long term experience with minoxidil given to a total of 248 patients with resistant hypertension frequently the result of, or complicated by, renal failure. Minoxidil was never used alone and doses varied according to the blood pressure response. It was agreed that minoxidil was effective in most cases. Side effects inevitably included *hypertrichosis, edema, pericardial effusion* (limited largely to patients with renal failure) and *ECG changes.* Other side effects reported included *gynecomastia, repigmentation* of previously white hair, temporary *coarsening of facial skin* and *nausea* and *abdominal fullness.* Effects on serum creatinine varied – in some patients it was improved and in others made worse.

Another study, again of open label design, describes an Asian patient who developed *darkening of his skin* especially around the eyes (70[c]). Yet another open study of long term minoxidil given to 25 patients reports edema, hypertrichosis and pericarditis, the latter occurring in two patients who were already uremic (71[C]).

A study comparing minoxidil with a similar compound, carprazidil, in open crossover fashion in 18 patients, reported hypertrichosis and fluid retention occurring with both compounds. No details are given of the possible magnitude of carryover effects related to the design of the trial (72[c]).

There are three further reports of pericardial effusion in the literature (73[C], 74[C], 75[c]).

There is a further report of a man developing chest pain, SGOT elevation and T-wave inversion on ECG while taking minoxidil (76[C]).

In a fascinating report, Wilkin and Kirkendall (77[C]) describe a patient who was a welder. This man was taking minoxidil and developed *facial hirsutism and bullae* on the dorsum of both hands. The bullae turned out to be due to welding sparks but the man was investigated for porphyria which the syndrome closely resembled. Finally, a case of bilateral *optic neuritis* is reported in a patient who had already had a renal transplant for which he was taking prednisone and azathioprine.

No details are given regarding the patient's blood pressure control while taking minoxidil nor were other causes of optic neuritis excluded (78[c]).

Nitroprusside

Two interesting developments in the use of nitroprusside have been reported in the last 12 months. The first of these is its place in the acute early management of myocardial infarction (79[C], 80[C]). The end point of these studies had been mortality. The evidence is at present not conclusive. Under study conditions, nitroprusside was well tolerated. Side effects reported were *flushing, drowsiness, nausea, dizziness, exacerbation of migraine* and *severe hypotension.*

The other new concept is the concurrent use of sodium thiosulphate with nitroprusside to prevent *cyanide toxicity.* The pharmacokinetics of cyanide accumulation in the presence of thiosulfate infusions are described by Ivankovich et al in volunteers and patients undergoing cholecystectomy (81[C]). A similar study involving patients undergoing surgery requiring controlled hypotension is described by Pasch et al (82[C]). The second study demonstrates that sodium thiosulphate lowers plasma concentrations of cyanide. This observation is not so convincing in the first study. One obvious flaw in both studies is that details of renal and hepatic function are not given. Since patients in renal failure are generally considered to be most at risk from nitroprusside therapy, it would be of interest to see how this group fared given sodium thiosulphate.

Within the context of cyanide toxicity, a 43-year-old man is described who was treated for hypertension complicated by renal failure with nitroprusside for 14 days. During this time he suffered 3 respiratory and 1 cardiac arrests. During the course of his illness, he lapsed into a coma and subsequently died never having regained consciousness. At autopsy, cystic lesions were found in the globus pallidus on both sides along with other lesions throughout the brain. The authors point out that this type of lesion in the globus pallidus is characteristic of cyanide poisoning and is likely to have been related to nitroprusside therapy (83[C]).

Tolmesoxide

This is a new vasodilating agent. Single doses given to hypertensive patients as part of a dose finding study produced complaints of facial flushing, nausea, headache, palpitations and postural dizziness (84[C]).

DRUGS INTERFERING WITH THE SYMPATHETIC NERVOUS SYSTEM

Alpha-methyldopa

Alpha-methyldopa continues to be widely used and a number of adverse reactions have again been reported. A study comparing single versus twice daily dosing regimens of a combination of alpha-methyldopa and hydrochlorothiazide showed both regimens to be equally effective (85[C]). Unfortunately, the investigators gave the single daily dose in the morning, thereby enhancing complaints of drowsiness and orthostatic dizziness. Had the methyldopa been taken before going to bed, the single dose may have proved more acceptable.

In another study (86[c]), methyldopa and pindolol are compared. The outcome is messy since two protocols are reported out together. In the one, methyldopa or pindolol were given separately. In the other, methyldopa or pindolol were combined if necessary with hydralazine, hydrochlorothiazide or guanethidine. Abnormalities in serum liver enzyme concentrations occurred in one patient taking methyldopa alone and in 8 patients taking methyldopa in combination, although details of the combination are not given. Four of these patients also developed Coombs positivity and 6 developed erythrocyte antibodies. Further, antinuclear antibodies were found in 16 of 32 patients taking methyldopa and in 10 of 32 taking pindolol. This incidence seems extremely high and one must query the specificity of the assay and the patient inclusion criteria. Again details are not given as to whether methyldopa was being taken alone or in combination.

Hemolytic anemia has again received attention. Schubothe et al (87[C]) review 11 patients with methyldopa-induced hemolysis and come to the following conclusions. The dose needed is extremely variable. The onset was diagnosed 2–52 months after induction of therapy and hemolysis took 4–16 weeks to resolve after suspension of therapy. Antibodies took 4–12 months to disappear. The authors postulate that inhibition of methyldopa-sensitive suppressor T-cells may initiate the disturbance of immune tolerance. Jaffé (88[C]) reports a 70-year-old woman developing a hemolytic anemia after having taken methyldopa for 18 months. This was accompanied by positive direct and indirect Coombs tests, a strongly positive test for antinuclear antibody and a grossly elevated serum lactic dehydrogenase level. All abnormalities resolved promptly on suspension of methyldopa treatment.

Two patients are described (89[C], 90[C]) who developed both *chronic active hepatitis* and *auto-immune hemolytic anemia* while taking methyldopa.

A case of *lupus like syndrome* related to methyldopa has been reported (91[C]).

The patient was a 48-year-old woman who developed malaise, generalized weakness, arthralgia, morning stiffness and Raynaud's phenomenon while taking methyldopa 250 mg 3 times daily. Direct Coombs test, LE cell preparations, antinuclear, antithyroid microsome and anti-single-stranded DNA antibody tests were all positive. The symptoms resolved within 2 weeks of stopping methyldopa therapy. Abnormal laboratory tests resolved over a 3 month period with the exception of a persistent positive LE cell preparation.

There is also a single case report of a black woman who developed *thrombocytopenic purpura* while taking methyldopa 500 mg twice daily and hydrochlorothiazide 50 mg daily. This resolved when methyldopa was suspended. In vitro clot retraction was inhibited by the patient's serum in the presence of methyldopa, but not in the presence of serum alone. The Coombs test was negative (92[C]).

Two cases of *drug fever* related to methyldopa have been reported (93[C], 94[C]). In one case (94[C]), serum hepatic transaminase levels also became slightly abnormal. Both cases showed no evidence of underlying infection and resolved promptly when methyldopa was suspended.

Ramsay et al (95[C]) report on a 68-year-old patient who developed *pancreatitis* while taking methyldopa 1000 mg and one Moduretic (hydrochlorothiazide 50 mg and amiloride 5 mg) daily.

There was no history of diabetes mellitus, pancreatic disease, biliary tract disease or alcohol abuse. What is of interest is that he presented after 4 weeks of therapy in diabetic ketoacidosis and had severe diarrhea. Methyldopa was stopped although Moduretic was continued and he recovered and remained well enough requiring oral hypoglycemic agents. However on rechallenge with methyldopa he developed epigastric pain and a worsening of his glucose intolerance. Methyldopa was again stopped, but 7 months later he represented with full blown steatorrhea and X-ray changes of chronic pancreatitis.

There was a further report of myocarditis possibly attributable to the drug (96[C]).

Finally, there is a letter to the Lancet (97[C]) written in response to the article by Cockburn et al (98[C]) declaring methyldopa to be safe in pregnancy. This latter study has been previously discussed (SEDA-7, 241). The authors claim that 3 infants whose mothers were given methyldopa in pregnancy had very low cerebrospinal fluid levels of noradrenaline. However, the control data came from babies over 1000 g heavier. It would be of interest to see the results from these 3 infants compared to more appropriate controls before leaping to any conclusions regarding methyldopa's ability to denervate the newborn.

Clonidine hydrochloride

A number of overdoses with clonidine (SEDA-7, 237) have again been reported. Gossinger et al describe 31 patients admitted for clonidine poisoning (99[cR]). Subjects ranged from infants to adults and symptoms of overdose were sometimes seen after ingestion of only a few clonidine tablets. The authors make the point that, once the clinical syndrome is fully developed, gastric lavage is of little benefit because the drug is rapidly absorbed. The most frequently encountered syndrome was of cardiovascular depression. Respiratory depression, hypertension and alterations of myocardial conduction were less frequent. Patients were treated with fluids, dopamine, phentolamine and atropine as indicated and routine supportive therapy.

Anderson et al (100[c]) report 6 cases of clonidine overdose. These patients again presented with either hyper- or hypotension, brady- or tachycardia and varying degrees of respiratory and conscious level suppression. Some of these patients had other severe illnesses which contributed to their clinical picture, in particular a diabetic who presented with extremely high blood sugar levels.

Ory et al (101[C]) report a woman admitted extremely hypertensive after a clonidine overdose who was successfully treated with tolazoline. It is worth remembering that tolazoline is only likely to be of value in the hypertensive clonidine overdose syndrome where clonidine is probably stimulating post- rather than presynaptic alpha-adrenoreceptors.

Artman (102[C]) reports 4 young children aged between 21 and 24 months who took unknown quantities of clonidine. All became hypotensive and comatose. One infant developed stridor. All were treated with fluids and vasopressors and recovered uneventfully.

Hattner et al (103[C]) report on 2 patients who became hypotensive after taking clonidine as part of a diagnostic test for pheochromocytoma. Both patients had been taking clonidine but had stopped the drug 4 and 7 days previously. The authors interpret this as an increased sensitivity to clonidine. However, a relatively large single dose of clonidine (0.3 mg) was used in the presence of other antihypertensive agents and the response may well be what would be expected.

Effects on insulin secretion As one of the above cases of overdosage (132[C]) reminds us, clonidine can *suppress insulin output* and raise blood sugar levels. There is a case report (145[C]) of a 63-year-old man whose blood sugars rose to unacceptable levels while he was taking clonidine 0.3 mg daily. His glucose intolerance became considerably easier to manage, albeit with insulin, once clonidine was suspended.

Mania Ahsanuddin (104[c]) reports a patient with Tourette syndrome who was doing well taking clonidine for control of his tics until he developed a *manic syndrome* accompanied by delusions. This occurred after 8–9 months of therapy and resolved once clonidine was stopped.

Withdrawal Lilja et al (105[C]) report their open study on abrupt cessation of clonidine therapy. Four patients who ceased a dose of 0.3 mg three times daily and were switched 12 hours later to atenolol all developed symptomatic withdrawals. Halving the dose of clonidine before withdrawal prevented side effects. Beta-adrenoceptor antagonists are generally accepted as making clonidine withdrawals worse and it may be that the relatively rapid switch from clonidine to atenolol contributed to the development of symptoms and signs.

Another publication relating to clonidine withdrawal reports a study of clonidine in ordinary and slow release formulations (106[C]). In this case clonidine was only given for 3 days in a maximum dose of 0.3 mg daily and no clinical signs of withdrawal were observed.

Lofexidine

Lofexidine is a new imidazoline derivative which is being advocated for the treatment of hypertension and opiate withdrawals (107[R]). The interim report of a large double-blind study comparing lofexidine and clonidine (108[C]) suggests that clonidine was slightly more potent on a milligram basis. It also caused more side effects (29% compared to 13%), though it is not clear from the paper whether complaints were volunteered or sought using a questionnaire. Major side effects attributable to lofexidine were drowsiness, fatigue and other CNS symptoms, dryness of the mouth, gastrointestinal upsets and unspecified cardiovascular effects.

In another publication (109[C]) combining data from several studies, the main side effects attributed to lofexidine were dryness of the mouth, tiredness, dizziness, headaches, blocked nose, depression, nausea, dyspnea, sexual disorders and tachycardia. Again, it is not clear whether these side effects were spontaneous or elicited complaints.

A small volunteer study of the comparative pharmacology of clonidine and lofexidine (110[C]) again suggested that lofexidine was less potent than clonidine on a milligram basis in terms of fall in blood pressure and inhibition of salivary flow and had a shorter duration of action. The two compounds appeared similar in terms of the sedation they produced, but the study is probably not large enough to produce a meaningful result in these terms.

Guanidinium derivatives *(SEDA-6, 204; SEDA-7, 238)*

Guanfacine has been submitted to a number of large multicenter trials. In one open study, it was given to 48 hypertensives (111[C]) in a dose of 1–3 mg for 6 weeks. Most side effects were mild and transient and only 2 patients abandoned therapy. Most frequent side effects recorded were dry mouth (10.5%), sedation (6.3%), constipation (2.8%), bitter taste, dizziness, headache, palpitations, polyuria and thirst.

Several other recent studies point to the same pattern of adverse effects as reported earlier (112[C]–114[C]). One double-blind crossover study in 7 volunteers and 7 hypertensives (115[C]) assessed side effects from single doses of clonidine and guanfacine. Variables measured were maximal salivary output, sedation, dry mouth and arterial pressure. Clonidine was considerably more potent than guanfacine in terms of all variables assessed. The authors conclude that single doses of guanfacine in excess of 2 mg do not increase the hypotensive effect but are associated with increasing side effects.

There is a single report of guanfacine overdose characterized by sedation, bradycardia and hypotension. It was treated with isoprenaline infusions (116[C]).

Guanabenz A guanabenz/hydrochlorothiazide combination has been compared with hydrochlorothiazide alone in a double-blind parallel group study involving 204 hypertensive outpatients, of whom 122 completed the study. Guanabenz produced an excess of complaints of dry mouth (52%), drowsiness (38%) and weakness (22%) all of which were transient. Patients taking hydrochlorothiazide alone had similar complaints although not as frequently (117[C]).

In another study (118[C]) guanabenz was compared with methyldopa in a double blind crossover design, separated by a 2 week washout period. Doses were adjusted according to blood pressure response. Only volunteered side effects were recorded. In the guanabenz group 21% stopped therapy because of side effects and were moved on to the washout period. No patients in the methyldopa group stopped therapy. The overall complaint rate was 76% for guanabenz and 50% for methyldopa. Major complaints related to guanabenz were dry mouth, drowsiness, diarrhea, dizziness, nausea and vomiting.

Guanadrel Guanadrel has been compared with methyldopa in a 2-year open study involving 547 hypertensives (119[C]). Drug dosages were adjusted against arterial pressure response. Side effects were elicited with a questionnaire. 276 patients received guanadrel, and 265 patients completed the study. Side effects accounted for 10.9% of the dropouts in the guanadrel group. Major elicited side effects given as the reason for discontinuation were orthostatic faintness, faintness unrelated to posture, impotence, decreased libido, diarrhea, drowsiness and retrograde ejaculation. Of those men completing the study, 5.6% complained of impotence. Other complaints were drowsiness, dizziness, diarrhea and disturbances of ejaculation.

Reserpine

There is a single case report (120[C]) of an 85-year-old woman who became *manic* after suspension of reserpine therapy which she had been taking for 20 years. This occurred during a hospital admission for diverticulitis and a urinary tract infection. The syndrome settled a week after reserpine was restarted. The authors postulate that dopamine receptors supersensitivity secondary to reserpine therapy may have been the underlying cause of the psychotic episode.

Trimethaphan

The effect of trimethaphan on *renal function* has been assessed in 15 healthy young patients undergoing maxillofacial surgery (121[C]). Patients were evaluated before, during and after trimethaphan-induced hypotension. Creatinine clearance and urinary sodium reabsorption decreased reversibly during arterial hypotension.

Beta-adrenoceptor antagonist/diuretic combinations

A number of publications regarding trials of beta-blocker-diuretic combinations have appeared in the last year. These have not always been easy to assess reliably for reported side effects. This seems a shame, since large scale patient trials are generally the only opportunity available to a manufacturer to assess accurately the incidence rate of side effects, or indeed to assess whether complaints can be genuinely considered side effects at all. This is of particular importance to this class of compounds which are generally marketed as a means of improving patient compliance. While single tablet dosing regimens may contribute to improved compliance, greater tolerance of a fixed dose combination may also be of considerable importance.

When side effects are reported, the method of collection of those complaints is generally not given. The method of collection, be it the noting of spontaneous complaints, or complaints made in response to a general inquiry or the use of a questionnaire, will influence the incidence rate and also possibly the nature of those complaints. Of recent papers eligible for review in this section, in fact, only two make any statement as to the method of collection of symptomatic side effects.

A further problem lies in the size of such patient trials. Frequently small studies involving, say, 20 or 30 patients, are uninterpretable since they will not differentiate out genuine drug effects from the background prevalence of such symptoms. Other faults in trial design such as drug comparisons using open, single-blind and crossover studies without any attempt at washout periods complicate the issue further. The use of the statement that complaints are not reported because they are not considered to be drug-related must be deplored. The criteria by which their relationship to drug is assessed are never given. It cannot be considered right to ignore data, since it may only be in the accumulation of data from numerous patient trials that rare or unusual side effects may become apparent.

Moducren

Moducren (timolol/hydrochlorothiazide/amiloride) has been given to a large number of patients in several different studies. Parry et al (122[C]) gave Moducren or a cyclopenthiazide/potassium combination to 641 patients in an open study in general practice. Details of elicitation of side effects are not given, nor are individual complaints. Moducren produced twice as many central nervous system and four times as many cardiovascular/respiratory complaints as the diuretic. There is no statement regarding the statistical significance of these findings.

Woollard and Cooper (123[C]) report an open study comparing Moducren with propranolol in 104 patients. Adverse symptoms were inquired for at each visit in the study, and at the end patients assessed their wellbeing on a visual analog scale. At doses which controlled blood pressure, patients reported side effects more frequently with propranolol than with Moducren. Overall this did not reach statistical significance except for complaints of cold extremities which occurred much more frequently with propranolol than with Moducren.

Atenolol

Three studies involving atenolol have been reported. In one (124[C]), atenolol 100 mg, indapamide 2.5 mg and a combination of the two at the same dosage are compared in groups of 20 patients. The study was apparently open. It is not clear whether complaints were spontaneous or actively sought. In the atenolol group, 5 patients complained of fatigue, 3 of dizziness, 2 of gastrointestinal upsets and one of headache. Three patients developed a bradycardia. In the indapamide group, there was 1 complaint of fatigue, 5 of leg cramps and 2 of gastrointestinal upsets. Four patients developed hypokalemia and 1 hyperuricemia. In the combined group, 1 patient complained of tiredness and 1 of lack of energy. Reams of laboratory data are given, analyzed unfortunately by multiple student t-tests rather than by analysis of variance and therefore not making interpretation any easier for the reader. However, it would seem that the combination is capable of partly preventing hypokalemia brought on by indapamide alone.

Douglas-Jones and Tweed (125[C]) compared atenolol/chlorthalidone with pindolol/clopamide given for 4 weeks each to 40 patients in a single-blind, possibly balanced, crossover study with no washout period. Side effects reported on an invention to treat basis and variously described as evoked or volunteered were what one would expect of beta-blockers and diuretics. There were 19 complaints in the atenolol/chlorthalidone period and 32 in the pindolol/clopamide period. There are real problems in the assessment of this study, not only in its single-blindness but also that in not knowing about the adequacy of the balance of the design and there being no washout period, an excess of subjective complaints may be due to carryover effects from one treatment period to the next.

Acebutolol

A double-blind crossover study without a washout period was carried out in 32 patients, comparing acebutolol 400 mg daily with the same dose of acebutolol combined with a hydrochlorothiazide/amiloride preparation (126[C]). Each treatment period was for 6 weeks. Side effects were infrequent and were not broken down by treatment period. Of interest is the observation that 2 patients developing dyspnea while taking acebutolol improved when switched to the combination product.

Nadolol

Nadolol in varying doses and hydrochlorothiazide 50 or 100 mg were given by open label to 32 patients for 2 years (127[C]). Six patients are reported as developing symptoms considered related to nadolol. These complaints were dizziness in 3, fatigue in 1, dyspnea and paresthesiae in 1 and gastrointestinal intolerance, impotence and paresthesiae in 1. An additional patient developed a sino-atrial dysrhythmia which resolved spontaneously while treatment continued.

Sotazide

There is a single case report (128[C]) of a patient developing severe hypokalemia (serum potassium 2.4 mEq/l) while taking Sotazide (sotalol 160 mg and hydrochlorothiazide 25 mg). This resolved when the patient was switched to propranolol, hydralazine and Moduretic and recurred on rechallenge with sotazide. The diagnosis of hyperaldosteronism was investigated and excluded.

MISCELLANEOUS

Indapamide

An unfortunate example of a study, the presentation of which renders it impossible to interpret the results fully, is one in which indapamide was given by open label to 2497 evaluable patients for 3 months in a general practitioner study (129[C]). Of these, 1202 took indapamide alone and the rest various combinations of drugs.

Individual side effects data are not given for indapamide only. The group as a whole reported dizziness in 3%, headache in 1.5%, nausea in 1.2% and fatigue in 2.6%. Serum potassium, blood glucose and serum uric acid levels showed no consistent changes in response to therapy.

Indapamide has also been given by open label to 13 patients with impaired renal function (130[C]). Two complained of moderately severe symptoms, nervousness and palpitations. Other minor complaints were dizziness, nasal congestion, insomnia, gastrointestinal intolerance, coldness and pruritus.

Metolazone

There is a single case report of a 75-year-old woman who had been taking multiple therapy for ischemic heart disease, congestive cardiac failure, hypertension and diabetes mellitus (131[C]). She also had a history of a hemolytic anemia secondary to methyldopa and a rash due to hydralazine. Two weeks after commencing metolazone, she developed generalized pains and a raised nodular eruption on the trunk. On biopsy, these proved to be a necrotizing arteritis. Her ESR was 91 mm/hr and she had elevated antinuclear antibody titres and low C_3 and C_4 fractions. Metolazone and the reserpine which she had also been taking were stopped and the rash and high ESR slowly resolved without further therapy.

REFERENCES

1. Castelli WP, Doyle JT, Gordon T et al (1977) HDL cholesterol and other lipids in coronary heart disease. The Cooperative Lipoprotein Phenotyping Study. *Circulation, 55,* 767.
2. Rhoads GG, Gulbrandsen CL, Kagan A (1976) Serum lipoproteins and coronary heart disease in a population study of Hawaiian Japanese men. *N. Engl. J. Med., 294,* 293.
3. Miller NE, Førde OH, Thelle DS et al (1977) The Tromsø Heart Study. High density lipoprotein and coronary heart disease. A prospective case-control study. *Lancet, 1,* 965.
4. Gordon T, Castelli WP, Hjortland MC et al (1977) High density lipoprotein as a protective factor against coronary heart disease. The Framingham Study. *Am. J. Med., 62,* 207.
5. Johnson BF (1982) The emerging problem of plasma lipid changes during antihypertensive therapy. *J. Cardiovasc. Pharmacol., 4, Suppl. 2,* S213.
6. Leren P, Eide I, Foss OP et al (1982) Antihypertensive drugs and blood lipids: The Oslo study. *J. Cardiovasc. Pharmacol., 4, Suppl. 2,* S222.
7. Parker M, Atkinson J (1982) Withdrawal syndromes following cessation of treatment

with antihypertensive drugs. *Gen. Pharmacol.*, *13*, 79.
8. Moore MP, Redman CWG (1982) The treatment of hypertension in pregnancy. *Curr. Med. Res. Opin.*, *8*, *Suppl. 1*, 39.
9. Paykel ES, Fleminger R, Watson JP (1982) Psychiatric side effects of antihypertensive drugs other than reserpine. *J. Clin. Psychopharmacol.*, *2*, 14.
10. Editorial (1983) Captopril: five years on. *Br. Med. J.*, *287*, 851.
11. Ram CVS (1982) Captopril. *N. Engl. J. Med.*, *307*, 58.
12. Christensen HR, Kampmann JP, Svendsen TL (1983) Severe hypotension after captopril. *Ugeskr. Laeg.*, *145*, 1686.
13. Veterans Administration Co-operative Study Group on Antihypertensive Agents (1982) Racial differences in response to low-dose captopril are abolished by the addition of hydrochlorothiazide. *Br. J. Clin. Pharmacol.*, *14*, 97S.
14. Weinberger MH (1982) Comparison of captopril and hydrochlorothiazide alone and in combination in mild to moderate essential hypertension. *Br. J. Clin. Pharmacol.*, *14*, 127S.
15. Havelka J, Boerlin HJ, Studer A et al (1982) Long-term experience with captopril in severe hypertension. *Br. J. Clin. Pharmacol.*, *14*, 71S.
16. Raine AEG, Ledingham JGG (1982) Clinical experience with captopril in the treatment of severe drug-resistant hypertension. *Am. J. Cardiol.*, *49*, 1475.
17. Fernandez-Cruz Jr A, Otero ML, Pinilla CF, Claros NM (1982) Captopril in the treatment of mild essential hypertension. *Br. J. Clin. Pharmacol.*, *14*, 117S.
18. Icasas-Cabral E, Roa C, Mendoza-Wi J et al (1982) Efficacy and safety of an angiotensin converting enzyme inhibitor in the treatment of severe hypertension. *Philipp. J. Intern. Med.*, *20*, 173.
19. Ectors M, Staroukine M, Demanet J-C (1982) Long term captopril treatment of severe hypertension resistant to tritherapy. *Acta Clin. Belg.*, *37*, 59.
20. Chatterjee K, Rouleau J-L, Parmley WW (1982) Captopril in congestive heart failure: improved left ventricular function with decreased metabolic cost. *Am. Heart J.*, *104*, 1137.
21. Dahlström U, Karlberg BE (1982) Short and long-term effects of treatment with low dose captopril in patients with severe congestive heart failure. *Br. J. Clin. Pharmacol.*, *14*, 231S.
22. Awan NA, Mason DT (1982) Vasodilator therapy of severe congestive heart failure: the special importance of angiotensin-converting enzyme inhibition with captopril. *Am. Heart J.*, *104*, 1127.
23. Steingo L, Pocock WA, Flax H et al (1982) Long-term captopril therapy in severe refractory congestive heart failure. *Br. J. Clin. Pharmacol.*, *14*, 203S.
24. Aurell M, Delin K, Herlitz H, Mulec H (1982) Captopril treatment in hypertensive dialysis patients. *Scand. J. Urol. Nephrol.*, *16*, 251.
25. Wizemann A (1983) Nekrotisierende Blepharitis nach Captopril-induzierter Agranulozytose. *Klin. Monatsbl. Augenheilk.*, *182*, 82.
26. Christeler A, Waeber B, Brunner HR, Delacrétaz J (1982) Pemphigus superficial induit par le captopril. *Schweiz. Med. Wochenschr.*, *112*, 1483.
27. Reinhardt LA, Wilkin JK, Kirkendall WM (1983) Lichenoid eruption produced by captopril. *Cutis*, *31*, 98.
28. Solinger AM (1982) Exfoliative dermatitis from captopril. *Cutis*, *29*, 473.
29. Luderer JR, Lookingbill DP, Schneck DW et al (1982) Captopril-induced skin eruptions. *J. Clin. Pharmacol.*, *22*, 1151.
30. Palla R, Marchitiello ME, Sassano P, Salvetti A (1982) Effect of captopril on renal function in patients with essential hypertension. *Am. J. Cardiol.*, *49*, 1577.
31. Textor SC, Gephardt GN, Bravo EL et al (1983) Membranous glomerulonephropathy associated with captopril therapy. *Am. J. Med.*, *74*, 705.
32. Hymes LC, Warshaw BL (1983) Captopril. Long-term treatment of hypertension in a preterm infant and in older children. *Am. J. Dis. Child.*, *137*, 263.
33. Aurell M, Delin K, Herlitz H (1982) Captopril in treatment-resistant essential and renal hypertension. *Scand. J. Urol. Nephrol.*, *16*, 243.
34. Hooke D, Walker RG, Walter NMA et al (1982) Repeated renal failure with use of captopril in a cystinotic renal allograft recipient. *Br. Med. J.*, *285*, 1538.
35. Chrysant SG, Dunn M, Marples D, DeMasters K (1983) Severe reversible azotemia from captopril therapy. Report of three cases and review of the literature. *Arch. Intern. Med.*, *143*, 437.
36. Hricik DE, Browning PJ, Kopelman R et al (1983) Captopril-induced functional renal insufficiency in patients with bilateral renal-artery stenoses or renal-artery stenosis in a solitary kidney. *N. Engl. J. Med.*, *308*, 373.
37. Creager MA, Faxon DP, Halperin JL et al (1982) Determinants of clinical response and survival in patients with congestive heart failure treated with captopril. *Am. Heart J.*, *104*, 1147.
38. Marichal JF, Faller B (1982) Leucopénie transitoire chez un hypertendu hémodialysé: responsabilité du captopril? *J. Méd. Strasbourg*, *13*, 613.
39. Albertazzi A, Del Rosso G, Cappelli P et al (1982) Clinical experience with captopril in the treatment of severe and resistant hypertension. *Drugs Exper. Clin. Res.*, *8*, 529.
40. Panel Discussion (1982) Selection of patients for treatment (including side effects of captopril). *Br. J. Clin. Pharmacol.*, *14*, 113S.
41. Editorial (1983) Captopril associated neutro-

penia. Who is at risk? *Arch. Intern. Med., 143,* 659.

42. De Ligny BH, Mariot A, Kessler M et al (1982) Hépatite au cours d'une polythérapie associant le captopril. *Thérapie, 37,* 689.
43. Ryckelynck, J-Ph, Batho J-M, Peny J, Beuvemery P (1982) Hépatite au captopril. *Nouv. Presse Méd., 11,* 1950.
44. Kallenberg CGM, Hoorntje SJ, Smit AJ et al (1982) Antinuclear and antinative DNA antibodies during captopril treatment. *Acta Med. Scand., 211,* 297.
45. Silberbauer K, Stanek B, Templ H (1982) Acute hypotensive effect of captopril in man modified by prostaglandin synthesis inhibition. *Br. J. Clin. Pharmacol., 14,* 87S.
46. Cressman MD, Vidt DG, Acker C (1982) Renal glycosuria and azotaemia after enalapril maleate (MK-421). *Lancet, 2,* 440.
47. Barnes JN et al (1983) Rash eosinophilia and hyperkalaemia associated with enalapril. *Lancet, 2,* 41.
48. Kronzon I, Cohen M, Winer HE (1982) Adverse effect of hydralazine in patients with primary pulmonary hypertension. *J. Am. Med. Ass., 247,* 3112.
49. McKelvie GM, Bayliff CD, Gaska JA, Linkewich JA (1982) Adverse reaction reviews. Drug-induced liver diseases: part 3, illustrative cases. *Hosp. Pharm., 17,* 562.
50. Von Roschlau G, Baumgarten R, Winter H (1982) Hepatitis mit konfluierenden Nekrosen durch Depressan. *Dtsch. Gesundheitswes., 37,* 709.
51. Freestone S, Ramsay LE (1982) Transient monoclonal gammopathy in hydralazine-induced lupus erythematosus. *Br. Med. J., 285,* 1536.
52. Aylward PE, Tonkin AM, Bune A (1982) Cardiac tamponade in hydrallazine-induced systemic lupus erythematosus. *Aust. N.Z. J. Med., 12;* 546.
53. Portanova JP, Rubin RL, Joslin FG et al (1982) Reactivity of anti-histone antibodies induced by procainamide and hydrallazine. *Clin. Immunol. Immunopathol., 25,* 67.
54. Lin M-S, McNay JL, Shepherd AM et al (1983) Increased plasma norepinephrine accompanies persistent tachycardia after hydralazine. *Hypertension, 5,* 257.
55. Packer M, Meller J, Medina N et al (1981) Provocation of myocardial ischemic events during initiation of vasodilator therapy for severe chronic heart failure. *Am. J. Cardiol., 48,* 939.
56. Mäntylä R, Mannistö P, Nykänen S et al (1983) Pharmacokinetic interactions of timolol with vasodilating drugs, food and phenobarbitone in healthy human volunteers. *Eur. J. Clin. Pharmacol., 24,* 227.
57. Koch H (1983) Endralazine mesylate. *Drugs Today, 19,* 18.
58. Kirch W, Axthelm T (1982) Endralazine, a new peripheral vasodilator – a randomized cross-over trial dihydralazine. *J. Cardiovasc. Pharmacol., 4,* 562.
59. Zacest R, Reece PA (1983) Endralazine and sexual arousal. *Lancet, 1,* 1221.
60. Ruzicka T, Ring J (1983) Hypersensitivity to prazosin. *Lancet, 1,* 473.
61. Kokubu T, Itoh I, Kurita H et al (1982) Effect of prazosin on serum lipids. *J. Cardiovasc. Pharmacol., 4, Suppl. 2,* S228.
62. Lithell H, Waern U, Vessby B (1982) Effect of prazosin on lipoprotein metabolism in premenopausal, hypertensive women. *J. Cardiovasc. Pharmacol., 4, Suppl. 2,* S242.
63. Velasco M, Silva H, Morillo J et al (1982) Effect of prazosin on blood lipids and on thyroid function in hypertensive patients. *J. Cardiovasc. Pharmacol., 4, Suppl. 2,* S225.
64. Von Sprenger KBG, Bundschu D, Von Sprenger-Klasen I et al (1982) Behandlung des therapieresistenten renalen Hypertonus mit Minoxidil. *Nieren-Hochdruckkrankh., 11,* S61.
65. Von Kindler J, Glockner WM, Vaith P, Sieberth HG (1982) Antihypertensive Langzeitbehandlung mit Minoxidil bei therapierefraktärer Hypertonie. *Nieren-Hochdruckkrankh., 11,* S25.
66. Von Demers HG, Wessely W., Höffler D (1982) Minoxidil bei schwer einstellbarer Hypertonie: 6-jährige Erfahrung mit einem neuen Vasodilator. *Nieren-Hochdruckkrankh., 11,* S15.
67. Von Brodersen H-P, Sack K (1982) Klinische Erfahrungen mit Minoxidil. *Nieren-Hochdruckkrankh., 11,* S36.
68. Von Meurer KA, Wambach G, Böttcher W et al (1982) Langzeittherapie der akzelerierten Hypertonie mit Minoxidil. *Nieren-Hochdruckkrankh., 11,* S45.
69. Von Buhler G, Ismadi K, Albert FW (1982) Ergebnisse der Behandlung schwerster renaler und renalisierter Hypertonien mit dem Vasodilator Minoxidil. *Nieren-Hochdruckkrankh., 11,* S51.
70. Bannan LT, Beavers DG, Shapiro LM (1982) Clinical and echocardiographic studies of minoxidil in resistant hypertension. *Ir. Med. J., 75,* 192.
71. Hagstam KE, Lundgren R, Wieslander J (1982) Clinical experience of long-term treatment with minoxidil in severe arterial hypertension. *Scand. J. Urol. Nephrol., 16,* 57.
72. Bianchetti MG, Weidmann P, Boehringer K et al (1982) Comparative evaluation of the new vasodilator carprazidil and minoxidil in the treatment of moderate to severe hypertension. *Eur. J. Clin. Pharmacol., 23,* 483.
73. Von Feldhoff CM, Pistor K, Bachmann H (1982) Langzeitbehandlung mit Minoxidil bei einem Kind mit hämolytisch-urämischen Syndrom. *Nieren-Hochdruckkrankh., 11,* S75.
74. Zaruba K, Rohacek M, Grauer W (1982) Flüssigkeitsretention mit Perikarderguss unter Behandlung mit Minoxidil. *Dtsch. Med. Wochenschr., 107,* 984.
75. Webb DB, Whale RJ (1982) Pleuropericardial effusion associated with minoxidil administration. *Postgrad. Med. J., 58,* 319.

76. Bennion SD (1982) Chest pain and abnormal electrocardiogram associated with minoxidil. *Mil. Med., 147,* 367.
77. Wilkin JK, Kirkendall WM (1982) Porphyria mimicked during minoxidil therapy. *Cutis, 31,* 61.
78. Gombos GM (1983) Bilateral optic neuritis following minoxidil administration. *Ann. Ophthalmol, 15,* 259.
79. Durrer JD, Lie KI, Van Capelle JL, Durrer D (1982) Effect of sodium nitroprusside on mortality in acute myocardial infarction. *N. Engl. J. Med., 306,* 1121.
80. Cohn JN, Franciosa JA, Francis GS et al (1982) Effect of short-term infusion of sodium nitroprusside on mortality rate in acute myocardial infarction complicated by left ventricular failure. Results of a Veterans Administration Cooperative Study. *N. Engl. J. Med., 306,* 1129.
81. Ivankovich AD, Braverman B, Stephens TS et al (1983) Sodium thiosulfate disposition in humans: relation to sodium nitroprusside toxicity. *Anesthesiology, 58,* 11.
82. Pasch T, Schulz V, Hoppelshäuser G (1983) Nitroprusside-induced formation of cyanide and its detoxication with thiosulfate during deliberate hypotension. *J. Cardiovasc. Pharmacol., 5,* 77.
83. Kim YH, Foo M, Terry RD (1982) Cyanide encephalopathy following therapy with sodium nitroprusside. Report of a case. *Arch. Pathol. Lab. Med., 106,* 392.
84. O'Boyle CP, Laher M, O'Brien ET et al (1982) The clinical pharmacology of tolmesoxide. A new vasodilator antihypertensive agent. *Eur. J. Clin. Pharmacol., 23,* 93.
85. Noveck R, McMahon FG, Jain AK (1982) Treatment of elevated blood pressure with a simplified methyldopa-hydrochlorothiazide treatment regimen. *Curr. Ther. Res., 32,* 822.
86. Carr AA, Mulligan OF, Sherrill LN (1982) Pindolol versus methyldopa for hypertension: Comparison of adverse reactions. *Am. Heart. J., 104,* 479.
87. Schubothe H, Maas D, Weber S et al (1982) Methyldopainduzierte autoimmunhämolytische Anämien. Verlaufs- und Langzeitbeobachtungen an 11 Patienten. *Immun. Infekt., 10,* 230.
88. Jaffé ER (1982) Methyldopa-induced hemolytic anemia. *Med. Grand Rounds, 1,* 136.
89. Shalev O, Mosseri M, Ariel I, Stalnikowicz R (1983) Methyldopa-induced immune hemolytic anemia and chronic active hepatitis. *Arch. Intern. Med., 143,* 592.
90. Breland BD, Hicks Jr GS (1982) Hepatitis and hemolytic anemia associated with methyldopa therapy. *Drug. Intell. Clin. Pharm., 16,* 489.
91. Dupont A, Six R (1982) Lupus-like syndrome induced by methyldopa. *Br. Med. J., 285,* 693.
92. Polk OD, Kletter GG, Smith J, Castro O (1982) Impaired clot retraction in thrombocytopenia due to methyldopa. *South. Med. J., 75,* 374.
93. Jain A, Sanders CV, Nicolle FI (1982) Drug fever during treatment of pulmonary edema. *South. Med. J., 75,* 1140.
94. Sawa H, Miyazaki M, Kato K et al (1981) Febrile reaction during treatment with alpha-methyldopa. *Mie Med. J., 31,* 189.
95. Ramsay LE, Wakefield VA, Harris EE (1982) Methyldopa-induced chronic pancreatitis. *Practitioner, 226,* 1166.
96. Jauslin P-A (1983) Myocardite par hypersensibilité, d'origine médicamenteuse (méthyldopa). *Rev. Med. Suisse Romande, 103,* 163.
97. Bodis J, Sulyok E, Ertl T et al (1982) Methyldopa in pregnancy hypertension and the newborn. *Lancet, 2,* 498.
98. Cockburn J, Moar VA, Ounsted M, Redman CWG (1982) Final report of study on hypertension during pregnancy: the effects of specific treatment on the growth and development of the children. *Lancet, 1,* 647.
99. Gössinger H, Hruby K, Haubenstock A et al (1983) Die Intoxikation mit Clonidinhydrochlorid im Kindes- und Erwachsenenalter. *Wien. Klin. Wochenschr., 95,* 232.
100. Anderson RJ, Hart GR, Crumpler CP, Lerman MJ (1981) Clonidine overdose. Report of six cases and review of the literature. *Ann. Emerg. Med., 10,* 107.
101. Ory J-P, Delorme N, Laprevote-Heully M-C et al (1981) Effet paradoxal hypertenseur de la clonidine. Réflexions à propos d'une intoxication. *J. Toxicol. Med., 1,* 211.
102. Artman M, Boerth RC (1983) Clonidine poisoning. A complex problem. *Am. J. Dis. Childh., 137,* 171.
103. Hattner RS, Engelstad BL, Roizen MF, Huberty JP (1982) Complications of clonidine suppression test for pheochromocytoma. *N. Engl. J. Med., 307,* 756.
104. Ahsanuddin K (1982) Side effects of clonidine. *Am. J. Psychiatry, 139,* 1083.
105. Lilya M, Jounela AJ, Juustila HJ, Paalzow L (1982) Abrupt and gradual change from clonidine to beta blockers in hypertension. *Acta Med. Scand., 211,* 375.
106. Planz G, Beckenbauer U, Bundschu HD (1982) Response of plasma catecholamines and blood pressure to clonidine and to sudden withdrawal of the drug in subjects with essential hypertension. *Int. J. Clin. Pharmacol. Ther. Toxicol., 20,* 474.
107. Anon (1982) Lofexidine. *Drugs Today, 18,* 586.
108. Beitman RE, Kuzma RJ, McMahon FG et al (1982) Comparative efficacy and safety of lofexidine and clonidine given alone or concomitantly with hydrochlorothiazide in hypertensive outpatients. *Arzneim. Forsch., 32,* 988.
109. Aigner A, Schmidt U (1982) Lofexidine, a new antihypertensive imidazoline derivative. *Arzneim. Forsch., 32,* 976.
110. Dollery CT, Reid JL (1982) Double-blind comparison of the hypotensive, sedative and

salivary flow effects of lofexidine and clonidine in normal subjects. *Arzneim. Forsch.*, *32*, 984.
111. Westelinck K, Michotte Y (1982) Low dose guanfacine once a day for the treatment of hypertension in general practice: a multi-centre pilot study. *Curr. Med. Res. Opin.*, *7*, 631.
112. Chaudron JM, Daubresse JC, Lauwers Ph et al (1982) Le traitement de la maladie hypertensive par la guanfacine. Etude multicentrique de 100 cas. *Ars Med.*, *37*, 471.
113. Schäfer N, Knaup G (1982) Antihypertensive Therapie mit Guanfacin. Ein Multizenter-Studie mit Estulic-Wander 1 mg. *Münch. Med. Wochenschr.*, *124*, 249.
114. Efstratopoulos AD, Spantideas A, Sakopoulou-Pipi H et al (1982) Treatment of arterial hypertension. Trial of a new antihypertensive agent guanfacine (Estulic). *Clin. Trials J.*, *19*, 129.
115. Chierichetti SM, Fiorella G, Vibelli C et al (1982) Double-blind comparison between acute guanfacine and clonidine administrations on hypotensive activity and side effects in healthy volunteers and hypertensive patients. *Curr. Ther. Res.*, *31*, 588.
116. Granier P, Arsec P, Debru JL (1982) Intoxication par la guanfacine. *Nouv. Presse Méd.*, *11*, 1636.
117. Walker BR, Deitch MW, Gold JA, Levey BA (1982) Evaluation of guanbenz added to hydrochlorothiazide therapy in hypertension. *J. Int. Med. Res.*, *10*, 131.
118. Rosendorff C (1982) Guanabenz versus methyldopa in the therapy of mild to moderate hypertension. *S. Afr. Med. J.*, *62*, 435.
119. Nugent CA, Palmer JD, Ursprung JJ (1982) Guanadrel sulfate compared with methyldopa for mild and moderate hypertension. *Pharmacother.*, *2*, 378.
120. Kent TA, Wilber RD (1982) Reserpine withdrawal psychosis: the possible role of denervation supersensitivity of receptors. *J. Nerv. Ment. Dis.*, *170*, 502.
121. Behnia R, Martin A, Koushanpour E, Brunner EA (1982) Trimethaphan-induced hypotension: effect on renal function. *Can. Anaesth. Soc. J.*, *29*, 581.
122. Parry EE, Young J, Arr S (1982) Comparison of timolol/hydrochlorothiazide/amiloride (Moducren) with cyclopenthiazide/potassium in mild to moderate hypertension. *Curr. Med. Res. Opin.*, *8*, 253.
123. Woollard ML, Cooper WD (1983) Moducren and propranolol as initial therapies in essential hypertension. *Clin. Trials J.*, *20*, 89.
124. Messin R, De Smedt J (1982) Etude de l'action hypotensive d'une nouvelle association médicamenteuse le SF-979. *Ars Med.*, *37*, 943.
125. Douglas-Jones AP, Tweed JA (1982) Randomized trial of two beta-blocker/diuretic combinations (atenolol/chlorthalidone and pindolol/clopamide) in mild to moderate hypertension. *Acta Ther.*, *8*, 345.
126. Khalil SI, El Zein O, Bella MEM (1982) A double-blind crossover study of acebutolol and hydrochlorothiazide/amiloride diuretic in Sudanese patients with essential hypertension. *Curr. Med. Res. Opin.*, *8*, 39.
127. El-Mehairy MM, Shaker A, Ramadan M et al (1982) Long-term treatment of essential hypertension with nadolol and hydrochlorothiazide. A two-year follow-up. *J. Int. Med. Res.*, *10*, 87.
128. Skehan JD, Barnes JN, Drew PJ, Wright P (1982) Hypokalaemia induced by a combination of a beta-blocker and a thiazide. *Br. Med. J.*, *284*, 83.
129. Wheeley MSG, Bolton JC, Campbell DB (1982) Indapamide in hypertension: a study in general practice of new or previously poorly controlled patients. *Pharmatherapeutica*, *3*, 143.
130. Brennan L, Wu MJ, Laquer VJ (1982) A multicenter study of indapamide in hypertensive patients with impaired renal function. *Clin. Ther.*, *5*, 121.
131. Weinrauch LA, Belok SS, Gauvin GP, D'Elia JA (1982) Palpable acute necrotizing arteritis secondary to metolazone. *Cutis*, *30*, 83.
132. Webster Jr WB, McConnaughey MM (1982) Clonidine and glucose intolerance. *Drug Intell. Clin. Pharm.*, *16*, 325.

E.J. Buurke

22 Diuretic drugs

Acute interstitial nephritis with thiazide and triamterene

With today's intensive use of medicaments acute interstitial nephritis due to a hypersensitivity reaction is not uncommon. Such drug-induced acute interstitial nephritis may also occur with diuretics, especially with thiazides and triamterene. The overall incidence of this kind of nephrotoxic reaction to these drugs is unknown but remarkable in a study by Magil (1[C]). In order to gain immuno-pathogenetic insight into this process renal biopsy specimens of 9 patients with drug-induced acute interstitial nephritis were studied. 8 of these 9 patients had used triamterene and/or a thiazide. 4 patients had been treated with both triamterene and thiazide without other drugs, 2 patients received this diuretic-combination together with other drugs. The remaining 2 patients had received hydrochlorothiazide with metoprolol tartrate and triamterene with frusemide respectively. Renal insufficiency developed approximately 4 to 10 weeks after initiation of drug therapy. In all cases withdrawal of the drug(s) with or without steroid therapy resulted in restoration of normal or near-normal renal function. Based upon this combined histological immunopathological and ultrastructural study of the renal biopsy specimens the author provides evidence for participation of cell-mediated immunity in the pathogenesis of at least some cases of this drug-induced acute interstitial nephritis.

Plasma lipoproteins and chlorthalidone *(SED-9; SEDA-7)*

Although the clinical relevance of the finding remains unclear it is well known that thiazides may induce small but significant elevations of both triglycerides and cholesterol, whereas thiazide and loop diuretics can alter (unfavorably) the ratio between low-density and high-density lipoproteins in hypertensive patients. A new feature of this phenomenon is presented by Boehringer et al (2[C]) who studied 22 premenopausal and 18 postmenopausal women during single-blind placebo-controlled treatment with chlorthalidone, 100 mg/day for 6 weeks. Women taking estrogen-containing preparations were excluded and other diuretic or beta-blocking medications were discontinued. Lipoprotein fractions were isolated by sequential ultracentrifugation. Total serum cholesterol, low-density lipoprotein-cholesterol and apoprotein B increased in the postmenopausal but not in the premenopausal women. Other lipoprotein fractions and free fatty acids were not significantly altered during treatment with chlorthalidone in either group of women.

The findings in the postmenopausal women were comparable with those reported in diuretic-treated men. Apparently premenopausal women may often be protected from these diuretic-induced biochemical side effects. The authors consider the possibility that certain diuretics may interfere with metabolic pathways of lipoproteins in men and in postmenopausal women who are somewhat estrogen deficient.

Electrolytes *(SED-9, 342; SEDA-4, 158; SEDA-5, 227; SEDA-7, 246)*

Hypokalemia, and its relation to cardiac arrhythmias in digitalized and non-digitalized patients, has been dealt with in previous SEDA editions. Extensive studies by Haalboom and Struyvenberg on the mechanism underlying chlorthalidone-induced hypokalemia indicate hyperaldosteronism as the main causal factor (3[C]). Accordingly such diuretic-induced hypokalemia cannot be corrected by potassium chloride suppletion

Side Effects of Drugs Annual 8
M.N.G. Dukes, editor

ISBN 0 444 90339 9
$0.80 per article per page (transactional system)
$0.20 per article per page (licensing system)

but requires administration of spironolactone, triamterene or amiloride (4[C], 5[C]).

However, controversy persists as to the need for and safety of such potassium repletion. The possibility could be raised that not hypokalemia alone but hypokalemia in combination with hypomagnesemia is a significant risk factor for the development of cardiac arrhythmias. Little attention has been paid to this possibility although diuretic-induced magnesium depletion with or without low serum concentrations was documented earlier (6[C], 7[C]).

Sheehan and White (8[C]) report their findings in 40 diuretic-treated patients with symptoms suggestive of *magnesium depletion*, i.e. depression, muscle weakness, refractory hypokalemia and rapid atrial fibrillation despite vigorous digoxin treatment. 21 of these 40 patients were found to have appreciable hypomagnesemia. 9 patients had hypokalemia despite copious oral supplements. 5 patients had uncontrollable atrial fibrillation. Treatment with intramuscular boluses of 4–8 mmol of magnesium sulfate resulted in prompt improvement of all symptoms in all cases. Oral supplementation with magnesium salts was dose-limited by diarrhea. Dietary supplementation with bananas was useful. In 6 patients a magnesium-sparing property of spironolactone was noted; amiloride and triamterene were not used in this study. Sheehan's observations clearly indicate the necessity for further studies on diuretic-induced magnesium-depletion and on the effects of magnesium treatment both on clinical symptoms (including arrhythmias) and on potassium depletion with hypokalemia.

As regards urinary magnesium excretion, Reyes' observations in healthy volunteers may be relevant (9[C]). After single-dose oral administration of 100 mg chlorthalidone the time-courses of volume, potassium, sodium and chloride coincided whereas the urinary magnesium (and zinc) excretions proceeded at significantly slower rates, suggesting endocrine mechanisms for the latter.

INDIVIDUAL COMPOUNDS

Furosemide

A hitherto unknown pediatric complication of furosemide was reported in premature infants treated with the drug in doses of at least 2 mg/kg/day for at least 12 days (10[C]). In the course of 4 years 10 of such infants developed *renal calcifications.* They proved to have calcium excretion rates 10–20 times those in normal, age-matched premature infants in the same nursery. An important complication of the stone formation was sepsis secondary to urinary tract infections. Additive treatment with chlorothiazide resulted in a decrease in calcium excretion and in radiographic diminution or disappearance of the calcifications. The authors warn against long-term use of *furosemide* in premature infants because of the risk of *stone formation* consequent on such drug-induced hypercalciuria.

Xipamide

Xipamide is a new, non-thiazide diuretic. It has its main site of action on the distal convoluted tubule and can be used in patients with hypertension and edema of differing origin. In normal subjects 20 mg xipamide has similar diuretic and natriuretic activity to 40 mg furosemide but the long duration of action of xipamide resembles that of the thiazides.

In an open crossover trial 15 patients with edema and renal disease were treated with xipamide 40 mg/day and furosemide 40 mg/day (11[C]). Both renal impairment and degree of proteinuria ranged widely. Edema diminished on both drugs, slightly more on xipamide. There were no adverse reactions to furosemide. 3 patients experienced side effects on xipamide: *nausea* and a *syncopal attack, muscular cramps* disappearing after dose reduction and *headache* disappearing after discontinuation of treatment. *Lowest serum potassium values* were 3.6 and 3.7 mmol/l, both during xipamide treatment. No data on magnesium are given.

Xipamide was compared with cyclopenthiazide in a randomized crossover trial in 14 patients with uncomplicated, mild to moderate hypertension (12[C]). Both drugs were effective in lowering blood pressure and no adverse effects were found. However, *plasma potassium was reduced* markedly, and more after both 10 mg and 20 mg xipamide than after cyclopenthiazide 0.5 mg. In 13 of 14 patients on xipamide plasma potassium concentrations fell to 3.5 mmol/l or below versus 6 of 14 on cyclopenthiazide.

This study too fails to present data on the patients' magnesium status.

Interaction between nonsteroidal anti-inflammatory agents and diuretics

In addition to the data reported in SEDA-7 (p. 248), Favre et al have presented information on this interaction (13[C]). 24 normal subjects on a constant sodium intake were studied during treatment with furosemide, hydrochlorothiazide, triamterene or spironolactone, both without and after pretreatment with indomethacin. The diuretic-induced stimulation of plasma renin activity and urinary aldosterone was blunted after indomethacin which also suppressed urinary antidiuretic hormone. After pretreatment with indomethacin urinary prostaglandins were significantly inhibited in all patients but the natriuresis was reduced only after furosemide and spironolactone.

The authors therefore conclude that prostaglandins contribute to the natriuretic effects of furosemide and spironolactone but not to those of hydrochlorothiazide and triamterene. They stress the clinical relevance of their study: combined use of nonsteroidal antiinflammatory drugs and certain diuretics, among which furosemide and spironolactone, may cause *drug resistance.*

REFERENCES

1. Magil AB (1983) Drug induced acute interstitial nephritis with granulomas. *Human Pathol., 14,* 36.
2. Boehringer K, Weidmann P, Mordasini R et al (1982) Menopause-dependent plasma lipoprotein alterations in diuretic-treated women. *Ann. Intern. Med., 97,* 206.
3. Haalboom JRE, Struyvenberg A (1982) The mechanism underlying chlorthalidone-induced hypokalaemia: effects of sodium restriction, potassium suppletion, spironolactone and triamterene. *Ned. Tijdschr. Geneesk., 25,* 184.
4. Chaudhurry PK, Mac Lennan WJ, Peterson S (1982) Thiazide and potassium sparing diuretics in the elderly. *J. Clin. Exp. Gerontol., 5,* 43.
5. Marende RF, Milgrom M, Vlachakis ND, Chan L (1983) Response of thiazide-induced hypokalemia to amiloride. *J. Am. Med. Assoc., 249,* 237.
6. Duarte CG (1968) Effects of ethacrynic acid and frusemide on urinary calcium, phosphate and magnesium. *Metabolism, 17,* 867.
7. Lim P, Jacob E (1972) Magnesium deficiency in patients on long-term diuretic therapy for heart failure. *Br. Med. J., 111,* 620.
8. Sheehan J, White A (1982) Diuretic-associated hypomagnesaemia. *Br. Med. J., 285,* 1157.
9. Reyes AJ, Leary WP (1982) Urinary magnesium and zinc excretions after monodosing healthy volunteers with chlorthalidone. *Curr. Ther. Res., 32,* 128.
10. Hufnagle KG, Khan SN, Penn D et al (1982) Renal calcifications: a complication of long-term furosemide therapy in preterm infants. *Pediatrics, 70,* 360.
11. Mihindukulasuriya J, Lee HA (1982) Effect of xipamide in oedema of renal disease with varying degrees of renal insufficiency: a comparative trial with furosemide. *Curr. Med. Res. Opinion, 8,* 208.
12. MacGregor G, Banks RA, Markandu MD, Roulston J (1982) Xipamide and cyclopenthiazide in essential hypertension – comparative effects on blood pressure and plasma potassium. *Br. J. Clin. Pharmacol., 13,* 859.
13. Favre L, Glasson Ph, Riondel A, Valloten MB (1983) Interaction of diuretics and nonsteroidal anti-inflammatory drugs in man. *Clin. Sci., 64,* 407.

C. Reinicke

23 Metals

Aluminium

Antacid-induced *calcium loss* has been discussed in a recent editorial (1[R]). Aluminium contained in antacids combines with phosphate in the intestine, resulting in inhibition of intestinal phosphate absorption and therefore in a notable increase in fecal phosphate excretion. The phosphate depletion syndrome and osteomalacia in association with the intake of large amounts of aluminium-containing antacids has been known since the late sixties (SED-9, 368). In addition to hypophosphaturia, hypophosphatemia, and hypercalciuria, other symptoms of phosphorus depletion are bone pain, debility, muscle weakness, anorexia, and malaise. Recently, it has been demonstrated that even small doses (90–120 ml/day) of commonly used aluminium-containing antacids can lead to adverse effects on calcium and phosphorus metabolism similar to those earlier shown to be induced by large doses. There is an increase in both urinary and stool calcium resulting in a negative calcium balance. During long-term antacid therapy, a considerable loss of calcium may occur resulting in skeletal demineralization. A high intake of phosphate during antacid therapy may counteract the increase in urinary and fecal calcium and thus reduce the loss of calcium. The aluminium-containing antacid of choice in terms of the integrity of bone metabolism would be aluminium phosphate. In summary, the use of antacids should be considered as one of the causative factors in bone disease of unknown etiology. Clear instructions should be given to the patient regarding the dose and duration of antacid intake in order to prevent the development of severe bone pain and substantial bone loss within some years of instituting therapy, as a result of uncontrolled long-term use of the medication.

Aluminium possesses *hepatotoxic properties* which become manifest if it accumulates in high concentrations in the liver (2[Cr]). Aluminium was present in massive amounts in the lipofuscin granules of hepatocytes and was associated with severe lesions of most hepatic cells in a female patient who died from dialysis encephalopathy with aluminium intoxication.

Direct evidence of the *neurotoxic effects* of aluminium could be obtained in rabbits following the injection of aluminium chloride into the cisterna magna (3). Acute disorganization of the axonal and peripheral dendritic skeleton, with resultant accumulation of neurofilaments, was the prominent feature of aluminium intoxication of the central nervous system. It is not clear, however, whether these same mechanisms are involved in aluminium encephalopathy in man (SEDA-4, 163; SEDA-5, 232; SEDA-6, 216; SEDA-7, 251).

Arsenic

Non-cirrhotic *portal hypertension* has been suggested as a late consequence of administration of inorganic arsenic in a patient who had participated 20 years earlier in a trial of arsenical drugs in multiple sclerosis (4[c]).

Suinat et al (5[c]) report a modern case of severe arsenic-induced *polyneuritis* and deplore the still existing possibility of involuntary arsenic intoxication due to misuse of arsenic-containing tonic elixirs, which in France are sold over the counter.

Bismuth

Two years ago, the question was raised as to whether bismuth would retain a place in this yearly review (SEDA-6, 217). So far it does; 5 new cases of bismuth *encephalopathy* were reported in 1982 (6[c], 7[CR],

Side Effects of Drugs Annual 8
M.N.G. Dukes, editor

ISBN 0 444 90339 9
$0.80 per article per page (transactional system)
$0.20 per article per page (licensing system)

8[CR], 9[c]). Curiously enough, one of these patients, reported from France, kept in stock sufficient amounts of a bismuth preparation which had earlier been withdrawn from the market, to supply herself with the drug for about 4 years (6). One case reported from Spain showed features of a sensimotor *polyneuropathy* that has not been referred to in earlier cases of bismuth encephalopathy (8[CR]).

Calcium

Soft tissue calcification in the forearm developed in a newborn infant one week after paravenous injection of 300 mg of 10% calcium gluconate solution (10[C]). The condition proved to be spontaneously reversible over a period of 11 weeks.

White et al (11[Cr]) have pointed to the risks of rendering an infant formula diet hypertonic by adding medication to it, a hitherto underestimated problem involving infants in intensive care nurseries. Addition of calcium glubionate in elixir form (sorbitol and sugar mixed with high concentrations of calcium lactobionate and calcium gluconate) to formula feeding was thought to have contributed to the development of necrotizing enterocolitis in a premature infant. The authors suggest that any medication with high osmolality should probably only be given undiluted with extreme caution to infants who are at risk for necrotizing enterocolitis. Drug manufacturers might well include information about osmotic strength on the product information sheets and produce oral formulations of lower osmolality for infants.

Gold

Gold in rheumatoid arthritis The introduction of chrysotherapy more than 50 years ago made a major contribution to the management of rheumatoid arthritis (RA). Although its mechanism of action is not yet understood and undesirable adverse effects frequently necessitate the premature interruption of treatment, gold remains indispensable to every rheumatologist caring for RA patients. In a literal sense, rheumatologists have to live with the adverse effects of gold. Although this is no unique situation in drug treatment, modern pharmacotherapy does not offer many parallels to the role which gold plays in rheumatology.

As a very oldtimer among the drugs of today, gold might be expected to be devoid of major unknown side effects. Nevertheless, there is no end to communications pointing to hitherto unsuspected adverse reactions in association with chrysotherapy. This flood of data is probably due to the abovementioned situation in anti-rheumatic drug treatment, which does not leave many alternatives. Many current papers reexamine special aspects of well-known side effects of gold. Others newly describe rare complications and compare them with earlier case reports. Now and then, a paper provides truly new insights, e.g. into mechanisms or time-dependence of adverse gold reactions, safety of long-term treatment, prediction or treatment of severe complications and suchlike. In the present state, any serious contribution promising an advance as regards the safety of chrysotherapy deserves notice, as for instance the finding of a probable association between the antigen constellation B8-DR3 and the risk of thrombocytopenia and chrysonephropathy (12[Cr], 13[CR], SEDA-7, 253); such new departures are however few and far between.

Reliable data on the frequency of adverse gold reactions and their relationship to the duration of chrysotherapy is difficult to obtain. Controlled prospective clinical trials of sufficiently large size and duration are lacking. It has been suggested that mucocutaneous and renal toxicity is more common in the first 3–6 months, whilst hematological complications may occur at any moment in the course of chrysotherapy (SEDA-5, 234). This suggestion obtains some confirmation from two recent papers which analyze the reasons for termination of gold in patients with RA (14[Cr], 15[Cr]). Sambrook et al (14[Cr]) used the life-table method with termination of gold sodium thiomalate therapy as the endpoint to assess the incidence of significant reactions. The major reasons for stopping gold by the end of 1 year were mucocutaneous reactions (26%) and proteinuria (11%). Terminations due to rash tended to reach a plateau at about 45% of all patients after 40 months, whereas proteinuria reached a plateau level of 15% after 18 months. On the other hand, withdrawals due to hematological adverse reactions gradually increased over a longer period attaining 7% after 32 months. The time required to reach the relatively safe treatment period was thus longer than that suggested above.

Halla et al (16[CR]) performed a follow-up study on 90 patients with RA who had received courses of gold followed by penicillamine treatment. Patients with gold-induced proteinuria appeared to be at a higher risk of developing proteinuria during penicillamine therapy, whilst other adverse reactions to gold did not, according to these authors, predispose patients to the corresponding reactions under the influence of penicillamine.

Respiratory *(SEDA-5, 236; SEDA-7, 251)* A further 4 cases of diffuse *interstitial lung disease* due to gold have been reported (17[cr], 18[Cr], 19[CR]). Two patients presented with life-threatening *respiratory insufficiency* that progressed despite discontinuation of gold. In both cases, dramatic improvement occurred following corticosteroid administration (19[CR]).

Nervous system *(SEDA-4, 170; SEDA-6, 222) Polyneuropathy* is an uncommon but well-recognized complication of gold therapy, which has been observed following the use of sodium gold thiomalate, gold thioglucose and sodium gold thiopropanol sulfonate (20[Cr], 21[CR], 22[CR], 23[Cr]). The clinical features are either those of predominantly distal, mixed-sensory and motor neuropathy or an acute polyneuropathy of the Guillain-Barré type. The duration of gold therapy in the majority of cases reported was between 2 and 3 months. The onset of symptoms was mostly followed by a fairly rapid progression over the course of 10–14 days. Patients who developed the Guillain-Barré syndrome had in addition a variable degree of cranial nerve involvement. Complete recovery, albeit sometimes with persistent areflexia, was the usual outcome. Differentiation from rheumatoid vasculitis or lupus-associated neuropathy is possible, as these other causes occur in a setting of a patient who is systemically ill and becoming progressively more so. The physician needs to evaluate the patient for exposure to unusual toxins or the use of medications associated with neuritis before the diagnosis of gold neuropathy can be made with confidence. Therapy is supportive but may include the use of BAL in an attempt to accelerate gold excretion (22[CR]).

Myokymia, also known as 'chorée fibrillaire de Morvan', after the first physician to describe this syndrome, consists of continuous vermicular twitching of a few muscle fibres within single muscles, excessive sweating, insomnia and other mental symptoms. The muscle movements can be distinguished from fasciculations, usually being more prolonged. This unusual condition has previously been reported almost exclusively in the French literature, primarily in association with chrysotherapy. It may or may not occur concomitantly with peripheral neuropathy (21[CR], 22[CR]). Carbamazepine has been found to be useful in some cases (21[CR]). Damage to the peripheral motor axons resulting in terminal motor neuropathy has been suggested as the cause of myokymia.

Endocrine Gold does not influence endogenous hormone secretion. Chipman et al (24[CR]) did not find significant changes in the secretion of cortisol, dehydroepiandrosterone sulfate, human growth hormone, luteinizing hormone or follicle stimulating hormone under the influence of gold sodium thiomalate treatment in 13 patients with juvenile RA.

Hematological Hematological complications remain critical events in association with chrysotherapy. However, the prognosis of gold-induced thrombocytopenia has recently been assessed more optimistically than in the past (SEDA-4, 170; SEDA-7, 253). Gottlieb et al (25[c]) even feel that this might also apply to gold-induced granulocytopenia. In an ARA abstract, these authors describe the full recovery of 6 patients, without granulocyte transfusions or use of chelating agents, from severe granulocytopenia due to conventional aurothioglucose treatment. Chrysotherapy was abandoned permanently. The suggestion made by these authors that gold-associated agranulocytosis is a brief self-limited process which may be successfully treated without chelating agents perhaps appears presumptuous at the moment, but lends support to the cautious optimism referred to above. According to Gottlieb et al, gold chelators should be reserved for patients whose peripheral granulocyte counts do not improve after several weeks of conservative management.

The opposite point of view concerning the management of hematological complications due to gold has been expressed by Godfrey et al (26[CR]). These investigators postulate that early treatment with very high doses of intravenous N-acetylcystein as a gold chelator and SH-donor, may improve recovery of hematological parameters, even in cases of pancytopenia, by reversing enzyme inhibition due to gold. The results of 12 patients are presented. Two of 4 patients with pancytopenia died; the other 2 survived but without full recovery of the hematological parameters. N-Acetylcystein treatment was only instituted late in the patients who succumbed. This paper is noteworthy in spite of the bias likely to have been created by the incidence of spontaneous recovery in such cases (cf 25[c]).

The suggestion based upon 2 case observations that changes associated with hypothyroidism may predispose patients to acute thrombocytopenia in the course of chrysotherapy (27[cr]) appears speculative.

The significance of eosinophilia as a marker of impending more severe adverse reactions to gold has possibly been overestimated (SED-9, 372). In a recent communication, gold sodium thiomalate and auranofin were only found to be associated with a low prevalence of eosinophilia; the presence of eosinophilia did not aid in predicting toxicity (28[Cr]).

Liver *(SEDA-5, 238; SEDA-6, 222; SEDA-7, 251) Jaundice* and *hepatic dysfunction* occurred in a 3-year-old boy with juvenile RA following two injections of sodium gold thiomalate (29[CR]). Although acute hepatic dysfunction has been reported in patients with RA, the authors found the diagnosis of gold-induced hepatotoxicity were compatible with the clinical features of the present case.

Gastrointestinal *(SEDA-6, 222; 31[CR])* Another case of severe *pseudomembranous and ulcerative colitis* during gold therapy has been described (30[CR]). Many months elapsed before full recovery.

Urinary system *(SEDA-7, 252)* Newton et al (32[Cr]) discuss the problem as to when gold should be permanently withdrawn in cases where proteinuria develops. Heavy proteinuria (2–9.1 g/day) developed in 10 of 118 patients starting on gold sodium thiomalate therapy. This complication led to discontinuation in 3 cases. None of the patients in this series developed permanent renal impairment.

Eyes *(SEDA-7, 253)* A conjunctival biopsy specimen was obtained from a patient with clinical *chryseosis corneae* 2 years after finishing a treatment course with 5.5 g of gold sodium thiomalate (33[CR]). Intra- and extracellular deposits of refractile material could be shown at all levels of the epithelium and also in the superficial stroma. There was no evidence of any inflammatory reaction, and the tissue architecture was not otherwise disrupted. Sometimes the deposits were within lysosomes and often they were associated with lipids. The mostly benign character of chryseosis corneae, which is only rarely associated with ulcerating keratitis (SED-9, 373), is again underlined.

Skin *(SED-9, 373) Chrysiasis* resulting from gold therapy in RA has been reviewed by Beckett et al (34[CR]) on the basis of a case of their own. The patient had received a total of 20.8 g aurothioglucose over 12 years. She developed a blue-grey discoloration of the skin of her face, neck, and hands. Light microscopy of skin biopsy tissue revealed deposits of gold in macrophages. On electron microscopy, the particles were found in the lysosomes of the cells. The rarity of this complication today in patients with RA who are receiving gold therapy is thought to be due to the smaller gold doses used as compared with those used in the past, especially when gold was given to tuberculous patients.

Interactions Sambrook et al (2[c]) found that concurrent corticosteroid administration had no significant influence on the incidence of adverse reactions serious enough to justify termination of chrysotherapy. This casts further doubt on the older view that glucocorticoid treatment increased the toxicity of gold.

In a letter to the J. Am. Med. Assoc., one physician sought confirmation of his impression that coadministration of hydroxychloroquine induced rapid healing of gold-induced mouth ulcers. It seems very doubtful whether this is indeed the case (35).

Oral gold: auranofin

Auranofin [(2,3,4,6-tetra-O-acetyl-1-thio-β,D-glucopyranosato-S)gold(triethylphosphine)] has been used in clinical trials for the treatment of RA over the past 7–8 years but in most parts of the world it is still regarded as an experimental agent. Nevertheless, much seems to favor its early introduction as a new 'remission inducing drug' in RA. Experience with auranofin has been gained from the treatment of more than 2000 (some sources say 3000) patients according to the conditions set by various protocols. These are remarkable numbers, especially if the difficulties of conducting long-term clinical trials, lasting for at least 6 months, are considered. Many centers have patients under observation who have received auranofin for 4 years or more, but most of the available therapeutic experience relates to treatment periods which are comparatively short as compared with the natural history of RA. The caution adopted towards its widespread introduction into medicine at the moment is therefore understandable.

Recent reviews in English and German have surveyed the present state of knowledge of auranofin in the treatment of RA (36[R], 37[R], 38[R], 66[R]). Due to its lipid solubility, auranofin is adequately absorbed from the gastrointestinal tract (25%). Despite important physicochemical, pharmacologic, toxicologic, immunologic and pharmacokinetic differences between auranofin and conventional parenteral gold compounds such as sodium gold thiomalate and aurothioglucose (39–46), oral and parenteral gold apparently have a congruent therapeutic profile in RA, and both exhibit a delayed onset of action. Auranofin is effective in doses between 2 and 6 mg daily (47); 1 mg was found too low and 9 mg too high (48). Most of the recently published clinical trials were performed with 6 mg (49–55), occasionally up to 8 mg daily (56). Stable serum gold levels are reached after 12 weeks of treatment (44). As with parenteral gold, no relationship seems to exist between serum gold levels (which show a considerable interindividual range of deviation) and the outcome of therapy in the individual case (57, 58, 49). Whether this also applies to adverse effects is not yet clear, although it seems likely. Very recently, Hafström from Sweden suggested that there is no correlation between the occurrence or severity of adverse reactions and serum gold concentrations in auranofin-treated RA patients (59[cr]). However, the number of patients in his open 12-month study was too small to justify a definite conclusion (n = 18).

Review of recent clinical trials *The adverse reaction pattern of auranofin clearly differs from that of parenteral gold compounds. All investigators agree that severe symptoms of gold toxicity are much less frequent with auranofin than with traditional chrysotherapy. The assessment of auranofin made in SEDA-6 (p. 233) thus still holds good, but the view can now be based upon a much greater number of clinical reports (47–56, 59, 61–65).*

Placebo-controlled trials of a sufficiently large size and duration will provide the most relevant information on incidence and pattern of side effects of drugs. Studies of this kind have only rarely been performed on patients with rheumatoid arthritis, mainly for ethical reasons; however, thanks to Katz et al (50[CR]), the results of a 6-month double-blind clinical trial of auranofin versus placebo in RA patients have become available. 289 patients entered this multicentre study which was carried out in the USA. In the auranofin group, 7 of 139 patients dropped out because of complications or adverse effects (rash and diarrhea each in 2 cases, 1 proteinuria, 1 reversible thrombocytopenia of 55,000/mm^3 noted after about 18 weeks, and 1 taste abnormality). For comparison, 1 patient dropped out from the placebo group (n = 150) because of proteinuria. All except 1 of the withdrawals had been treated for more than 3 months. Complications not necessitating patient withdrawal developed in 57.6% (80/139) of patients on auranofin compared with 26.7% (40/150) on placebo (Table 1).

In 13 gold-treated patients the reactions were considered severe enough to lower the doses. Diarrhea was the major adverse effect occurring in 31.7% of the auranofin group versus 6% in the placebo group. In 10 patients the severity of diarrhea required a decrease in auranofin dosage. Diarrhea occurred as a single episode in 16 patients and was considered mild in 19, moderately severe in 20 and severe in 6 occurrences. Other adverse reactions requiring a reduction in dosage or interruption of treatment were similar in both groups. They included other gastrointestinal problems, abnormalities of the skin and mucous membranes. There were no changes in renal or liver function. Besides the aforementioned case of thrombocytopenia, which was reversible within 2 weeks after withdrawal, no other hematological abnormalities were attributable to auranofin.

Table 1. Total complications in 289 patients during treatment with auranofin (A) (6 mg/day) or placebo (P)

Type of complication	Treatment group	No. of complications	Patients with complications
Diarrhea	A	45	44
	P	6	6
Lower GI tract	A	20	20
	P	6	6
Upper GI tract	A	16	16
	P	12	12
Skin	A	18	17
	P	16	15
Mucous membrane	A	9	7
	P	7	7
CNS	A	0	0
	P	0	0
Miscellaneous	A	6	5
	P	6	6

Number of patients on A: 139; number with complications: 80. Number of patients on P: 150; number with complications: 40.
Adapted from Katz et al (50).

Three patients developed proteinuria while taking auranofin, but the total incidence of proteinuria was actually higher in the placebo group. Regrettably, this important and interesting point has not further been substantiated. The number of adverse effects involving the upper gastrointestinal tract, skin and mucous membranes was equal in the auranofin and placebo groups. This was most likely due to the trial protocol, which allowed stable doses of salicylates or a single nonsteroidal antiinflammatory drug concomitant with auranofin and placebo. There have been objections to this protocol since it did not involve 'true' placebo treatment. However, it is impossible to leave patients with active RA without any medication for several months. The compromise allowing concomitant symptomatic treatment is therefore inevitable, even though, as in the case of proteinuria, difficulties may arise attributing to auranofin or to the comedication those side effects which are common to both (50[CR]).

Valuable data on the adverse effects of auranofin has been derived from blind or open controlled clinical trials comparing different daily doses of auranofin (47[CR], 48[C]), or comparing auranofin with parenteral gold, mostly with sodium gold thio-

Table 2. Adverse effects and withdrawals in 273 patients during treatment with 2 mg (n = 134) or 6 mg (n = 139) auranofin per day (47)

Adverse effect	No. of patients	2 mg	6 mg	No. of withdr.
Anemia	1	–	1	1
Thrombocytopenia	3	2	1	3
Proteinuria	2	–	2	2
Gastrointestinal				
Diarrhea	78	30	48	4
Lower GI tract	52	21	31	4
Upper GI tract	62	34	28	1
Skin	105	51	54	9
Mucous membranes	33	20	13	4
CNS	6	4	2	0

Table 3. Adverse reaction data compiled from 4 recent controlled clinical trials comparing auranofin (AF) with sodium gold thiomalate (SGTM) in RA. In general, treatment periods were 6 months or longer. The AF dosage was 6 mg (3 mg b.i.d.) daily. SGTM was administered according to the classical dosage regimen (50 mg weekly for 20 weeks followed by 50 mg monthly)

Adverse reaction	*Ménard et al (52)*		*Schattenkirchner et al (53)*		*Smith et al (54)*		*Barraclough et al (55)*	
	AF n = 87	*SGTM n = 83*	*AF n = 52*	*SGTM n = 51*	*AF n = 26*	*SGTM n = 36*	*AF n = 13*	*SGTM n = 11*
			(adv. reactions/pts)					
Mucocutaneous								
Skin rash			13/9	28/23	7	17	0	3
Pruritus			17/12	26/19				
Stomatitis					1	3	0	2
Not differentiated	28	42						
Gastrointestinal								
Upper GI (nausea, vomiting, indigest.)	12	4			3	0	0	2
Lower GI (diarrhea, loose stools)	28	5	29/15	14/9	5	0		
Not differentiated			14/13	9/9				
Hematological								
Leukopenia					2	1	0	2
Thrombocytopenia					0	2		
Cytopenia (not specified)	0	9						
Renal								
Proteinuria								
mild	0	2			5	6	0	1
significant					0	1		
severe	1	0						
Hematuria (intermittent)					5	5		
Miscellaneous								
Alopecia			5/4	3/1				
Conjunctivitis			5/5	6/5				
Not specified	18 (one possible gold lung each)	21						
Total	87	83	83/58	86/66	28	35	2	8
Withdrawals	4[a]	8[b]	5[c]	8[d]	0	5[e]	0	5[f]

Reasons for withdrawal: (a) 2 diarrheas, 1 proteinuria, 1 possibly gold lung; (b) not specified (1 possibly gold lung, else probably hematological); (c) 3 severe exanthemata, 1 exanthema with stomatitis, 1 herpes zoster; (d) 1 exanthema and pruritus, 1 exanthema and stomatitis, 2 severe systemic reactions on inject., 2 marked eosinophilias, 1 dysuria, 1 hepatic dysfunct., 1 osteomyelosclerosis; (e) 3 mucocutan. react., 1 proteinuria, 1 'blood disorder'; (f) 2 rashes, 1 stomatitis, 2 leukopenias.

malate (52[C], 53[Cr], 54[Cr], 55[C], 65[C]). The adverse effects observed by Bernhard et al (47[CR]) in a double-blind multicentre study comparing daily doses of 2 and 6 mg auranofin, respectively, are summarized in Table 2. Diarrhea and bowel problems were the most frequent symptoms; they appeared to be dose-dependent and rarely resulted in discontinuation of the study medication.

Thrombocytopenia resolved spontaneously with cessation of auranofin. Proteinuria was less than 2.5 g/24 hr and also cleared spontaneously when the drug was discontinued. No significant abnormalities of liver

Table 4. Adverse reactions of auranofin (AF, total n = 59) versus sodium gold thiomalate (SGTM, total n = 62), recorded in the Austrian-German double-blind comparative multicentre study

Adverse reaction	Treatm. group	Patients with A.R. No.	Patients with A.R. %	No. of A.R.	Severity mild	Severity mod.	Severity severe	Severity not spec.
Diarrhea	AF	20	34	34	17	11	3	3
	SGTM	11	18	12	9	2	1	–
Other gastrointestinal symptoms	AF[1]	20	34	21	10	7	0	4
	SGTM[2]	11	18	12	9	2	1	–
(Aphthous) stomatitis	AF	13	22	17	6	8	1	2
	SGTM	14	23	19	7	8	1	3
Rash	AF	10	17	15	8	4	3	
	SGTM	26	42	32	12	14	2	4
Pruritus	AF	15	25	23	12	4	3	4
	SGTM	27	43	32	17	12	3	–
Alopecia	AF	5	9	5	4	1		
	SGTM	4	7	7	3	1	2	1
Conjunctivitis	AF	5	9	5	4	1		
	SGTM	7	11	7	2	3	2	0
Other	AF			72	26	26	12	8
	SGTM			57	23	16	10	8
Total	AF			192	83	62	24	23
	SGTM			177	80	57	21	19

[1]Including abdominal pain, anorexia, dyspepsia, flatulence, gastritis, nausea, irregular bowel movement, and vomiting.
[2]Including abdominal pain, anorexia, constipation, flatulence, and nausea.
Adapted from Rau et al (65).

function or other parameters of renal function were observed (47[CR]).

Calin et al (48[C]), also in a double-blind multicenter study, compared two patient groups receiving 1 mg (n = 70) and 9 mg (n = 67) auranofin daily for a period of 6 months. Significantly fewer patients on 1 mg (7%) required reduced dosage or dropped out because of adverse reactions than did those on high dose (27%). All drop-outs (2 in the low, 3 in the high dosage group) were due to skin rash, whereas dose reduction was related to diarrhea (1 patient on 1 mg, 13 cases on 9 mg/day). One patient on the low dose developed mild leukocytopenia after 12 weeks of treatment, which spontaneously normalized after dose reduction. One patient on high dose experienced epigastric pain.

The adverse reactions observed in 4 recent comparative trials with auranofin versus sodium gold thiomalate in the treatment of RA are summarized in Table 3. All in all, 178 patients received auranofin and 181 gold sodium thiomalate. The total number of adverse effects was 200 for auranofin and 212 for sodium gold thiomalate. Several patients exhibited more than one adverse effect or several occurrences of the same side effect during the treatment course. Table 3 shows that mucocutaneous reactions are more common with the parenteral gold compound, whereas gastrointestinal disorders preponderate with auranofin. This finding emerged from all studies except that in Australia (55[C]), where gastrointestinal upset was only observed in association with sodium gold thiomalate. However, the number of cases presented in the Australian report was too small to substantiate possible geographical differences with respect to the occurrence of adverse effects. This also applies to further differences between the four studies. A relatively high incidence of renal complications, which has not been observed by other authors, was found in the South African trial both in the auranofin and sodium gold thiomalate groups (54[Cr]). In the same study, 2 cases of transient leukopenia were recorded. Ménard et al (52[C]) from Canada reported 1 case of severe proteinuria and 1 possible case of gold lung in association with auranofin. Alopecia and conjunctivitis were only reported from Western Germany and Austria (53[Cr]). Alopecia was more common during auranofin treatment, whilst conjunctivitis occurred with equal frequency in both groups. A separate synopsis of the adverse effects data of the Austrian-German study taken from a second report of this group on a recent gold workshop held at Munich may be found in Table 4. This study is one of the most relevant trials on auranofin, since it was conducted in a strictly double-blind way using even placebo injections in order to mask the identity of the gold product which was being given. The reasons for withdrawal are listed in Table 5.

The authors of this study (65[C]) conclude that both forms of treatment induce clinical improvement in RA. This improvement seems to occur earlier in the sodium gold thiomalate-treated group. Gastrointestinal side effects, in particular diarrhea, are twice as frequent in the auranofin group. However, mucocutaneous adverse reactions are twice as frequent in patients treated with sodium gold thiomalate. Withdrawals are more often reported in the sodium gold thiomalate group.

The results of several uncontrolled prospective trials performed in Japan (51[C]), Sweden (59[C]), and a multicentre study from Switzerland, Austria and Western Germany (49[C], 63[C]), are in accordance with those of the controlled trials referred to above. Possible new facets of the adverse reaction pattern of auranofin are edemas, which have hitherto only been reported from Japan (51[c]), and the development of increasing titres of antinuclear factors observed in a Swedish patient (59[c]). Whether these observations are meaningful remains to be seen. Recently, membranous glomerulonephritis has been attributed to auranofin (67[Cr]).

Final comment *Auranofin treatment appears to be relatively safe. However, several complications severe enough to necessitate withdrawal may be associated with auranofin treatment. Besides the well-known side effects localized to the lower gastrointestinal tract, which rarely require the interruption of treatment, these conditions can include mucocutaneous (rash, stomatitis, taste abnormalities), hematological (anemia, thrombocytopenia) and renal (proteinuria) adverse reactions. Furthermore, leukopenia, hematuria, and perhaps gold lung and reactivation of quiescent infections (herpes zoster) may occur and should carefully be looked for. Both over- and underestimation of risks is possible at the present state of affairs. Most of the reports still have an interim character. However, although further trials appear necessary, auranofin and its place in the treatment of RA can now more reliably be assessed.*

Table 5. Reasons for exclusions from study (65)

Adverse reaction	*AF oral (n = 59)*	*SGTM parenteral (n = 62)*
Mucocutaneous reactions	*7*	*4*
Eosinophilia	*0*	*1*
Injection reactions	*0*	*3*
Pathological hepatic data	*0*	*1*
Inefficacy	*0*	*1*
Hemorrhagic cystitis	*1*	*0*
Herpes zoster	*1*	*0*
Dysuria	*0*	*1*
Osteomyelosclerosis	*0*	*1*
Dropout	*1*	*3*
Total	*10*	*15*
Adverse reaction	*9*	*11*
Inefficacy	*0*	*1*
Dropout	*1*	*3*

Iron

Parenteral iron A gradual but significant decrease in the levels of serum inorganic phosphorus, accompanied by increased urinary phosphate clearance and decreased tubular reabsorption of phosphate, was reported by a Japanese group in 9 patients with iron deficiency treated with intravenous injections of saccharated iron oxide (71[Cr]). The changes were reversible in all patients after the discontinuation of iron injections, although in some cases recovery took several weeks. Parathormone and other electrolytes showed no significant changes. The mechanism of this hitherto unknown side effect is not clear. Since iron oxide saccharate is in use in many countries, more observations and in-depth investigations should become available.

The opposite effects, namely hyperphosphatemia and hypophosphaturia, have been observed in the presence of excessive and protracted iron overload in hypertransfused thalassemic patients (72^{Cr}). The gradual changes in parathyroid function, ranging from initial hyperparathyroidism (possibly depending on vitamin D deficiency) in young patients, through an intermediate stage characterized by normocalcemic hyperphosphatemia, and then slowly evolving into overt hypoparathyroidism in advanced thalassemia, are assumed to be due to an increasing hemochromatosis of the parathyroid glands.

R Iron overload

The possible negative effects of nutrient iron fortification, iron prophylaxis and/or uncontrolled therapy remain topics of current concern (SED-9, 374; SEDA-4, 171; SEDA-5, 239; SEDA-6, 224). The potentially noxious effects of surplus iron are now generally acknowledged, although the relationship between parenchymal iron deposition and associated tissue damage is by no means a simple one (68^R). Other factors are often involved, which mostly remain unknown.

Most of the present knowledge about iron overload has been derived from clinically important iron-loading conditions such as idiopathic hemochromatosis, thalassemia major and other iron loading anemias, transfusional iron overload etc., but relatively little is known about the contribution of long-term prophylactic or supplementary surplus iron. The classical storage organs in iron overload are the liver, pancreas, heart, and endocrine glands. Moreover, also the spleen and bone marrow are involved in several conditions associated with diffuse iron overload. Parenterally administered hemoglobin-iron is apparently less toxic than iron absorbed from the intestine.

In an extensive review, which was mainly based on electronmicroscopic findings in thalassemic children, Iancu (69^R) has summarized current knowledge about iron overload. The discussion of this paper is mainly focussed on the above-mentioned major iron-overloading diseases, but the role of pharmaceutical surplus iron has – albeit marginally – also been considered.

The amount of iron deposited in various tissues and organs is highly variable and probably related to the iron-turnover and certain biological attributes of each cell type. The cell exposed to excessive iron reacts on several levels: it increases the iron storing capacity of its individual ferritin molecules, but also increases the number of ferritin molecules available within the cytosol. If these changes go on, the cell reaches the state of cytosiderosis. During iron overload a large amount of ferritin and hemosiderin is segregated within membrane-bound vesicles or bodies (siderosomes) by the process of autophagocytosis. Degraded ferritin molecules may provide most of the non-heme iron present in hemosiderin of endogenous origin. As the process of overload continues, the number of iron containing particles increases constantly until the 'end-stage' of the disease has been reached. Important ultrastructural differences exist between various cell lines not only with respect to the concentration of ferritin particles in the cytosol, but also in regard of the morphology of iron-laden bodies. Siderosomes in the parenchymal cells of the liver are different from those of the Kupffer cells, which are also distinguished from those of the endothelial sinusoidal lining cells, and so on. These observations lead to the concept of cell-line specific lysosomes, which seems at least to apply to the handling of surplus iron.

Thanks to their capacity to segregate large amounts of storage iron, lysosomes have actually been thought to possess a protective function in the early stages of iron overload. In later stages, when this capacity has been saturated, cell damage by lysosomal enzymes is conceivable. However, the mechanisms by which hemosiderin may damage the lysosomal membrane have not yet been clarified. Increased lipid peroxidation initiated by iron overload, with concomitant or secondary vitamin E deficiency, has been postulated as a major mechanism in the liver cell damage which must underlie the development of hepatic cirrhosis, a condition frequently encountered in the advanced stages of iron overload diseases.

Information about the fate of 'fortified' and supplementary iron in the organism and its contribution to iron overload is scarce. Iancu (69^R) classifies excessive iron intake (iatrogenic, dietary) as one of the conditions associated with asymptomatic iron load, i.e. conditions in which excess iron has been documented or is suspected to be present, without deleterious effects related

Table 6. Side effects of iron fortification or prolonged iron therapy (69[R])

A. Promotion of iron overload by increased absorption in:
1. Idiopathic hemochromatosis, homozygotes and heterozygotes
2. Porphyria cutanea tarda
3. Iron-loading anemias:
thalassemia
sideroblastic anemias
pernicious anemia
hereditary spherocytosis
pyruvate-kinase deficiency
4. Congenital atransferrinemia
5. Alcoholism: in the Bantu
in sweet wine drinkers
in association with liver disease of variable origin
6. Chronic pancreatitis, pancreatic insufficiency
B. Masking of anemia in gastrointestinal cancer
C. ? Infection-promoting effect of iron ?
D. ? Tumor-enhancing effect of surplus iron ?

to its presence. However, this classification, which seems to be adequate for a 'healthy' population, may not hold good for risk groups, where additional iron intake means a potential danger. Population groups at risk of side effects due to iron fortification or supplementation are listed in Table 6.

An involvement of iron overload in the pathogenesis of porphyria cutanea tarda has recently been suggested (70[C]).

From the presently available data, it is difficult to conclude whether and to what extent iron fortification is a significant infection-promoting factor, and whether the successful prevention of iron-deficiency anemia outweighs the dangers associated with long-standing iron administration, if real. The controversy is still unsettled. The same applies to the possible role of iron in carcinogenesis. Although adult patients with hemochromatosis show an increased frequency of hepatoma (hepatocarcinoma), it is not clear to what extent this complication is the direct result from iron overload or secondary to cirrhosis and/or other factors. Evidence, clinical or experimental, showing that iron, protein bound or ionic, is indeed a significant factor in carcinogenesis, is up to the present still lacking (69[R]).

Total-dose infusion of iron dextran

Total-dose infusion of iron dextran is a technique of iron administration which delivers the total necessary amount of iron in a single administration rather than intermittently. Whenever possible, other routes or methods of iron dextran administration should be considered. Particularly careful monitoring is necessary in the elderly. In one series of 40 patients receiving total-dose infusions of iron dextran, 9 had an immediate adverse reaction (2 cases of anaphylaxis, the others with gastrointestinal reactions, epistaxis, chest pain, and hypotension) (73[Cr]). Patients who experienced adverse reactions were older than those who did not.

A unique case of protracted polyarthritis, mainly of the large joints, following total-dose iron dextran infusion has been reported by Brighton and De la Harpe (74[Cr]). Clinical recovery which required prolonged glucocorticoid treatment occurred after 6 months. This case report is noteworthy as it recalls the relationship earlier suspected between iron administration and exacerbations of arthritis (cf. SEDA-7, 254). This is the first description of the induction by iron of a condition bearing a resemblance to rheumatoid joint disease, though no immunological changes typical of an immune disease developed. The authors mention a second patient with no evidence of RA or ankylosing spondylitis who developed an acute polyarthritis following a total-dose iron dextran infusion.

Infusions of large doses of iron dextran may lead to serum discoloration for a few days, which should not be mistaken for evidence of hemolysis. This misinterpretation occurred in a case reported by Simon et al (75[cr]). The patient had received an iron-dextran infusion followed by a blood transfusion before she developed an episode of shaking chill, fever and generalized pruritus. The laboratory evaluation for a transfusion reaction was negative. The Gomori iron stain of the serum gave a blue color indicating the presence of excess iron in the posttransfusion specimen.

Temporary topical lipomyodystrophy followed a 50 mg dose of intramuscular iron dextran in a 6-month-old child. Local changes were not observed up to 1 month after injection, when a dimple occurred at the injected buttock. The dimple gradually disappeared within about 7 months (76[Cr]).

Mercury

The case of a 22-year-old woman has been reported, who presented with a nephrotic syndrome due to membranous glomerulonephritis induced by the daily ingestion of a laxative containing mercurous chloride (calomel) (77[CR]). The poisoning was confirmed by urinary mercury assay. This case adds to previous intoxications due to calomel-containing laxatives and underlines the need to abandon calomel as an ingredient of drugs (SED-9, 377; SEDA-6, 225).

Problems associated with allergic reactions to mercury present in amalgam dental fillings have been discussed by Duxbury et al (78[cR]).

Zinc *(SEDA-4, 172; SEDA-6, 225)*

Wray (79[cr]), in a double-blind crossover study, could demonstrate no beneficial effects of zinc sulfate over 3 months in recurrent aphthous stomatitis. The dosage was 220 mg t.i.d. in capsule form per os. Four patients had to discontinue the zinc therapy because of severe abdominal discomfort, consisting of abdominal cramping and nausea. In addition, 2 patients had frank vomiting, and 1 patient in addition noticed 'increased skin sensitivity'.

Metal implants and prostheses *(SEDA-6, 225; SEDA-7, 256)*

Using the leukocyte migration inhibition test, Hierholzer and Hierholzer (80[CR]) investigated metal allergy in association with osteosyntheses. They found that patients bearing metallic implants without infection showed the same rate of metal allergy as patients without implants. Patients bearing metallic implants with infection showed an increased rate of allergy to cobalt and nickel as compared to persons without implants and to patients bearing metallic implants without infection. They were sensitive to one of the three tested metals (cobalt, chromium, nickel) more than twice as often as patients with aseptic osteosynthesis. The authors recommend the removal of metallic devices in cases of substantiated manifest allergy, i.e. patients with a positive migration index and positive skin test. A possible alternative is the use of titanium implants. If only the migration index is positive, the decision must depend on the clinical findings.

REFERENCES

1. Editorial (1983) Antacid-induced calcium loss. *Arch. Intern. Med., 143,* 657.
2. Galle P, Giudicelli CP (1982) Toxicité de l'aluminium pour l'hépatocyte. Localisation ultrastructurale et micro-analyse des dépôts. *Nouv. Presse Méd., 11,* 1123.
3. Troncoso JC, Price DL, Griffin JW, Parhad IM (1981) Neurofibrillary axonal pathology in aluminium intoxication. *Ann. Neurol., 12,* 278.
4. Robertson DAF, Low-Beer TS (1983) Long term consequences of arsenical treatment for multiple sclerosis. *Br. Med. J., 286,* 605.
5. Suinat JL, Leon A, Vallee D, Rendoing J (1982) Polynévrite arsenicale iatrogène. *Nouv. Presse Méd., 11,* 3800.
6. Stahl JP, Gaillat J, Leverve X et al (1982) Encéphalites aux sel insoluble de bismuth. Toujours d'actualité. *Nouv. Presse Méd., 11,* 3856.
7. Mattle H, Henn V, Baumgartner G (1982) Akutes Delir bei Wismut-Intoxikation. *Schweiz. Med. Wochenschr., 112,* 1308.
8. Cervelló MA, Alfaro A, Antolin MA, Penarrocha M (1982) Encefalopatía mioclónica busmútica: a propósito de dos nuevas observaciones clínicas. *Med. Clin. (Barcelona), 79,* 137.
9. Hasking GJ, Duggan JM (1982) Encephalopathy from bismuth subsalicylate. *Med. J. Aust., 2,* 167.
10. Propst-Proctor SL, Jones RB, Nagel DA (1982) Iatrogenic soft-tissue calcification in an extremity. *J. Bone Jt. Surg., 64-A,* 449.
11. White KC, Harkavy KL (1982) Hypertonic formula resulting from added oral medications. *Am. J. Dis. Child., 136,* 931.
12. Wooley PH, Griffin J, Panayi GS et al (1980) HLA-DR antigens and toxic reactions to sodium aurothiomalate and D-penicillamine in patients with rheumatoid arthritis. *N. Engl. J. Med., 303,* 300.
13. Ewald RW, Mayer M, Römer W (1983) HL-A-Antigene und gold-induzierte Nebenwirkungen bei Patienten mit chronischer Polyarthritis *Aktuel. Rheumatol., 8,* 25.
14. Sambrook PS, Browne CD, Champion GD et al (1982) Terminations of treatment with gold sodium thiomalate in rheumatoid arthritis. *J. Rheumatol., 9,* 932.
15. Rainer F, Ulreich A (1982) Ursachen für den Therapieabbruch bei 499 Polyarthritikern. *Therapiewoche, 32,* 5892.
16. Halla JT, Cassady J, Hardin JG (1982) Sequential gold and penicillamine therapy in rheumatoid arthritis. *Am. J. Med., 72,* 423.
17. Richards AM (1982) Gold lung. *N.Z. Med. J.,*

95, 897.
18. Schapira D, Lorber M, Rubin A (1982) Lung injury due to gold therapy (Hebrew). *Harefuah, 102,* 284.
19. Levinson ML, Lynch III JP, Bower JS (1981) Reversal of progressive, life-threatening gold hypersensitivity pneumonitis by corticosteroids. *Am. J. Med., 71,* 908.
20. Dougados M, Amor B (1982) Polyradiculo-névrite de la chrysothérapie. *Nouv. Presse Méd., 11,* 1878.
21. Mitsumoto H, Wilbourn AJ, Subramony SH (1982) Generalized myokymia and gold therapy. *Arch. Neurol., 39,* 449.
22. Weiss JJ, Thompson GR, Lazaro R (1982) Gold toxicity presenting as peripheral neuropathy. *Clin. Rheumatol., 1,* 285.
23. Dick DJ, Raman D (1982) The Guillain Barre syndrome following gold therapy. *Scand. J. Rheumatol., 11,* 119.
24. Chipman JJ, Boyar RM, Fink CW (1982) Anterior pituitary adrenal function of gold-treated patients with juvenile rheumatoid arthritis. *J. Rheumatol., 9,* 63.
25. Gottlieb NL, Buchoff HS, Vidal AF et al (1982) The course of severe gold-associated granulocytopenia. *Clin. Res., 30,* 659A.
26. Godfrey NF, Peter A, Simon TM, Lorber A (1982) IV N-Acetylcysteine treatment of hematologic reactions to chrysotherapy. *J. Rheumatol., 9,* 519.
27. Hunter JA, Capell HA (1982) Does hyperthyroidism predispose to gold-induced thrombocytopenia? *Scott. Med. J., 27,* 247.
28. Edelman J, Davis P, Owen ET (1983) Prevalence of eosinophilia during gold therapy for rheumatoid arthritis. *J. Rheumatol., 10,* 121.
29. Howrie DL, Gartner JC (1982) Gold-induced hepatotoxicity: case report and review of the literature. *J. Rheumatol., 9,* 727.
30. Reinhart WH, Kappeler M, Halter F (1983) Severe pseudomembranous and ulcerative colitis during gold therapy. *Endoscopy, 15,* 70.
31. Nagler J, Paget SA (1983) Nonexudative diarrhea after gold salt therapy: case report and review of the literature. *Am. J. Gastroenterol., 78,* 12.
32. Newton P, Swinburn WR, Swinson DR (1982) Proteinuria with gold therapy: when should gold be permanently stopped? *Br. J. Rheumatol., 22,* 11.
33. Kincaid MC, Green WR, Hoover RE, Schenck PH (1982) Ocular chrysiasis. *Arch. Ophthalmol., 100,* 1791.
34. Beckett VL, Doyle JA, Hadley GA, Spear KL (1982) Chrysiasis resulting from gold therapy in rheumatoid arthritis. *Mayo Clin. Proc., 57,* 773.
35. Manshady BM, McCarty DJ (1982) Gold toxicity. *J. Am. Med. Assoc., 247,* 2155.
36. Bernhard GC (1982) Auranofin therapy in rheumatoid arthritis. *J. Lab. Clin. Med., 100,* 167.
37. Bandilla KK, Berg D, Böttcher I (1982) Auranofin: ein orales Goldpräparat zur Behandlung der rheumatoiden Arthritis. *Therapiewoche, 32,* 4070.
38. Zeidler H (1982) Vergleich von oraler und parenteraler Goldtherapie. *Aktuel. Rheumatol., 7,* 184.
39. Sadler PJ (1982) The comparative evaluation of the physical and chemical properties of gold compounds. *J. Rheumatol., 9, Suppl. 8,* 71.
40. Walz DT, Dimartino J, Griswold DE (1982) Comparative pharmacology and biological effects of different gold compounds. *J. Rheumatol., 9, Suppl. 8,* 54.
41. Payne BJ (1978) The toxicity of three gold-containing compounds in laboratory animals. *Vet. Pathol., 15, Suppl. 5,* 1.
42. Lorber A, Jackson WH, Simon TM (1982) Effects of chrysotherapy on cell mediated immune response. *J. Rheumatol., 9, Suppl. 8,* 37.
43. Walz DT, Dimartino MJ, Griswold DE (1982) Mechanisms of action of auranofin: effects on humoral immune response. *J. Rheumatol., 9, Suppl. 8,* 32.
44. Gottlieb NL (1982) Comparative pharmacokinetics of parenteral and oral gold compounds. *J. Rheumatol., 9, Suppl. 8,* 99.
45. Blocka K, Furst DE, Landaw E et al (1982) Single dose pharmacokinetics of auranofin in rheumatoid arthritis. *J. Rheumatol., 9, Suppl. 8,* 110.
46. Herrlinger JD, Alsen C, Beress R et al (1982) Distribution of gold in serum erythrocytes and white blood cells after in vitro incubation and during chrysotherapy with different gold compounds. *J. Rheumatol., 9, Suppl. 8,* 81.
47. Bernhard GC (1982) Auranofin treatment for adult rheumatoid arthritis. Comparison of 2 mg and 6 mg daily dose. *J. Rheumatol., 9, Suppl. 8,* 149.
48. Calin A, Saunders D, Bennett R et al (1982) Auranofin: 1 mg or 9 mg? The search for the appropriate dose. *J. Rheumatol., 9, Suppl. 8,* 146.
49. Bandilla K, Gross D, Herrlinger JD et al (1982) Oral gold therapy with auranofin (SK&F 39 162). A multicenter open study in patients with rheumatoid arthritis. *J. Rheumatol., 9, Suppl. 8,* 154.
50. Katz WA, Alexander S, Bland JH et al (1982) The efficacy and safety of auranofin compared to placebo in rheumatoid arthritis. *J. Rheumatol., 9, Suppl. 8,* 173.
51. Homma M, Abe T, Akizuki M et al (1982) Interim results of a multicenter open study with auranofin in Japan. *J. Rheumatol., 9, Suppl. 8,* 160.
52. Ménard HA, Beaudet F, Davis P et al (1982) Gold therapy in rheumatoid arthritis. Interim report of the Canadian multicenter prospective trial comparing sodium aurothiomalate and auranofin. *J. Rheumatol., 9, Suppl. 8,* 179.
53. Schattenkirchner M, Kaik B, Müller-Fassbender H et al (1982) Auranofin and sodium

aurothiomalate in the treatment of rheumatoid arthritis. A double-blind, comparative multi-center study. *J. Rheumatol., 9, Suppl. 8,* 184.
54. Smith PR, Brown GMM, Meyers OL (1982) An open comparative study of auranofin vs. gold sodium thiomalate. *J. Rheumatol., 9, Suppl. 3,* 190.
55. Barraclough D, Brook A, Brooks P et al (1982) Comparative study of auranofin, gold sodium thiomalate, and D-penicillamine in rheumatoid arthritis: a progress report. *J. Rheumatol., 9, Suppl. 8,* 197.
56. Champion GD, Bieri D, Browne CD et al (1982) Auranofin in rheumatoid arthritis. *J. Rheumatol., 9, Suppl. 8,* 137.
57. Finkelstein AE, Walz DT, Batista V et al (1976) Auranofin. New oral gold compound for treatment of rheumatoid arthritis. *Ann. Rheum. Dis., 35,* 251.
58. Berglöf FE, Berglöf K, Walz DT (1978) Auranofin: an oral chrysotherapeutic agent for the treatment of rheumatoid arthritis. *J. Rheumatol., 5,* 68.
59. Hafström J (1983) Auranofin (SK&F D-39 162) in the treatment of rheumatoid arthritis. *Clin. Trials J., 20,* 25.
60. Weisman MH, Hannifin DM (1979) Management of rheumatoid arthritis with oral gold. *Arthritis Rheum., 22,* 922.
61. Weisman MH, Hanninen DM, Guerra J et al (1982) Analysis of auranofin as a rheumatoid remitting agent. *J. Rheumatol., 9, Suppl. 8,* 132.
62. Giannini EH, Brewer EJ, Person DA (1983) Auranofin in the treatment of juvenile rheumatoid arthritis. *J. Pediatr., 102,* 138.
63. Bandilla KK, Baumgarten F, Berg D et al (1983) Long-term treatment of rheumatoid arthritis with auranofin: open studies. *Rheumatology, 8,* 148.
64. Blodgett Jr RC (1983) Auranofin: clinical studies in the United States of America. *Rheumatology, 8,* 158.
65. Rau R, Kaik B, Müller-Fassbender H et al (1983) Auranofin (SK&F 39 162) and sodium aurothiomalate in the treatment of rheumatoid arthritis. *Rheumatology, 8,* 162.
66. Zeidler H (1983) Comparison of oral and parenteral gold therapy. *Rheumatology, 8,* 175.
67. Plaza JJ, Herrero G, Barat A et al (1982) Membranous glomerulonephritis as a complication of oral gold therapy. *Ann. Intern. Med., 97,* 563.
68. Bothwell TH, Charlton (1979) Current problems of iron overload. *Recent Results Cancer Res., 69,* 87.
69. Iancu TC (1982) Iron overload. *Mol. Aspects Med.,* 1.
70. Ivanov E, Adjarov D, Kerimova M, Naidenova E (1982) Rare cases of porphyria cutanea tarda associated with additional iron overload. *Dermatologica, 164,* 127.
71. Okada M, Imamura K, Iida M et al (1983) Hypophosphatemia induced by intravenous administration of saccharated iron oxide. *Klin. Wochenschr., 61,* 99.
72. Brezis M, Leibel B, Dagan I, Ben-Ishay D (1982) The spectrum of parathyroid function in thalassemia subjects with transfusional iron overload. *Miner. Electrolyte Metab., 8,* 307.
73. Shimada A (1982) Adverse reactions to total-dose infusion of iron dextran. *Clin. Pharm., 1,* 248.
74. Brighton SW, De la Harpe AL (1982) Development of an inflammatory synovitis following total-dose infusion of iron-dextran. *S. Afr. Med. J., 62,* 141.
75. Simon SD, Kuriyan MA, Kim HC (1982) 'Pseudo-hemolytic' transfusion reaction caused by intravenous iron-dextran therapy. *Transfusion, 22,* 341.
76. Amitai I, Acker M (1982) Adverse effects of intramuscular iron injection. *Acta Haematol., 68,* 341.
77. Faux N, Taillandier J, Charpentier B et al (1983) Un accident des laxatifs: La néphropathie glomérulaire mercurielle. *Rev. Méd., 24,* 591.
78. Duxbury AJ, Watts DC, Wastell EA (1982) Allergie au mercure dans l'amalgame dentaire. *Méd. Hyg., 40,* 3416.
79. Wray D (1982) A double-blind trial of systemic zinc sulfate in recurrent aphthous stomatitis. *Oral Surg., 53,* 469.
80. Hierholzer S, Hierholzer G (1982) Untersuchungen zur Metallallergie nach Osteosynthesen. *Unfallchirurgie, 8,* 347.

R.H.B. Meyboom

24 Metal antagonists

Penicillamine

An interesting review of recent information on penicillamine, with special reference to side effects and the possible relation with genetic determinants, has been presented in the report of a workshop in Perth, April 1982 (see below) (1[CR]).

When considering the merits and the side effects of penicillamine and other second-line drugs in rheumatology, one should take into account, as has been pointed out by Scott et al (60[CR]), that it remains unproven that these drugs do reduce the rate of joint destruction.

A further study has provided evidence that with low doses (300 mg or less) the efficacy of penicillamine declines, whereas side effects continue to occur, although less frequently (SEDA-7, 258; 72[CR]). Polymyositis (54[C]) and pemphigus (40[C]) have been reported in patients taking only 250 mg penicillamine daily.

Penicillamine and the HLA system Garlepp et al (2[CR], 47[CR]) have compared the HLA type of patients with penicillamine-associated *myasthenia gravis* with patients having rheumatoid arthritis but no myasthenic reactions, patients with genuine myasthenia gravis and a group of controls. Although the numbers were small, patients with myasthenic reactions to penicillamine appear to differ genetically from the other groups. BW35, DR1 and the combination thereof were more frequent, whereas the high proportion of DR4 usually found in rheumatic patients was absent. Despite the clinical similarity, there was a reduction in DR3 in cases of penicillamine-induced myasthenia instead of the increase found in genuine myasthenia gravis.

It is of interest that in another study the antigens B8, B18 and BW35 were each present in 3 of 7 patients with penicillamine-induced *polymyositis or dermatomyositis* (3[CR]). It remains, however, to be determined whether this complication has an immunogenetic basis.

Following on the work of Panayi and Wooley the results of Stockman et al (4[CR]) indicate that the antigens B8 and DR3 predispose to the development of *proteinuria*, whereas the presence of DR2 seems to be a protecting factor. There was no significant difference of HLA antigens between patients with mild and severe proteinuria. In patients with *thrombocytopenia* there was a decrease in DR2, whereas A1 and DR4 occurred in increased frequencies. It has been suggested (5[CR]) that partial C4 deficiency may be a risk factor and that there is a supratype associated with thrombocytopenia, i.e. BW44 Bf5 C4A3 C4BQO DR4. There was no difference in frequencies of HLA antigens as between mild and severe thrombocytopenia (4[CR]). Preliminary data from Japan show low frequencies of proteinuria (7[CR]). Since the antigens B8 and DR3 are very infrequent in Japanese people, further Japanese studies are awaited with much interest.

Little information is available on the HLA characteristics of patients with penicil-

Table 1. *Penicillamine-induced effects and associated HLA C4 phenotype*

High penicillamine binding	– B62, DR4; A1, B8, DR3
Low penicillamine binding	– A3, B7, DR2; A11, BW35, DR1
Antimuscle antibodies	– A3, B7
Proteinuria	– B8, DR3
Thrombocytopenia	– BW44, C4A3, C4BQ0, DR4
Myasthenia gravis	– BW35, DR1
Polymyositis/dermatomyositis	– B8, B18 or BW35
IgA deficiency (70[R])	– A3, B40
SLE	– A11, B15

Adapted from Zilko and Dawkins (8[R]).

Side Effects of Drugs Annual 8
M.N.G. Dukes, editor

ISBN 0 444 90339 9
$0.80 per article per page (transactional system)
$0.20 per article per page (licensing system)

lamine-induced pemphigus and more should be collected in future studies (6[r]).

3 of 6 patients with SLE reactions on penicillamine had the HLA antigen A11, whereas B15 was found in as many as 5 of these patients (69[C]). In a control group of 20 patients not experiencing complications on penicillamine, 3 had A11 and 8 had B15.

Frequency of reactions; risk factors Several trials have again demonstrated the high frequency of adverse reactions in patients on penicillamine.

Lyle (30[CR]) has presented an important review comparing the frequency of various adverse reactions in patients treated for different conditions. Interesting findings are that thrombocytopenia develops very rarely in patients with cystinuria as compared with rheumatoid arthritis and Wilson's disease. Proteinuria on the other hand appears to be particularly frequent in cystinuria; it may occur in up to 50% of cystinuric patients and 30% of patients with rheumatic disease when doses exceed 600 mg.) Gastrointestinal intolerance is rare in patients with Wilson's disease and cystinuria (less than 1%) but more frequent (4%) in rheumatic patients, perhaps reflecting the influence of analgesic drugs in the latter.

Pemphigus (40[C]), myasthenia gravis (SEDA-7, 260) and lupus erythematosus (69[C]) each developed in approximately 2% of patients on penicillamine; this figure is probably more realistic than those cited by Lyle (0.51%, 0.55% and 0.19% respectively).

Influence of food and iron Recent work has confirmed that the absorption of penicillamine is impaired when taken with *food* (14[CR]). The bioavailability, which is otherwise about two-thirds of the dose (15–17), is decreased by approximately 50%. For a valid comparison of different trials as regards efficacy and adverse reactions, it is therefore important to know whether the drug has been taken with or between meals.

It has been known for some time that concomitant *iron* intake, too, considerably reduces the absorption of penicillamine (SEDA-1, 192). Iron supplements are frequently taken without the knowledge of the rheumatologist. As demonstrated by Harkness and Blake (18[CR]), on withdrawal of the iron preparation a sudden increase in penicillamine absorption occurs and severe reactions, including renal damage, may ensue.

Penicillamine and previous gold treatment It has been thought that penicillamine, in patients who had been treated with gold, would mobilize a considerable proportion of the stored gold with a subsequent risk of recurrence of gold reactions. Recent reviewers, however, consider that the effect on protein-bound gold is probably of little importance (9[R], 10[R]).

In previous editions the possibility has repeatedly been discussed that the prior occurrence of adverse reactions to gold or even the mere previous use of gold might predispose to reactions to penicillamine (SEDA-5, 244; SEDA-7, 258). Although this issue is difficult to investigate, the data now available indicate that with the exception of proteinuria (which appears more frequently in the case of previous proteinuria on gold) the prior use of gold with or without toxic reactions has no influence on the subsequent occurrence of reactions to penicillamine (11[CR], 12[CR], 13[R], 71[CR]).

It would seem reasonable to assume that genetic factors (see above) rather than the successive use of these drugs are responsible for the increased occurrence of certain complications to both drugs in the patients concerned.

Respiratory *(SEDA-6, 230; SEDA-7, 259)* Camus (19[CR]) has reviewed penicillamine-related pulmonary disorders and discussed 10 published cases of *pneumonitis*. Besides generalized micro-nodular infiltrates alveolar lesions have also been documented. Fever and eosinophilia can occur. Rare cases of penicillamine-induced *bronchospasm* are on record (19). A rare but life-threatening complication is *Goodpasture's syndrome*, characterized by progressive hemorrhagic pneumonitis associated with glomerulonephritis (see below, Urinary system).

The alleged association between penicillamine and *bronchiolitis obliterans* has for several years been the subject of controversy (SEDA-7, 259; 20[R]). and has recently been reviewed by Epler and Colby (25[R]).

Although there are now many well documented cases of obliterative bronchiolitis in patients on penicillamine, its occurrence in patients who have never received penicillamine is also increasingly being reported (21[CR]–24[CR]). Probably this condition is a previously unrecognized expression of rheumatic lung disease rather than a complication of penicillamine (26[CR], 27[CR]).

Nervous system Whereas in SEDA-7 (p. 260) a case of *toxic polyneuropathy* was described, Mayr et al (28[CR]) have now described a patient with *immunoallergic polyneuropathy* induced by penicillamine.

Within 6 weeks after starting penicillamine this patient presented with bilateral oculomotor palsy and axonal polyneuropathy of the motor and sensory nerves. Simultaneously antinuclear antibodies, antibodies against native DNA, proteinuria and increased alkaline phosphatase had developed. Biopsy of the nervus suralis revealed the presence of vasculitis.

Withdrawal of penicillamine and the use of 10 mg prednisone daily was followed by rapid improvement. It is concluded that in this case neuropathy was part of a pseudo-lupus syndrome.

Liver One further case has been described of *cholestatic hepatitis* induced by penicillamine (SEDA-6, 231; SEDA-7, 259; 29[CR]). Interestingly, the reaction occurred acutely after four years use of the drug. Antinuclear factor and antibodies against DNA were detected in the serum.

The differential diagnostic considerations in arthritic patients presenting with liver symptoms have been reviewed by Mills and Sturrock (57[CR]).

Urinary system In a series of 185 patients on penicillamine for rheumatoid arthritis for more than 12 months, 22% had *proteinuria* greater than 0.5 g/24 hr and 12.4% had proteinuria greater than 1 g/24 hr (71[CR]). In cystinuria, proteinuria appears to be even more frequent and approaches 50% (30[CR], 73[CR]).

The pathological lesion is *membranous glomerulonephritis*, of the immune-complex type (SEDA-5, 247; 71[R]), as again illustrated by two reports from Spain (31[C], 32[C]). Proteinuria can proceed to the *nephrotic syndrome*, the latter occurring in only a few per cent of the patients on penicillamine (30[C]). Successful rechallenge with lower dosage of penicillamine, without relapse proteinuria, occurred in 4 out of 7 patients who had over 2 g proteinuria per day. With less than 1 g per day all rechallenged patients were able to continue penicillamine (71[CR]). *Extramembranous glomerular involvement* mainly occurs in the case of an SLE reaction or in the rarely occurring Goodpasture's syndrome.

In addition, Banfi et al (33[CR]) have recently described the occurrence of severe extramembranous glomerulonephritis in association with *renal vasculitis* (necrotizing lesions of small arteries, anuria) and purpura. In this patient, who improved after stopping penicillamine (2 g daily for rheumatoid arthritis), no features of SLE or Goodpasture's syndrome were found.

Renal vasculitis with impaired renal function, attributed to penicillamine, has been described previously (SEDA-4, 178; 34[C]). One of a number of patients with penicillamine-induced SLE described by Chalmers et al (69[CR]) similarly had proliferative glomerulonephritis with vasculitis. Swainson et al (35[CR]) have reported on the 8th case of penicillamine induced Goodpasture's syndrome.

The complication presented with frank hemoptysis, uremia, proteinuria and hematuria. Renal biopsy showed focal proliferative and necrotizing glomerulonephritis. Immunofluorescence revealed scanty granular depositions of fibrin and C_3 in capillary walls. *Indirect* immunofluorescence to IgG demonstrated bright staining around cell nuclei but no linear staining of the basal membrane. Moribund on admission, the patient recovered on daily plasma exchange, immunosuppression and the stopping of penicillamine.

Skin and appendages The varied spectrum of skin reactions to penicillamine has been reviewed by Barrière and Dreno (36[CR]).

In different case reports recently 5 further patients with penicillamine-induced *pemphigus* (SEDA-7, 260) have been described (36[CR]–39[CR]). Direct immunofluorescence was positive in all 4 patients tested; circulating pemphigus antibodies (indirect fluorescence) were present in 3, absent in 1 and not tested in the remaining patient.

In addition McGirr and York (40[CR]) have observed 5 patients with *pemphigus foliaceus* in a total of 280 patients on penicillamine, i.e. approximately 2%. Ruocco et al (41[CR]) have postulated that penicillamine-associated pemphigus is related to the drug's ability to interfere with the process of keratinization. The level of blistering might reflect characteristics of the antigen concerned. The authors prefer to speak of pericellular rather than intercellular antigen.

Fellner et al (42[CR]) found transient circulating pemphigus antibodies in 3 out of 6 patients with drug eruptions *other than pemphigus* (mainly caused by penicillin derivatives) and suggest that drug eruptions, in analogy with skin burns, can be associated with altered antigenicity of the skin.

In another article from the same group (43[C]), 2 patients are presented with pemphigus, apparently triggered by ampicillin and carbenicillin respectively. This observation renews the interest in the unsolved question whether penicillin and related antibiotics can under certain conditions produce significant amounts of penicillamine, can provoke a relapse in penicillamine hypersensitive patients (SEDA-5, 249) and can perhaps cause penicillamine-like reactions (SEDA-5, 244).

In this respect recent literature on penicillin-induced granulocytopenia, which presumably is caused by metabolites rather than penicillin itself (44[CR]), may be of interest.

Since the case report by Troy et al (SEDA-7, 260), 2 further patients have been described with *bullous pemphigoid* apparently induced by penicillamine (40[C]); both patients had severe skin disease.

Raymond et al (45[CR]) have presented detailed information on the ultrastructural changes in penicillamine-induced *elastosis perforans serpiginosa.* Their findings are in accordance with earlier studies (SEDA-2, 216; SEDA-5, 248; SEDA-6, 232). Both elastin, showing characteristic budding of the fibers, and collagen (in which many fibers are altered in shape and sometimes enormously enlarged) appeared to be grossly abnormal.

Not previously reported in this series is the 1976 case study of Klingberg et al (46[CR]), describing the concomitant occurrence in a patient on penicillamine of pronounced *parakeratotic lesions* of the skin at pressure points, *alopecia,* mild *granulocytopenia, keratitis* and *scotoma.* The patient, a 14-year-old boy with Wilson's disease, recovered on zinc supplements and continuation of penicillamine and it was concluded that zinc deficiency had been responsible for the abnormalities.

Genital system In SEDA-5 (p. 248) a review has been given of the remarkable gigantism of the breasts in women, an apparently very rare complication of penicillamine. Although since then no new cases have been reported, the first case of *gynecomastia* has now been published, which receded after stopping penicillamine (58[C]). One other case of gynecomastia has been reported to the UK Committee on Safety of Medicines (58[r]). In both patients the lesion was unilateral, as is often seen in drug-related gynecomastia.

Musculoskeletal system The relation between HLA types and penicillamine-induced *myasthenia gravis* has been studied by Garlepp et al (47[CR]), as discussed above. The differences in HLA antigens which they found between patients on penicillamine and others support the view that myasthenia gravis in patients on penicillamine is not coincidental but truly drug induced. The controversy as to whether there are significant differences between the antibodies against acetylcholine receptors in penicillamine-related myasthenia as compared to idiopathic myasthenia gravis has not yet been settled. The lesser cross reactivity found in penicillamine-related cases, may either be characteristic for penicillamine (SEDA-5, 250; 48[CR]) or may simply relate to myasthenia gravis of early onset (49[CR], 50[CR]).

Not only the anti-acetylcholine receptor antibodies but also the characteristics of the acetylcholine receptor itself have recently been studied. It was already known that acetylcholine receptor (of electric fish) has two well characterized reducible disulfide bonds (51[R]). Bever et al (51[C]) have found that penicillamine becomes covalently linked to the alpha and gamma subunits of acetylcholine receptor (*Torpedo californica*), probably by mixed disulfide bond formation. As a result, penicillamine alters acetylcholine binding, presumably by decreasing high-affinity ligand binding and cooperativity.

It was shown some years ago that chronic treatment of guinea pigs with high doses of penicillamine decreased the amplitudes of miniature endplate potentials and that application of penicillamine to rat neuromuscular junctions decreased the amplitude and the frequency of endplate potentials (51[R]). A direct toxic effect on the acetylcholine receptor has also been suggested in 1 human observation of rapid onset of muscular weakness after administration of penicillamine (SEDA-4, 178, ref. 39). Bever et al conclude that penicillamine presumably alters the antigenic configuration of acetylcholine receptor with the subsequent formation of auto-antibodies.

In a myasthenic patient recently studied by Fawcett et al (52[CR]), acetylcholine receptor antibody titers decreased steeply after the stopping of penicillamine.

One patient has been reported with *polymyositis and myasthenia gravis* at the same time and in association with several other reactions to penicillamine (59[C]) (see below, Multiple reactions).

Since the case study and comprehensive review by Wouters et al (53[CR]), a case of fulminant polymyositis apparently induced by penicillamine has been described (54[CR]). This patient, who only used 250 mg penicillamine daily, was the second to die from myocardial involvement.

In addition, Carroll et al (3[cR]) reported in their review upon 6 new cases of myositis. These authors emphasize the likelihood of a causative role of penicillamine in the development of polymyositis.

Arthropathy, a side effect which is difficult to assess in rheumatic patients, occurred in 5 out of 32 patients receiving penicillamine for cystinuria (73[C]).

Special senses The exact pathophysiology of the temporary *taste loss* which is so characteristic for penicillamine in adults (SED 8, 536) has remained obscure. The issue of taste disturbance induced by penicillamine and other drugs has recently been reviewed by two authors (55[R], 56[R]). Interestingly, taste disturbance has been observed in association with a number of different drugs, all having in common a sulphydryl group, i.e. penicillamine, captopril, propylthiouracil, methimazole and carbimazole.

Lupus erythematosus Chalmers et al have now presented details of the 6 patients, referred to earlier (SEDA-7, 261), with SLE reactions during treatment with penicillamine (69[CR]). Their HLA typing is noted above. Pleuropulmonary symptoms are frequent and the lupus syndrome may be associated with central (69[CR]) and peripheral (28[CR]) neurologic manifestations and with renal vasculitis. Chalmers et al confirmed the occurrence of antibodies against double-stranded DNA and noted the presence of hypocomplementemia.

Immunodeficiency *(SEDA-5, 250)* The influence of penicillamine on IgA antibodies has been reviewed by Stanworth (70[CR]). IgA deficiency (0–0.36 g/l) developed in 3 patients on penicillamine and 3 other patients on gold out of a series of 65 patients with rheumatoid arthritis. The condition is frequently associated with recurrent upper respiratory tract infections. Interestingly, the onset of IgA deficiency was in 5 of these 6 patients associated with a marked improvement in rheumatoid disease activity and, again in 5 patients, occurred together with other side reactions (e.g. rash, thrombocytopenia, proteinuria). Reduced serum levels of IgA have also been observed in 6 out of 40 patients with Wilson's disease (70[r]).

Multiple reactions It is a matter of interest that several patients have been described who presented with more than 1 major adverse reaction to penicillamine, occurring simultaneously or in succession. Thyroiditis has for example occurred concomitantly with myasthenia gravis (SEDA-2, 218), whereas in another patient myasthenia developed together with hepatitis (SEDA-4, 178).

Essigman (59[C]) has even observed a patient in whom, on 500 mg penicillamine daily for rheumatoid arthritis, as many as 5 serious reactions had developed, i.e. polymyositis and myasthenia gravis, nephropathy, systemic lupus erythematosus and erythema annulare centrifugum.

Other metal or cystine antagonists

Because of the toxicity of penicillamine several alternative drugs are in development. Some of these are discussed in other chapters because they have alternative uses. In addition, several new routes or regimens for the management of acute or chronic metal intoxications are subject to study. Current knowledge of the side effects of these drugs has been reviewed in SED-10; it is clearly still very incomplete.

Deferoxamine, vitamin C and iron

Evidence from different sources has indicated that there exists a complex interaction between iron, vitamin C and deferoxamine (61[CR], 62[CR], 63[R]). It is known that vitamin C can increase the excretion of iron by deferoxamine.

Interestingly, vitamin C deficient Bantu people in South Africa with long-standing dietary iron storage disease have been found to be relatively insensitive to the deleterious effect of iron on the heart. In contrast to other forms of iron overload, the heart (and several endocrine organs) in these patients have been shown to be largely free of iron, most of the iron being deposited in reticulo-endothelial cells (spleen, liver). In addition, nearly normal serum levels of iron and of transferrin saturation were found, which however increased when vitamin C supplements were given. Observations in patients with thalassemia have provided evidence that the concomitant use of vitamin C and deferoxamine can cause arrhythmia and cardiac failure; fatal cases have been reported.

Since hypovitaminosis C seems to protect against the complications of iron overload, vitamin C supplements, and even orange juice as a source of potassium, are contra-indicated in these patients. If vitamin C is however needed, it should be given only after adequate serum levels of deferoxamine have been achieved.

Two further cases of anaphylactic reactions to deferoxamine have been briefly referred to by Davies et al (68[C]). They have also reported on their experiences with extremely high doses of intravenous deferoxamine, in an effort to cope with cardiac complications in thalassemia. 2 out of 4 patients developed substantial loss of vision, which rapidly but not completely recovered after stopping the drug.

In 1 patient, who received a total amount of 9.16 g deferoxamine per kg body-weight over a 50-day period, damage to the rods predominated with inability to see in dim light, and bilateral annular scotoma resulting in tunnel vision. There was stippled retinal pigmentation. In addition, the patient had posterior lens opacity in both eyes.

In the other patient, after 1.65 g deferoxamine per kg body-weight in 8 days, cone function was mainly disturbed, with severely impaired color vision and bilateral central scotoma. No lens opacities or retinal pigmentation was seen.

The pathophysiology of the ocular damage remains obscure.

Sodium calcium edetate and dimercaprol were given concomitantly for 5 days in a series of 130 children with subclinical lead-poisoning (64[CR]). Acute renal failure developed in 4 patients and biochemical evidence of renal damage in another 13% of the children, within a period of 4–8 days after discontinuation of the treatment.

Trientine (triethylene tetramine dihydrochloride) has been found to be effective in Wilson's disease. So far the main disadvantage has been that iron absorption is impaired and deficiency may develop when no iron supplements are given (65[CR]). Teratogenic effects have not been observed (65[R]).

Mercaptopropionylglycine has been used as an alternative to penicillamine in cystinuria. The drug is chemically related to penicillamine and has been implicated in the development of *urticaria, fever* and *lymphadenopathy* (67[r]). The development of the *nephrotic syndrome* has been reported in 2 children receiving high doses of mercaptopropionylglycine (80 and 100 mg/kg/day) for cystinuria (67[C]). The disorder rapidly recovered when the drug was discontinued and lower doses were later on well tolerated. One case has been described of *myopathy* which rapidly resolved after stopping penicillamine (66[C]).

REFERENCES

1. Dawkins RL, Christiansen FT, Zilko PJ (Eds.) (1982) *Immunogenetics in Rheumatology; Musculoskeletal Disease and d-Penicillamine.* Excerpta Medica, Amsterdam.
2. Garlepp MJ, Christiansen FT, Dawkins RL (1982) Myasthenia gravis induced by d-penicillamine. In: 1, p 317–321.
3. Carroll GJ, Peter JB, Garlepp MJ (1982) d-Penicillamine-induced dermatomyositis and polymyosistis. In: 1, p 326–330.
4. Stockman A, Flory E, Tait B et al (1982) Genetics of d-penicillamine induced renal disease in Caucasians. In: 1, p 336–340.
5. McClusky J, Kay P, Zilko PJ et al (1982) Genetics of d-penicillamine induced thrombocytopenia. In: 1, p 350–354.
6. Carrano JA, Zolko PJ, Dawkins RL (1982) Autoantibodies induced by d-penicillamine. In: 1, p 362–367.
7. Sekiguchi S, Nishikai M, Takata H, Ito S (1982) Gold and d-penicillamine induced renal disease in Japanese. In: 1, p 341–343.

8. Zilko PJ, Dawkins RL (1982) D-penicillamine – immunogenetics of effects and side effects; overview and summary. In: 1, p 373–375.
9. Kean WF, Lock CJ, Howard-Lock HE, Buchanan WW (1982) Prior gold therapy does not influence the adverse effects of d-penicillamine in rheumatoid arthritis. *Arthritis Rheum.*, *25*, 917.
10. Champion GD, Sambrook PN, Browne CD et al (1982) Influence of previous gold on penicillamine toxicity. In: 1, p. 311–315.
11. Smith PJ, Swinburn WR, Swinson DR, Stewart IM (1982) Influence of previous gold toxicity on subsequent development of penicillamine toxicity. *Br. Med. J.*, *285*, 595.
12. Halla JT, Cassady J, Hardin JG (1982) Sequential gold and penicillamine therapy in rheumatoid arthritis. *Am. J. Med.*, *72*, 423.
13. Editorial (1983) Toxicity of penicillamine with respect to prior gold therapy: conflicting opinions. *Pharmacy Int.*, *6*,
14. Schuna A, Osman MA, Patel RB et al (1983) Influence of food on the bioavailability of penicillamine. *J. Rheumatol.*, *10*, 95.
15. Kukovetz WR, Beubler E, Kreuzig F et al (1983) Bioavailability and pharmacokinetics of d-penicillamine. *J. Rheumatol.*, *10*, 90.
16. Perrett D (1981) The metabolism and pharmacology of d-penicillamine in man. *J. Rheumatol.*, *8*, *Suppl. 7*, 41.
17. Van der Korst JK, Van de Stadt RJ, Muijsers AO et al (1981) Pharmacokinetics of penicillamine in rheumatoid arthritis. In: Maini RN, Berry R (Eds.) *Modulation of Autoimmunity and Disease*, p 165–174.
18. Harkness JAL, Blake DR (1982) Penicillamine nephropathy and iron. *Lancet*, *2*, 1368.
19. Camus Ph (1982) Manifestations respiratoires associées aux traitements par la d-pénicillamine. *Rev. Fr. Mal. Respir.*, *10*, 7.
20. Jaffe IA (1982) Influence of underlying disease on d-penicillamine induced side effects. In: 1, p 301–305.
21. Bégin R, Massé, Cantin A et al (1982) Airway disease in a subset of nonsmoking rheumatoid patients. *Am. J. Med.*, *72*, 743.
22. Turton CW, Williams G, Green M (1982) Cryptogenic obliterative bronchiolitis in adults. *Thorax*, *36*, 805.
23. Seggev JS, Mason UG, Worthen S et al (1983) Bronchiolitis obliterans. *Chest*, *83*, 169.
24. McCann BG, Hart GJ, Stokes TC, Harrison BDW (1983) Obliterative bronchiolitis and upper-zone pulmonary consolidation in rheumatoid arthritis. *Thorax*, *38*, 73.
25. Epler GR, Colby TV (1983) The spectrum of bronchiolitis obliterans. *Chest*, *83*, 161.
26. Jansen HM, Elema JD, Hylkema BS et al (1982) Progressive obliterative bronchiolitis in a patient with rheumatoid arthritis. *Eur. J. Respir. Dis.*, *63*, *Suppl. 121*, 43.
27. Pieters R, Martens J, Dequeker J (1982) Rheumatoid arthritis associated with bronchiolitis obliterans and immunoblastic sarcoma. *Clin. Rheumatol.*, *1*, 35.
28. Mayr N, Graninger W, Wessely P (1983) Polyneuropathie bei chronischer Polyarthritis unter D/Penicillamin, medikamentös induziert? *Wien. Klin. Wochenschr.*, *95*, 86.
29. Job-Deslandre C, Delrieu F, Rondier J et al (1982) Hépatite cholestatique et anticorps anti-DNA induits par la d-pénicillamine. *Nouv. Presse Méd.*, *11*, 2356.
30. Lyle WH (1982) Influence of underlying disease on d-penicillamine induced side effects. In: 1, p 306–310.
31. Prieto Carles C, Gutiérrez Millet V, Barrientos A et al (1982) Nefropatia membranosa por d-penicilamina. *Med. Clin. (Barcelona)*, *79*, 164.
32. Becares Lozano M, Pascual Izuel JM, Mateos Sanchez A et al (1982) Glomerulonefritis membranosa por d-penicilamina. *Rev. Clin. Esp.*, *164*, 411.
33. Banfi G, Imbasciati E, Guerra L et al (1983) Extracapillary glomerulonephritis with necrotizing vasculitis in d-penicillamine-treated rheumatoid arthritis. *Nephron*, *33*, 56.
34. Halverson PB, Kozin F, Bernhard GC, Goldman AL (1978) Toxicity of penicillamine. *J. Am. Med. Assoc.*, *240*, 1870.
35. Swainson CP, Thomson D, Short ALK, Winney RJ (1982) Plasma exchange in the successful treatment of drug-induced renal disease. *Nephron*, *30*, 244.
36. Barrière H, Dreno B (1982) Les accidents curanés induits par la d-pénicillamine. *Ouest Méd.*, *35*, 881.
37. Barety M, Ortonna J-P, Chichmanian RM et al (1982) Pemphigus et traitement par la d-pénicillamine. *Therapie*, *37*, 471.
38. Fye KH, Tanenbaum L (1982) Penicillamine-induced pemphigue vulgaris in psoriatic arthritis. *J. Rheumatol.*, *9*, 331.
39. Benito Urbina S, Chavez Calvo M, Riesco Diaz M et al (1982) Pénfigo inducido por d-penicillamina. *Rev. Clin. Esp.*, *166*, 249.
40. McGirr EE, York J (1982) Pemphigus and pemphigoid associated with d-penicillamine. In: 1, p 352–354.
41. Ruocco V, De Luca M, Pisani M et al (1982) Pemphigus provoked by d-penicillamine. *Dermatologica*, *164*, 236.
42. Fellner MJ, Moshell A, Mont MA (1981) Pemphigus vulgaris and drug reactions. *Int. J. Dermatol.*, *20*, 115.
43. Fellner MJ, Mark AS (1981) Penicillin- and ampicillin-induced pemphigus vulgaris. *Int. J. Dermatol.*, *20*, 392.
44. Neftel K, Müller M, Hauser S et al (1983) Wie atoxisch sind Penicilline? *Schweiz. Med. Wochenschr.*, *113*, 446.
45. Raymond JL, Stoebner P, Zambelli P et al (1982) Penicillamine induced elastosis perforans serpiginosa: an ultrastructural study of two cases. *J. Cutan. Pathol.*, *9*, 352.
46. Klingberg WG, Prasad AS, Oberleas D (1976) Zinc deficiency following penicillamine therapy.

In: Prasad AS (Ed.) *Trace Elements in Human Health and Disease*. Academic Press, New York.
47. Garlepp MJ, Dawkins RL, Christiansen FT (1983) HLA antigens and acetylcholine receptor antibodies in penicillamine induced myasthenia gravis. *Br. Med. J., 286,* 338.
48. Garlepp MJ, Dawkins RL, Christiansen FT (1983) HLA antigens and acetylcholine receptor antibodies in penicillamine induced myasthenia gravis. *Br. Med. J., 286,* 442.
49. Vincent A, Newson-Davis JE (1982) Acetylcholine receptor antibody characteristics in myasthenia gravis. II. Patients with penicillamine-induced myasthenia or idiopathic myasthenia of recent onset. *Clin. Exp. Immunol., 49,* 266.
50. Vincent A, Newsom-Davis JE (1983) HLA antigens in penicillamine induced myasthenia gravis. *Br. Med. J., 286,* 893.
51. Bever CT, Hai Won Chang, Penn AS et al (1982) Penicillamine-induced myasthenia gravis: effects of penicillamine on acetylcholine receptor. *Neurology, 32,* 1077.
52. Fawcett PR, McLachlan SM, Nicholson LVB, Mastaglia FL (1982) D-penicillamine-associated myasthenia gravis: immunological studies. *Muscle Nerve, 5,* 328.
53. Wouters JMGW, Van de Putte LBA, Renier WO, Joosten EMG (1982) D-penicillamine-induced polymyositis. *Neth. J. Med., 25,* 159.
54. Doyle DR, McCurley TL, Sergent JS (1983) Fatal polymyositis in d-penicillamine-treated rheumatoid arthritis. *Ann. Intern. Med., 98,* 327.
55. Schiffman SS (1983) Taste and smell in disease. *N. Engl. J. Med., 308,* 1275.
56. Willoughby JMT (1983) Drug-induced abnormalities of taste sensation. *Adverse Drug Reactions Bull., 100,* 368.
57. Mills PR, Sturrock RD (1982) Clinical association between arthritis and liver disease. *Ann. Rheum. Dis., 41,* 295.
58. Reid DM, Martynoga AG, Nuki G (1982) Reversible gynaecomastia associated with d-penicillamine in a man with rheumatoid arthritis. *Br. Med. J., 285,* 1083.
59. Essigman WK (1982) Multiple side effects of penicillamine therapy in one patient with rheumatoid arthritis. *Ann. Rheum. Dis., 41,* 617.
60. Scott DL, Coulton BL, Chapman JH et al (1983) The long-term effects of treating rheumatoid arthritis. *J. Royal Coll. Physicians London, 17,* 79.
61. Nienhuis AW (1981) Vitamin C and iron. *N. Engl. J. Med., 304,* 170.
62. Cohen A, Cohen IJ, Schwartz E (1981) Scurvy and altered iron stores in thalassemia major. *N. Engl. J. Med.,304,* 158.
63. Nienhuis AW (1977) Safety of intensive chelation therapy. *N. Engl. J. Med., 296,* 114.
64. Moel DI, Kumar K (1982) Reversible nephrotoxic reactions to a combined 2,3-dimercapto-1-propanol and calcium disodium ethylenediaminetetra-acetate acid regimen in asymptomatic children with elevated blood lead levels. *Pediatrics, 70,* 259.
65. Walshe JM (1982) Treatment of Wilson's disease with trientine (triethylene tetramine) dihydrochloride. *Lancet, 1,* 643.
66. Hales DSM, Scott R, Lewi HJE (1982) Myopathy due to mercaptopropionylglycine. *Br. Med. J., 285,* 939.
67. Rizzoni G, Pavanello L, Dussini N et al (1979) Nephrotic syndrome during treatment with alpha-mercaptopropionylglycine. *J. Urology, 122,* 381.
68. Davies SC, Marcus RE, Hungerford JL et al (1983) Ocular toxicity of high-dose intravenous desferrioxamine. *Lancet, 2,* 181.
69. Chalmers A, Thompson D, Stein H, Reid G, Patterson C (1982) Systemic lupus erythematosus during penicillamine therapy for rheumatoid arthritis. *Am. Intern. Med., 97,* 659.
70. Stanworth DR (1982) D-penicillamine induced immunodeficiency. In: 1, p 358–361.
71. Stockman A, Flory ED, Muriden KD (1982) Renal disease induced by penicillamine. In: 1, p 331–335.
72. Nissilä M, Nuotio P, Von Essen R, Mäkisara P (1982) Low-dose penicillamine treatment of RA. *Scand. J. Rheumatol., 11,* 161.
73. Halperin EC, Thier SO, Rosenberg LE (1981) The use of d-penicillamine in cystinuria: efficacy and untoward reactions. *Yale J. Biol. Med., 54,* 439.

G. Reybrouck

25 Antiseptic drugs and disinfectants

ACIDS

Boric acid *(SED-9, 392; SEDA-6, 236)*

Although boric acid has little or no therapeutic value, it is still contained in some antiseptic powders, mouthwashes, eye drops, vaginal preparations, foot powders, denture adhesives and detergents. Schillinger et al (1[Cr]) have described the striking skin manifestations observed in a case of acute boric acid intoxication: the erythema was very intense, creating a 'boiled lobster' appearance, and there were massive areas of desquamation, clinically resembling the staphylococcal 'scalded skin syndrome'. On the 10th day the patient developed a patchy alopecia of the scalp which progressed to alopecia totalis within a few days.

Sorbic acid

Sorbic acid is used as a preservative in foods, and contact urticaria has been recognized for years. Clemmensen and Schiødt (2[c]), however, were unable to produce urticarial reactions on the buccal mucosa in normal subjects, or in patients with skin diseases without mucosal involvement and without a history of urticaria or atopy. Even a 20-min intrabuccal patch test with 10% sorbic acid in water produced only an overall erythema; a slight infiltration, mimicking urticaria, was seen in 1 patient, but a concentration of 10% is 100 times higher than that normally allowed in foods. These findings confirm the clinical impression that when used as a food additive the preservative is not urticariogenic.

Side Effects of Drugs Annual 8
M.N.G. Dukes, editor

ISBN 0 444 90339 9
$0.80 per article per page (transactional system)
$0.20 per article per page (licensing system)

ALCOHOLS

Benzyl alcohol *(SEDA-7, 265)*

Benzyl alcohol is sometimes employed as a preservative in vials of physiological saline or water for injection (known as bacteriostatic saline or water). It has earlier caused a fatal toxic syndrome in premature infants, but generally only when used to flush i.v. catheters: in this case the volume of fluid used is large, and the risk for the infant is therefore greater than with the administration of i.v. medications containing benzyl alcohol (3[R]).

Feasby et al (4[c]) have now, however, reported a case illustrating the toxicity of bacteriostatic water used as a solvent for intrathecal injections.

A 64-year-old man rapidly developed a flaccid paraplegia after intrathecal injection of cytarabine which was dissolved in 5 ml of bacteriostatic water containing 1.5% benzyl alcohol. Rinsing the cerebrospinal-fluid space with saline reversed the neurological deficit. Autopsy 6 months later showed fibrosis of the cauda equina with a patchy distribution of thinly myelinated fibers in the dorsal and ventral roots, indicative of repaired segmental demyelination. The same histologic findings were produced in rats by the intrathecal injection of 0.05 ml bacteriostatic water.

Chlorobutanol

In a case reported by De Christoforo et al, an unexpected complication of a high-dose morphine infusion (up to 6.8 mg/kg body weight/hr) in a patient with Ewing's sarcoma was excessive somnolence, which was attributed to the 0.5% chlorobutanol preservative in the morphine; the dose of chlorobutanol administered (90 mg/hr) indeed exceeded the sedative threshold, but it is clear that the morphine itself could also have caused this effect (5[C]).

Methylated spirits

Any substance which comes into contact with the skin of preterm babies, e.g. alcohol used for disinfection, is rapidly absorbed into the blood stream (SEDA-6, 236). In addition the delicate skin of these newborns is easily damaged; burns can for example be caused by the extensive application of isopropyl alcohol (SEDA-7, 266), another case of this now having been reported by Harpin and Rutter (6[C]).

A 27-week-gestation infant developed haemorrhagic skin necrosis on the back and buttocks after umbilical arterial catheterization; industrial methylated spirits (95% ethanol and 5% wood naphtha consisting of at least 60% methanol) had been used for skin cleaning and disinfection. Even 18 hours after disinfection, the blood ethanol level was still 259 mg/dl and the blood methanol level 26 mg/dl; it is likely that the maximum level reached was in the potentially fatal range.

ALDEHYDES

Formaldehyde *(SED-9, 391; SEDA-6, 236; SEDA-7, 266)*

Intravesical instillation of a formaldehyde solution (formalin) appears to be the method of choice for the control of massive hematuria following radiation cystitis, but Capen et al (7[C]) have now reported a fatal case of intraperitoneal spillage of formalin.

A 74-year-old woman had been treated with radiation therapy for cervix cancer. Mild hematuria and moderate rectal bleeding occurred 3 years later and were due to radiation cystitis and proctosigmoiditis; a biopsy specimen was taken from the dome of the bladder. One week later she was hospitalized for massive hematuria, due to diffuse bleeding in the bladder as cystoscopy revealed. Formaldehyde solution (100 ml of 10% formalin) was instilled intravesically, but when after 15 min the Foley catheter was unclamped, there was no return of the formalin solution. Laparotomy, 40 min after the instillation, revealed a bladder perforation at the site of the previous biopsy; there was little bowel or peritoneal reaction due to the formalin. Extensive irrigation was performed and sump drains placed. Arterial blood gases at that time demonstrated a marked metabolic acidosis with a pH of 7.1 as a result of formic acid absorption. Serum glucose levels of 600 mg/dl present within the first 4 hours were attributed to the stress and the acidosis but also to the direct effect of formic acid; up to 150 units of insulin per day were required in the first week. Hypocalcemia (6.3 mg/dl) developed within 24 hours. Severe peritonitis and intra-abdominal distention occurred. An elevated serum creatinine (4.7 mg/dl) on the 4th postoperative day was due to acute tubular necrosis: the patient was oliguric for 24 hours. There were several episodes of hypotension. At the time of death, 4 weeks after surgery, most problems were resolved, but there was no evidence of bowel function; gastrograph studies showed no activity of the stomach and the contrast material placed in the rectum at the time of the laparotomy was still present. The death of the patient appeared to be due to cardiac arrest.

The acute renal tubular necrosis observed in this case could have been related to the absorption of intravesically instilled formalin through the hyperemic bladder mucosa (8[c]).

CHLORINE COMPOUNDS

Hypochlorite *(SEDA-6, 237)*

With a view to obtain more lustre and brightness housewives often mix domestic cleaning agents, but this is not entirely without risk. Mixing solutions of ammonia and household bleach (hypochlorite) produces acrid chloramine fumes. Although there are no reported cases of serious injury from inhaling the fumes, respiratory distress and pneumonitis can require admission to hospital (9[C]). Pulmonary function tests are particularly helpful in diagnosing the pneumonitis, since radiographic signs appear only later, around the 3rd day after exposure.

CHLORHEXIDINE *(SED-9, 394; SEDA-5, 254; SEDA-7, 266)*

During a study of the evaluation of the antiplaque effect of some chlorhexidine rinses, Ainamo et al (10[C]) observed that *bleeding of the gingival margin* occurred more often after chemical treatment with chlorhexidine than after mechanical oral hygiene measures.

A more methodical study of the same volunteers 18 months later confirmed this finding: gingival bleeding after gentle massage of the margin with the side of a periodontal probe occurred in 1.3% of all gingival units after mechanical cleaning of the teeth, but in 5.4% after rinsing with a 0.2% chlorhexidine solution twice daily. The reason for this observation is not clear and the bleeding was not of clinical significance.

Another rare side effect of 0.2% chlorhexidine mouthwash is the occurrence of severe desquamative reactions of the oral mucosa (11[C]); it has been suggested that one should dilute the solution, since 0.1% chlorhexidine did not affect the oral mucosa and it provides adequate treatment. Use of this lower concentration does not eliminate the occurrence of *allergic reactions* such as contact eczema; these are, however, extremely rare (12[c]).

HEXETIDINE *(SED-9, 394)*

Hexetidine is a pyrimidine derivative used mainly as a fungicide in gargles. Merk et al (13[c]) refer to a case of *allergic contact dermatitis* due to the use of hexetidine in a person without a history of allergy.

IODOPHORS

Poloxamer-iodine

The same strain of *Pseudomonas aeruginosa* was isolated from 4 cases of peritonitis and 1 of wound infection at the catheter site in outpatients on chronic peritoneal dialysis (14[C]). An identical strain was present in unopened bottles of the poloxamer-iodine solution used for disinfection of the catheter tubing connection and of the skin at the catheter insertion site. This incident recalls the contamination of povidone-iodine solutions by *Pseudomonas cepacia* leading to pseudobacteremia (SEDA-7, 267); whenever a common source of hospital infection is suspected, samples of all the fluids in use, even disinfectants and chemotherapeutic agents, should be cultured; it is too often forgotten that they are not self-sterilizing.

Povidone-iodine *(SED-9, 400; SEDA-5, 256; SEDA-6, 237; SEDA-7, 267)*

In recent years some concern has arisen as regards alterations in thyroid function due to the local application of iodine-containing agents, especially povidone-iodine (PVP-I), to wounds or burns and (in newborns) even to the intact skin (15[C]). Schönberger and Grimm (16[C]) examined prospectively 350 neonates, which were not seriously ill, for hypothyroidism, and in the majority of them the blood level of thyroxin (T4) and TSH and the iodine excretion in urine were determined. Only 15 of them developed a transient hypothyroidism, which was observed between the 3rd and 16th day of life; in 14 of these cases there was no history of surgical intervention or of urography and in these the T4 level ranged between 1.3 and 5.0 μg/dl (normal value 5.0 μg/dl or more), and the TSH blood level between 21.4 and 171.3 μIU/ml (normal value less than 20 μIU/ml).

During the first study period, when PVP-I was used in the ward, only 11 out of the 95 patients (no operation or radiography with contrast media) showed normal iodine values in the urine. During the second period all iodine-containing disinfectants were removed from the ward; even then 39 out of the 55 patients showed iodine urine levels above 30 μg/dl; the reason for this finding is unclear, but iodine may well have been used prior to admission to the ward. In this group, however, no clinical cases of hypothyroidism were observed. It was notable that T4 values decreased significantly during the first few postoperative days, irrespective of whether alcohol of PVP-I had been used for skin disinfection; relatively low T4 values were also observed in preterm newborns and in infants with the respiratory distress syndrome (15[C]).

Habermann et al (17[C]) investigated thyroid function in 12 patients with second- or third-degree burns; iodine sources comprised an i.v. urography usually performed on the first day, and local treatment with PVP-I cream and solution (Betaisodona). Every 4 days the parameters for thyroid function were measured. The initial decrease of the thyroxine binding globulin (TBG) was attributed to the loss of proteins due to the burn injury. The decrease of the T3/TBG and T4/TBG ratios during PVP-I treatment induced a minor but significant increase of the basal TSH levels. The authors concluded that in normal thyroids, autoregulatory mechanisms are able to prevent iodine-induced hyperthyroidism.

The allergic potential of PVP-I must be less than that of an iodine-iodide mixture, since in the former case no free iodide is present. Patch testing with 3% iodine-potassium iodide showed positive reactions in 35 out of 104 patients (22 cases with ulcera crurum and 82 patients with infectious skin diseases or skin tumours). Hyperreactivity to PVP-I ointments occurred in 12 patients, and to PVP-I solutions in 29 patients. Allergic skin reactions must be expected in 2–9% of all patients using PVP-I ointments, but in 6–25% of patients known to be allergic to iodine; in the case of PVP-I solutions, these figures are 12–20% and 34–60% respectively (18[C]).

MERCURY COMPOUNDS *(SED-9, 394; SEDA-5, 257; SEDA-7, 268)*

Mercury compounds are easily absorbed through wounds and burns and can rapidly produce organic damage. In a case reported by Steen, *local* application of merbromin to second-degree burns covering 34% of the body surface for only 36 hours produced clinical symptoms of injury of the tubular epithelium of the kidneys, of the gastrointestinal mucosae and of the central nervous system, with fatal outcome (19[C]).

In another patient, irrigation of the bowel ends and the adjacent peritoneum with a 0.2% mercuric chloride solution during a hemicolectomy produced acute renal failure, which required haemodialysis for 12 days before the renal function recovered. Renal failure was followed by adynamic ileus, wound disruption and a severe peritoneal reaction (20[Cr]).

Mercury compounds can be absorbed even through the normal oral mucosae.

A 7-month-old female was hospitalized for Morbus Hirschsprung. As a sop during the preoperative anemia, the comforter was dipped into a formulation of phenylmercuric borate (Glycero-Merfen) as often as 10 times a day for 16 days. The practice was stopped one week after the intervention. Mercury blood levels reached 180 mg/l on the day of the operation (urine: 100 mg/l); one week after the intervention 50 mg/l mercury was still present in the blood and 150 mg/l in the urine; after 3 weeks less than 10 mg/l (normal value) was present in the blood, and 30 mg/l (normal level less than 20 mg/l) in the urine. There were no clinical features of intoxication (21[Cr]).

PARABENS *(SED-9, 393; SEDA-6, 238)*

Kaminer et al (22[C]) have described what they consider to be the first reported case of *immediate hypersensitivity to parabens in oral preparations.* In one reported case, within 36 hours after the substitution of a methylparabens-containing haloperidol syrup for the haloperidol tablets previously used, a urticarial maculopapular rash appeared over the entire body of the patient, except for his face. The macrophage migration inhibition test was positive to the mixtures containing the preservative.

PHENOLIC COMPOUNDS

Neonatal jaundice has been associated with the use of phenolic disinfectants in nurseries, not only when used in excessive concentrations (SEDA-4, 182), but also when applied in the recommended dilution (SEDA-5, 258). Vitkun et al (23[Cr]) found in 2 unrelated premature infants in the same hospital nursery contemporaneously exhibited features of an acute Heinz body hemolytic anemia (HBHA), probably associated with cleaning of the inside of isolettes by a too highly concentrated phenolic disinfectant. However, it did not prove possible to induce HBHA experimentally in cats, rats, mice, or in human adult or infant cord blood; HBHA is therefore thought to be highly specific for the intact human premature infant. It may be that the hyperbilirubinemia reported earlier in infants exposed to these compounds was of erythrocytic rather than hepatic origin.

SULFITES

Sodium bisulfite and metabisulfite are used as preservatives in many foods, but also in some medications as isoetharine, hydrocortisone, isoproterenol hydrochloride. The physician must be aware that the administration of such drugs can lead to anaphylactoid symptoms in asthmatic patients who are allergic to bisulfites or metabisulfites, e.g. as suggested by a history of repeated adverse reactions to foods (24[C]).

REFERENCES

1. Schillinger BM, Berstein M, Goldberg LA et al (1982) Boric acid poisoning. *J. Am. Acad. Dermatol.*, *7*, 667.
2. Clemmensen OJ, Schiødt M (1982) Patch test reaction of the buccal mucosa to sorbic acid. *Contact Dermatitis*, *8*, 341.

3. Lovejoy FH (1982) Fatal benzyl alcohol poisoning in neonatal intensive care units. *Am. J. Dis. Child.*, *136*, 974.
4. Feasby TE, Hahn AF, Gilbert JJ (1983) Neurotoxicity of bacteriostatic water. *N. Engl. J. Med.*, *308*, 966.
5. DeChristoforo R, Corden BJ, Hood JC et al (1983) High-dose morphine infusion complicated by chlorobutanol-induced somnolence. *Ann. Intern. Med.*, *98*, 335.
6. Harpin V, Rutter N (1982) Percutaneous alcohol absorption and skin necrosis in a preterm infant. *Arch. Dis. Child.*, *57*, 477.
7. Capen CV, Weigel JW, Magrina JF et al (1982) Intraperitoneal spillage of formalin after intravesical instillation. *Urology*, *19*, 599.
8. Melekos M, Lalos J (1983) Intravesical instillation of formalin and its complications. *Urology*, *21*, 331.
9. Gapany-Gapanavičius M, Molho M, Tirosh M (1982) Chloramine-induced pneumonitis from mixing household cleaning agents. *Br. Med. J.*, *285*, 1086.
10. Ainamo J, Asikainen S, Paloheimo L (1982) Gingival bleeding after chlorhexidine mouthrinses. *J. Clin. Periodontol.*, *9*, 337.
11. Skoglund LA, Holst E (1982) Desquamative mucosal reactions due to chlorhexidine gluconate. *Int. J. Oral Surg.*, *11*, 380.
12. Staab W, Gängler P (1982) Allergische Reaktion auf Chlorhexidindiglukonat. *Stomatologie D.D.R.*, *32*, 700.
13. Merk H, Elbert L, Goerz G (1982) Allergic contact dermatitis due to the fungicide hexetidine. *Contact Dermatitis*, *8*, 216.
14. Parrot PL, Terry PM, Whitworth EN et al (1982) Pseudomonas aeruginosa peritonitis associated with contaminated poloxamer-iodine solution. *Lancet*, *2*, 683.
15. Bucher H, Torresani T, Sobradillo B et al (1983) Führt PVP-Jod-Desinfektion von Neugeborenen zur transienten Hypothyreose? *Schweiz. Med. Wochenschr.*, *113*, 671.
16. Schönberger W, Grimm W (1982) Transiente Hypothyreosen durch jodhaltige Desinfizientien bei Neugeborenen. *Dtsch. Med. Wochenschr.*, *107*, 1222.
17. Habermann J, Pickardt CR, Scriba PC et al (1982) Veränderungen der Schilddrüsenfunktion bei Behandlung von Brandwunden mit Polyvinylpyrrolidon-Jod-Komplex. *Unfallheilkunde*, *85*, 253.
18. Kunze J, Kaiser HJ, Petres J (1983) Relevanz einer Jodallergie bei handelsüblichen Polyvidon-Jod-Zubereitungen. *Z. Hautkr.*, *58*, 255.
19. Steen M (1983) Quecksilberintoxikation durch Lokalbehandlung einer Verbrennung mit Merbromin (Mercurochrom). *Unfallheilkunde*, *86*, 34.
20. Lai K-N, Pugsley DJ, Black RB (1983) Acute renal failure after peritoneal lavage with mercuric chloride. *Med. J. Aust.*, *1*, 37.
21. Schaad UB, Kehrer BH (1983) Phenylmercuriborat in Glycerin (Glycero-Merfen) im Kleinkindesalter: unerwünschte Quecksilberresorption auch bei intakter Mundschleimhaut. *Schweiz. Med. Wochenschr.*, *113*, 148.
22. Kaminer Y, Apter A, Tyano S et al (1982) Delayed hypersensitivity reaction to orally administered methylparaben. *Clin. Pharm.*, *1*, 469.
23. Vitkun SA, Smith RP, French EE et al (1983) Heinz body hemolytic anemia in newborns and failure of laboratory studies to implicate a phenolic disinfectant. *Pediatrics*, *71*, 352.
24. Twarog FJ, Leung DYM (1982) Anaphylaxis to a component of isoetharine (sodium bisulfite). *J. Am. Med. Assoc.*, *248*, 2030.

T. Midtvedt

26 Penicillins, cephalosporins and tetracyclines

TRIALS – OR ERRORS?

The large number of new beta-lactams launched in the last few years has led to a tremendous number of clinical trials. These trials, most often initiated and paid for by the companies responsible for these new drugs, are sometimes well conceived, but more often badly planned and dubiously performed.

One of the main criticisms of such trials is that they may include patients who are not truly infected (1[R]). By infection we usually mean that the patient shows the adverse effects of microorganism multiplication in the body. In the absence of isolation of a possible agent, it may be difficult to differentiate between a microbial infection and other causes of local symptoms such as swelling or tenderness or of general symptoms such as fever. Even with the results of a bacteriological examination to hand, it is far from easy to differentiate between infection and mere colonization.

When an infection is established and therapy started, the assessment of whether and to what extent a patient is responding to therapy may also be difficult. However, gone should be the days of 'good' and 'poor' response. Depending on where the infection is located, the response should be judged by more precise criteria. These can be as simple as the presence or absence of the infecting pathogen in the urine, or involve a more sophisticated scoring system such as that newly reported for sepsis (2[R]).

Most of the trials are reported in terms of 'X number of patients treated with the new drug magicomycin....'. The number of comparative investigations is remarkably low. Where a comparison is made, the new drug is sometimes compared with an old drug and not with the regimen currently accepted as the best one. Very often, the conclusions are couched in positive and optimistic terms. Readers should indeed be aware that the (decisive) step from 'meningitis can be treated with magicomycin' to 'meningitis should be treated with magicomycin' has to be based upon a great number of well planned and acceptably performed investigations.

In the meantime, we all have to remember that the flow of badly planned clinical trials is still increasing; some of us may drown in the flood of papers to come.

Side Effects of Drugs Annual 8
M.N.G. Dukes, editor

ISBN 0 444 90339 9
$0.80 per article per page (transactional system)
$0.20 per article per page (licensing system)

Interaction of penicillin with HLA-A and -B antigens

In 1978 it was reported that patients treated with penicillin may have a transient loss of HLA antigens (3[C]), and the authors assumed that penicillin could change HLA antigens in vivo. Recently, the influence of penicillin G, carbenicillin and ticarcillin on the interaction between HLA antigens and their specific antisera has been tested (4[C]). Many individual HLA-A and -B specificities were investigated with lymphocytotoxicity and platelet fluorescence. Penicillin G and carbenicillin reacted in a similar way, whereas no effect was reported when ticarcillin (and cotrimoxazole) were investigated. When lymphocytes from healthy donors were incubated with penicillin and washed before HLA typing, the cytotoxic reactivity of some typing sera with their corresponding antigens was blocked. When penicillin was added to the cytotoxic assay at different times, competition between penicillin and alloantiserum for binding on or near the same epitope on the HLA molecule could be observed. The authors divide HLA antigen into the following three groups: (1) antibody reactivity blocked by penicillin (Bw35); (2) antibody reactivity not blocked by penicillin (B14); (3) antibody reactivity blocked by penicillin in some donors but not in others (A2).

In general, some penicillins – as well as other members of the beta-lactam group of antibiotics – seem to be able to react with many structures on the cell membrane, of which the HLA antigens are only a minority. The present findings may have some practical implications for HLA typing, as addition of penicillin to multispecific antisera may change these sera into useful monospecific typing sera. The present findings may also have some consequences for cellular typing. If the tissue culture contains penicillin, the drug present may interfere with typing.

CEPHALOSPORINS *(SEDA-4, 187; SEDA-5, 263; SEDA-6, 242; SEDA-7, 274)*

New cephalosporins and new problems

Few – if any – will contest the view that the newer cephalosporins represent an important advance in chemotherapy. They represent a logical follow-up in antibiotic engineering, starting with the development of penicillinase-resistant penicillins more than 30 years ago. Since then, most of us have held the simplistic view that hydrolysis was the sole function of bacterial beta-lactamases. Following that line, it was reasonable to assume that any modification of a cephalosporin (or another beta-lactam) that rendered it insusceptible to bacterial beta-lactamases, without reducing its ability to penetrate the bacterial cell wall and to bind to target protein, would be a proper goal for any pharmaceutical company and a sure basis for future commercial success. The third-generation cephalosporins, and even some of the second-generation compounds and other beta-lactams, fulfill these criteria.

However, there are clouds on the horizon. The disturbing features have been summarized as follows (5[R]): (1) rapid development of bacterial resistance; (2) failure of routine susceptibility tests to detect such resistance; (3) antagonism between beta-lactam antibiotics.

As recently stated (5[R]), the main source of these problems can be traced to one characteristic of the new cephalosporins initially thought to be their most desirable – namely, their stability in the presence of beta-lactamases. Delineation of several recently recognized interactions between beta-lactam antibiotics and beta-lactamases reveals how enzyme stability has conferred unanticipated disadvantages upon these new antibiotics.

In the good old days, emergence of resistance during appropriately administered therapy with beta-lactam antibiotics was a rare event. Although still the exception rather than the rule, emergence of resistance has been observed in up to one-third of the patients treated with some of these new cephalosporins (6[C], 7[C]). In fact, the greatest risk of emergence of resistance appears to exist in patients who (1) have a serious infection with an organism possessing inducible beta-lactamases, and (2) are debilitated or otherwise compromised. By bad luck, these are the same patients for whom the new cephalosporins were especially developed.

Even worse things seem to be following. A recent report (8[C]) indicates the emergence of cross-resistance to aminoglycosides during therapy with latamoxef (moxalactam). There seems to be no reason to believe that an emergence of this type of resistance is limited to latamoxef. If this holds true, the use of the newer cephalosporins should indeed be limited.

Bleeding complications from cephalosporins

Serious infections are often associated with bleeding disorders. Any bleeding disorder associated with antimicrobial therapy is therefore especially serious; such a disorder might easily be attributed in error to the infection itself and not to the drug therapy.

Antibiotics may interfere with cellular and humoral coagulation factors in several ways. The beta-lactams in particular are often associated with platelet disorders (9[R], 10[R]). At least in the case of the penicillins, the effects on the platelets seem to comprise an interference with the secondary wave of aggregation and a depressed primary aggregation response to an ADP stimulus

(11[C]). Findings in a case rechallenged with nafcillin indicated that the alteration of platelet function may be dependent either upon the dose administered or upon time-related exposure of the platelets to the antibiotics. It is important to remember that the duration of the platelet dysfunction may vary from 2–21 days after treatment is discontinued (11[C], 12[C], 13[C], 14[C], 15[C]).

If a patient is on warfarin or some related anticoagulant, the prothrombin time may be lengthened by a direct interaction. At therapeutic concentrations warfarin is 97% bound to plasma albumin, and only 3% is active. Displacement of 3% of the bound drug results in a 100% increase in free and active warfarin. The potentiation of the anticoagulant effect of warfarin by some antimicrobials, such as nalidixic acid (16[R]) and some sulfonamides (17[C]), is most probably caused by competition at these albumin binding sites.

Other antimicrobials, such as chloramphenicol (18[C]), metronidazole (19[R]) and rifampin (20[C]), may interact with the anticoagulant effects of some drugs (warfarin, dicumarol, phenprocumon) by interfering with the hepatic metabolism of these drugs. Chloramphenicol as well as co-trimoxazole can cause bone marrow suppression and reduction in platelet numbers to bleeding levels (21[C]).

Antibiotic-associated hypoprothrombinemia has been known for several years. One of the first reports was from Ham (22[C]), who found hypoprothrombinemia in 5 patients treated with parenteral ampicillin (plus kanamycin in one). On administration of vitamin K, prothrombin times became normal.

Pineo et al (23[C]) reported on 15 patients with a prolonged prothrombin time; all but one had received broad-spectrum antibiotics and intravenous fluids. Some of the newer cephalosporins are often involved in prolongation of prothrombin time. Such a disturbance of hemostasis has been reported after cephazolin, cephamandol, cefoperazone, latamoxef and cefmetazole (9[R], 24[R], 25[C], 26[R], 27[C]–29[C], 57[R], 58[r], 61[r]), but not, to date, after cefotaxime (30[R]). This hypoprothrombinemia is usually thought to be related to a disturbance in the normal bowel flora by the antibiotics which interferes with the microbial production of vitamin K in the intestine. However, this hypothesis might indeed be questioned. Udall (31[C]) showed nearly 20 years ago that vitamin K instilled in the cecum of patients was apparently not absorbed, and animals have to practise coprophagy in order to utilize their own microbial intestinal production of vitamin K (32[R]). Total starvation combined with antibiotic therapy (unspecified but 'affecting the intestinal flora') induced vitamin K deficiency in man after 3–4 weeks (31[C]). In contrast, the hypoprothrombinemia observed after administration of cephalosporins usually occurs within the first week of therapy. It is therefore likely that the hypoprothrombinemia found after cephalosporin therapy is caused, not by a disturbed microbial intestinal production of vitamin K or by an inhibition of the absorption of the vitamin, but by some influence on vitamin-K dependent production of prothrombin by the hepatocytes (29[C]).

These cephalosporins, except for cephazolin, have a methyltetrazole side chain at position 3 of the molecule. Neu (33[R]) has suggested that this side chain might be responsible for the disulfiram-like effects as well as for the bleeding often associated with these compounds, and Lipsky has provided experimental evidence for this (59). However, the precise action of the methyltetrazole part of the molecule upon the hepatic production of prothrombin is still obscure. The prolonged prothrombin time associated with cephazolin therapy also remains unexplained. Other mechanisms are still being studied (60[cr]).

To sum up: any bleeding disorder found in a patient receiving antibiotics should be suspected to be caused by the drug itself and not by the infection. Patients receiving the newer cephalosporins with a methyltetrazole side chain should probably have their prothrombin time monitored, especially if they are elderly.

Interaction between newer cephalosporins and ethanol

Disulfiram-like reactions to *alcohol* in patients treated with some of the newer cephalosporins are well known (SEDA-5; SEDA-6). Inspection of the molecular structure of the cephalosporins reveals that several, including cefamandole, cefoperazone, latamoxef, cefametazole and cefmenoxime contain a methyltetrazole side chain on the 3-position of the beta-lactam nucleus. This side chain closely resembles part of the disulfiram molecule and it is postulated that these antibiotics inhibit acetaldehyde dehydrogenase in the same manner that disulfiram does (33[R], 34[R]). Animal studies support such a hypothesis (35[R]). The fact that disulfiram-like reactions have not been reported for cephalosporins that lack the methyltetrazolium side chain makes a strong case for this explanation of the phenomenon. Clearly, several important pieces of data are, as usual, still lacking. It is not known how long the inhibition of the acetaldehyde dehydrogenase persists and it is anticipated, although not proven, that these antibiotics do not exhibit their inhibitory effect unless they are administered prior to ingestion of alcohol. So far, it would seem advisable to put the patient strictly on the 'water-waggon' as long as he receives these new cephalosporins.

Cefoperazone – antibiotic or laxative?

Cefoperazone is a new third-generation cephalosporin characterized by a broad antibacterial spectrum including *Pseudomonas aeruginosa.* Unlike most other beta-lactam antibiotics, its main excretory pathway is through the liver, leading to a very high concentration of cefoperazone in the bile (36[R]). Data to date indicate that it may not be necessary to adjust the normal dosage of cefoperazone even in the presence of severe renal impairment. The compound has undergone worldwide clinical investigation over the past 3 to 4 years and its value in clinical medicine is well established (37[C]).

However, the results concerning the incidence of *intestinal side effects* are somewhat puzzling. The first clinical studies were performed in Japan where the tolerability of the drug was reported to be very good, with a frequency of diarrhea of less than 0.5% in a series of more than 450 cases (38[C]). In multi-center trials from Europe and Latin-America, however, diarrhea or loose stools have been reported in 7% of more than 350 patients (39[C]). In a worldwide survey covering more than 4000 patients diarrhea or loose stools were found in 3.4% of the patients (37[C]). The diarrhea was usually mild or moderate and only rarely required discontinuation of therapy.

Unfortunately, these low averages mask some much higher figures from individual studies. In 2 German reports diarrhea occurred in approximately 30% of the cases (40[C], 41[C]). In most cases the diarrhea was considered to be of mild or moderate severity. In Sweden the situation may be even worse. In a pharmacokinetic study on volunteers 3 out of 10 experienced diarrhea after an intravenous bolus dose of 1 g of cefoperazone and 6 out of 10 after a dose of 2 g (42[C]). In a clinical study, diarrhea occurred in 12 out of 52 patients treated with cefoperazone 2 g twice daily (50 patients) or 1 g twice daily (2 patients) (25[C]). Furthermore, 11 patients had stools with a consistency subjectively regarded as looser than normal and defecation 2 or 3 times daily. In 5 of the former patients *Cl. difficile* or its toxin was found as well as in another 3 patients in the latter group. There was no evidence of an epidemic spread of *Cl. difficile* and no other cases of *Cl. difficile*-associated diarrhea in other patients treated at the clinic occurred during the 6-month study.

There are various ways of approaching puzzling data like these, and the Swedish data have indeed been questioned (43[R]). However, even if there should be a somewhat higher incidence of diarrhea in cefoprazone therapy as compared to the use of the other new cephalosporins, it might sometimes be a price worth paying, especially in patients with bacterial infections in the biliary system. The final answer can only be expected from carefully planned and well performed clinical studies.

TETRACYCLINES

Doxycycline – in memory

R

A call for new investigations before the observation is forgotten.

The use of antibiotics that block protein synthesis, or of other inhibitors of protein synthesis, to study memory function is a well known approach in general physiology (44[R]). In humans, it has been reported that a combination of selective REM-sleep deprivation and doxycycline administration impaired memory retention. For some reason or another, this observation was nearly forgotten, but the experiments which led to it have now been repeated and extended (45[C]).

In a carefully designed and well per-

formed double-blind study, 32 volunteers were given either doxycycline (200 mg/day) or placebo at bedtime. After 2 nights for adaptation in the laboratory, 16 formed a group which was subjected to deliberate deprivation of REM sleep (REM-dep group), while the others were each allowed 15 min of REM sleep (REM-15 group). All the volunteers then had to learn a 40 words sentence which was to be recalled at intervals during the night. The results indicated that doxycycline impaired memory function in both the REM-dep and REM-15 group.

This observation might have more than an academic interest. It may be true that few patients normally have to learn 40 word sentences and recall them during the night – or in other ways stress their memory functions to a comparable extent. However, doxycycline as well as the other tetracycline derivatives are given – for long periods of time – to young patients for the treatment of acne vulgaris. These are patients who need all their capacity for learning and memory. It would therefore seem to be important to test whether – and to what extent – tetracycline and doxycycline interfere with memory function.

Minocycline and black thyroid

Minocycline has been reported to cause skin and conjunctival pigmentation in man (SEDA-6, 244; SEDA-7, 277), and thyroid pigmentation has been reported in laboratory animals receiving minocycline (46[R]). At autopsy, Attwood and Dennett (47[C]) found a black thyroid in a 69-year-old man who had received 100 mg of minocycline twice daily for pulmonary disease (total dose 36.5 g). For good reasons, no thyroid function testing had been performed.

Recently, 3 new reports of black thyroids in patients have appeared. White and Besanceney report a black thyroid found at autopsy (after an accident) in a 21-year-old man, who had received 732 g of tetracycline hydrochloride and 68 g minocycline (48[C]). During the last 2 months of life he had taken 400 mg of minocycline per day for his acne vulgaris. Microscopically, a granular brown pigment was found in the cytoplasm of the follicular epithelial cells. Microscopic examination of all other visceral organs failed to demonstrate any unusual pigment.

Bilano et al (49[C]) found a uniformly black thyroid in a 37-year-old woman who was operated upon after demonstration of a right-lobe nodule at thyroid uptake scan. The patient had received a total dose of nearly 250 g minocycline over a period of 5 years. Histological examination showed dark-brown, granular, cytoplasmic pigment in the follicular epithelial cells.

Saul et al (50[C]) have described a black thyroid found in a 61-year-old man who was operated upon after demonstration of a solitary nodule in the left thyroid lobe. The patient had a long history of acne rosacea, for which he had been treated intermittently with various oral and topical antibiotics, including minocycline. He received minocycline in 1973–1974, 1976, 1979–1980. The nodule was found to be a typical adenoma devoid of pigment. The surrounding macroscopically black thyroid tissue showed follicular cells containing multiple round, golden to dark-brown bodies, sometimes extending from the follicular cells into the adjacent colloid. The results of several histochemical stains indicated that the pigment was melanine or a melanine-like substance.

The ability of thyroid to concentrate minocycline has been demonstrated in rats and dogs (51[R]). In vitro, minocycline can easily be oxidized to an insoluble black pigment (51[R]), and Benitz et al (46[R]) consider that minocycline can interfere with an iodine peroxidase and is oxidized in the thyroid into a black, nonfluorescent pigment. Saul et al (50[C]) state that the pigment found was not unlike the pigment seen spontaneously in the thyroid gland of homozygous Gunn rats and in the lysosomes of hepatozytes of patients with Dubin-Johnson syndrome. They stress the well-known fact that substances similar to melanine can be produced in cells lacking melanosomes. Their own results indicate that the pigment was melanine or melanine-like.

Both mechanisms rely on the preferential concentration of minocycline by the thyroid gland. Whether minocycline causes an aberration in human thyroid function and whether this function should be monitored in patients taking minocycline for months is still unclear.

Tetracyclines and theophylline; an interaction?

Several drugs, including such antibiotics as the *macrolides* (SEDA-7, 283), have been shown capable of interacting with the kinetics of theophylline. Data now provided by Pfeifer et al (52^C) indicate an increase in elimination half-life and a decrease in body clearance in 6 out of 9 subjects receiving theophylline and tetracycline concomitantly. In an earlier study, the same authors noted an increased incidence of side effects when the 2 drugs were given together (53^C).

In a recent study on healthy male volunteers receiving tetracycline 250 mg 4 times daily for 1 week and theophylline 5 mg/kg as an intravenous infusion over a 15-min period on day 0 and day 7, no statistically significant change in the kinetics of theophylline was observed (54^C). The probability of missing a 25% change in the kinetic value (type II error) was calculated to be less than 6%.

At least in young men, it may be justifiable to conclude that the 'data do not offer reasons for any major concern about the concomitant use of theophylline and tetracycline' (54^C). Whether this conclusion is also valid for older patients has yet to be demonstrated.

Tetracyclines and fatty liver *(SEDA-7, 276)*

Tetracyclines are known to induce fatty liver degeneration in experimental animals (55^R). A prominant feature of tetracycline-induced fatty liver degeneration in humans is that it occurs most frequently during pregnancy, especially in the third trimester.

Prompted by the observation that the tetracycline-induced degeneration displays features that closely resemble those of the fatty liver of pregnancy itself – and experimental evidence obtained in rats – Gwee (56^R) has recently put forward the hypothesis that a precipitous fall in maternal liver choline concentration towards the end of pregnancy could lead to a severe reduction in the lipotropic activity of the liver. In this state the liver will be at a much greater risk of developing fatty degeneration, especially if it is exposed to hepatotoxic agents such as tetracyclines.

REFERENCES

1. Editorial (1983) Some tribulations of antibiotic trials. *Lancet, 1,* 337.
2. Elebute EA, Stoner HA (1983) The grading of sepsis. *Br. J. Surg., 78,* 29.
3. Majsky A, Todoroviicova H (1978) The transient loss of HLA antigens on lymphocytes in patients following administration of penicillin and tetracycline. *Folia Haematol., 4,* 502.
4. Claas FHJ, van Nieuwkoop RR, van der Berge W et al (1982) Interaction of penicillin with HLA-A and -B antigens. *Hum. Immunol., 5,* 83.
5. Sanders CC (1983) Novel resistance selected by the new expanded-spectrum cephalosporins: A concern. *J. Infect. Dis., 147,* 585.
6. Winston DJ, Busuttil RW, Kurtz TO et al (1981) Moxalactam therapy for bacterial infections. *Arch. Intern. Med., 141,* 1607.
7. Platt R, Ehrlich SL, Afarian J et al (1981) Moxalactam therapy of infections caused by cephalothin-resistant bacteria: influence of serum inhibitory activity on clinical response and aquisition of antibiotic resistance during therapy. *Antimicrob. Agents Chemother., 20,* 351.
8. Preheim LC, Penn RG, Sanders CC et al (1982) Emergence of resistance to beta-lactam and aminoglycoside antibiotics during moxalactam therapy of *Pseudomonas aeruginosa* infections. *Antimicrob. Agents Chemother., 22,* 1037.
9. Editorial (1983) Antimicrobials and haemostasis. *Lancet, 1,* 510.
10. Alanis A, Weinstein AJ (1983) Adverse reactions associated with the use of oral penicillins and cephalosporins. *Med. Clin. North. Am., 67,* 113.
11. Alexander DP, Russo ME, Fohrman DE et al (1983) Nafcillin-induced platelet dysfunction and bleeding. *Antimicrob. Agents Chemother., 23,* 59.
12. Andrassy K, Ritz E, Hasper B et al (1976) Penicillin-induced coagulation disorder. *Lancet, 2,* 1039.
13. Brown III CH, Natelson EA, Bradshaw MW et al (1974) The homeostatic defect produced by carbenicillin. *N. Engl. J. Med., 291,* 265.
14. Brown III CH, Bradshaw MW, Natelson EA et al (1976) Defective platelet function following the administration of penicillin compounds. *Blood, 47,* 949.
15. Natelson EA, Brown III CH, Bradshaw MW et al (1976) Influence of cephalosporin antibiotics on blood coagulation and platelet function. *Antimicrob. Agents. Chemother., 9,* 91.
16. Sellers EM, Koch-Weser J (1970) Displacement of warfarin from human albumin by diazoxide and ethacrynic, mefenamic and nalidixic acids. *Clin. Pharmacol. Ther., 11,* 524.
17. Sioris LJ, Weibert RT, Pentel PR (1980) Potentiation of warfarin anticoagulation by sulfisoxazole. *Arch. Intern. Med., 140,* 546.
18. Christensen LK, Skovsted L (1969) Inhibition

of drug metabolism by chloramphenicol. *Lancet, 2,* 1397.

19. Dean RP, Talbert RL (1980) Bleeding associated with concurrent warfarin and metronidazole therapy. *Drug Intell. Clin. Pharm., 14,* 864.

20. Bockhout-Mussert RJ, Bieger R, Van Brummelen P et al (1974) Inhibition by rifampin on the anticoagulant effect of phenprocoumon. *J. Am. Med. Assoc., 229,* 1903.

21. Böttiger LE, Westerholm B (1972) Drug-induced thrombocytopenia. *Acta Med. Scand., 191,* 541.

22. Ham JM (1971) Hypoprothrombinemia in patients undergoing prolonged intensive care. *Med. J. Aust., II,* 716.

23. Pineo GF, Gallus AS, Hirsh J (1973) Unexpected vitamin K deficiency in hospitalized patients. *Can. Med. Assoc. J., 109,* 880.

24. Beam TR (1982) The third generation of cephalosporins, part II. *Rational Drug Ther., 16,* 1.

25. Carlberg H, Alestig K, Nord CE et al (1982) Intestinal side effects of cefoperazone. *J. Antimicrob. Chemother., 10,* 483.

26. Funk EA, Strausbaugh LJ (1982) Antimicrobial activity, pharmacokinetics, adverse reactions, and therapeutic indications of cefoperazone. *Pharmacotherapy, 2,* 185.

27. Pakter RL, Russell TR, Mielke CH et al (1982) Coagulopathy associated with the use of moxalactam. *J. Am. Med. Assoc., 248,* 1100.

28. Clancy CM, Glew RH (1983) Hypoprothrombinemia and bleeding associated with cephamandole. *Lancet, 1,* 250.

29. Bruch K (1983) Hypoprothrombinemia and cephalosporins. *Lancet, 1,* 1983.

30. Carmine AA, Brogden RN, Heel RC et al (1983) Cefotaxime. A review of its antibacterial activity, pharmacological properties and therapeutic use. *Drugs, 25,* 223.

31. Udall JA (1965) Human sources and absorption of vitamin K in relation to anticoagulation stability. *J. Am. Med. Assoc., 194,* 127.

32. Gustafsson BE (1980) Vitamin K deficiency in germfree rats. *Nutr. Rev., 38,* 344.

33. Neu HC (1982) The in vitro activity, human pharmacology and clinical effectiveness of new betalactam antibiotics. *Ann. Rev. Pharmacol. Toxicol., 22,* 599.

34. Platt R (1982) Adverse effects of third-generation cephalosporins. *J. Antimicrob. Chemother., 10, Suppl. C,* 135.

35. Buening MK, Wold JS, Israel KS et al (1981) Disulfiram-like reactions to beta-lactams. *J. Am. Med. Assoc., 245,* 2027.

36. Lode H (1983) Pharmacokinetics of new cephalosporin antibiotics: cefotaxime, cefoperazone, moxalactam. *Intern. Med., 2,* 7.

37. Ueda Y (1983) Clinical and bacteriological efficacy of cefoperazone sodium in worldwide studies of 4,485 adults and pediatric patients. *Intern. Med., 2,* 15.

38. Ueda J, Ohmori M, Saito A et al (1979) Clinical studies of cefoperazone (T-1551) in the field of internal medicine in Japan. *11th Int. Congress Chemotherapy, Boston 1979,* Abstract 401.

39. Gordon AJ, Lahon H, Pfyfferoen M (1980) A review of cefoperazone in clinical use. *Proc. 2nd Intern. Symp. Cefoperazone Sodium, at the XVth Intern. Congr. Internal Medicine, Hamburg.*

40. Brewer W, Franke D (1980) Clinical experience with cefoperazone in the treatment of surgical infections. *Proc. 2nd Intern. Symp. Cefoperazone Sodium, at the XVth Intern. Congr. Internal Medicine, Hamburg.*

41. Kemmerich B, Lode H (1980) Clinical experience with cefoperazone in respiratory tract infections. *Proc. 2nd Intern. Symp. Cefoperazone Sodium, at the XVth Intern. Congr. Internal Medicine, Hamburg.*

42. Norrby R, Alestig K (1981) High frequency of gastrointestinal adverse reactions to single doses of cefoperazone in healthy volunteers. *Lancet, 2,* 1417.

43. Gibbs DL, Hakes JL, Ando G (1983) Intestinal side effects of cefoperazone, in perspective. *J. Antimicrob. Chemother., 10,* 559.

44. Springer AD, Schacht J, Agranoff BW (1976) The effect of memory blocking antibiotics and their analogs on acetylcholinesterase. *Pharmacol. Biochem. Behav., 5,* 1.

45. Idzikowski C, Oswald I (1983) Interference with human memory by an antibiotic. *Psychopharmacology, 79,* 108.

46. Benitz K, Roberts GS, Usa A (1967) Morphologic effects of minocycline in laboratory animals. *Toxicol. Appl. Pharmacol., 11,* 150.

47. Attwood H, Dennett X (1976) A black thyroid and minocycline treatment. *Br. Med. J., 2,* 1109.

48. White SW, Besanceney C (1983) Systemic pigmentation from tetracycline and minocycline therapy. *Arch. Dermatol., 119,* 1.

49. Bilano RA, Ward WQ, Little WP (1983) Minocycline and black thyroid. *J. Am. Med. Ass., 249,* 1887.

50. Saul SH, Dekker A, Lee RE et al (1983) The black thyroid. Its relation to minocycline use in man. *Arch. Pathol. Lab. Med., 107,* 173.

51. Kelly RG, Kanegis LA (1967) Metabolism and tissue distribution of radioisotopically labeled minocycline. *Toxicol. Appl. Pharmacol., 11,* 171.

52. Pfeifer H, Greenblatt D, Friedman P (1979) Effects of three antibiotics on theophylline kinetics. *Clin. Pharmacol. Ther., 26,* 36.

53. Pfeifer H, Greenblatt D (1978) Clinical toxicity of theophylline in relation to cigarette smoking: a report from the Boston Collaborative Drug Surveillance Program. *Chest, 72,* 455.

54. Mathis JW, Prince RA, Weinberger MM et al (1982) Effect of tetracycline hydrochloride on theophylline kinetics. *Clin. Pharm., 1,* 446.

55. Seto JT, Lepper MH (1954) The effect of chlortetracycline, oxytetracycline, and tetracycline administered intravenously on hepatic fat content: a quantitative method of study including failures of some vitamins and other drugs to mitigate the effect. *Antimicrob. Agents Chemother., 4,* 666.
56. Gwee MCE (1982) Can tetracycline-induced fatty liver in pregnancy be attributed to choline deficiency? *Med. Hypothesis, 9,* 157.
57. Editorial (1983) Latamoxef and haemorrhage. *Reactions, 9 September,* 10.
58. Ferres H, Nunn B (1983) Penicillin metabolites and platelet function. *Lancet, 2,* 226.
59. Lipsky JJ (1983) N-Methylthiotetrazole inhibition of the gamma carboxylation of glutamic acid: possible mechanism for antibiotic-associated hypoprothrombinemia. *Lancet, 2,* 192.
60. Wold JS, Buening MK, Hanasono GK (1983) Latamoxef-associated hypoprothrombinaemia. *Lancet, 2,* 408.
61. Anon (1983) Moxalactam boxed warning about bleeding problems. *FDA Drug Bull., 13,* 16.

T. Midtvedt

27 Miscellaneous antibiotics

R Antibiotics and oral contraceptives

Various drugs, including antibiotics, may cause failure of oral contraceptives (OC) and induce menstrual disorders. However, it is far from easy to demonstrate clearly that an antibiotic has been responsible for an oral contraceptive failure. The infection itself – for which the drug is prescribed – may also interact with the menstrual cycle. At least theoretically, the antibiotic may interfere with the action of OC by: (1) reducing the amount of steroid absorbed or reabsorbed from the gut, (2) stimulating their hepatic degradation, (3) increasing their urinary excretion, (4) displacing them from their biologic receptor site, or (5) opposing their action through some physiologic effect.

In 1971 it was reported that rifampicin seemed to cause a high incidence of breakthrough bleeding (1[C]). Later reports, covering the period from 1973 to 1977 implicated rifampicin as the cause of 17 pregnancies in women taking OC (2[R]). Rifampicin (like barbiturates and phenytoin) may cause an induction of the formation of hepatic microsomal enzymes also capable of breaking down OC. A similar mechanism may also be involved in the OC failures attributed to sulfonamides and chloramphenicol (3[R], 4[R]). An increased incidence of breakthrough bleeding has been reported in patients taking OC together with phenoxymethylpenicillin, neomycin and nitrofurantoin (5[R]). Ampicillin, given during pregnancy to non-infected women, caused a reduction in maternal plasma and urinary estriol (6[R]) which has been assumed to be brought about by an interference of ampicillin with the enterohepatic circulation of estriol (7[R]).

Recently certain cases of breakthrough bleeding in patients simultaneously receiving OC and cefalexin have been reported (8[C]), and 2 pregnancies while on OC seem also to have occurred as a result of concurrent use of this antibiotic (8[C], 9[C]).

Failures of OC have also been recorded in patients receiving various tetracyclines (10[R]). This interaction is thought to be caused by an interference with the intestinal flora, thereby reducing the amount of steroid absorbed – or reabsorbed – from the gut.

As recently underlined (10[R]), OC and antibiotics have been used concurrently by tens of thousands of women over a considerable number of years, and yet it is only relatively recently that adverse reactions have been suspected. This of course may indicate a low incidence of interactions between OC and antibiotics. However, if doctors became more aware of this potential problem, the incidence of breakthrough bleeding and unwanted pregnancies could be reduced further. It might be wise to follow a rule saying that 'any patient on oral contraception for whom a new drug is being prescribed should be warned, and extra precautions should be given in any cycle during which antibiotics are administered' (8[C]).

MACROLIDES

Macrolides and carbamazepin

An interaction between troleandomycin (TAO) and carbamazepin (CBZ) is well established (SEDA-6, 247), and now two more macrolides seem to share this risk with TAO.

A clinical picture similar to that reported by Dravet et al (11[C]) in their patients on TAO and CBZ (dizziness, nausea, vomiting), has now been described by Straughan (12[C]) in 2 children receiving CBZ for epilepsy when erythromycin was introduced. The

Side Effects of Drugs Annual 8
M.N.G. Dukes, editor

ISBN 0 444 90339 9
$0.80 per article per page (transactional system)
$0.20 per article per page (licensing system)

symptoms disappeared after withdrawal of erythromycin.

A comparative study of the pharmacokinetics of CBZ in 10 subjects receiving the drug alone or associated with josamycin showed an increased half-life and decreased plasma levels of CBZ while josamycin was given (13[C]).

Although the clinical implications of these findings have yet to be evaluated, it seems wise to act as if all macrolides might interact with CBZ, i.e. use of macrolides should be avoided in patients receiving CBZ.

Erythromycin-induced digoxin toxicity

Although therapeutically known since 1785, digitalis and its derivatives are still able to raise new and unexpected problems. Recently, the first recognized case of erythromycin-induced digoxin toxicity was described (14[C]).

A 71-year-old woman underwent a heart operation and was put on digoxin 0.25 mg/day. Steady state digoxin levels obtained periodically over a 10-month period ranged between 1.4 and 1.7 ng/ml. Four days before admission to hospital, she developed cough and wheezing, and erythromycin was prescribed. Because of nausea, which occurred only after she ingested the medication, she stopped taking erythromycin after only 4 tablets. Two days later she was hospitalized. Shortly after admission, she developed severe nausea and vomiting. An electrocardiogram at that time showed an A-V junctional rhythm; the digoxin level was 2.6 ng/ml. After stopping digoxin, nausea abated and sinus rhythm returned. Subsequently, digoxin was resumed at a lower dosage. One month later, digoxin 0.25 mg/day, was resumed and the steady-state digoxin level was 1.3 ng/ml.

This patient thus developed elevation of digoxin levels associated with ECG and gastrointestinal toxicity 3–4 days after receiving 1 gram of erythromycin. The changes occurred even though she had been taking the same dosage of digoxin as before; toxicity did not recur when the same dosage of digoxin was resumed one month later. She did not demonstrate any changes in renal and hepatic functions. The author suggests that a small dose of orally administered erythromycin can alter gut flora substantially, resulting in an increase in the serum levels of digoxin to toxic values.

Erythromycin and interaction with warfarin

As also described in Chapter 26, many antibiotics may interact with normal hemostasis, particular interest having focussed on the newer cephalosporins with a methyltetrazole side chain at position 3 on their molecule. Now it is reported that erythromycin apparently interacts with warfarin (15[C]).

A 59-year-old woman (55 kg), on maintenance warfarin therapy (4 mg daily) for several months and having a prothrombin time (PT) twice the control value, was given erythromycin ethylsuccinate 400 mg 4 times daily for parotitis. On admittance to hospital 4 days later, her PT was 120 sec (control: 12 sec) and her activated partial thromboplastin time was 72 sec (control: less than 35 sec). After withdrawal of erythromycin her PT rapidly returned to baseline values and she was put on a maintenance therapy of 4 mg warfarin, with no subsequent problems.

The above authors also performed some experiments in rats. Their findings were consistent with inhibition of warfarin metabolism by erythromycin. Systemic warfarin clearance is governed by mixed function oxidases (MFOs) in the liver. Recently, another macrolide antibiotic (troleandomycin) has been shown to decrease the in vitro activity of the hepatic MFOs in rats (16[R]).

It is more than interesting – it is amazing – that two drugs available for general prescription for more than 25 years have only recently been identified as potentially serious interactants. The significance of – and the mechanism behind – this interaction should indeed be evaluated.

Erythromycin estolate and jaundice *(SED-9, 467)*

Another contribution to the long history of erythromycin estolate as a cause of jaundice has come from Inman's group at Southampton. Prescription/event monitoring of 12,208 patients treated with erythromycin estolate, erythromycin sterate or tetracycline led to the identification of 3 cases of antibiotic-related jaundice in erythromycin stearate patients; no case was attributable to the estolate (30[Cr]).

Josamycin and hepatotoxicity

The hepatic toxicity of various preparations of erythromycin has been known for a long time (SEDA-5, 250; SEDA-7, 283). Recently, another macrolide, josamycin, has been shown to be hepatotoxic (17[C]).

Messer and Willard gave josamycin in granule form, 50 mg/kg/day for 8–10 days, to 30 newborns. In all, 8 cases showed raised levels of alkaline phosphatases and one case showed a moderate rise in transaminases. The rise in the levels of alkaline phosphatases was stated to be moderate in 6 cases and marked in the 2 others. It is noteworthy that the levels of alkaline phosphatases were increased in 4 out of the 5 prematures receiving josamycin. The authors did not state when raised enzymatic levels returned to normal values.

Josamycin should clearly not be given to premature infants.

CHLORAMPHENICOL

Chloramphenicol toxicity in adults

The 'gray baby syndrome', occurring in neonates after receiving chloramphenicol, is very well known. The presumed mechanisms are decreased hepatic conjugation due to inadequate glucuronyl transferase activity combined with decreased glomerular filtration in the neonatal period. A similar vasomotoric collapse has, however, also been reported in older patients (18[C], 19[C]), and now also the teenagers have to be put on the list (20[C]).

A previously well 16-year-old girl was admitted to hospital and treated with chloramphenicol (approximately 100/mg/kg/day) for a rickettsial infection. During her stay in hospital she became progressively more ill and developed metabolic acidosis, peripheral vascular insufficiency and encephalopathy. On day 4, her chloramphenicol serum levels showed a trough of 122 μg/ml and a peak of 140 μg/ml (therapeutic levels 10–25 μg/ml). The chloramphenicol therapy was stopped on day 5 and the serum levels declined slowly; being 90 μg/ml on day 7 and 24 μg/ml on day 9. These results, among others, indicate reduced hepatic function. After chloramphenicol therapy was stopped, the clinical status of the patient gradually improved, and she left the hospital on day 11.

Rickettsial infections such as Rocky Mountain spotted fever can produce a somewhat similar clinical picture, but patients with severe rickettsial disease usually present their symptoms before treatment. The progressive worsening parallelling the rise in serum concentration of chloramphenicol and her improvement when the serum concentration of chloramphenicol declined strongly indicate that this was indeed a case of chloramphenicol-induced 'gray teenager syndrome'.

LINCOMYCIN AND CLINDAMYCIN

Clindamycin-induced cardiac arrest

As early as in 1968, Waisbren (21[C]) reported in 4 patients, an association between large doses of rapidly administered intravenous lincomycin and cardiac arrest. Without stating the dose and infusion rate, he noted that when similar doses were administered slowly, the drug was well tolerated. Intravenous lincomycin given rapidly in high doses to animals has resulted in hypotension, supraventricular arrhythmias, premature ventricular contractions, ventricular fibrillation and cardiac standstill (22[R]).

Clindamycin is structurally a lincosamine antibiotic very similar to lincomycin. The first case of cardiac arrest associated with rapid intravenous administration of clindamycin has now been reported (23[C]).

A 50-year-old woman was admitted to hospital for evaluation of crampy, abdominal pain and bloody diarrhea, starting after an elective aortobifemoral bypass. On admission there was no evidence of peritonitis or obstruction. Her symptoms persisted and, 12 days after admission, an X-ray showed free air in the abdomen. She was taken for surgery at which a perforated distal colon and a pelvic abscess were found. 45 min into the procedure, 600 mg of undiluted clindamycin phosphate was injected over 'several minutes' into a central intravenous line. Immediately after the drug was given, the patient developed ventricular bigeminy, second-degree heart block, and finally complete heart block in rapid succession, and the systolic blood pressure fell to 60 mg Hg. After immediate treatment with isoprotenerol, atropine sulfate and sodium bicarbonate the patient's electrocardiogram reverted from complete heart block to paroxysmal atrial tachycardia within 2 minutes. After two bolus injections of 0.5 mg of propranolol hydrochloride the heart returned to normal sinus rhythm.

Some days later, the patient received clindamycin, 600 mg every 6 hours, given intravenously over 30 min, and now without any cardiovascular complications. Thus it seems likely that the observed cardiovascular effects were not the results of hypersensitivity to the drug, but a toxic interaction directly related to the rapid infusion.

It might be mentioned that structural similarities between quinidine and the lincosame antibiotics have been noted, and quinidine has been reported to induce ventricular fibrillation (24[R]). Clindamycin can better not be injected undiluted intravenously and the infusion rate should not exceed 30 mg/min (25[R]).

Clindamycin and leukocytoclastic angiitis

There have been rather few reports on side effects associated with clindamycin therapy apart from intestinal disorders. Skin reactions consist mainly of various minor skin eruptions (SEDA-7, 389) and more severe reactions, as Stevens-Johnson syndrome, seem to be rare (26[C]). Now a case of leukocytoclastic angiitis, most probably induced by clindamycin, is reported (27[C]).

A 57-year-old man with a 17-year history of diabetes mellitus, was admitted to hospital for osteomyelitis. Blood cultures were positive for *Staphylococcus aureus,* and therapy with tobramycin (70 mg intravenously every 8 hours) and clindamycin (600 mg intravenously every 6 hours) was initiated. During the next few days the patient gradually improved, but on the 5th day he complained of generalized arthralgia, and on the 6th day he developed a diffuse, palpable, diffuse rash. Both antibiotics were discontinued and in the ensuing 3 days the pain in his joints subsided and the skin eruption diminished. Clindamycin, in the same dosage as before, was administered, and within 24 hours his symptoms and skin eruption reappeared. A skin biopsy specimen showed an inflammatory cell infiltrate (consisting of neutrophils, lymphocytes, and occasional plasma cells) in the upper dermis, centering around the small vessels which showed destruction on their walls, deposition of fibrin, leukocytoclasis, and extravasation of erythrocytes.

Clindamycin was discontinued, and once again the symptoms and rash disappeared. His osteomyelitis was then successfully treated with oxacillin and tobramycin.

Obviously, leukocytoclastic angiitis occurs only rarely during clindamycin therapy. As mentioned above, clindamycin therapy is most often associated with intestinal disorders, especially so-called antibiotic-associated colitis (AAC). Most of these cases are thought to be caused by toxins liberated from *Clostridium difficile*, but in some cases neither the bacteria nor its toxins can be demonstrated. If an angiitis similar to that found in the skin can also occur in the colon wall, the symptoms might be very similar to those found in difficile-associated AAC. A prominant feature in a case of AAC previously commented upon in SEDA (SEDA-5, 272) was indeed vasculitis in the colon wall. Time will show whether some cases of AAC might be caused by the drug itself and not by an interaction on the intestinal flora leading to formation of bacterial toxin(s).

AMINOGLYCOSIDES

Nephrotoxicity of the aminoglycosides

The nephrotoxicity of all aminoglycosides is well documented (SEDA-4, 192; SEDA-5, 272; SEDA-6, 250; SEDA-7, 282) but the 'battle of the renal toxicity level' is still going on. Every time a new aminoglycoside is introduced, results are presented showing this new compound to be less nephrotoxic than those already on the market. After a while, new reports usually appear, showing the new one to be nearly as toxic as the older ones or at least advancing important cautions (31[c]). A reason for these discrepancies might be the infection itself. Clinical experience shows clearly that aminoglycosides can be administered for long periods without any signs of nephrotoxicity to patients with localized infections, so long as they have no manifestations of systemic infection, or any underlying kidney disease. Such patients are often involved in the first clinical evaluation of a new drug. In contrast, the incidence of renal damage following aminoglycosides might be much higher in patients who are seriously ill. Such patients are usually involved in clinical trials only at a later stage than the first group.

The possibility that bacterial products (endotoxin etc), might potentiate the nephrotoxicity of aminoglycosides has recently been investigated (28[C]). In rats with an experimental *E. coli* pyelonephritis and treated with gentamicin (30–60 mg/kg for various periods of time) sensitive markers of early toxicity (enzymuria, proteinuria, osmolality and histology), and late markers (C_{INU}, C_{PAH} and T_{PAH}) were strikingly more disturbed in the infected group than in either the treated, infected or normal controls.

In rats given 0.05 to 0.50 mg of *E. coli* endotoxin followed 3 hours later by a 10 mg/kg dose of gentamicin, statistically more gentamicin was found to be present in the renal cortex and medulla compared to rats receiving gentamicin only. At doses of endotoxin above 0.25 mg, a marked effect on intrarenal pharmacokinetic parameters was found. The authors put forward the assumption that endotoxin, known to be capable of modifying the physiological status of the host and also known to focalize in mitochondria and lysosomes, might 'modify the permeability of renal components, explaining the observed unusual intrarenal pharmacokinetics of gentamicin. Its direct action in lysosomes, priviliged sites where aminoglycosides tend to concentrate, could have contributed to the increased susceptibility of the pyelonephrotic kidney to aminoglycosides'.

As recently stated by Klastersky (29[R]), it is believed that 'aminoglycosides should be a part of any initial therapy of severe gram negative infection, especially in the compromized host'. Particularly in these patients, the possibility of increased nephrotoxicity due to liberated endotoxin should be kept in mind. Avoiding both Scylla and Charybdis is as hard as ever.

REFERENCES

1. Reimers D, Jezek A (1971) The simultaneous use of rifampin and other antituberculous agents with oral contraceptives. *Prax. Klin. Pneumol., 25,* 225.
2. Beckenridge AM, Back DJ, Orme M (1979) Interactions between OCs and other drugs. *Pharmacol. Ther., 7,* 617.
3. Hempel E, Bohm W, Carrol W et al (1973) Medikamentose enzyminduktion und hormonale kontrazeption. *Zentralbl. Gynaekol., 95,* 1451.
4. Back DJ, Breckenridge AM (1978) Drug interactions with oral contraceptives. *IPPF Med. Bull., 12,* 1.
5. Stockley I (1976) Interactions with oral contraceptives. *Pharmaceutical J., 216,* 140.
6. Willman K, Pulkinen MO (1971) Reduced maternal plasma and urinary estriol during ampicillin treatment. *Am. J. Obstet. Gynecol., 109,* 893.
7. Tikkanen MJ, Pulkkinen MO, Adlercreutz H (1973) Effect of ampicillin treatment on the urinary excretion of estriol conjugates in pregnancy. *J. Steroid Biochem., 4,* 439.
8. Friedman M, Divon M, Peretz BA (1982) Cephalexin and Microgynon-30 do not go well together. *J. Obstet. Gynaecol., 2,* 195.
9. DeSano EA, Hurley SC (1982) Possible interactions of antihistamines and antibiotics with oral contraceptive effectiveness. *Fertil. Steril., 37,* 853.
10. Stockley I (1982) Tetracyclines and oral contraceptives. *J. Am. Acad. Dermatol., 7,* 279.
11. Dravet C, Mesdjian E, Roger J (1980) Triacetyloleandomycin et carbamazepine. *Concours Méd., 103,* 1980.
12. Straughan J (1982) Erythromycin-carbamazepine interaction? *S. Afr. Med. J., 61,* 420.
13. Albin H, Vincon G, Pehourco F et al (1982) Influence de la josamycine sur la pharmacocinétique de la carbamazepine. *Thérapie, 37,* 151.
14. Friedman HS, Bonventre MV (1982) Erythromycin-induced digoxin toxicity. *Chest, 82,* 202.
15. Schwartz J, Bachmann K, Perrigo E (1983) Interaction between warfarin and erythromycin. *South. Med. J., 76,* 91.
16. Pessayre D, Konstantinova-Mitcheva M, Descatoire V et al (1981) Hypoactivity of cytochrome P-450 after triacetyloleandomycin administration. *Biochem. Pharmacol., 30,* 559.
17. Messer J, Willard D (1982) Clinical trial of josamycin in a neonatology ward. *Drugs Exp. Clin. Res., 8,* 313.
18. Thompson WL, Anderson SE, Lipsky JJ et al (1977) Overdose of chloramphenicol. *J. Am. Med. Assoc., 234,* 149.
19. Graft AW, Brocklebank JT, Hey EN et al (1974) The 'grey toddler'. *Arch. Dis. Child., 49,* 235.
20. Brown RT (1982) Chloramphenicol toxicity in an adolescent. *J. Adolesc. Health Care, 3,* 53.
21. Waisbren BA (1968) Lincomycin in larger dose. *J. Amer. Med. Assoc., 206,* 2118.
22. Daubeck JL, Daughbety MJ, Petty C (1974) Lincomycin-induced cardiac arrest: a case report and laboratory investigations. *Anesth. Analg., 53,* 563.
23. Aucoin PA, Beckner R, Nelson MG (1982) Clindamycin-induced cardiac arrest. *South. Med. J., 75,* 768.
24. Selzer A, Wray HW (1964) Quinidine syncope: paroxysmal ventricular fibrillation occurring during treatment of chronic atrial arrhythmias. *Circulation, 30,* 17.
25. Upjohn Pharmaceuticals (1980) Cleocin phosphate package insert. Kalamazoo, Mich., April 1980.
26. Maulide T, Villar TG (1974) Therapeutic trials with clindamycin in non-tuberculosis infections of the respiratory tract. *Pneumologia, 5,* 79.
27. Lambert WC, Kolber LR, Proper SA (1982) Leukocytoclastic angiitis induced by clindamycin. *Cutis, 30,* 615.
28. Bergeron MG, Beauchamp D, Poirier A et al (1983) Increased gentamicin nephrotoxicity in the presence of pyelonephritis: the role of endotoxin. *Proc. 13th International Congress of*

Chemotherapy, Vienna.
29. Klastersky J (1983) Clinical effectiveness of aminoglycosides. *Proc. 13th International Congress of Chemotherapy, Vienna.*
30. Inman WHW, Rawson IVSB (1983) Erythromycin estolate and jaundice. *Br. med. J., 286,* 1954.
31. Bhattacharya BK, Gorringe H, Farr MJ (1983) Netilmicin and nephrotoxicity. *Lancet, 2,* 216.

A.V. Astahova

28 Antifungal drugs

GENERAL TOPICS

Since the publication of the last Annual, various new reviews on side effects of antifungal drugs have appeared in the literature (1[R], 2[R], 3[R]).

The review of Daneshmend and Warnock (1[R]) provides an overview of the pharmacokinetics of these drugs, their interactions and also of the relationship between their pharmacokinetics and unwanted effects. It is, for example, stressed that while *amphotericin B* invariably causes dose-related renal damage, this does not markedly alter its pharmacokinetics.

Since *flucytosine* is largely eliminated by renal excretion, serum concentrations are markedly increased in the presence of renal impairment, but the drug itself does not prove toxic to the kidneys. Although gastrointestinal, hepatic and hematological side effects of flucytosine are uncommon, there is some evidence to suggest that in certain patients these may be related to serum concentrations rather than to idiosyncrasy. Bone marrow toxicity is likely when serum flucytosine concentrations are 125 mg/l or more, and this is more likely in the presence of renal impairment. The bone marrow depression is usually reversible following reduction of serum flucytosine concentrations. However, 10 fatal instances of bone marrow suppression have been reported (4[R]).

The relationship between gastrointestinal and hepatic side effects and serum concentrations is even less well established. Present evidence suggests that the likelihood of toxicity is reduced if serum flucytosine concentration does not exceed 100 to 125 mg/l. This is well above the mean steady-state concentration range of 35 to 70 mg/l recommended as effective in antifungal chemotherapy.

For the treatment of various systemic fungal diseases it is advisable to combine flucytosine with amphotericin B. Amphotericin B, however, invariably causes a deterioration in renal function, thereby increasing flucytosine serum concentrations and half-life. This is probably the most common important drug interaction with flucytosine, although any drug which impairs renal function will similarly cause flucytosine toxicity. Flucytosine is competitively inhibited by cytarabine (cytosine arabinoside) and should therefore not be used in patients receiving the latter drug.

Serum concentrations of *miconazole* are higher in renal failure, but dosage adjustment is rarely necessary. As far as *ketoconazole* is concerned, absorption is decreased in renal failure (and when gastric acidity is reduced). Beyond this, renal and hepatic diseases do not appear to affect ketoconazole kinetics.

The antimicrobial and pharmacokinetic properties of the three classic antifungal agents and their side effects are also reviewed by Graybill and Graven (3[R]), who provide dosage guidelines designed to minimalize the risk of adverse reactions; these are summarized in Table 1.

INDIVIDUAL DRUGS

Amphotericin B *(SED-9, 475; SEDA-4, 201; SEDA-5, 275; SEDA-6, 253; SEDA-7, 287)*

Hematological *Thrombocytopenia* has occasionally been noted in patients receiving amphotericin B. However, because of concomitant chemotherapy, the presence of sepsis, or an underlying malignancy such as leukemia in relapse, a definite cause-and-effect relation between amphotericin B and thrombocytopenia could hitherto not be established.

Side Effects of Drugs Annual 8
M.N.G. Dukes, editor

ISBN 0 444 90339 9
$0.80 per article per page (transactional system)
$0.20 per article per page (licensing system)

Table 1. *Administration schedule for amphotericin B, flucytosine and miconazole*

Amphotericin B

1. Dilute drug in at least 200 ml of sterile dextrose and water (not sodium chloride solution)
2. Via peripheral vein, administer 1 mg over 1 to 2 hours
3. If no severe reaction, administer 10 mg over 2 to 4 hours shortly after initial 1 mg dose
4. If patient is acutely ill, proceed to give 0.3 to 0.5 mg/kg over next 2 to 4 hours. Maximum dose is 1 mg/kg/day
5. If patient is not acutely ill, dose may be increased by increments of 10 mg/day to full daily dose (0.3 to 1.0 mg/kg)
6. Because of slow clearance of amphotericin B, it may be preferable to give dose every other day
7. Monitor serum creatinine twice weekly and electrolytes (hypokalemia due to tubular renal acidosis may require K^+ replacement)

Flucytosine

1. If normal renal function, give 150 mg/kg/day orally in 4 divided doses
2. If renal function impaired, dosage should be monitored by blood levels to maintain serum level between 50 and 100 μg/ml
3. Monitor complete blood count for evidence of thrombocytopenia, leukopenia

Miconazole

1. Dilute each dose into at least 200 ml of sterile dextrose and water
2. Administer over a minimum period of 1 hour intravenously
3. Repeat dose every 8 hours. Maximum adult dose is 1200 mg 8-hourly
4. To administer intrathecally, withdraw 5 to 10 ml of CSF in syringe, mix with miconazole (up to 20 mg per dose) and reinstil. This can be done in a closed system using a 3-way stopcock for mixing, with 2 syringes and spinal needle attached

Chan et al (5^C) have now described a patient with acute leukemia in complete hematologic remission who developed reversible thrombocytopenia during two courses of amphotericin B for the treatment of hepatic candidiasis. The absence of other definable causes for thrombocytopenia and reversal when amphotericin B was stopped provide strong evidence for a causal relation.

During the first course of therapy the patient received amphotericin B concomitantly with 5-fluorocytosine. After 2 weeks of amphotericin B therapy (after receiving a total dose of 1.5 g), the patient developed fever and rigor which persisted despite the withdrawal of both antifungal agents. The platelet count declined from 240,000/mm³ during the early phase of amphotericin B therapy to 130,000/mm³ when the drugs were discontinued, finally reaching a level of 30,000/mm³. Bone marrow examination showed a virtual absence of megakaryocytes with normal maturation of the granulocyte and erythroid series. 10 days after discontinuation of the antifungal drugs, the platelet count had returned to normal.

During the second course of therapy, amphotericin was restarted without 5-fluorocytosine for fear that the latter was the cause of the thrombocytopenia. 2 weeks later, however, the platelet count again plunged to a low of 30,000/mm³. Bone marrow examination again showed marked megakaryocytopenia without evidence of leukemic relapse.

Amphotericin B was continued at a dose of 55 mg every other day with close monitoring of platelet count. The authors felt that amphotericin B should be discontinued only if the platelet count declined further or if bleeding complications occurred. Surprisingly, in this case the platelet count stabilized at the 30,000 to 80,000/mm³ level which permitted continuation of therapy for an additional 3 months until resolution of the clinical symptoms.

When amphotericin B therapy was stopped, the platelet count rapidly rose to 200,000/mm³ within 2 weeks.

Amphotericin B appears to have caused thrombocytopenia in this patient by suppressing platelet production rather than peripheral destruction of platelets. This is similar to the mechanism of anemia associated with amphotericin B (SED-9, 476). Thrombocytopenia induced by amphotericin B appears to be reversible despite prolonged use. The development of thrombocytopenia is not an absolute contraindication to continued amphotericin B therapy. However, caution should be taken to monitor closely platelet counts and clinical bleeding.

Mineral balance Gallar et al (6^C) have reported on 2 patients with mucormycosis and systemic candidiasis respectively who were treated with amphotericin B at doses of 925 mg in 30 days and 640 mg in 35 days. Both developed *hypokalemia* secondary to loss of potassium and *distal renal tubular acidosis* during the course of treatment. In the second case, the renal acidosis was incomplete, and the PCO_2 gradient between urine and plasma after bicarbonate administration was above 30 mm Hg, a fact which is considered characteristic of distal tubular acidosis induced by amphotericin B. This patient also presented with nephrogenic diabetes insipidus. Glomerular filtration rate remained within normal limits in both patients. In the first case renal functional alterations reverted 6 months after drug withdrawal, whereas in the second case they persisted 4 months after stopping the drug.

Weddington (7[Cr]) observed a 39-year-old man with disseminated histoplasmosis who developed *delirium and depression* after treatment with amphotericin B administered intravenously.

Following the first few injections the patient experienced chills and mild dysphoria. During the hospital stay the daily dosage of amphotericin B was progressively raised to 60 mg, but the patient became increasingly anxious and restless. This was attributed to the hospitalization and he was soon discharged. 8 hours after the first dosage of 60 mg amphotericin B as an outpatient, he developed a fever of 99.2°F (37.3°C) and emotional irritability. Additionally the patient manifested dysphoria, confusion, hyperverbal productions and suicidal thoughts during and after amphotericin B therapy. The dosage of amphotericin B was gradually reduced to 40 mg daily. The behavioral symptoms were controlled with haloperidol. 4 months after completing amphotericin B treatment, the patient had returned to normal. The author suggests that patients receiving amphotericin B be carefully monitored for any change in mental or behavioral status.

No similar cases appear to have been described before.

Nervous system 2 cases of *acute polyneuropathy* in young alcoholic women after oral administration of amphotericin B were reported by Audry et al (8[C]). Neuropathy extended to all 4 limbs and the face. These neurological manifestations are unusual and probably comprized an aggravation of preexistent neuropathy, but neuropathy or neurotoxicity have occasionally been described with amphotericin B before (SED-9, 475; SEDA-6, 254).

Whether *Parkinsonism* could be an adverse effect of amphotericin B or not remains very uncertain despite a report to this effect by Fisher and Dewald (9[C]). Their patient, as they point out themselves, was suffering from cryptococcal infection which may have involved the basal ganglia and for which treatment was instituted; this could provide a sufficient explanation of the complication.

THE IMIDAZOLES

Ketoconazole *(SEDA-5, 276; SEDA-6, 256; SEDA-7, 287)*

With the increasing usage of this drug it is not surprising to notice an accumulation of new findings and reviews (10[R], 11[R], 12[R]). One review concludes that patients tolerate up to 60 days of therapy with ketoconazole well (10[R]). The drug has been given continuously to patients for more than 2 years, but the small number receiving such therapy only allows a preliminary view of its long-term safety. Approximately 10% of patients treated with ketoconazole (most of them for weeks or months) have shown adverse reactions that include nausea, vomiting, headache, dizziness, constipation, diarrhea, somnolence, nervousness, and pruritus. The most frequent adverse reactions, nausea and pruritus, have been observed in approximately 3% of the patients. The gastrointestinal tract symptoms may usually be avoided by taking ketoconazole immediately before a meal.

Gynecomastia This seems to be a rare idiosyncratic reaction unrelated to estrogen or androgen effects and possibly caused by a direct effect of ketoconazole on breast tissue. Again, dosage, schedule, cumulative dose, and length of treatment do not seem to be determining factors. An incidence of 0.2% was cited in Annual 7 (2 cases in a series of 1361 treated).

Risk factors Since the drug is metabolized and excreted via both the renal and hepatic routes, it seems that the drug can safely be used in the face of renal failure. Because of the idiosyncratic hepatotoxicity it would not be prudent to use ketoconazole for patients with hepatic failure. Considering that some of the patients with hepatotoxicity had an antecedent history of hepatitis, it would seem wise, until more is known, to avoid prescribing ketoconazole to patients recovering from hepatitis.

Second generation effects Since the safety of ketoconazole has not been established in gestation, the drug, like most medications, should not be recommended for use during pregnancy. Until adequate information is available, the drug must be used cautiously, if at all, in lactating mothers and infants.

Safe dosage levels Hume and Kerkering (11[r]), who have reviewed the role of ketoconazole in antifungal chemotherapy, point out that most data on ketoconazole have been derived from uncontrolled open trials and case reports. Until well-controlled studies and long-term experience are available, ketaconazole should be used cautiously. Against the background of these remarks, the dosage recommendations of these authors are interesting. Their recommended daily dose of ketoconazole for adults is a single 200-mg tablet. For serious infections and inadequately responding mycoses, ketoconazole 400 mg may be administered in a single daily dose, according to the manufacturer. For children older than 2 years of age, the dosage is based on the following weights: ≤20 kg, 50 mg/day; 20–40 kg, 100 mg/day; >40 kg, 200 mg/day.

Dosage guidelines for the presence of renal and hepatic failure are not available (see above). The duration of treatment is not well defined. Therapy should be continued at least until the active infection has subsided. The manufacturer suggests a minimum of 1 to 2 weeks for candidiasis, while chronic mucocutaneous candidiasis in most cases required maintenance therapy. The minimum duration of treatment for the other indicated mycoses is 6 months.

Ketoconazole and the liver

The 3 cases of massive hepatic necrosis which triggered regulatory action in the USA in 1982 were reviewed in Annual 7 (p. 289) together with a number of other related reports.

The hepatotoxicity does not seem to relate to the daily dosage, the cumulative total dose, or the length of therapy. Its frequency is low: 10 cases have been identified from all the patients treated to date. Since the patients in question have generally been asymptomatic, and the toxicity initially manifests only as abnormal liver enzyme function, use of ketoconazole must be accompanied by proper clinical laboratory monitoring. Monthly testing is probably sufficient to detect evidence of developing hepatotoxicity.

It has been argued, probably rightly, that the drug should be discontinued if any clinical signs of symptomatic liver dysfunction occur (13[C]). Whether ketoconazole therapy should be discontinued in the presence of nonsymptomatic increases of liver enzyme concentration is less clear. In many of these patients abnormalities of liver function will resolve even when ketoconazole is continued. Withdrawal of ketoconazole remains a decision for the clinician based on an assessment of the likely benefit-to-risk ratio in the individual patient.

Of the 32 other cases of hepatic dysfunction known to the US FDA at the time regulatory action was taken (see SEDA-7, p. 292), one involved hepatic necrosis with recovery. Signs of liver function abnormalities include elevated transaminases, as well as jaundice, bilirubin and alkaline phosphatase, accompanied by symptoms of anorexia, nausea and/or malaise. In only 5 cases eosinophilia or fever was noted. Duration of ketoconazole therapy ranged from 11 to 110 days (mean duration 56 days) and daily doses from 100 mg to 400 mg (mostly 200 mg) daily. 23 of the cases were in females and 9 in males, and the mean age was 57 with a range of 35–83 years. It is notable that the indication for which the drug was used in most cases was a superficial topical infection.

The mechanism of hepatic dysfunction with ketoconazole is still unknown. All cases of liver function abnormalities occurred in normal therapeutic doses. Signs of hypersensitivity were present in 1 case as eosinophilia and in 2 cases as fever.

14 cases of liver function abnormalities associated with the use of ketoconazole were reported to the American Academy of Dermatology. 6 of these cases were symptomatic, i.e. malaise, loss of appetite or dark urine. All 14 cases exhibited abnormal liver function tests.

Trach and Rinaldi (14[C]) have reported on a second case of severe hepatitis associated with ketoconazole therapy in a child of 6 years with chronic mucocutaneous candidiasis.

Svejgaard and Ranek have described a case of biopsy-proven toxic hepatitis in a patient treated with ketoconazole (15[C]).

A 48-year-old physician was included in an open, multicenter study of ketoconazole for treatment of fingernail onychomycosis. The patient had no history of liver disease nor of excessive ethanol intake and took no other medications. Ketoconazole was administered in a single oral daily dose of 200 mg. Improvement of the nail infection was obvious after 8 weeks of therapy and a slight increase in serum ALT, although still within normal limits, was found. One month later, fatigue and nausea suddenly occurred, leading to cessation of therapy after 81 days. Laboratory studies showed markedly elevated ALT. This rise was further accelerated by intake of a single ketoconazole dose (200 mg) 48 hours before studies were done on day 86. At that time, icterus was present along with marked malaise.

In addition to ALT, serum bilirubin, alkaline phosphatase, and lactic dehydrogenase, were all markedly elevated. Viral hepatitis (types A and B) was excluded by serologic studies. Ultrasonic and computed tomographic scanning of the liver and pancreas showed no abnormalities. The patient refused a liver biopsy. Abnormal laboratory findings gradually subsided, and findings were within normal limits 2 months after the episode.

Kramer et al (16[C]) have described liver damage in a woman aged 24 years with a postulated dermatomycosis which was treated with ketoconazole.

The patient had no history of hepatology, had not used alcohol to excess and had used no other medication. 4 months after treatment was instituted, nausea and jaundice developed. Results of liver function tests were comparable with parenchymal liver damage. Biopsy of the liver revealed enlarged portal tracts with mononuclear cell infiltration and piecemeal necrosis. Serological testing for a possible viral cause gave negative results. After discontinuation of ketoconazole the symptoms subsided and liver function returned to normal 6 weeks later.

Toxic hepatitis caused by ketoconazole was also observed by Boëtius et al (17[C]) in 2 patients. After discontinuation of the use of this drug, one patient recovered spontaneously, while the other required a period of prednisone therapy.

A 1-year-old boy presented with recurrent infections of the fingers. At first, these were partially controlled by oral penicillin, but the condition progressively deteriorated, causing repeated shedding of the fingernails. At the age of 2 years, his parents noted the onset of repeated episodes of oral thrush which appeared as white plaques on the buccal mucosa. Liquid nystatin held in the mouth did not control the problem. At the age of 5 years, dermatologic consultation was requested, and the patient was subsequently treated with little success with nystatin, miconazole, cloxacillin, and clotrimazole.

At the age of 6 years, ketoconazole treatment was started with 100 mg taken orally once a day. After 5.5 months of ketoconazole therapy, the patient suddenly developed nausea, vomiting, and jaundice. Ketoconazole therapy was stopped. On physical examination he was afebrile and jaundiced. His liver was palpable 5 cm below the right costal margin. Laboratory values included the following: total bilirubin 10.4 mg/dl; direct bilirubin 7.8 mg/dl; indirect bilirubin 2.6 mg/dl; SGOT 2150 U/l; SGPT 1980 I.U./l; prothrombin time 93% of control; total protein 6.5 g/dl; albumin 4.4 g/dl.

The patient recovered 3 months after ketoconazole therapy was discontinued. The authors conclude that this patient had an adverse reaction to ketoconazole. This conclusion is based on the lack of evidence demonstrating an infectious cause. It is suggested that periodic liver function tests be performed when a child is on ketoconazole therapy to guard against the possibility of hepatitis.

5 patients described by Dijke (18[C]) developed parenchymatous hepatitis while using ketoconazole and recovered after discontinuation of the drug. No viral cause could be found, and 4 of the 5 patients used no other medication that may cause hepatitis, so that a causal relationship with the use of ketoconazole may be assumed.

Elevations of lactic dehydrogenase (LDH) and aspartate aminotransferase (AST) were noted by Strauss (19[C]) in a patient of 52, who had a long-standing history of persistent tinea pedis and onychomycosis of the toenails.

She had previously been treated with tolnafate, clotrimazole, and miconazole topically and griseofulvin orally without success. Potassium hydroxide preparations from her toenails were strongly positive, and Trichophyton rubrum was cultured from the toenails. She was treated with ketoconazole. At the beginning of treatment she received ketoconazole in daily doses of 200 mg (during 3 months), then 400 mg (during 2 months), and again 200 mg (during 2 months). It should be noted that there was a transient, relatively mild, elevation of the AST on the laboratory screen taken about 6 weeks after the drug was started. The LDH was also increased on this occasion. The AST gradually returned to normal while therapy was continued. No other elevations of the LDH were noted at this time. However, a second rise in the AST was noted after the therapy was stopped. This was progressive and marked; the AST reached a level of 346 I.U./l. The second rise in the AST continued to increase for at least a week after therapy was stopped. There was a slower increase in the LDH, but the rise was much less. After the drug was stopped, the abnormal laboratory values slowly returned to normal and remained normal throughout the last examination.

While no liver biopsy was performed in this case and there was no way to evaluate whether the patient could have had non-A, non-B hepatitis, it was felt that the abnor-

malities in the liver function tests probably reflected transient liver damage since they were temporarily associated with the use of ketoconazole. It should be noted that the changes in the enzyme levels followed a 60-day period when ketoconazole had been increased to 400 mg/day for 60 days, but the increase continued on the lower dosage of 200 mg/day. Because of the continued increase in the AST, the drug was stopped and, it was therefore not determined whether the liver enzyme elevation would have been reversed if ketoconazole had been continued.

The authors conclude that in spite of the low incidence of such abnormalities physicians should carefully monitor all patients who receive ketoconazole during long-term therapy in high doses.

Individual case histories of liver damage attributed to ketoconazole continue to appear, and no attempt will be made here to consider them all individually since some are very similar; the cases cited in detail above present a fair picture of the type of reactions which can occur. One paper by Pegram et al (20[C]) does, however, suggest that a patient with a history of alcoholism, apparently responsible for the presence of portal fibrosis with early bridging, may have been at greater risk of (reversible) hepatic derangement during ketoconazole treatment than would otherwise have been the case.

Janssen and Symoens (21[R]), representing the manufacturer of ketoconazole, have reviewed all the cases of silent and symptomatic hepatic reactions that had been reported during ketoconazole treatment down to March 1982. The pattern of silent hepatic reactions was investigated in detail in 1074 patients in whom laboratory investigations were performed during clinical studies. The patients, of both sexes and aged between 1 and 86 years, had been treated for various deep and superficial mycoses with daily doses of ketoconazole between 50 and 1000 mg (usually 200 mg) for various periods of time up to 15 months.

The liver enzyme data of these 1074 patients were systematically screened for elevations of 50% above the upper limit of the normal range of SGOT, SGPT, GT and/or alkaline phosphatase just before or at any time during ketoconazole treatment. 148 (14%) patients showed such elevations on one or more occasions before and/or during treatment. However, 8% of the patients had elevated enzyme levels before ketoconazole treatment, and this increased to 11% during treatment, while the elevations were somewhat more pronounced. Towards the end of treatment, the incidence of elevated enzyme levels (6%) dropped to pretreatment levels. The elevations of SGOT, which occurred at any time, were transient and tended to be less frequent towards the end of treatment. None of the observed changes was accompanied by any symptoms suggestive of hepatitis. The transient elevations of liver enzymes during treatment often paralleled the healing of the fungal disease.

By the same date, i.e. March 1982, 31 patients had been reported with either icteric signs (jaundice and/or dark urine and pale stools) or anicteric symptoms (fever, fatigue, weakness, malaise, anorexia, nausea, vomiting) during ketoconazole treatment. The majority of patients with reported symptomatic hepatic reactions had onychomycosis. It is not known what proportion of all patients who received ketoconazole had onychomycosis, but it is almost certainly much lower than 70%. The authors suggest that patients with onychomycosis may thus be more prone to develop symptomatic reactions to ketoconazole than patients with other mycotic infections, but other confirmatory evaluation is needed.

Of the 31 patients with reported hepatic reactions (18 women and 13 men) more than half were over 50 years of age. At least 9 of the patients with a symptomatic hepatic reaction while taking ketoconazole had a history of idiosyncrasy to other drugs; 8 had a previous history of hepatitis. At least 14 patients (45%) had been treated with griseofulvin before, usually for a year or more, and at least 19 had one or more concomitant treatments.

Symptoms usually occurred within the first few months of treatment: the median time of onset of icteric reactions was 6 weeks (extremes 1 and 20 weeks), and of anicteric reactions 11 weeks (extremes 3 and 24 weeks).

In conclusion: silent and symptomatic reactions have occurred during ketoconazole treatment. The silent reactions may occur at any time during ketoconazole treatment. Minor asymptomatic elevations of serum transaminase or alkaline phosphatase levels during ketoconazole treatment are in the manufacturer's view as a rule no reason to discontinue the medication, but each individual case should be evaluated, and the decision to continue therapy should be based upon total medical assessment.

Symptomatic hepatic reactions have occurred mainly during the first few months of treatment. The estimated incidence of symptomatic reactions is of the order of 1/10,000. The available data suggest that the phenomenon is reversible upon discontinuation of treatment. The authors conclude that if symptoms and signs of hepatic disorder are detected in a patient, it is sound medical practice to interrupt existing medications promptly. This applies not only to many drugs which induce liver reactions (e.g. isoniazid, diazepam, methyldopa, sulfonamides) but also to ketoconazole.

The clinical experience of Rollman and Loof (22[C]) with this agent in the treatment of onychomycosis fully confirms the necessity of vigilant supervision of liver function in patients on ketoconazole treatment. These authors, however, do not agree with Janssen and Symoens that asymptomatic increases in serum liver enzyme levels during ketoconazole therapy are harmless and no reason for withdrawing the drug. During an 8-month therapeutic trial of ketoconazole 4 of their 36 patients developed various types of liver reactions possibly induced by the drug. They demonstrated with the help of histopathological techniques that a hepatic lesion may be present even though liver-derived enzymes show only slight aberrations. Furthermore, they showed that it is not possible to predict from the first observed abnormal liver function tests whether a progressive liver reaction has been initiated.

KETOCONAZOLE AND HORMONES

Several articles on the effects of ketoconazole on hormone production have appeared since the publication of Annual 7.

The gynecomastia and loss of libido and of potency occasionally observed in men taking antifungal imidazole-ketoconazole (Nizoral) may, according to Schurmeyer and Nieschlag (23[C]), be related to a decrease in testosterone available to the target organs, despite the views of some workers to the contrary. Certainly, hormonal effects can and do occur.

5 healthy male volunteers treated by Schurmeyer and Nieschlag received a single oral dose of 400 mg ketoconazole. both serum and saliva testosterone concentrations fell sharply; the lowest values were found 4 to 6 hours after drug ingestion when serum and saliva levels had fallen to 30% and 34% of basal levels respectively, well within the range of values found in hypogonadal men. Pharmacokinetic studies revealed a reciprocal relationship between testosterone levels and ketoconazole levels.

Pointing out that the salivary testosterone concentration is a good index of serum free testosterone, these West German researchers conclude that the parallel decrease in serum and saliva testosterone indicates that the decrease in total serum testosterone is accompanied by a decrease in available testosterone at the target organs. In their view investigations of long-term effects of ketoconazole treatment on hormonal indices and fertility should be carried out in men receiving ketoconazole.

Pont et al (24[Cr]) have shown that ketoconazole is a potent inhibitor of testosterone synthesis in humans and unisolated rat Leydig cells. The development of gynecomastia in 2 patients prompted them to investigate the effect of the drug on testosterone production.

A 38-year-old man received 200 mg daily of ketoconazole, which was subsequently increased to 600 mg daily. Seven months after starting the therapy, painful bilateral gynecomastia developed. The serum testosterone concentration was 402 ng/dl 24 hours after a dose (normal, 300 to 1,100 ng/dl). 4 hours after this dose, however, the testosterone concentration was 91 ng/dl. The gynecomastia resolved spontaneously in 1 month despite continuation of ketoconazole therapy. At no time did the patient experience sexual dysfunction.

Primary cutaneous coccidioidomycosis in a 22-year-old man was treated with ketoconazole 200 mg daily, subsequently increased to 400 mg daily. There was a rapid resolution of all active disease. In 1 month of therapy gynecomastia developed. A breast biopsy specimen demonstrated ductal hyperplasia. The patient denied sexual dysfunction. Serum testosterone concentration was 260 ng/dl 4 hours after his ketoconazole dose, and 1,100 ng/dl 24 hours after dose.

Studies have also been performed in normal volunteers and in vitro in rat material to examine the effect of ketoconazole on testosterone levels. In men, 2 hours after a 600 mg dose, the testosterone level had declined significantly from 698 ± 314 to 287 ± 13 ng/dl. The testosterone level fell 30% to 73% in the 4 volunteers. The testosterone level remained depressed between

4 and 8 hours after the dose, and the nadir of testosterone concentration occurred between 4 and 12 hours after the dose. By 24 hours, the testosterone concentration was normal in 1 subject, and was minimally below the baseline value in the other 3. The testosterone level also fell in subjects who received 400 mg of ketoconazole. 8 hours after a 400 mg dose, the testosterone level appeared to be starting its return to baseline. In subjects who received 200 mg, the fall in testosterone level was initially less dramatic and appeared to be returning to baseline 4 hours later. The luteinizing hormone levels also rose modestly in all male volunteers. 8 hours after a 600 mg dose, the LH level had increased from 8.7 ± 1.5 to 13.1 ± 0.8 Imu/ml. 24 hours after the dose, the mean LH level was 13.3 ± 2.3 Imu/ml.

The exposure of rat Leydig cells to 0.5 mg/l ketoconazole, a serum concentration easily achieved in patients treated with the drug at currently recommended doses, dramatically reduced both basal and stimulated testosterone production, and totally inhibited both by increasing the ketoconazole concentration to 50 or 500 mg/l.

The authors conclude that the effect of ketoconazole on testosterone synthesis need not diminish its clinical usefulness. At currently recommended doses, patients tolerate the drug well and rarely manifest hormone-related side effects. However, it is clear that patients with resistant fungal diseases will sometimes be given the drug at higher doses and more frequently than once a day. Careful attention will then have to be paid to the possible development of side effects secondary to diminished testicular, ovarian, or adrenal steroid synthesis.

Engelhardt et al. (25[Cr]) have studied the influence of ketoconazole on the cortisol secretion in a patient with a cortisol producing adrenal adenoma. Repeated oral doses of ketoconazole (200 mg every 5 hr over a period of 48 hr) induced a reproducible, clear-cut fall of serum cortisol levels to below 2.5 μg/dl. The inhibitory effect on cortisol secretion could be detected for the first time 5 hr after the first dose, and 9 hr after the last dose. Moreover, the inhibitory effect of ketoconazole on cortisol secretion could be reproduced in vitro by incubating tissue slices of the excized adrenal tumor together with the antifungal agent in concentrations equivalent to therapeutic serum levels. These findings emphasize that patients with an autonomous cortisol production caused by an adrenal tumor are prone to dangerous hypoadrenalism if treated with ketoconazole.

High dose ketoconazole for fungal infections of the central nervous system

Previous reports of cerebrospinal fluid penetration of ketoconazole after oral doses of 200 and 400 mg have shown low or undetectable concentrations, and efficacy could generally not be evaluated. The apparent safety of this agent suggested that higher doses might provide effective cerebrospinal fluid drug levels without excessive toxicity. A study by Craven et al (26[c]) provides a systematic evaluation of the pharmacokinetics of ketoconazole in the cerebrospinal fluid during high-dose treatment of 6 young male patients with fungal infection of the central nervous system. The authors evaluated the ventricular and lumbar cerebrospinal fluid penetration of ketoconazole and the response to therapy in 2 patients receiving ketoconazole orally, 800 mg daily, and amphotericin B intraventricularly for meningeal and extrameningeal coccidioidomycosis. 5 patients received ketoconazole only (1200 mg): one had uncomplicated coccidioidal meningitis, one a histoplasmal brain abscess and 3 had obstructive hydrocephalus due to coccidioidal meningitis.

Clinical results in 5 patients with active coccidioidal meningitis suggest that treatment with 800 mg ketoconazole plus amphotericin B intraventricularly or 1200 mg ketoconazole alone, is effective. All patients responded to ketoconazole with clear improvement during 8 to 15 months of therapy.

Several consistent findings were observed in this study: ketoconazole was detected in the lumbar and ventricular fluid of all patients after the 800 or 1200 mg dose; ketoconazole could not be detected in the cerebrospinal fluid of any patient 24 hours after either dose; penetration from blood into cerebrospinal fluid was greater for lumbar fluid (5.4% ± 2.6%) than for ventricular fluid (1.9 ± 0.8%). This degree of lumbar fluid penetration is similar to that of penicillin in subjects with inflamed meninges. In both locations, cerebrospinal fluid concentrations were directly dependent upon serum levels in a linear manner, suggesting that higher doses of ketoconazole will result in further elevations of cerebrospinal fluid concentrations. Ketoconazole concentrations in cerebrospinal fluid were further augmented by elevated protein values, consistent with the high protein binding of ketoconazole.

Prolonged therapy with these high doses (up to 3 years thus far) appears to be well tolerated. 2 patients have tolerated combined regimens well, without gastrointestinal symptoms (except briefly after instillation of amphotericin B) or evidence of marrow, renal or hepatic toxicity, or gynecomastia.

Gynecomastia (1 patient, receiving 1200 mg ketoconazole alone during 15 months), a mild increase in nipple sensitivity (after 8 months of therapy with ketoconazole alone) and modest elevations in serum alanine aminotransferase, alkaline phosphatase, and γ-glutaryl transpeptidase (less than 3 times the normal value, after 24 months of therapy) have been the only adverse effects of ketoconazole in this series.

OTHER ADVERSE REACTIONS OF KETOCONAZOLE

Cox et al (27[c]) have reported their experience with ketoconazole in 19 patients with superficial dermatophyte infections. The patients were treated with 200 to 400 mg per day orally, which proved to be an effective dose level. Adverse reactions to ketoconazole developed in 6 patients. One patient developed a *generalized drug eruption* after the first dose of ketoconazole, and minor side effects were noted in 5; 3 patients complained of *nausea*, 1 of *increased appetite*, and 1 of transient *visual disturbance* (blurring). The latter complaint could not be substantiated on ophthalmologic examination. Therapy was discontinued only in the patient with generalized eruption. This side effect is uncommon (see SEDA-7, 290).

Clotrimazole *(SED-9, 477; SEDA-6, 258; SEDA-7, 287)*

A self-medication therapy with clotrimazole vaginal tablets, involving application of 2 tablets at bedtime on 3 consecutive days, was carried out to find out whether vulvo-vaginal mycoses could be treated more effectively and with fewer drop-outs when treatment is simpler and shorter (28[c]). The study included 41 patients. The results of this study suggest that this regimen of treatment is effective and particularly suited for primary infection. Only in 1 case was burning experienced after insertion of the vaginal tablet, so that treatment was discontinued; no other side effects were observed.

Miconazole *(SED-9, 478; SEDA-4, 202, 207; SEDA-5, 282; SEDA-6, 254; SEDA-7, 292)*

10 cases of drug *interactions* with miconazole have been reported by Loupi et al (29[C]): 4 interactions with oral anticoagulants, 3 with hypoglycemic sulfonamides and 3 with CNS drugs. The analysis of these reports showed that miconazole might increase pharmacological effects of these other drugs. The mechanism is thought to involve enzyme inhibition.

Flucytosine *(SED-9, 476; SEDA-4, 201; SEDA-6, 259; SEDA-7, 287)*

In published series, flucytosine has been estimated to cause *diarrhea* in approximately 6–10% of patients. A potentially fatal ulcerating *enterocolitis* has been reported in 4 patients. In none of these reports have radiologic or pathologic data been presented. A report by White and Traube (30[C]) is the first to describe radiographic and biopsy findings of flucytosine-associated ulcerative enteritis.

A 66-year-old man was admitted to hospital because of headache and confusion of 10 days' duration. The patient had a history of insulin-requiring diabetes and chronic liver disease of presumed alcoholic etiology. Cerebrospinal fluid and urine cultures eventually grew *Cryptococcus neoformans.* The patient received oral flucytosine, 7.0 g (150 mg/kg/day in 4 divided doses) and intravenous amphotericin B, 15 mg daily. At the end of 5 weeks of treatment, the patient developed abdominal discomfort and diarrhea. Physical examination revealed abdominal distention, without organomegaly, abdominal masses, or tenderness.

Small bowel X-ray revealed severe luminal narrowing of the distal half of the small bowel with ulceration and marked separation of loops of bowel. A biopsy specimen was obtained from the terminal ileum. Microscopic examination of this specimen revealed an erosive enteritis with many polymorphonuclear leukocytes, eosinophils, and mononuclear cells infiltrating the mucosa. There was disruption of the surface epithelium. Flucytosine and amphotericin B were discontinued. Over the following 2 weeks the patient improved clinically with resolution of diarrhea and abdominal bloating. A repeat small bowel X-ray demonstrated only minimal dilatation of the ileal lumen.

Although it is impossible to be certain that this syndrome resulted from flucytosine therapy alone, published experience with amphotericin B single-agent and combination therapy would support this conclusion.

Fond et al (31[C]) reported a fatal case of colitis during treatment with flucytosine; there were neither ulcerations nor pseudomembranes. The complications developed in a 60-year-old man with cryptococcus neuromeningitis after 37 days of flucytosine treatment (180 mg/kg/day). The histological data, with significant lesions, were consistent with a toxic-induced disorder of protein synthesis.

Shelley and Sica (32[c]) have reported their experience of using fluorocytosine in treating sporotrichosis. They found it helpful in 1 patient. Cure was achieved after 6 months of fluorocytosine treatment (8 g/day) in conjunction with amphotericin B (total 4.8 g). The flucytosine was continued for an entire year. The only complication was a marked *photosensitivity* associated with the flucytosine therapy. The patient first noted a pruritic dermatitis of the dorsum of his hands associated with exposure to sunlight. The photosensitivity gradually became worse, so that an acute exudative dermatitis of the superior helices of the ears as well as the face developed whenever he was in the sun for a few hours. This sensitivity persisted throughout his entire 12-month course of flucytosine and did not disappear until 12 months after the flucytosine was discontinued. This is the second case of such photosensitivity in the literature.

Griseofulvin *(SED-9, 474; SEDA-6, 259; SEDA-7, 293)*

The dermatological side effects of griseofulvin are now well known. Manifestations have included urticaria, photosensitivity eruptions, lichen planus, erythema, erythema multiforme, vesicular and morbilliform rashes, serum sickness-like reactions, and angioedema. There are a few reports of cases in which lupus erythematosus was unmasked or exacerbated. However, there are no previous reports of griseofulvin being associated with exacerbation of *leprosy* or with a downgrading reaction.

Shulman et al (33[C]) have now described the first case of a downgrading reaction associated with griseofulvin. The latter is a subtype of the type 1 (lepra) reaction and represents an acceleration of the spontaneous movement of untreated non-polar leprosy toward the lepromatous leprosy. It may involve a sudden decrease in cell-mediated immunity, resultant proliferation of bacilli, and the development of a vicious cycle with increased antigen load and decreased immunity. The authors observed a dramatic alteration from clinically subpolar tuberculoid leprosy toward subpolar lepromatous leprosy during griseofulvin therapy in a 29-year-old man with normal cell-mediated immunity. They suggested that this reaction was due to inhibition of polymorphonuclear leukocyte chemotaxis by griseofulvin.

REFERENCES

1. Daneshmend TK, Warnock DW (1983) Clinical pharmacokinetics of systemic antifungal drugs. *Clin. Pharmacokin., 8,* 17.
2. Koldin MN, Medoff G (1983) Antifungal chemotherapy. *Pediatr. Clin. of North Am., 30,* 49.
3. Graybill JR, Craven PC (1983) Antifungal agents used in systemic mycoses activity and therapeutic use. *Drugs, 25,* 41.
4. Scholer HJ (1980) Flucytosine. In: Speller (Ed.), *Antifungal Chemotherapy,* p. 35.
5. Chan CSP, Tuazon U, Lessin LS (1982) Amphotericin B-induced thrombocytopenia. *Ann. Intern. Med., 96,* 332.
6. Gallar P, Ruilope LM, Perez AJ et al (1982) Nefrotoxicidad inducida por anfotericina B. Presentacion de 2 casos. *Nefrologia, 2,* 133.
7. Weddington WW (1982) Delirium and depression associated with amphotericin B. *Psychosomatics, 23,* 1076.
8. Audry D, Marchal G, Lambery D, Guard O et al (1982) Neuropathie aiguë après prise orale

d'amphotericine B. *Lyon Méd., 14,* 67.
9. Fisher JF, Dewald J (1983) Parkinsonism associated with intraventricular amphotericin B. *J. Antimicrob. Chemother., 12,* 97.
10. Jones H (1982) Ketoconazole. *Arch. Dermatol., 118,* 217.
11. Hume AL, Kerkering TM (1983) Ketoconazole (Nizoral, Janssen Pharmaceutica). *Drug Intell. Clin. Pharm., 17,* 169.
12. Sohn CA (1982) Evaluation of ketoconazole. *Clin. Pharm., 1,* 217.
13. McNair AL, Gascoigne E (1981) Hepatitis and ketoconazole therapy. *Br. Med. J., 283,* 1058.
14. Trach JR, Rinaldi MG (1982) Severe hepatitis associated with ketoconazole therapy for chronic mucocutaneous candidiasis. *Cutis, 29,* 482.
15. Svejgaard E, Ranek L (1982) Hepatic dysfunction and ketoconazole therapy. *Ann. Intern. Med., 96,* 788.
16. Kramer NSM, Montnor LP, Berghuis PHE (1983) Toxische hepatitis tijdens gebruik van ketoconazol (Nizoral). *Ned. Tijdschr. Geneeskd., 127,* 343.
17. Boëtius G, Peeters JPC, Peters JH (1983) Toxische hepatitis door ketoconazol (Nizoral). *Ned. Tijdschr. Geneeskd., 127,* 341.
18. Dijke CPH (1983) Hepatitis tijdens gebruik van ketoconazol (Nizoral). *Ned. Tijdschr. Geneeskd., 127,* 339.
19. Strauss JS (1982) Ketoconazole and the liver. *J. Amer. Acad. Dermatol., 6,* 546.
20. Pegram PD et al (1983) Successful ketoconazole treatment of protothecosis with ketoconazole-associated hepatotoxicity. *Arch. Intern. Med., 143,* 1802.
21. Janssen PAJ, Symoens JE (1983) Hepatic reactions during ketoconazole treatment. *Am. J. Med., 18,* 80.
22. Rollman O, Lööf L (1983) Hepatic toxicity of ketoconazole. *Br. J. Dermatol., 108,* 376.
23. Schurmeyer TH, Nieschlag E (1982) Ketoconazole induced drop in serum and saliva testosterone. *Lancet, 2,* 1098.
24. Pont A, Williams PL, Azhar S et al (1982) Ketoconazole blocks testosterone synthesis. *Arch. Intern. Med., 142,* 2137.
25. Engelhardt D, Mann K, Hormann R et al (1983) Ketoconazole inhibits cortisol secretion of an adrenal adenoma in vivo and vitro. *Klin. Wochenschr., 61,* 373.
26. Craven PC, Graybill JR, Jorgensen JH et al (1983) High-dose ketoconazole for treatment of fungal infections of the central nervous system. *Ann. Intern. Med., 98,* 160.
27. Cox FW, Stiller L, South A, Stevens DA (1982) Oral ketoconazole for dermatophyte infections. *J. Am. Acad. Dermatol., 6,* 455.
28. Higashide K, Kawaguchi C, Tomoda Y (1983) Three-day clotrimazole therapy for vulvo-vaginal mycosis. I. *Intern. Med. Res., 11,* 21.
29. Loupi E, Descottes J, Leky N, Evreux JCl (1982) Interactions médicamenteuses et miconazole. A propos de 10 observations. *Thérapie, 37,* 437.
30. White CA, Traube J (1982) Ulcerating enteritis associated with flucytosine therapy. *Gastroenterology, 83,* 1127.
31. Fond B et al (1983) Colite introgène au cours d'un traitement par la flucytosine pour crytpococcose neuromeningée. *Sem. Hôp. Paris., 58,* 1187.
32. Shelley WB, Sica PA (1983) Disseminate sporotrichosis of skin and bone cured with 5-fluorocytosine: photosensitivity as a complication. *J. Am. Acad. Dermatol., 8,* 229.
33. Shulman DG, Wilkinson D, Nguyen N (1982) Leprosy downgrading reaction associated with griseofulvin. *Arch. Dermatol., 118,* 909.

I. Nir

29 Antiprotozoal drugs

ANTIMALARIAL DRUGS

Chloroquine *(SED-9, 482; SEDA-5, 278; SEDA-6, 261; SEDA-7, 294)*

Chloroquine, as well as continuing to be the drug of choice for malarial suppression and treatment, is also used for a wide spectrum of other indications. The diversity of the conditions, the enormous size of the populations treated and the prolonged periods for which this drug has been employed expose it to many forms of adverse events. Numerous somatic side effects and iatrogenic diseases, including gastrointestinal, neurological, dermatological, hematological and cardiovascular complications, have been attributed to it in the literature.

Moreover, the fact that this drug possesses an extremely long half-life renders it liable to accumulate in high concentrations in various tissues, including the brain, where it may precipitate *personality changes* and possibly lead to various *psychotic syndromes.* Delirious behavior and a state of fluctuating impairment of thinking, memory and perception is produced. This state of toxic psychosis may also take the form of irrational compulsive impulses or even a tendency to suicide. In their review dealing with behavioral toxicity, Good and Shader (1[R]) conclude that the mental status of patients receiving chloroquine should be carefully evaluated.

Poisoning and reportedly death have occurred with relatively mild overdosage, although these could be considered hypersensitivity reactions.

Acute intoxication A case of acute intoxication was presented (2[C]), in which a young woman swallowed 5 g of chloroquine. When first examined 13 hours after ingesting the drug she appeared conscious and normal. The first changes recorded were electrocardiographic, and ventricular fibrillation developed. Electrical shock was without effect and cardiac arrest occurred. The cardiac state improved with diazepam. In another case mentioned in the same report, a young man took 6 g of chloroquine. Here, too, the main symptoms were cardiac, as evidenced by ECG changes, and again the application of diazepam was beneficial and contributed to less fulminant development of the disease.

Incidence of adverse reactions Follow-up of 90 polyarthritic patients after prolonged use (up to 7 years) of relatively high doses (250–500 mg daily) of chloroquine together with other nonsteroidal antiinflammatory agents or corticosteroids showed rare and mild adverse reactions comprising 4 sleep disturbances, 2 incidences of dizziness and 1 case of photosensitivity on exposure to the sun. In some patients with highly active disease, leukopenia and lymphopenia were occasionally observed (low absolute figures of T and B lymphocytes) (3[C]).

Neuromyopathy Neuromyopathy was described in an 18-year-old girl who received 100 mg of chloroquine prophylactically for 6 days. She complained of losing the strength in her legs but had no pain. Muscular biopsy at the quadriceps level indicated denervation atrophy without signs of inflammation, whilst electromyographic tracing presented signs of neurogenic and myogenic changes (4[C]).

Pigmentation 10 young white patients who had been taking 150 mg of chloroquine daily, together with 15 mg pyrimethamine, and complained of hyperpigmentation, were found to have pigmentation of the gums over and between the teeth (5[C]). 5 patients had increased pigmentation of the lips and 4 over the whole body, including nail bases,

Side Effects of Drugs Annual 8
M.N.G. Dukes, editor

ISBN 0 444 90339 9
$0.80 per article per page (transactional system)
$0.20 per article per page (licensing system)

nipples and scars. Ophthalmological examination revealed no ocular lesions, but biopsy of the skin in 6 patients indicated melanin pigmentation in the epidermis. The total dosage ingested before pigmentation changes appeared ranged from 28 to 144 tablets within a period of several months. The pigmentation was still present and seemed unchanged 4 months after terminating pyrimethamine intake. It should be noted that pigmentation due to pyrimethamine is rare.

Eye lesions Of the toxic effects of chloroquine, eye lesions have been considered as the most serious since they can progress to an irreversible and disabling loss of visual acuity. A case of bilateral edema of the optic nerve following antiinflammatory therapy with chloroquine has now been described (6^C). The woman patient had been taking 200 mg of chloroquine daily for 2.5 months.

An unusual pattern of delayed onset and progression of a chloroquine maculopathy was reported in a man who had received the drug as antimalarial therapy for 2 years (7^C). When first seen 2 years after discontinuing chloroquine therapy, a granular macular appearance was noted with near normal vision. Progressive decreased central acuity was recorded during the following years, and 9 years after ceasing chloroquine therapy, vision had dropped to a level defined in law as blindness, with dense central scotomas. Fluorescein angiography revealed 'bull's eye' maculopathy compatible with chloroquine retinopathy. This case illustrates the possibility of progressive ocular damage despite discontinuance of the drug and a delayed sustained deleterious effect of chloroquine on the retina.

When corneal and retinal changes occur with chloroquine, it is usually with high dosages (300–500 mg daily). In malaria prophylaxis, where 300 mg weekly is given, retinopathy is rare (8^R). In recent years, however, a number of publications have indicated the possibility of retinopathy occurring after several years' prophylactic chloroquine treatment. It has been argued that in all these instances the drug was clearly over-dosed and that total intake must exceed 100 g before retinopathy can be observed (8^R). Certainly ocular toxicity with low chloroquine dosage is only seen very rarely, especially when administration of the drug is periodically interrupted (9^R), but the 100 g minimum is not absolute. In another report (10^R) retinopathy due to chloroquine was noted in 14 patients of a group receiving 250–750 mg daily during periods varying from 2 to 20 years; the total quantity consumed here varied between 45 and 3600 g. The pathology was studied in depth and classified into 3 categories according to the degree of lesions established.

Amodiaquine *(SED-9, 485; SEDA-7, 296)*

Diffuse *conjunctival and corneal changes,* which included intralysosomal membranous and amorphous inclusions in the epithelial cells, and *abnormal retinal tests* were observed in a 34-year-old man who had ingested 250 g amodiaquine HCl over a period of about a year (11^C). The drug was discontinued and a more than 2-year follow-up revealed a decrease in clinical and electron microscopic abnormalities, though retinal function tests continued to produce abnormal results. It was concluded that amodiaquine should be on the list of drugs capable of inducing a *phospholipidosis-like disorder.*

Out of 20 patients on amodiaquine therapy for onchocerciasis given 22–68 mg/kg body weight over 2 to 9 days, 12 suffered various side effects (12^C). The most striking adverse reactions were *gastrointestinal disturbances,* involving nausea, vomiting, diarrhea or constipation, and insignificant transient *granulocytopenia.* In the dosages used, the drug proved ineffective against adult worms and microfiliariae of *O. volvulus.*

Hydroxychloroquine

A white woman suffering from psoriatic arthropathy developed severe *exacerbation of psoriatic skin lesions* between the 2nd and 3rd week of hydroxychloroquine therapy. This report gives support to those who believe that patients with psoriatic arthropathy are more susceptible to severe skin reactions whilst on hydroxychloroquine therapy (13^C).

Mefloquine

A single 20 mg/kg body weight dose of mefloquine in children and 750 mg in adults is considered the treatment of choice for falciparum malaria resistant to 4-aminoquinolines (14^C). This single dose curative therapy is possible because of the long half-life (about 15 days) of this 4-quinoline-methanol derivative. When the above-mentioned dosages were used, the main adverse symptoms observed were *nausea, giddiness* and *vomiting.* When dosages were increased to 30 mg/kg in children and to 1000 mg in adults, a higher frequency of vomiting was recorded in the adults (14[C]).

Occasional nausea and vomiting with general *malaise* were observed in 8 African blacks treated with 1 g mefloquine on a single day; no other pathology was reported. Good clinical tolerance and effectiveness was also found in 44 patients of both sexes and various ages and ethnic origins given 1.25 to 1.5 g divided into 2–3 doses as a daily curative treatment (15[C]).

Oxamniquine

Several double-blind studies were carried out to evaluate the cure rate of schistosomiasis versus adverse reactions of oxamniquine as compared to placebo or other drugs used in treating this malady.

In Brazil, 48 children with chronic schistosomiasis mansoni were treated with a single oral dose of oxamniquine 20 mg/kg body weight (16[C]). Adverse reactions encountered, mainly on the day of treatment, were *drowsiness, nausea, dizziness, vomiting, abdominal pain, cough, ronchi* and *wheezing.* A significant *rise in blood eosinophils and SGPT* was found on day 30 post treatment. Transitory *urinary urobilinogen, bilirubin* and *proteinuria* were noted on first examination 10 hours after treatment. All abnormal laboratory findings thereafter became negative. Transitory *pulmonary changes* characterized by pulmonary condensation were present in 7 children on days 3 and 5 post treatment. These pulmonary X-ray changes receded spontaneously and none was present on day 30 post treatment. Good therapeutic efficacy was recorded.

Oxamniquine vs niridazole Another evaluation of the cure rate of schistosomiasis versus adverse effects was undertaken using oxamniquine 20 mg/kg/day for 3 consecutive days, comparing it with niridazole 25 mg/kg/day for 6 days (17[C]). Both drugs produced a high cure rate in adults, but in children niridazole was far more effective. *Fever* and *epigastric colic* were the most frequent adverse reactions in oxamniquine, while *headache, fever* and *CNS symptoms* (dizziness, withdrawn personality) were more common with niridazole. The total number of side effects was higher with niridazole (48% vs 26% with oxamniquine). Abnormal laboratory findings – *elevations in alkaline phosphatase* and *eosinophilia* – were equally frequent with both drugs. All symptoms and abnormal findings resolved after completing the therapy.

Oxamniquine vs praziquantel An additional double-blind study compared oxamniquine with praziquantel in the treatment of schistosomiasis using single oral doses of 20 and 65 mg/kg body weight respectively (18[C]). The 2 drugs, which have completely different chemical and pharmacological features, were both highly efficient, with similar tolerances. The patients in both treatment groups experienced side effects, among which *headache* and *giddiness* were associated more with oxamniquine and *abdominal distress* was significantly more common with praziquantel. All adverse reactions were mild to moderate and disappeared spontaneously. Similar results were recorded in a study in which oxamniquine 13–17 mg/kg and praziquantel 41–52 mg/kg were administered in single oral doses. The same adverse reactions as in the foregoing study were recorded with no differences between the drugs in parasitological cure rates(19[C]).

Piperaquine

This synthetic substance, 1,3-bis(1-(7-chloro-4′-quinolyl)-4-piperazinyl)propane, belonging to the 4-aminoquinoline group, has been used effectively against *Plasmodium falciparum.* Large field studies were undertaken in China to investigate the preventive effectiveness and tolerability in several thousands of people living in highly infected areas (20[R]). The subjects in the study were taking two 300 mg tablets of piperaquine monthly for several months. The drug, which brought about a marked decrease in malaria incidence, was fairly well tolerated. Adverse effects recorded were *headache, dizziness, vomiting* and diarrhea. In a few instances there were complaints of irregular menstruation which normalized after 2 months. It was suggested that this drug be used in cases of parasite resistance to chloroquine.

Proguanil (chlorguanide)

Serious hematological complications and other severe adverse reactions were reported in 2 male patients suffering from severe renal failure (21[C]). In one instance proguanil 200 mg/day was given for 6 weeks to a white American on vacation in Africa. He developed *anorexia, dizziness, vomiting, diarrhea, mouth ulceration* and *low white blood cell and platelet counts.* Bone marrow showed normal cellularity with gross megaloblastic changes but normal folate and B_{12} serum levels. Proguanil was not discontinued and the patient subsequently developed further hematological abnormalities. In the second instance the patient, an Anglo-Indian, had undergone bilateral nephrectomy for nephrotic syndrome and severe hypertension. Several years later he was given proguanil 100 mg daily. The patient developed an extensive *purpura* over the trunk, epistaxis and vomiting. Bone marrow examination showed hypoplasia and gross megaloblastic changes. Serum folate and B_{12} were normal, but platelet count was depressed. Although the adverse reactions observed in these 2 patients are common in advanced renal failure, Boots et al, the authors of the report, believe that in both patients proguanil treatment was responsible for the clinical and hematological abnormalities. It should be noted that megaloblastic anemia is unknown in proguanil therapy. However, the severe degree of renal failure could lead to retention and accumulation of the drug to toxic blood levels.

Pyrimethamine with sulfadoxine

Ectodermis pluriorificialis developed in a young Congolese 4 days after receiving 3 intramuscular injections of Quinimax and 2 tablets of pyrimethamine with sulfadoxine. Bilateral mucupurulent *conjunctivitis,* intense *photophobia, cutaneous lesions* and high *fever* were the main clinical features of the syndrome (22[C]). This appears to be a toxic reaction due to hypersensitivity.

A white man who took 1 tablet of pyrimethamine with sulfadoxine weekly for several weeks as antimalarial chemoprophylaxis developed severe *febrile malaise* with generalized bullous *skin rash*, diagnosed as *Stevens-Johnson syndrome.* The causative agent was shown by a specific lymphocytic transformation test to be the pyrimethamine component (23[c]). Fever and general malaise were also observed in 2 out of 9 subjects who had taken 4×1 tablet of pyrimethamine with sulfadoxine weekly, and another subject developed an extensive allergic reaction 5 days after the first tablet (24[c]). *Petechiae* and *ecchymosis* were observed in a young woman treated for acute toxoplasmic retinochoroiditis with pyrimethamine 75 mg 3 times a day for 8 days. A week later *metrorrhagia* with *pancytopenia* and *thrombocytopenia* developed. Colebunders and Mathijs, in reporting this case, suggest that treatment with high doses of pyrimethamine, a folic acid antagonist, be supplemented with folinic acid (25[c]).

Quinine *(SED-9, 485; SEDA-5, 280; SEDA-6, 263; SEDA-7, 296)*

A unique case of *acute quinine poisoning* in a young woman who had taken between 3.8 and 4.8 g quinine sulfate is described as observed at the initial stage of intoxication and 6 months later (26[C]). On day 1 general physical signs were unremarkable except for vision and hearing. The patient appeared drowsy but oriented. Biochemical tests, including electrolytes, were within normal limits. ECG showed mild Q-T interval prolongation and mild STT wave abnormalities, which resolved 9 days later. Ophthalmological examinations, including electroretinographic recordings, electro-oculograms and the pattern of visually evoked potentials, demonstrated various changes occurring at an early stage and permanent ones seen 6 months later. It was concluded that quinine exerted an early direct toxic effect on the retinal cells and caused early neural damage involving the inner nuclear layer.

Acute quinidine toxicity and pharmacokinetics were studied in 25 and 13 cases of cerebral and uncomplicated falciparum malaria respectively, following intravenous infusions of 10 mg/kg body weight of quinine hydrochloride every 8 hours (27[C]). In patients with cerebral malaria, plasma quinine concentrations consistently exceeded 10 mg/l, reaching a peak 60 ± 25 hours after treatment was begun. Total quinine clearance (Cl) and total apparent volume of distribution (Vd) were significantly lower in cerebral than in uncomplicated malaria, but no significant difference in elimination half-times (t½) or renal clearances (C_u) were evident between the groups. In a follow-up of 9 patients after recovery, Cl, Vd and C_u were significantly greater and t½ shorter than during the acute illness. Renal failure did not alter the disposition kinetics in cerebral malaria. There was no clinical or electrocardiographic evidence of cardiotoxicity and no permanent neurotoxicity. The opinion is expressed that quinine toxicity in cerebral malaria has probably been over-emphasized and that the benefits of high plasma concentrations in the acute phase of the life-threatening disease appear to outweigh the risks. The results obtained in this study should also be of assistance in adjusting quinine infusion procedures to obtain an optimal effect with minimal toxicity in cerebral and uncomplicated malaria.

DRUGS ON TRIAL

Artemether

Studies have been undertaken with artemisininelactol methyl ether, a newly synthesized antimalarial derived from artemisinine (ginghaosu) isolated from the Chinese herb *Artemisia annua L.* Falciparum malaria and vivax (829 and 259 cases respectively) were treated with intramuscular injection of an oil solution of artemether for 3 days at a total dose of 0.48–0.64 g. Most of the patients became afebrile and negative for the asexual stage within 2 or 3 days. Adverse reactions were not observed and no toxic cardiac, liver or kidney changes were evident. The dose required for 90% suppression of parasite infection (SD_{90}) was found to be 1.02 to 1.16 mg/kg given intramuscularly. LD_{50} in mice was 263 mg/kg. A reference to limited acute and short-term toxicity studies in mice, rats, dogs and monkeys is also made in the report; in the dosages used, the main pathology appears to be fatty degeneration in liver cells and weight loss (28[r]).

BRL 2-6231

BRL 2-6231 is the code name for 4,6-diamino-1,2-dihydro-2,2-dimethyl-1-(2,4,5-trichlorophenoxypropyloxy)-1,3,5-triazine hydroxychloride which has been proposed for use as an antimalarial. This substance has been found effective in mice against *P. berghei* (N. strain), which is highly resistant to pyrimethamine and cycloguanil. Preliminary clinical studies, however, indicated that the drug is poorly tolerated orally (29[r]).

DRUGS USED IN THE TREATMENT OF OTHER PROTOZOAL INFECTIONS

Metronidazole *(SED-9, 489; SEDA-4, 205; SEDA-5, 281; SEDA-6, 263; SEDA-7, 297)*

Several interesting reviews of the pharmacokinetic properties, mechanism of action and adverse effects, including mutagenicity and carcinogenicity, of metronidazole have recently been published (30[R], 31[R]). The pharmacokinetic data are of particular interest in conjunction with the recorded adverse reactions and should be helpful when estimating appropriate dosages for various clinical conditions in order to minimize unwanted effects.

When given orally, metronidazole reaches peak serum concentrations after about an hour and its bioavailability approaches 100%, not being affected either by food intake or enteric diseases. Repeated 6 to 8 hourly dosage results in some drug accumulation. Rectal administration by suppository results in peak serum concentrations after 4 hours which reaches approximately half those following equivalent oral doses. The systemic absorption of intravaginal metronidazole is extremely slow, with low peak serum concentrations (about one-fifth those obtained by oral administration), attained after 8 to 24 hours.

Metronidazole is capable of penetrating the blood-brain barrier and CSF concentration approximates 100% of serum level. The concentration in breast milk appears to be 50% or more of the concurrent serum level. The pharmacokinetics of the drug in neonates, children and pregnant women do not appear to differ significantly. In renal failure the serum half-life of metronidazole remains unchanged, although some differences may be found in that of some of the metabolites. In hepatic failure a definite trend towards longer elimination half-time has been established. Hemodialysis effectively removed both metronidazole and its hydroxy metabolites.

On the usual dose regimens of 2 g/day the adverse reactions recorded comprise: *nausea, vomiting,* mild *gastrointestinal complaints, metallic taste* and *mild diarrhea.* Occasionally the drug may produce *leukocytopenia,* usually associated with prolonged therapy with high doses. With such a regimen *neurological* side effects, including ataxia, dizziness, confusion, as well as peripheral neuropathy, have also been reported to occur.

Various studies in animal models and bacterial systems have demonstrated evidence of potential *dysmorphogenicity, tumorigenicity* and *mutagenicity* of metronidazole and some of its metabolites. However, some of these studies have been considered scientifically invalid, and population studies have not shown increased incidence of the corresponding complications. Further studies are necessary to define better the mechanism of action of metronidazole in order to improve our understanding of its potential cellular toxicity (30[R]).

The compilation of all recorded adverse reactions and their assessment, provided by Tally and Sullivan in their review, is of similar value to those using this drug (31[R]).

An evaluation of the safety of intravenous use of metronidazole as an antimicrobial drug was carried out in 72 patients receiving dosages of 500 mg every 8 hours for 48 hours or 8 days. Acute tolerance of the drug was very good and no immediate reactions were recorded. Later on, however, adverse effects including *gastrointestinal* (nausea, vomiting, diarrhea, dyspepsia), *CNS* (dizziness, confusion, drowsiness, anxiety) and *cardiovascular* (palpitation, tachycardia, chest pain) events, and several incidents of *phlebitis* in the infusion vein were recorded. Laboratory abnormalities due to the underlying microbial disease generally improved during treatment (32[C]).

Although a single, 2 g dose of metronidazole has been approved for the treatment of *vaginal trichomoniasis,* this regimen has not gained general acceptance. Aubert and Sesta (48[c]) compared the single 2 g dose with the regimen of 250 mg administered 3 times daily for 7 days. 263 women with vaginal trichomoniasis were treated. 170 returned for follow-up, 96 of whom received the single 2 g dose and 74 the 7-day treatment. The cure rates were 93.8% and 97.3% respectively, and were not significantly different. The side effects were minimal and occurred with greater frequency in the group receiving the single 2 g dose. 4 patients in this group (4.1%) reported side effects: 2 experienced nausea and vomiting, the others nausea only. None of the women treated with the standard regimen reported side effects. The authors recommend the 2 g regimen for the treatment of vaginal trichomoniasis.

CNS toxicity Convulsions and seizures due to metronidazole therapy have been described previously.

A case report has now been presented of a 56-year-old man in Guam who was given a 10-day course of metronidazole 750 mg p.o., t.i.d., on suspicion of hepatic amebic abscess. The patient had a 2-month history of intermittent fever, a 16-kg weight loss and right upper quadrant abdominal pain. He had a high hemagglutination inhibition titer for antiamebic antibody. The symptoms and the abnormality did not change after metronidazole therapy and after confirmation of the diagnosis a second similar course was started. On day 6 of this regimen the patient had a single generalized seizure. Neurological, biochemical and EEG examinations and brain scan did not indicate any pathology. Metronidazole treatment was stopped and no more seizures occurred.

On the basis of this and previous other reports, it could be implied that high doses of metronidazole may cause CNS toxicity, and convulsions should be regarded as a potential complication of such treatment (33[C]).

Seizures and prolonged *neurological abnormalities* following intravenous administration of metronidazole were reported in a 12-year-old boy who received a total of 4 g (250 mg every 6 hours) postoperatively. Clinical symptoms were of grand mal seizures over a period of 3 hours, followed by a comatose mental state, high fever and elevated blood pressure. Laboratory examinations, including blood, CSF chemistry and computed tomographic brain scan, were all normal just after his seizures. Bailes et al in concluding their report, suggest that the neurologic toxic effects of metronidazole given intravenously need further exploration, and that caution should be exerted in its future use in children (34[C]).

Serious *mental confusion, hallucinations* and *agitation* in a 65-year-old man following intravenous administration of 2 g of metronidazole has been reported by Schentag et al (35[C]). Serum concentrations of metronidazole and its hydroxy metabolite were elevated at the time of the mental status changes. Symptoms resolved within 24–48 hours after stopping the drug. No such effect was seen at a daily dose of 500 mg. The mental status of patients receiving metronidazole appeared to be associated with a relationship between the dose and the serum concentration.

Neurological function tests were carried out in 42 patients with Crohn's disease who were given metronidazole in addition to long-standing treatment with corticosteroids and salazosulfapyridine. After several months' metronidazole therapy 5 patients developed a light *polyneuropathy* with hypalgesia and hypasthesia and light paresis and occasionally, in some of them, motor NLG reduction in N. tibialis. Abnormal electrodiagnostic findings were also present in 2 patients who had no clinical symptoms (36[c]).

Tumorigenicity Long-term experimental dosing with metronidazole was found by Sloan et al in Canada to be associated with the production of an increased number of tumors in a laboratory rat model for colonic neoplasia. It was not suggested that this would happen in clinical use. However, when deciding about the application of metronidazole in Crohn's disease or ulcerative colitis, where the colon is sensitized and metronidazole given for an extended length of time, this finding should be borne in mind. Further elucidation of the metabolism of metronidazole in the rat and in human gut would be of interest (37[C]).

Benzoylmetronidazole (benznidazole) *(SEDA-5, 282; SEDA-7, 298)*

1-(2-(Benzoyl)ethyl)-2-methyl-5-nitro-1H-imidazole is a new synthetic compound recommended for use in urogenital trichomoniasis, all forms of amebiasis, giardiasis and anaerobic infections. Unpleasant *bitter taste, furred tongue, nausea, vomiting* and *gastrointestinal disturbances* are the most frequent adverse effects. *Drowsiness, dizziness, headache* and *ataxia* are rare. *Skin rashes, pruritus* and *dark urine* have also been recorded. With prolonged treatment and/or high doses, transient peripheral *neuropathy* and epileptiform *seizures* may occur. It may interact with other drugs including certain anticoagulants and with alcohol. It should not be given in pregnancy and if it is administered for more than 10 days, regular clinical and biochemical surveillance is advisable (38[r]).

Ornidazole

Mild transient side effects consisting of *nausea, headache* and *gastric discomfort* occurred in 10 out of 50 patients given two 500 mg tablets of ornidazole daily for 5 days. Parasitological cure rate was 90% (39[c]).

Tinidazole *(SED-9, 489; SEDA-4, 207; SEDA-5, 282; SEDA-6, 265; SEDA-7, 298)*

10 patients with amebic colitis and 20 with liver abscesses were treated intravenously with tinidazole 800 mg b.i.d. for up to 5 days. The drug was very well tolerated with only mild *nausea* occurring in 5 patients. The cure rate was 90% in colitis and 100% in liver abscesses (40[C]).

From an extensive review made by Carmine et al on antibacterial activity, therapeutic efficacy and pharmacological properties of intravenous tinidazole, it also appears to be very well tolerated. The main adverse features mentioned were *thrombophlebitis, nausea, diarrhea* on intravenous administration; *metallic taste, nausea* and *rash* when taken orally. As far as its genetic toxicity is concerned tinidazole should be assumed to resemble the other nitroimidazoles (41[R]).

OTHER COMPOUNDS

N-Methylglucamine antimonate

Autoimmune *hemolytic anemia* was diagnosed in a 74-year-old man with leishmaniasis after having been given N-methylglucamine antimonate 0.1 mg/kg intramuscularly for 5 days (42[C]).

Arsenobenzol

Administration of adrenaline as preventive and curative measures against the development of *encephalopathy* and other toxic effects associated with arsenobenzol treatment for trypanosomiasis was found very successful, producing a 92–100% recovery of patients with hemorrhagic encephalopathy (43[C]).

Difetarsone

This pentavalent arsenical, which has been known for many years to be useful for treating intestinal amebiasis and trichuriasis, has been considered generally innocuous, causing only rare minor reactions such as rashes, nausea, abdominal pain and reversible changes in liver function tests. However, a case has been described of generalized angioedema in a man with *Entamoeba histolytica* who had been given difetarsone 500 mg t.i.d. for 10 days. On the 8th day of treatment slight *fever* developed and after the ingestion of another tablet of difetarsone *'water blister' lesions* appeared, which spread rapidly and covered about 30% of his body. On the 9th day he stopped taking the medication, but his wrists, hands, feet and lips became markedly swollen and he complained of a 'dry' sensation in his oropharynx. The edema and other symptoms subsided within a few days with antihistamine treatment. The same patient had been unsuccessfully treated with metronidazole and furamide but without any adverse reactions (44[c]).

Furazolidone *(SED-9, 507)*

5 days' furazolidone treatment of giardiasis in children was found to be a failure when compared with the standard 10-day regimen with the same drug. One or more adverse reactions, comprising mainly *dark urine, abdominal pain* and *vomiting,* were recorded in about half of the 20 children treated. Most effects were mild and transient, except in one instance, where medication had to be stopped because of abdominal pain and vomiting (45[c]).

Nifurtimox

Acute *polymyositis* and toxic *erythema purpura* developed in a young woman treated with nifurtimox for Chagas disease. The patient died because of respiratory and renal failure (46[c]).

Hycanthone mesilate *(SED-9, 490, 540; SEDA-4, 207; SEDA-5, 283; SEDA-6, 265)*

From Ethiopia comes a case report of fatal *hepatic necrosis* in a 30-year-old woman, following intramuscular injection of a rather exaggerated dose of hycanthone mesilate against schistosomiasis. The patient developed persistent vomiting a few hours after injection and 3 days later became jaundiced; before the injection, liver function tests had been normal. An association of the drug with her acute illness was strongly suggested (47[c]).

REFERENCES

1. Good MI, Shader RI (1982) Lethality and behavioral side effects of chloroquine. *J. Clin. Psychopharmacol., 2,* 40.
2. Hoang PTD, Pourriat JL, Larmignat P et al (1982) Intoxications aiguës à la chloroquine traitement par le diazépam. *Ann. Fr. Anesth. Reanim., 1,* 321.
3. Jajić I (1983) Wertung der biologischen und klinischen Parameter bei Kranken mit chronischer Polyarthritis die mit Chloroquin behandelt wurden. *Aktuel. Rheumatol., 8,* 6.
4. Eizenbaum JF, Mas JL (1983) Neuromyopathie Iatrogène. *Concours Méd., 105,* 757.
5. Levy H (1982) Chloroquine-induced pigmentation. *S. Afr. Med. J., 62,* 735.
6. Huismans H (1982) Bilaterales (toxisches?) Papillenödem bei Chloroquintherapie wegen primär chronischer Polyarthritis. *Klin. Mbl. Augenheilk., 181,* 36.
7. Sassani JW, Brucker AJ, Cobbs W, Campbell C (1983) Progressive chloroquine retinopathy. *Ann. Ophthalmol., 15,* 19.
8. Trojan HJ (1982) Augenschäden bei Langzeitprophylaxe der Malaria mit Chloroquin. *Klin. Mbl. Augenheilk., 180,* 232.
9. Arrigoui-Martelli E (1982) Antirheumatic drugs. *Drugs Today 18,* 461.
10. Alio DJ, Sayagues O, Lopez Bartolozzi L et al (1982) Retinopatia cloroquinica: criterios diagnosticos. *Arch. Soc. Esp. Oftal., 43,* 49.
11. Hirst LJ, Sanborn G, Green WR et al (1982) Amodiaquine ocular changes. *Arch. Ophthalmol., 100,* 1300.
12. Kale OO (1982) Clinical trials of amodiaquine in onchocerciasis. *Bull. WHO, 60,* 929.
13. Luzar MJ (1982) Hydroxychloroquine in psoriatic arthropathy exacerbations of psoriatic skin lesions. *J. Rheumatol., 9,* 462.
14. Tin F, Hlaing N, Laserre R (1982) Single-dose treatment of falciparum malaria with mefloquine: field studies with different doses in semi-immune adults and children in Burma. *Bull. WHO, 60,* 913.
15. Davis M, Felix H, Brucker G et al (1982) Traitement curatif du paludisme a plasmodium falciparum, p. vivax et p. ovale par la mefloquine. *Med. Trop., 42,* 427.
16. Lambertucci JR, Greco DB, Pedroso ERP

et al (1982) A double-blind trial with oxamniquine in chronic schistosomiasis mansoni. *Trans. Roy. Soc. Trop. Med. Hyg., 76,* 751.
17. Kilpatrick ME, El Masry NA, Bassily S, Farid Z (1982) Oxamniquine versus niridazole for treatment of uncomplicated schistosoma mansoni infection. *Am. J. Trop. Med. Hyg., 31,* 1164.
18. Katz N, Rocha RS (1982) Double-blind clinical trial comparing praziquantel with oxamniquine in schistosomiasis mansoni. *Rev. Inst. Med. Trop. São Paulo, 24,* 310.
19. Branchini MLM, Pedro RJ, Dias LCS, Deberaldini ER (1982) Double-blind clinical trial comparing praziquantel with oxamniquine in the treatment of patients with schistosomiasis mansoni. *Rev. Inst. Med. Trop. São Paulo, 24,* 315.
20. Lin C, Feng-yi Q, Yan-chang Z (1982) Field observations on the antimalarial piperaquine. *Chin. Med. J., 95,* 281.
21. Boots M, Phillips M, Curtis JR (1982) Megaloblastic anemia and pancytopenia due to proguanil in patients with chronic renal failure. *Clin. Nephrol., 18,* 106.
22. Menez B, Delrieu J (1982) A propos de deux cas d'ectodermose pluri-orificielle avec manifestations oculaires chez deux jeunes congolais. *Med. Trop., 42,* 565.
23. Hornstein OP, Ruprecht KW (1982) Fansidar-induced Stevens-Johnson syndrome. *N.E.J. Med., 307,* 1529.
24. Lelijveld J (1982) Problems with pyrimethamine/sulfadoxine malaria prophylaxis. *Lancet, 1,* 915.
25. Colebunders R, Mathijs R (1982) Ocular toxoplasmosis treated with pyrimethamine. *Am. J. Ophthalmol., 93,* 371.
26. Zahn JR, Brinton GF, Norton E (1981) Ocular quinine toxicity followed by electroretinogram, electro-oculogram and pattern visually evoked potential. *Am. J. Optom., 58,* 492.
27. White NJ, Looareesuwan S, Warrell DA et al (1982) Quinine pharmacokinetics and toxicity in cerebral and uncomplicated falciparum malaria. *Am. J. Med., 73,* 564.
28. Ru-yun J (1982) Artemether. *Drugs Future, 7,* 716.
29. Thorpe PJ (1982) BRL-6231. *Drugs Future, 7,* 724.
30. Ralph ED (1983) Clinical pharmacokinetics of metronidazole. *Clin. Pharmacokin., 8,* 43.
31. Tally FP, Sullivan CE (1981) Metronidazole in vitro activity, pharmacology and efficacy in anaerobic bacterial infections. *Pharmacotherapy, 1,* 28.
32. Van der Auwera P, Collier J, Goris RJA et al (1982) A comparison of metronidazole and clindamycin for the treatment of intra-abdominal anaerobic infection: a multicentre trial. *J. Antimicrob. Chemother., 10,* 57.
33. Halloran TJ (1982) Convulsions associated with high cumulative doses of metronidazole. *Drug Intell. Clin. Pharm., 16,* 409.
34. Bailes J, Willis J, Priebe C, Strub R (1983) Encephalopathy with metronidazole in a child. *Am. J. Dis. Child., 137,* 290.
35. Schentag JJ, Ziemniak JA, Greco JM et al (1982) Mental confusion in a patient treated with metronidazole – a concentration related effect? *Pharmacotherapy, 2,* 384.
36. Flugel KA, Sturm U, Druschky K-F, Riemann JF (1982) Untersuchungen zur Nervenleitfunktion unter Metronidazol – Behandlung des Morbus Crohn und bei Patienten mit Metronidazol-Polyneuropathie. *Z. EEG – EMG, 13,* 192.
37. Sloan D, Fleiszer D, Richards GK et al (1983) Increased incidence of experimental colon cancer associated with long-term metronidazole therapy. *Am. J. Surg., 145,* 66.
38. Owen RT (1982) Benzoylmetronidazole. *Drugs Today 18,* 357.
39. Huggins D (1981) Clinical trials with R07-0207, ornidazole, in the treatment of chronic intestinal amebiasis. *Folha Med., 82,* 445.
40. Nava C (1983) Tinidazol I.V. en el tratamiento de protocolitis aguda y absceso hepático amibiano. *Invest. Med. Int., 10,* 56.
41. Carmine AA, Brogden RN, Heel RC et al (1982) Tinidazole in anaerobic infections: a review of its antibacterial activity, pharmacological properties and therapeutic efficacy. *Drugs 24,* 85.
42. De Pablos Gallego JM, Caberra Torres A, Almagro M et al (1982) Kala-azar y anemia hemolítica autoimmune. A propósito de un caso de evolución fatal por hepatotoxicidad del antimonato de N-metilglucamina. *Rev. Clin Esp., 164,* 417.
43. Sina GC, Triolo N, Cramet B, Suh Bandu M (1982) L'adrénaline dans la prévention et le traitement des accidents de l'arsobalthérapie. *Med. Trop., 42,* 531.
44. McIntyre L, Krajden S, Keystone JS (1983) Angioedema due to diphetarsone and a review of its toxicity. *Trop. Geogr. Med., 35,* 49.
45. Murphy TV, Nelson JD (1983) Five *v* ten days' therapy with furazolidone for giardiasis. *Am. J. Dis. Child., 137,* 267.
46. Shaw M, Petroue J, Iglesias D et al (1982) Polimiositis aguda por nifurtimox. *Arch. Argent. Dermat., 32,* 191.
47. Mengistu M (1982) Fatal liver toxicity due to hycanthone (etrenol) in a patient with pre-existing liver disease: a case report. *Ethiop. Med. J., 20,* 145.
48. Aubert SM, Sesta HJ (1982) Treatment of vaginal trichomoniasis. Single 2-gram dose of metronidazole as compared with a 7-day course. *J. Reprod. Med., 27,* 743.

J. Tuomisto and J.E. Idänpään-Heikkilä

30 Miscellaneous antibacterial and antiviral drugs

NITROFURANTOIN

Pulmonary hypersensitivity reactions and the apparent differences in their incidence in various countries have been thoroughly discussed earlier in this series (SEDA-6, 268; SEDA-7, 301). 3 cases of chronic lung reactions were reported from South Africa (2[C]) and another 4 cases from Australia (3[C]). Responding to the manufacturer's comment (4), the authors of the former paper estimated that the South African rate of chronic reactions is, according to their limited data, probably closer to the high Swedish incidence than to the lower British incidence (5).

2 other rare reactions have been reported which may be due to some type of nitrofurantoin hypersensitivity mechanism, namely *parotitis* and *focal nodular hyperplasia of the liver.* The case of parotitis was clearly shown by rechallenge to be due to nitrofurantoin, a 50 mg dose producing a prominent swelling of the parotid gland within 4 hours (6[C]). This sort of reaction has been sporadically reported with α-methyldopa, oxyphenbutazone and phenylbutazone. It is of interest that all these drugs also cause liver and/or bone marrow toxicity which is attributed to toxic intermediates of metabolism binding covalently to cellular macromolecules. The causal relationship of the focal nodular hyperplasia (FNH) of the liver to nitrofurantoin is far less convincingly documented (7). An asymptomatic palpable liver tumor developed in a 6-year-old girl some 7 months after commencement of prophylactic nitrofurantoin therapy. The tumor was resected and the pathological findings were typical for FNH of the liver.

Neurotoxic effects of nitrofurantoin are well known. A rare case of *lateral rectus muscle palsy* without any other symptoms has now been reported (8[c]): previously this particular paresis has been described in a patient taking furaltadone, a related compound (9).

SULFONAMIDES AND TRIMETHOPRIM *(15[R])*

Some 15 years ago the long-acting sulfonamides fell in disfavor because they were suspected of causing an undue number of *Stevens-Johnson* and *Lyell* syndromes (10). Sulfonamides still seem to be an important cause of these serious and generalized hypersensitivity reactions. Aberer et al (11[C]) report having seen 11 patients over a period of 4 years with either Stevens-Johnson syndrome or toxic epidermal necrolysis (Lyell). In 8 of these patients sulfonamides were the most probable causative agent, although only in 3 patients sulfonamide-trimethoprim was the only medicament. It is very intriguing that (obviously because of changed prescribing habits) the long-acting sulfonamides do not occupy a prominent place in this series, only 3 of the patients having received sulfamethoxydiazine, and none sulfadimethoxine nor sulfamethoxypyridazine (11), the drug which dominated the statistics 15 years ago (10). 7 of the present 8 patients had received a sulfonamide-trimethoprim combination, 4 sulfamethoxazole and 3 sulfametrol; one had received sulfamethoxydiazine alone and 2 in addition a sulfamethoxazole-trimethoprim combination. Hence it seems that the particular sulfonamides are represented according to their frequency of use rather than an agent-specific risk. Co-trimoxazole was also an important suspect in another

Side Effects of Drugs Annual 8
M.N.G. Dukes, editor

ISBN 0 444 90339 9
$0.80 per article per page (transactional system)
$0.20 per article per page (licensing system)

series of cases of drug-induced Lyell's syndrome (12[C]). Among the total of 9, 3 patients had received cotrimoxazole.

Another severe generalized *multisystem allergic reaction* was reported in a 16-month-old infant following the use of co-trimoxazole (13[c]). An *acute interstitial nephritis* requiring dialysis treatment developed during the 3rd week.

All these serious side effects clearly speak against an indiscriminate use of sulfonamides or cotrimoxazole. Since most of the side effects of the combination have been attributed to the sulfonamide component (14), the discussion about the indications for trimethoprim alone continues (see SEDA-5, 287). Brumfitt and Hamilton-Miller have expressed their preferences as follows (14[r]): 'Trimethoprim alone is preferable in urinary tract infections and it may also be appropriate in respiratory infections, prostatitis, typhoid fever and prophylaxis in a compromized host, but further controlled studies are needed. In pneumocystis carinii infections, gonorrhea and brucellosis, co-trimoxazole is clearly superior'.

OTHER URINARY ANTISEPTICS

Nalidixic acid and congeners

Fatal acute *immune hemolytic anemia* caused by nalidixic acid has been described (16). Previously hemolytic anemia after nalidixic acid has been described only in patients with G6PD deficiency. In the case now published the patient had previously had several recurrent episodes of hemolytic anemia, and after the first 1000 mg dose of nalidixic acid prescribed for dysuria and pollakisuria she suffered a serious attack of hemolysis and died after a few hours.

Cinoxacin, which is chemically related to nalidixic acid and oxolinic acid, seems to have a somewhat similar pattern of side effects, most often nausea, abdominal discomfort, central nervous system effects (such as headache, insomnia, paresthesias, photophobia), skin eruptions and hypersensitivity reactions (17[c], 18, 19[R]).

Beeley (1[c]) has described a severe *anaphylactoid reaction* in a diabetic patient, 1 hour after a 660 mg dose of nalidixic acid. Chlorpheniramine was given and recovery followed within a few hours.

Pipemidic acid and norfloxazin

These 2 compounds were compared in 2 double-blind studies in cystitis and in complicated urinary tract infections (20[c], 21[c]). Among the total of 280 patients on each drug, side effects were reported in 10 patients on pipemidic acid and 7 patients on norfloxazin; they were generally limited to slight *gastrointestinal disorders*. In another open study on 151 patients pipemidic acid caused side effects in 6, and in 3 of these cases the treatment had to be stopped because of *allergy* or gastrointestinal symptoms (22[c]).

Bailey (32[C]) has described 2 adult male patients with immunosuppression and poorly functioning renal transplants who developed incapacitating *tendinitis* during long-term treatment with norfloxacin.

ANTIVIRAL DRUGS

Acyclovir

Acyclovir causes *renal damage* in experimental animals, and this is also of major concern in humans (23). Since animal studies suggest that impairment of renal function is due to crystal formation in the renal tubules and/or the collecting ducts (24), the dosage and route of administration may have a major influence on their incidence. When the drug is given by slow intravenous infusion, the otherwise high incidence of raised plasma urea and creatinine (25[r]) is considerably reduced (24[C]). Adequate hydration of the patient and adjustment of dosage in patients with pre-existing impaired renal function are also reported to be of importance (24).

In children too, renal toxicity is the most important adverse effect (25); here, as in adults, the use of a slow intravenous infusion over 1 hour seems to decrease the risk (26, 27[C]) and dosage should be reduced in the presence of renal impairment (27).

Since acyclovir for injection has a relatively high pH (9.0 to 11.0), *local irritation* is another typical side effect (25) and extravasation should be carefully avoided.

High-dose acyclovir has been tried in cytomegalovirus pneumonia (28[c]) and in chronic hepatitis B (29[c]). The treatments were not successful and some *bone marrow toxicity, neurotoxicity, renal toxicity* and *urticaria* were observed in these open trials.

In a prospective study on 3 patients treated with acyclovir for herpes simplex encephalitis, evidence of *megaloblastic hemopoiesis* was found in all patients (30[c]). Even if no hematological problems develop in association with the bone marrow changes, the potential for them seems to be present.

Topical treatment with acyclovir in genital herpes did not cause any treatment related side effects in a controlled, double-blind trial on 188 patients (31[c]). The safety and efficacy of acyclovir have been extensively reviewed (33[R]).

Cytarabine (cytosine arabinoside, Ara-C)

As pointed out previously (SEDA-7, 305), both topical and high-dose systemic use of cytarabine may cause *corneal lesions.* Gressel and Tomsak report 4 patients with bilateral keratitis after i.v. cytarabine and warn against using corticosteroids as a treatment (34[c]); since the mechanism is assumed to involve inhibition of corneal cell replication, corticoids might actually exacerbate this self-limiting condition. Some other authors still recommend the prophylactic use of a topical corticosteroid for the prevention of the severe keratitis associated with systemic high-dose therapy (35[c]). The usefulness of prophylactic corticosteroid therapy for corneal toxicity of cytarabine was confirmed in a placebo-controlled randomized study of 11 patients with leukemia (36[c]).

Fulton et al (37[c]) used intrathecal cytarabine (administered by lumbar puncture or a sc. reservoir connected to the ventricular system) to treat metastatic neoplasms in the ventricular system or subarachnoid space. The treatment was relatively safe. One patient out of 32 experienced *headache, fever* and *meningismus* after each injection, and in one patient a *meningitis/ventriculitis* developed.

Interferon

Human leukocyte interferon therapy for cancer, melanoma, leukemia or laryngeal papillomatosis has been used in several trials (38[c], 39[c], 40[c]). The typical pattern of side effects emerges from these limited studies (altogether 30 patients). *Fever* and *chills* are seen in the majority of all treated patients, usually only at the beginning of the treatment, but in some cases prolonged and even requiring interruption of the therapy. *Fatigue, malaise* and *anorexia* are also common but usually of minor importance, and as compared to chemotherapy, interferon is well tolerated. In some cases a mild *rise in the SGOT* has been observed (39, 40) as well as *depression of white cell counts* (39, 40). With human lymphoblast or fibroblast interferon the side effects were reported to be much the same as above with fever, chills, malaise, anorexia, reversible hepatic and renal dysfunction and leukopenia (41[c], 42[c], 43[c], 44[c]). Some *central nervous system toxicity,* usually manifested by drowsiness, confusion, disorientation and visual hallucinations, has been reported with all interferon preparations (41).

In one study interferon-alfa was administered intrathecally to 5 severely disabled patients with chronic progressive multiple sclerosis. Fever was seen in all patients 6 to 8 hours after the lumbar puncture and another peak of fever from 40 to 48 hours after the injection (45). The fever was resistant to conventional antipyretics and was associated with an obvious transient deterioration in physical signs. In earlier studies interferon-beta given intrathecally appeared to be fairly non-toxic, although a febrile response was reported (46). The difference in the interferon preparation used may not explain the difference in response since the fevers noted after intramuscular human leukocyte interferon-alfa and human fibroblast interferon-beta seem to be similar. A more likely explanation is that only severely disabled patients were selected for the interferon-alfa trial discussed earlier (45).

On in vitro grounds it has been suggested that interferon *potentiates radiation injury,* hence careful monitoring of dosage and timing of irradiation may be necessary if both treatments are used (47).

REFERENCES

1. Beeley L (1983) Personal communication to the Editor of the SED Annual.
2. Wilcox PA, Maze SS, Sandler M et al (1982) Pulmonary fibrosis following long-term nitrofurantoin therapy. *S. Afr. Med. J., 61,* 714.
3. Robinson BWS (1983) Nitrofurantoin-induced interstitial pulmonary fibrosis. *Med. J. Aust., 1,* 72.
4. Rensburg W (1982) Pulmonary fibrosis following long-term nitrofurantoin therapy. *S. Afr. Med. J., 62,* 716.
5. Wilcox PA, Benatar SR (1982) Pulmonary fibrosis following long-term nitrofurantoin therapy. *S. Afr. Med. J., 62,* 717.
6. Pellinen TJ, Kalske J (1982) Nitrofurantoin-induced parotitis. *Br. Med. J., 285,* 344.
7. Anttinen H, Ahonen A, Leinonen A et al (1982) Diagnostic imaging of focal hyperplasia of the liver developing during nitrofurantoin therapy. *Acta Med. Scand., 211,* 227.
8. Mesaros MP, Seymour J, Sadjadpour K (1982) Lateral rectus muscle palsy associated with nitrofurantoin (macrodantin). *Am. J. Ophthalmol., 94,* 816.
9. Smith JL, Creighton JB Jr (1961) Sixth nerve palsy due to furaltadone (Altafur). *Arch. Ophthalmol., 65,* 61.
10. Carroll OM, Bryan PA, Robinson RJ (1966) Stevens-Johnson syndrome associated with long-acting sulfonamides. *J. Am. Med. Assoc., 195,* 691.
11. Aberer W, Stingl G, Wolff K (1982) Stevens-Johnson-Syndrom und toxische epidermale Nekrolyse nach Sulfonamideinnahme. *Hautarzt, 33,* 484.
12. Gerard A, Roche G, Presles O et al (1982) Syndromes de Lyell médicamenteux. *Thérapie, 37,* 475.
13. Kraemer MJ, Kendall R, Hickman RO et al (1982) A generalized allergic reaction with acute interstitial nephritis following trimethoprim-sulfamethoxazole use. *Ann. Allergy, 49,* 323.
14. Brumfitt W, Hamilton-Miller JMT (1982) Co-trimoxazole or trimethoprim alone? *Drugs, 24,* 453.
15. Wormser GP, Keusch GT, Heel RC (1982) Co-trimoxazole (trimethoprim-sulfamethoxazole). *Drugs, 24,* 459.
16. Tafani O, Mazzoli M, Landini G et al (1982) Fatal acute immune haemolytic anaemia caused by nalidixic acid. *Br. Med. J., 285,* 936.
17. Sabbour MS, El Bokl MA, Osman L et al (1982) A comparative study of the safety and efficacy of cinoxacin and oxolinic acid with nalidixic acid in the treatment of urinary tract infections (U.T.I.). *Chemioterapy, 1,* 364.
18. Schneider RE (1982) Single-blind comparison of cinoxacin and nitrofurantoin in the treatment of urinary tract infection. *Clin. Ther., 4,* 390.
19. Scavone JM, Gleckman RA, Fraser DG (1982) Cinoxacin: mechanism of action, spectrum of activity, pharmacokinetics, adverse reactions, and therapeutic indications. *Pharmacotherapy, 2,* 266.
20. Kamidono S, Tomioka O, Hikosaka K et al (1982) A comparative double-blind study of norfloxacin (AM-715) and pipemidic acid in the treatment of acute simple cystitis. *Chemotherapy (Tokyo), 30,* 1159.
21. Kamidono S, Tomioka O, Hikosaka K et al (1982) A comparative double-blind study of norfloxacin (AM-715) and pipemidic acid in the treatment of complicated urinary tract infections. *Chemotherapy (Tokyo), 30,* 1182.
22. Bischoff W (1982) Pipemidsäure – eine Alternative in der oralen Behandlung von Harnwegsinfektionen und Prostatitis. *Fortschr. Med., 100,* 2234.
23. Selby PJ, Powles RL, Jameson B et al (1979) Parenteral acyclovir therapy for herpesvirus infections in man. *Lancet, 2,* 1267.
24. Brigden D, Rosling AE, Woods NC (1982) Renal function after acyclovir intravenous injection. *Am. J. Med., 73,* 182.
25. Keeney RE, Kirk LE, Brigden D (1982) Acyclovir tolerance in humans. *Am. J. Med., 73,* 176.
26. McGill J, MacDonald DR, Fall et al (1983) Intravenous acyclovir in acute herpes zoster infection. *J. Infection, 6,* 157.
27. Gould JM, Chessells JM, Marshall WC et al (1982) Acyclovir in herpesvirus infections in children: experience in an open study with particular reference to safety. *J. Infection, 5,* 283.
28. Wade JC, Hintz M, McGuffin RW et al (1982) Treatment of cytomegalovirus pneumonia with high-dose acyclovir. *Am. J. Med., 73,* 249.
29. Smith CI, Scullard GH, Gregory PB et al (1982) Preliminary studies of acyclovir in chronic hepatitis B. *Am. J. Med., 73,* 267.
30. Amos RJ, Amess JAL (1983) Megaloblastic haemopoiesis due to acyclovir. *Lancet, 1,* 242.
31. Corey L, Nahmias AJ, Guinan ME et al (1982) A trial of topical acyclovir in genital herpes simplex virus infections. *N. Engl. J. Med., 306,* 1313.
32. Bailey RR et al (1983) Norfloxazin. Tendinitis: first report. *N. Z. Med. J., 96,* 590.
33. The Medical Letter: (1983) Intravenous acyclovir (Zovirax). *25,* 33.
34. Gressel MG, Tomsak RL (1982) Keratitis from high dose intravenous cytarabine. *Lancet, 2,* 273.
35. Lazarus HM, Herzig RH, Herzig GP et al (1981) Central nervous system toxicity of high dose systemic cytosine arabinoside. *Cancer, 48,* 2577.
36. Lass JH, Lazarus HM, Reed MD, Herzig RH (1982) Topical corticosteroid therapy for corneal toxicity from systemically administered cytarabine. *Am. J. Ophthalmol., 94,* 617.
37. Fulton DS, Levin VA, Gutin PH et al (1982)

Intrathecal cytosine arabinoside for the treatment of meningeal metastases from malignant brain tumors and systemic tumors. *Cancer Chemother. Pharmacol., 8,* 285.

38. Einhorn N, Cantell K, Einhorn S et al (1982) Human leukocyte interferon therapy for advanced ovarian carcinoma. *Am. J. Clin. Oncol., 5,* 167.

39. Hill NO, Pardue A, Khan A et al (1982) Human leucocyte interferon trials in leukaemia and cancer. *Drug Exp. Clin. Res., 8,* 677.

40. Goepfert H, Gutterman JU, Dichtel WJ et al (1982) Leukocyte interferon in patients with juvenile laryngeal papillomatosis. *Ann. Otol. Rhinol. Laryngol., 91,* 431.

41. Rohatiner AZS, Prior PF, Burton AC et al (1983) Central nervous system toxicity of interferon. *Br. J. Cancer, 47,* 419.

42. Retsas S, Priestman TJ, Newton KA, Westbury G (1983) Evaluation of human lymphoblastoid interferon in advanced malignant melanoma. *Cancer, 51,* 273.

43. Quesada JR, Gutterman JU, Hersh EM (1982) Clinical and immunological study of beta interferon by intramuscular route in patients with metastatic breast cancer. *J. Interferon Res., 2,* 593.

44. Ezaki K, Ogawa M, Okabe K et al (1982) Clinical and immunological studies of human fibroblast interferon. *Cancer Chemother. Pharmacol., 8,* 47.

45. Ruutiainen J, Panelius M, Cantell K (1983) Toxic effects of interferon administered intrathecally. *Br. Med. J., 286,* 940.

46. Jacobs L, O'Malley J, Freeman A, Murawski J, Ekes R (1982) Intrathecal interferon in multiple sclerosis. *Arch. Neurol., 39,* 609.

47. Dritschilo A, Mossman K, Gray M et al (1982) Potentiation of radiation injury by interferon. *Am. J. Clin. Oncol., 5,* 79.

J. Elis

31 Drugs uscd in tuberculosis and leprosy

DRUGS USED IN TUBERCULOSIS

Two excellent reviews of the clinical pharmacology of antitubercular drugs (1[R]) and their adverse effects (2[R]) have been published during the past year. Both papers analyze the frequency, severity, type, clinical manifestations and management of adverse reactions after a single as well as after combined administrations of antitubercular drugs in adults and/or in children.

Isoniazid (INH)

Hepatotoxicity This adverse reaction which is far from being rare and sometimes even ends fatally, still receives considerable attention. Alexander et al (3[R]) have summarized present knowledge of INH-associated hepatitis. The disease resembles viral hepatitis biochemically and histologically as well as clinically. Its onset is usually overt during the first 3 months of INH administration. Acetylhydrazine, an INH metabolite, is presumed to be responsible for the liver lesion. The monitoring of serum transaminase levels at regular intervals is the best method for detection (and hence for prevention) of liver damage. The incidence of the disease varies considerably, from less than 1% to more than 30%, depending on the patient population studied and the definition of hepatitis. On the average, when biochemical tests are routinely conducted, the hepatitis is estimated to develop in 18.4% of patients. Advancing age and regular and/or excessive alcohol consumption are the main risk factors. The majority of clinical studies lead to the conclusion that the risk of hepatotoxicity during INH treatment with or without rifampicin is not dependent on the acetylator status of the patient.

The last of the above conclusions is indeed widely accepted, but it should be pointed out that a group of German authors (4[R]) consider that slow acetylators treated with a combination of INH and rifampicin have a higher risk of hepatic injury.

Interaction INH is a well-documented inhibitor of the metabolism of many drugs (e.g. *alcohol, vitamin D, bishydroxycoumarin, levodopa* and *carbamazepine* (5[C]). Recently, a further case of inhibition has been reported. The blood level of *phenytoin* was significantly increased in a patient temporarily treated with a combination of INH and pyrazinamide. INH affects phenytoin metabolism through interference with phenytoin parahydroxylation which is the first and rate-limiting step in the detoxication and elimination of the drug. As a consequence, clinical signs of phenytoin intoxication appeared in the patient (6[c]).

Some observations have shown that INH may induce, not only inhibition, but also stimulation of drug metabolism. Thompson et al (7[C]) have described an interaction in which the effect of INH upon *theophylline* may represent a case of increased metabolism. Administration of an oral dose of 300 mg INH for 6 consecutive nights to their patient increased the mean theophylline clearance by 16%. The authors presume that INH may have an inductive effect upon the P_{448} microsomal enzymatic system, which may be responsible for the theophylline metabolism.

Mazze et al (8[C]) found that INH treatment significantly enhanced *enflurane* defluorination in about half of the surgical patients whom they studied. The authors assume that rapid acetylator phenotype is

Side Effects of Drugs Annual 8
M.N.G. Dukes, editor

ISBN 0 444 90339 9
$0.80 per article per page (transactional system)
$0.20 per article per page (licensing system)

the decisive factor for increased anesthetic defluorination.

Rifampicin (RMP)

Intravenous administration The parenteral form of RMP represents a therapeutic advance in the treatment of critically ill or comatose patients and also in patients with gastrointestinal or absorption problems. In a review presented by Kissling et al (9[R]), 237 tuberculous and non-tuberculous patients were treated with the usual daily dose of 450–600 mg of RMP. 80% of the patients in whom assessment of efficacy was possible showed favorable clinical results. A total of 31 unwanted effects were reported in 31 of 237 patients (13%). In 5 (2.1%) patients the treatment had to be stopped because of side effects. Thrombophlebitis occurred in 4.2% of patients, practically always in those treated for a period of more than 30 days. The results indicate that i.v. RMP is a useful and in some critically ill patients even a life-saving drug.

Other effects Very good tolerance and efficacy of RMP in tuberculous as well as in non-tuberculous infections has been demonstrated in pediatric patients (10[C]).

Miyachi et al (11[c]) observed a case of severe *hemolytic anemia* and acute *renal failure* after re-administration of rifampicin. The authors recommend a direct antiglobin test using whole blood-drug mixture as a simple screening test.

Liver dysfunction was reported by Japanese authors in 11.1% of patients treated with rifampicin containing regimens (14[C]). In the majority of cases liver dysfunction was already found in the early stage of chemotherapy while the elevation of serum transaminases was mild.

Nigan et al (15[C]) reported on 2 patients treated with rifampicin who developed *eosinophilia.* Withdrawal of the drug led to a decrease of the eosinophil count, which increased again on administration of rifampicin.

The induction of hepatic microsomal enzymes by rifampicin is believed to be the cause of *vitamin K deficiency* which has led to hemorrhagic disturbances in pregnant women and their newborns. It is proposed that vitamin K should be given prophylactically to all mothers and their offspring when the mother has received rifampicin during pregnancy. It is recommended that blood coagulation studies should be repeated in both of them (17[C], 18[c]).

It is well known that rifampicin and its metabolites may cause *body fluids* such as sweat, urine, feces, saliva and tears to turn orange. Liggett et al (16[c]) observed a yellow tinge of the cerebrospinal fluid in 2 patients treated with the drug. Shortly after discontinuation of therapy the cerebrospinal fluid was clear and colourless.

Elansary et al have observed an adrenal crisis precipitated by rifampicin (39[c]).

Another 2 cases of rifampicin-prednisolone *interaction* have been described first in SEDA-4 (p. 216). The effectiveness of prednisolone was considerably reduced when the two drugs were used in combination. 7 patients were included in the study aimed at assessment of the effect of rifampicin on the pharmacokinetics of prednisolone. Overall, rifampicin increased the plasma clearance of prednisolone by 45% and reduced the amount of drug available to the tissues by 66% (19[C]).

A further case (SEDA-6, 235) of a substantial decrease in the serum *digitoxin* level on addition of rifampicin to the therapeutic regimen has been observed (20[C]).

Within 3 weeks from the start of a continuous daily INH-rifampicin therapy, 2 patients developed acute *renal failure* (12[c], 13[C]).

Renal biopsy demonstrated quite different pictures. In the first case lesions characteristic of rapidly progressive glomerulonephritis with minor interstitial changes were found (12). The second patient's renal biopsy revealed acute interstitial nephritis, normal glomerular histology, effacement of glomerular epithelial cell foot processes and electron-dense deposits in the mesangial matrix and at subendothelial as well as in paramesangial sites (13).

Ethambutol

To delineate the risk of *ocular* toxicity, Lal and Gupta (21[C]) performed a clinical study in 680 ethambutol-treated patients. The dose of ethambutol was 25 mg/kg per day for 60 days followed by 15 mg/kg per day until 18 months from the start of therapy. The study of 81 patients, of whom only 24 complained of any visual disturbance, revealed a definite change in the visual pattern in the form of a diminution of visual acuity and a change in the green color field of vision.

Because the optic nerve changes once produced are not reversible, except in mild and early cases, methods for the detection of early signs of optic nerve damage have been searched for intensively. The method of visual evoked potentials seems to be a promising means of an early detection of subclinical optic nerve disease (22[C]).

Pyrazinamide

Combined therapy with INH, rifampicin and pyrazinamide was administered to 84 tuberculosis patients. All the patients who received pyrazinamide showed *serum uric acid level increase* which in 75 patients (90%) was twice as high as that found before treatment. Arthralgia was observed in 5 (14.3%) of 35 patients who received pyrazinamide daily for 2 months, and in 11 (22.4%) of 49 patients who received pyrazinamide daily for 6 months. Soon after discontinuation of the drug, the serum uric acid level returned to normal and the arthralgia disappeared (23[C]).

Thiacetazone

Two cases of generalized *hypertrichosis* due to thiacetazone treatment have been reported. The mechanism of drug-induced hypertrichosis is unknown. This kind of side effect has not been reported after thiacetazone administration so far (24[c]).

Short course regimens (SCR)

Teo has published a review on the development of the drug therapy of pulmonary tuberculosis during the last 30 years (27[R]), pointing out that present therapeutical trends are aimed at developing suitable and effective regimens of short duration (SCR), i.e. not longer than 6 to 9 months. The strategy of treatment is based on an effective combination of 2, but mostly 3 or 4 bactericidal drugs, in order to kill both the quickly multiplying bacilli and the slowly growing strains known as persisters.

Several large and carefully designed clinical studies have been carried out in East Africa, Hong Kong, Madras and Singapore. Attempts were made to solve gradually all related problems in order to find the most effective and least toxic therapeutic regimens. The studies are still in progress (25[C]), but to date the incidence of side effects in patients has been estimated to be 20–25%, though the offending drugs had to be discontinued in only about 5% of cases. Adverse reactions usually comprise mild cutaneous, gastrointestinal and vestibular disturbances. Cases of severe exfoliative dermatitis are extremely rare. Hepatitis, usually described as abnormalitics in liver function, has been found in about 1–2%. In regimens containing pyrazinamide, the patients suffer more often from arthralgia, and their serum uric acid concentration may be increased. Adverse reactions are reported more frequently in regimens containing both streptomycin and pyrazinamide. Ethambutol regimens are usually associated with the lowest incidence of unwanted events.

The usefulness of SCR has been corroborated by further clinical studies performed by research groups in Korea (28[C]), in the United States (26[C]), India (29[c]) and Argentina (30[C]). In other countries SCR are still under investigation (31[c]).

In a clinical study oral polyunsaturated phosphatidylcholine given in combination with RMP, INH and streptomycin, reduced the incidence of raised transaminase levels by approximately 50% as compared to a control group treated with antituberculous drugs only (32[c]). Polyunsaturated phosphatidylcholine is recommended for the prevention of early gastrointestinal complications of antituberculous therapy.

DRUGS USED IN LEPROSY

Dapsone (4,4′-diaminodiphenyl sulfone)
(SED-9, 532; SEDA-7, 299, 313)

Sinha et al (33[C]) reported a case of marked *erythema of the labium majus* with slight purulent discharge after a week of dapsone treatment. The symptoms disappeared within 10 days after drug withdrawal.

Prolonged *cyanosis* associated with severe *methemoglobinemia* and delayed *sulfhemoglobinemia* has been described by Lambert et al (34[C]) in patients after a single massive (3 g) ingestion of dapsone.

Serious and unexpected adverse reactions may develop even after a low dose of dapsone administered for other diseases than leprosy. A patient with chronic eczematous skin eruptions, treated with 150 mg of dapsone daily, exhibited an infectious *mononucleosis-like syndrome*, accompanied by atypical cell displaying T-cell characteristics with markedly increased spontaneous tritiated thymidine uptake (35[c]).

Mild hemolytic anemia was found in a breast-fed infant and its mother who had continuously been taking 100–150 mg dapsone daily. Dapsone and its metabolite monacetyl dapsone were identified in the infant's serum (40[c]).

Peripheral motor *neuropathy* due to excessive dapsone intake was described in a young man. The patient started with a dosage of 50 mg daily, increasing it himself to 400 mg and occasionally up to 800 mg. *Atrophy of various muscles* appeared with reduced strength of dorsiflexion of the wrists and feet, but most reflexes remained normal. The condition improved significantly on reducing dapsone intake to a maximum of 300 mg per week. The patient was found to be a slow acetylator. In their report on the case Rosen and Sörnäs recommend that the acetylation capacity of patients be determined before starting long-term dapsone treatment (41[C]).

Clofazimine

Ichthyosis, which is a frequent side effect after clofazimine administration in doses higher than 100 mg/day, may be substantially alleviated by local application of 25% urea in emollient lotion (36[cr]).

Given in high doses over a long period, clofazimine may accumulate in the tissues and precipitate as a solid. Enteropathy may develop if crystals are stored in the lamina propria of the jejunal mucosa and in the mesenteric lymph nodes. After drug withdrawal, the drug precipitates slowly regress (37[C]).

Maloprim

Maloprim is a combined drug (dapsone and pyrimethamine) used primarily for malarial prophylaxis. In a 23-year-old woman its administration caused *agranulocytosis* and *red-cell hypoplasia* which spontaneously remitted over a period of 4 weeks (38[c]).

REFERENCES

1. Reed MD, Blumer L (1983) Clinical pharmacology of antitubercular drugs. *Ped. Clin. North Am., 30,* 177.
2. Girling DJ (1982) Adverse effects of antituberculosis drugs. *Current Therap., 23,* 101.
3. Alexander MR, Louie SG, Guernsey BG (1982) Isoniazid-associated hepatitis. *Clin. Pharm., 1,* 148.
4. Munsch E, Eichelbaum M, Wang JK et al (1982) Hepatotoxizität der tuberkulostatischen Kombination INH + RMP + EMB in Beziehung zum Arzneistoffwechsel der Leber. *Med-Welt Bd., 33,* 23/911.
5. Fischer PR, Stanberry LR, Glasgow LA (1982) Carbamazepine-isoniazid interaction. *Pediatrics, 69,* 494.
6. Sandyk R (1982) Phenytoin toxicity induced by antituberculosis drugs. *S. Afr. Med. J., 61,* 382.
7. Thompson JR, Burckart GJ, Self TH et al (1982) Isoniazid-induced alterations in theophylline pharmacokinetics. *Current Therap. Res., 32,* 92.
8. Mazze RI, Woodruff RE, Heerdt ME (1982) Isoniazid-induced enflurane defluorination in humans. *Anesthesiology, 57,* 5.
9. Kissling M, Bergamini N, Xilinas M (1982) Parenteral rifampicin in tuberculous and severe non-mycobacterial infections. *Chemotherapy, 28,* 229.
10. Bassetti D, Ciravegna B, Viscoli C (1982) Rifampicin's tolerance in paediatrics. *Drugs Exp. Clin. Res., 8,* 255.
11. Miyachi S, Kosuda T, Hisatomi T et al (1982) A case of severe hemolytic anemia and acute renal failure caused by RFP. *Kekkaku, 57,* 263.
12. Hirsch DJ, Bia FJ, Kashgarian M, Bia MJ (1983) Rapidly progressive glomerulonephritis during antituberculous therapy. *Am. J. Nephrol., 3,* 7.
13. Neugarten J, Gallo GR, Baldwin DS (1983) Rifampin-induced nephrotic syndrome and acute interstitial nephritis. *Am. J. Nephrol., 3,* 38.
14. Kutsukake F, Murakami T, Sasaki Y et al (1982) Liver dysfunction induced by rifampicin. *Kekkaku, 57,* 257.
15. Pranesh Nigam, Goyal BM, Saxena HN (1981) Eosinophilia as a result of rifampicin therapy. *J. Indian Med. Assoc., 77,* 158.
16. Liggett SB, Berger JR, Hush J (1982) Cerebrospinal fluid xanthochromia with rifampin. *Ann. Neurol., 12,* 228.
17. Chouraqui JP, Bessard G, Favier M, Kolodie L, Rambaud P (1982) Hémorragie par avitaminose K chez la femme enceinte et le nouveau-né. *Thérapie, 37,* 447.
18. Lissens J, Shih H, Verbist L et al (1983) Hemorragische ziekte bij boorling van een met rifampicine behandelde moeder. *Tijdschr. Geneeskd., 39,* 277.
19. McAllister WAC, Thompson PJ, Al-Habet SM, Rogers HJ (1983) Rifampicin reduces effectiveness and bioavailability of prednisolone. *Br. Med. J., 286,* 923.
20. Poor DM, Self TH, Davis HL (1983) Inter-

action of rifampin and digitoxin. *Arch. Intern. Med., 143,* 599.
21. Lal BB, Gupta RL (1982) Visual pattern in ethambutol treated tubercular patients. *Ind. J. Tub., 29,* 222.
22. Aiannikas C, Walsh JC (1982) The use of visual evoked responses in the detection of subclinical optic neuritis secondary to ethambutol. *Neurology, 32,* Part. 2, PP214.
23. Ishiguro S (1982) Arthralgia and uricemia produced by pyrazinamide. *Kekkaku, 57,* 483.
24. Nair LV, Sugathen P (1982) Thiacetazone induced hypertrichosis. *Indian J. Dermatol. Venereol. Lepr., 48,* 161.
25. Aquinas M (1982) Short-course chemotherapy. *S. Afr. Med. J. Spec. Issue, 62,* 12.
26. Spagnolo AV, Raven JM (1982) Nine-month chemotherapy for pulmonary tuberculosis. *South Med. J., 75,* 134.
27. Teo SK (1982) Tuberculosis chemotherapy a review of current treatment regimens. *Singapore Med., 23,* 55.
28. Myoung Hae Lee, Sung Koo Han, Young Soo Shim, Yong Chul Han (1981) Clinical experience of short-course chemotherapy for pulmonary tuberculosis. *Tuberculosis Respir. Dis., 28,* 145.
29. Purohit SD, Sobhawat VS, Bhutra BL et al (1982) Short course chemotherapy with rifampicin. *Indian Med. Gazette, 116,* 321.
30. Gonzalez Montener LJ, Dambrosi A, Manassero M, Dambrosi Vilar y Maria L (1982) Adverse effects of antituberculosis drugs causing changes in treatment. *Tubercle 63,* 291.
31. Brändli O, Häcki MA, Scheel A, Stiefel M (1983) Die Chemotherapie der Tuberkulose-Compliance, Nebenwirkungen und Rezidivhäufigkeit. *Schweiz. Med. Wschr., 113,* 92.
32. Djuric-Milosavlijevic O (1982) Impiego delle fosfatidilcolina polinsatura (EPL) per la prevenzione delle lesione epatiche in corso di terapia antitubercolare. *Epat 28,* 3.
33. Sinha MR (1982) Fixed genital drug eruption due to dapsone. *Leprosy 54,* 152.
34. Lambert M, Sonnet J, Mahieu P, Hassoun A (1982) Delayed sulfhemoglobinemia after acute dapsone intoxication. *J. Toxicol.-Clin. Toxicol., 19,* 45.
35. Gan TE, Van Der Weyden B (1982) Dapsone-induced infectious mononucleosis-like syndrome. *Med. J. Aust., 1,* 350.
36. Caver CV (1982) Clofazimine-induced ichthyosis and its treatment. *Cutis, 29,* 341.
37. De Micco C, Boutboul R, Devaux J et al (1982) Entéropathie à la clofazimine. *Ann. Pathol., 2,* 149.
38. Nicholls MD, Concannon AJ (1982) Moloprim-induced agranulocytosis and red-cell aplasia. *Med. J. Aust., 2,* 564.
39. Elansary EH, Earis JE (1983) Rifampicin and adrenal crisis. *Br. Med. J., 286,* 186.
40. Sanders SW, Zone JJ, Foltz RI et al (1982) Hemolytic anemia induced by dapsone transmitted through breast milk. *Ann. Int. Med., 96,* 465.
41. Rosen J, Sörnäs R (1982) Peripheral motor neuropathy caused by excessive intake of dapsone (avlosulfon). *Arch. Psychiatr. Nervenkr., 232,* 63.

M.N.G. Dukes

32 Anthelminthic drugs

Albendazole

Albendazole, as noted in SEDA-7 (p. 316) is a well-tolerated congener of mebendazole, and has the advantage of oral administration. A report from Costa Rica shows that its good tolerance is also evident in children; 50 children took a single 400 mg oral dose. Three of the patients developed slight headache. In 4 instances there was a transient increase in the transaminases, affecting only patients with pre-existent anemia and hypoproteinemia (1[C]).

℞ Difetarsone

Difetarsone is an arsenical which has been used quite widely to treat intestinal amebiasis since its efficacy against cysts of Entamoeba histolytica was first reported in 1953. That it has consistently escaped mention in these volumes reflects the fact that it has generally been reported to have excellent tolerance.

In the course of the years one finds a range of investigators commenting upon the absence of adverse reactions; Boyce et al did so in 1974 (2[r]), Desser and Yang in 1976 (3[C]), Limbos et al in 1968 (4[r]), Schnieder in 1957 (5[C]) and Lenczner in 1972 (6[Cr]). Writing also in 1972, O'Holohan and Hugoe-Matthews concluded that in all the years that difetarsone had been used in France and its former French-speaking colonies, chiefly for intestinal amebiasis, no significant toxic effects had been reported in the literature (7[CR]).

It would be somewhat surprising if this picture were to be confirmed by broader experience. The nature of the compound (1,2-di(4-arsonophenylamino)ethane decahydrate), a polar pentavalent arsenical, probably undergoing conversion to an active arsenoxide which inhibits sulfhydryl enzymes, is not such that one would expect it to be entirely innocuous as compared with others in its class. Although the literature refers only to occasional vomiting, gastrointestinal distress, skin rash and a transient rise in SGOT, little or no methodical human safety work appears to have been performed.

Like many older drugs, this one has now been looked at critically by a large and experienced clinical research unit, anxious to determine if it is indeed as safe as it is reputed to be. The Tropical Disease Unit at Toronto General Hospital brought the drug experimentally into routine use in all patients reporting with T. trichuria, E. histolytica or non-pathogenic amebiasis requiring treatment. They received 500 mg thrice daily for 10 days. With this dose, which proved to be an effective lever, side effects were observed in 9 of 89 patients treated; they comprised nausea or flatulence (3×), lightheadedness (2×), diarrhea (2×), swelling of the mouth (1×) and headache (1×). None was sufficiently severe to warrant interruption of treatment.

No changes occurred in the blood, blood chemistry or renal function, but 5 patients had transient elevations of SGOT, alkaline phosphatase or both, all these changes being transient and symptomless (8[CR]).

The present indications are therefore that difetarsone is reasonably well tolerated, but a single study on this number of people is not sufficient for a firm verdict; in the absence of data on the many patients who are reported to have been treated with difetarsone in the field, one must await further studies. As a group the arsenicals do cause encephalopathy, visual changes, dermatitis and polyneuritis, and one has to be very sure that these things do not happen to a significant extent with difetarsone before turning back to a family of drugs which have largely receded into the background.

Side Effects of Drugs Annual 8
M.N.G. Dukes, editor

ISBN 0 444 90339 9
$0.80 per article per page (transactional system)
$0.20 per article per page (licensing system)

Flubendazole

In SEDA-6 (p. 281) the impression was noted that flubendazole may be another relatively well tolerated member of the benzimidazole family. Another report to this effect is based on a comparison with diethylcarbamazine in Mexican patients with onchocerciasis. Given a 750 mg i.m. dose weekly for 5 weeks, flubendazole produced little in the way of side effects except for considerable inflammation at the injection site. Ocular complications (limbitis, punctate keratitis and uveitis) were common in the DEC group, but of patients taking flubendazole only 1 out of 10 developed a new punctate opacity at the 4th day. The main problem with this drug is its poor local tolerance and the fact that it cannot be given orally because of poor absorption (9[Cr]).

Ivermectin

Ivermectin is a chemical modification of one of a series of naturally occurring substances designated as avermectins, which are macrolide-like compounds with a broad range of activity against various sorts of parasite. Initial clinical studies in Senegal, involving 52 subjects, concluded that ivermectin was effective in *Onchocerca volvulus* infection (river blindness). Transient pruritus was observed in 2 of 8 subjects on a medium dose (30 μg/kg given once) and 4 of 8 on the highest dose (50 μg/kg given once). There were no abnormal laboratory findings (10[Cr]).

Levamisole

In view of the hematological problems which have beset the use of levamisole in rheumatology, attempts are still being made to find a more acceptable approach to the rheumatological use of this drug. Ristori et al (11[C]) attempted to assess the safety of a single weekly dose of 150 mg per os in 29 patients, comparing them with 26 taking injected gold. During the 6 months of the study, 9 patients on levamisole and 7 on gold experienced adverse effects sufficient to justify withdrawal of treatment. Of the 9 reactions in the levamisole group, one comprised acute renal failure with hematuria and proteinuria in a man of 70, occurring after the 4th dose and proving fatal within a week; the cause and effect relationship was unclear. There were 4 incidents of neutropenia, 1 of eosinophilia, 2 of headache and 1 of nausea and vomiting. Particularly since these same effects were also seen in a high proportion of other patients in a milder form where they did not justify withdrawal of the drug, the therapy was abandoned. This paper shows quite clearly that the hematological problems with levamisole in rheumatic patients can occur in a very high proportion of patients, no less than 10 individuals here being affected in a group of 29, though some only to a mild degree.

In passing it may be noted that the manufacturer's scientific staff have reviewed 46 controlled studies of adjuvant levamisole treatment in cancer with attention focused on efficacy and the incidence of agranulocytosis. They found 38 cases of agranulocytosis (in a total of more than 100 patients treated). The patients apparently at highest risk of developing agranulocytosis were those with breast cancer as a diagnosis who were receiving a treatment scheme involving taking levamisole on 2 consecutive days each week. Looking at the material another way, it was striking that no less than 21 of these cases developing agranulocytosis came from Finland, i.e. they belonged to a population which since the events surrounding clozapine (SED-9, 83) has been suspected by some of having a greater predisposition than others to develop this complication. The impression was also gained that agranulocytosis was more prone to occur in women than in men, but this could not be confirmed because of missing data on the sex distribution of the population treated (12[R]).

Mebendazole

In view of the almost legendary safety of mebendazole, any careful documentation of its adverse effects is of interest. Kern (13[CR]) used the drug in a 50 mg/kg daily dose prospectively in 23 patients with cystic alveolar echinococcus. In cases of cystic echinococcus, the drug was given for 1 month, with consolidation courses during the follow-up period. In alveolar cases, the intermittent scheme was also applied, but later the drug was given continuously.

One patient developed a toxic depression of granulopoiesis during the 5th cycle of mebendazole on the intermittent scheme; the condition was reversible when the drug was withdrawn. The same patient had developed an alopecia during the 1st treatment cycle.

Hemorrhages in an additional patient with renal insufficiency were interpreted as possible side effects to the continuous therapy, but later evidence strongly suggested that the marrow hypoplasia was due to the renal disease.

Allergic lung disease was observed in 4 patients with lung cysts shortly after the start of mebendazole treatment; it was almost certainly due to the release of parasitic material from the ruptured cysts, and not to the drug.

That even a safe drug can cause problems indirectly when parasites disintegrate is again evident from a Kenyan report on glomerular changes (characterized as mesangiocapillary 'glomerulonephritis') in 7 patients with hydatid disease who had been treated with mebendazole. The accepted way of treating hydatid disease has until recently been surgical removal of intact cysts; the fact that mebendazole is now being used and results in disintegration of the cysts with the release of parasitic antigens probably explains this new complication (14[Cr]).

One effect which mebendazole may have is to inhibit lactation; in a 24-year-old woman the start of mebendazole treatment using a 100 mg dose twice daily for 3 days was followed by a sudden decline in milk production; within a week lactation had ceased completely and did not return, though the drug was no longer being given. There was no other obvious cause (15[c]).

Phenylene diisothiocyanate (bitoscanate, Jonit)

Jonit has been tested in man at least since 1969, primarily in South-East Asia as an anti-hookworm agent. Abadi and Sasabone from Indonesia provide both an overview of findings to date and a study of their own on the treatment of 60 patients aged 5–50 years. The single dose treatment (50–150 mg per os, depending on body weight) was generally effective. Side effects such as nausea, diarrhea, vomiting, abdominal discomfort and dizziness were mild and transient, and none occurred in more than a third of the patients (16[CR]).

Praziquantel

Ching-Yu and Wei-Chuan Hsieh in Taiwan (17[C]) have provided an overview of the incidence of adverse effects to praziquantel in a series of 67 patients with *Clonorchiasis sinensis* infection who received the drugs in a dose of 3 times 25 mg either on 1 or 2 days. The duration of treatment did not affect the incidence of adverse reactions, which were mild and transient. The highest percentages recorded were for dizziness (36%), nausea (24%), lassitude (19%), abdominal distress (15%), diarrhea (10%), headache (10%) and epigastralgia (9%), with lower rates of anorexia, low back pain, myalgia and abdominal cramp. Liver function changes were found in 3% (2 cases) and renal function changes in 1. These figures must however be viewed against their findings regarding the symptoms of the primary disease, which showed loose stools or indigestion in 30% of cases, a similar incidence of epigastric pain, gastrointestinal disorders or hypochondralgia, and in lesser proportions of patients most of the other symptoms later reported as side effects in the same series. Whilst there is little doubt that there was in some instances a true adverse effect, the reactions as a whole were, in view of the general state of the patients, negligible.

From France, Gentilini et al (18[Cr]) report on a series of 182 patients treated with praziquantel for urinary or biliary bilharzia, a single dose of 40 mg/kg being given. Adverse reactions occurred in 25% of cases but they were mild, primarily consisting of digestive upsets, headaches and sensations of vertigo.

Pyrantel embonate

Hypersensitivity reactions to pyrantel are not generally known, but a brief Australian report describes the sudden onset of stridor – apparently due to angioedema – in a 6-year-old girl who had taken a 250 mg dose some hours previously. There was a suggestion of a virus infection, and the case hardly provides firm proof that the complication can indeed occur (19[c]).

Thiabendazole

An unusual report related to an 18-year-old man with Down syndrome who, 24 hours after starting a twice-daily course of thiabendazole (1,000 mg oral doses) developed generalized convulsions. There was no prior history of convulsions and no obvious alternative cause for them. There was complete recovery, and phenytoin was given briefly. Two weeks later, because of renewed chronic diarrhea, thiabendazole was restarted and within 2 days he developed another generalized convulsion (20[Cr]).

Although there is a known association between Down's syndrome and epilepsy (21[R]) it may be noted that thiabendazole has previously been suspected to have some epileptogenic potential, on the grounds of anecdotal reports submitted to the manufacturer (20[r]) and this paper rather suggests that the risk can become a real one in predisposed individuals.

REFERENCES

1. Cortés RL Solano Sánchez ME, Duarte Espinoza G, Quesada Morales V (1982) Albendazol en helmintiasis de niños. *Comp. Invest. Clin. Latinoamer., 2,* 63.
2. Boyce JMH, Fitzgerald TC, Gregg R (1974) Diphetarsone ('Bemarsal') and other antihelminthic drugs in the treatment of *Trichuris trichiura* (whipworm) infestation in a subnormality hospital. *Br. J. Psychiatry, 124,* 160.
3. Desser SS, Yang JY (1976) *Dientamoeba fragilis* in idiopathic gastrointestinal disorders. *Can. Med. Assoc. J., 114,* 290.
4. Limbos P, De Muynck A, Janssens PG (1968) Traitement de la trichocephalose par la diphetarsone. *Acta Gastro-Enterol. Belg., 31,* 492.
5. Schneider J (1957) Le traitement de l'amibiase intestinale et des colites ambiennes. *Sem. Hôp. Thér., 33,* 610.
6. Lenczner MM (1972) Treatment of trichuriasis. *Trans. R. Soc. Trop. Med. Hyg., 66,* 510.
7. O'Holohan DR, Hugoe-Matthews J (1972) Diphetarsone (Bemarsal) in the treatment of *Trichuris trichiura* infestations. *Southeast Asian J. Trop. Med. Public Health, 3,* 576.
8. Keystone JS, Proctor E, Glenn C, McIntyre L (1983) Safety and efficacy of diphetarsone in the treatment of amoebiasis, non-pathogenic amoebiasis and trichuriasis. *Trans. R. Soc. Trop. Med. Hyg., 77,* 84.
9. Dominguez-Vazquez, A, Taylor HR, Greene BM et al (1983) Comparison of flubendazole and diethylcarbamazine in the treatment of onchocerciasis. *Lancet, 1,* 139.
10. Aziz MA, Diallo S, Diop IB et al (1982) Efficacy and tolerance of ivermectin in human onchocerciasis. *Lancet, 2,* 171.
11. Ristori JM, Bussiere JL, Sauvezie B et al (1983) Traitement de la polyarthrite rhumatoïde par la lévamisole à dose unique hebdomadaire. *Rev. Rhum., 50,* 57.
12. Amery WK, Butterworth BS (1983) Review/commentary. The dosage regimen of levamisole in cancer: Is it related to efficacy and safety? *Int. J. Immunopharmacol., 5,* 1.
13. Kern P (1983) Human echinococcosis: Follow-up of 23 patients treated with mebendazole. *Infection, 11,* 21.
14. Kung'U A (1982) Glomerulonephritis following chemotherapy of hydatid disease with mebendazole. *East Afr. Med. J., 59,* 404.
15. Rao TS (1983) Does mebendazole inhibit lactation? (letter). *N. Z. Med. J., 96,* 589.
16. Abadi K, Sasabone PH (1981) Phenylene diisothiocyanate (1,4) or Jonit in the treatment of hookworm infections in Ujung Pandang, South Sulawesi, Indonesia. *Health Stud. Indones., 9,* 25.
17. Chen C-Y, Hsieh W-C (1982) Clinical investigation of praziquantel in the treatment of clonorchiasis sinensis. *J. Formosan Med. Assoc., 81,* 1434.
18. Gentilini M, Brucker G, Danis M et al (1982) Traitement de la bilharziose urinaire et intestinale par praziquantel. A propos de 182 observations. *Bull. Soc. Pathol. Exot., 75,* 523.
19. Del Mar C (1982) Angio-oedema after combantrin in a six-year-old. *Med. J. Aust., 2,* 117.
20. Tchao P, Templeton T (1983) Thiabendazole-associated grand mal seizures in a patient with Down syndrome. *J. Pediatr., 102,* 317.
21. Veall RM (1974) The prevalence of epilepsy among mongols related to age. *J. Ment. Defic. Res., 18,* 99.

C.P.H. van Dijke

33 Enzymes and enzyme inhibitors

L-Asparaginase

Blood *(SEDA-6, 283; SEDA-7, 320)* The majority of recent articles on side effects of L-asparaginase concern abnormalities of hemostasis.

The Children's Cancer Study Group (U.S.A.) has reported on 18 children with *thrombotic or hemorrhagic complications* during treatment with L-asparaginase, vincristine and prednisone (2.1% of similarly treated patients) (1^C). 5 children had intracranial thrombosis, 5 intracranial hemorrhage and 4 probably a hemorrhagic brain infarction. 5 other patients developed leg vein thrombosis, in 1 case accompanied by intracranial hemorrhage. In an addendum a fatal case of cerebral venous thrombosis with hemorrhagic brain necrosis is mentioned.

An accompanying paper (2^C) describes a prospective study of hemostatic function in 12 children treated using the same protocol. In nearly all patients a marked decrease of plasma antithrombin, plasminogen and fibrinogen was found, while the plasma clotting times were increased. These effects diminished after the discontinuation of L-asparaginase but before the end of treatment with the other drugs.

In 2 prospective studies (3^C, 4^C) in adults on treatment with L-asparaginase and other cytostatics, a decrease of both antithrombin III and fibrinogen was found in all patients.

As one of the studies stated, '(these) hemostatic abnormalities occur in nearly every patient receiving L-asparaginase, but only a few develop thrombosis or hemorrhage. Preventing these complications will depend on our ability to determine which hemostatic lesion is most important, and to predict the patients in whom the lesion will occur' (2^C).

4 children who had received a local or systemic reaction to L-asparaginase (presumably from *E. Coli*) and had been switched to *Erwinia* asparaginase developed *hemolytic anemia* (5^c). The indirect antiglobin test was positive when erythrocytes were incubated with both forms of L-asparaginase, pointing to an immunological mechanism.

Pancreatitis *(SEDA-4, 222)* Another case of hemorrhagic pancreatitis during treatment with L-asparaginase has been reported (6^C) in a patient who also received prednisone and vincristine. The authors point to several important aspects of this side effect: the condition may be rapidly fatal and an acute abdomen may not be present; routine amylase estimations may not give a warning of impending pancreatitis (possibly due to a relative hypoamylasemia induced by the enzyme), and the accompanying hyperglycemia may divert attention from the hemorrhagic pancreatitis.

Glutaminase-asparaginase *(SEDA-6, 284)*

The glutaminase-asparaginase enzyme from *Acinetobacter* was found to have a broader spectrum of in vitro antitumor activity than *E. Coli* asparaginase, without the induction of resistance. In a recent Phase II trial (7^c) the drug was administered to 13 adult patients with acute leukemia or chronic myelocytic leukemia in blast crisis. Generally the initial daily dose was 300 IU/m^2/day, increased by 100 IU/m^2/day every 2–3 days to the highest tolerated level.

With this dosage regime, no patient achieved complete or partial remission. However, severe *CNS toxicity* developed in 8 patients: 5 became comatose and 3 developed a marked encephalopathy. Other side effects were *respiratory alkalosis* (occurring in all patients), *nausea* and vomiting. One

Side Effects of Drugs Annual 8
M.N.G. Dukes, editor

ISBN 0 444 90339 9
$0.80 per article per page (transactional system)
$0.20 per article per page (licensing system)

patient developed severe *hyperglycemia* with subsequent coma, renal failure and disseminated intravascular coagulation. The study was discontinued because of these side effects and the authors recommend that further trials be limited to short courses, possibly with the addition of antimetabolites or amino acid analogs.

Chymopapain *(SEDA-4, 223)*

The efficacy of intradiscal injection of chymopapain for the treatment of herniated lumbar disk was recently demonstrated in a double-blind randomized trial (8[c]). At 6 weeks the enzyme was effective in 75% of 55 patients and placebo (saline injection) in 45% of 53 patients. The side effect most commonly experienced was *back spasm*, occurring in 36% of treated patients and 2% of controls. In addition, 15% of the patients receiving drug complained of *back pain* or ache.

In a survey of 120 patients who were treated by chemonucleolysis (9[c]) the following side effects were observed: acute *bronchospasm* in 2 patients, skin *rashes* in 3 others (occurring after 1 week) and 1 possible case of *aseptic discitis*. Although the observed side effects in this study were moderate and easily reversible, severe anaphylactic reactions to chymopapain have been reported and the authors stress that one must be prepared to treat these emergencies promptly.

REFERENCES

1. Priest JR, Ramsay NKC, Steinherz PG et al (1982) A syndrome of thrombosis and hemorrhage complicating L-asparaginase therapy for childhood acute lymphoblastic leukemia. *J. Pediatr., 100,* 984.
2. Priest JR, Ramsay NKC, Bennett AJ et al (1982) The effect of L-asparaginase on antithrombin, plasminogen, and plasma coagulation during therapy for acute lymphoblastic leukemia. *J. Pediatr., 100,* 990.
3. Liebman HA, Wada JK, Patch MJ et al (1982) Depression of functional and antigenic plasma antithrombin III (AT-III) due to therapy with L-asparaginase. *Cancer, 50,* 451.
4. Barbui T, Rodeghiero F, Meli S et al (1983) Fatal pulmonary embolism and antithrombin III deficiency in adult lymphoblastic leukaemia during L-asparaginase therapy. *Acta Haematol., 69,* 188.
5. Weetman RM, Coates TD, Griep JA (1982) Asparaginase induced immune hemolytic anemia. Proceedings of the *Am. Soc. Clin. Oncol.,* 18th meeting, 25.
6. McLean R, Martin S, Lam-Po-Tang PRL (1982) Fatal case of L-asparaginase induced pancreatitis. *Lancet, 2,* 1401.
7. Warrell RP, Arlin ZA, Gee TS et al (1982) Clinical evaluation of succinylated Acinetobacter glutaminase-asparaginase in adult leukemia. *Cancer Treatm. Rep., 66,* 1479.
8. Javid MJ, Nordby EJ, Ford LT et al (1983) Safety and efficacy of chymopapain (chymodiactin) in herniated nucleus pulposus with sciatica. *J. Am. Med. Assoc., 249,* 2489.
9. Benoist M, Deburge A, Heripret G et al (1982) Treatment of lumbar disc herniation by chymopapain chemonucleolysis. A report on 120 patients. *Spine, 7,* 613.

B. Hofman and H.P. Lansberg

34 Immunological preparations

Editorial note *Interferon is dealt with in Chapter 30.*

GENERAL

The side effects of various types of vaccinations with advice as to how to deal with them have been usefully summarized by Adler (1[r]). Fenichel has provided an extensive review of *neurological complications* after immunization with pertussis-, influenza- and live virus vaccines (2[r]), an article which has been extensively commented upon by Poser (3[r]).

Remy et al have described a *hypersensitivity Angiitis* appearing after TAB DT vaccine administration just after a sore throat had been treated by penicilline V (4[c]). Giroud et al report *thrombopenic purpura* after DT TAB vaccination (5[c]).

Slater et al describe 3 children in whom painful subcutaneous nodules developed 1–2 years after injection of adsorbed DTP vaccine. The diagnosis of *Aluminium hydroxide granuloma* was established by ultrastructural examination with X-ray microanalysis (6[c]). Orlans et al, in a paper dealing with skin reactions to triple vaccine, note modulation (of a minor nature and persisting for less than 9 months) only after the use of adsorbed vaccine (7[c]).

Hirtz et al found in 1.4% of a large series of children with seizures a history of immunization within the previous 14 days. Both in their clinical presentation and their generally benign outcome these immunization-related seizures closely resemble febrile seizures, which are common in early childhood (8[r]).

Side Effects of Drugs Annual 8
M.N.G. Dukes, editor

ISBN 0 444 90339 9
$0.80 per article per page (transactional system)
$0.20 per article per page (licensing system)

INDIVIDUAL PREPARATIONS

Animal immune sera

In a brief communication Kheirbek et al report 4 cases in which *malignant lymphoma* developed in renal transplant recipients treated with antithymocyte globulin (9[c]).

Diphtheria

The bioelectric activity of the brain after DT vaccination was studied in healthy children by Cizewska et al (19[r]). EEG investigation showed significant changes in 13 out of 17 children, which disappeared within 3 weeks.

Hepatitis B

Hepatitis B vaccine (Hepatavax-B), produced by Merck Sharp and Dohme, is a subunit vaccine which contains the surface antigen of hepatitis B virus. The reason for looking very carefully at its safety in the long run is the fact that pooled human plasma is used in its preparation, and the possibility can not be excluded that infectious agents might be transferred in this way, e.g. the agent thought to be responsible for the acquired immune deficiency syndrome, though the procedures used to prepare and inactivate the vaccine would in all probability also inactivate these viruses. To date there is no evidence at all that the acquired immune deficiency syndrome does occur in vaccinated populations more commonly than in control populations, despite the fact that up to 20,000 persons were involved in the clinical trials with this vaccine, and that ten times as many have received it as a commercial product in the United States alone. There have been occasional cases of raised liver enzymes, erythema multiforme, aseptic meningitis, seizures, transverse myelitis and Guillain-Barré syndrome, but in a population of this size these incidents could have been coincidental. As the authors of a recent review point out, long-term follow-up will however be needed to prove that the vaccine really is as safe as present evidence suggests it to be (35[R]).

Herpes

Evidence from 900 patients vaccinated with a herpes virus vaccine showed that 75% had an *erythematous reaction* with *swelling* at the vaccination site. 6 vaccinations were followed by a transient '*flue-like*' syndrome. The vaccine which gave rise to these mild reactions was prepared from the troisbell strain of herpes simplex virus cultivated on MRC 5 human embryo lung cells, inactivated with formaldehyde (20[c]).

Influenza

Comparison of two influenza vaccine preparations containing complete antigens, which in one vaccine were adsorbed onto aluminium oxide and in the other were present in an aqueous solution, showed that the slight reactions, such as *reddening, pain, headache and temperature elevation,* which occurred in about 9% of the 180 vaccinees were equally distributed over both groups of vaccinees (21[r]).

Another study, comparing the results of two polyvalent Tween-Ether split influenza vaccines in 131 medical students, showed that the group receiving the antigens absorbed onto $AL(OH)_3$ showed more reactions than those who received the aqueous preparations. Swelling, warmth, redness, local pain and restriction of arm movements tended to be more frequent in the former group (22[r]).

A case of bilateral *optic nerve atrophy* and *blindness* developing 3 weeks after vaccination with swine influenza virus vaccine in 1976 has been described. The patient was not treated with steroids and the blindness was irreversible (23[c]).

Measles

A study in a rural area in India, where 206 children received attenuated live measles vaccine (Schwartz strain) and 206 in the same age group served as controls, showed that the incidence of *fever* was higher in the immunized group, whereas the incidence of loose motions, cough and upper respiratory tract infections did not differ. Moreover, in the immunized group one child developed an *encephalitis* from which it recovered gradually. It was difficult to say if this complication was due to the vaccination. A third child had a *rash* which lasted for 2–3 days (24[C]).

A 14-year-old boy, who had received a killed measles vaccination at 2 years of age, received a live measles vaccine because of a local outbreak of the infection. After a few days a swelling developed at the injection site and this gradually progressed. After some months the face, feet and hands were affected. The general condition deteriorated and he finally died 20 months after the vaccination. The diagnosis of the lesions was *panniculitis.* In many respects there was similarity with the findings in SSPE. The authors present evidence for the conclusion that there must have been a relationship between the vaccination and this fatal disease (25[c]).

Even 14 years after administration of killed measles vaccine the *atypical measles syndrome* can occur. The clinical course of this disease in 17 adolescents has been described. All had peripheral dermatitis and 15 showed the characteristic pulmonary infiltrations. Extensive laboratory investigations showed that killed vaccine, although promoting hemagglutinin antibody, lacks the ability to give rise to hemolysin antibodies. Cell to cell spread of measles virus can therefore occur after an infection with unattenuated measles virus, thus giving rise to this clinical picture (26[c]).

Pertussis

The continuing debate on risk versus benefit has been extensively reviewed by Miller et al (30[R]); other relevant papers are those by Cockrell (31[r]), Pollock (32[r]) and Preston (33[r]).

The sudden infant death syndrome in relation to pertussis vaccination continues to be discussed, with Bernier et al (36[R]) and Torch (37[r]) coming to opposite conclusions.

Bellman et al in London (42[C]) have provided a case-control analysis of 269 cases of infantile spasms reported to Britain's National Childhood Encephalopathy Study. No significant association was found between infantile spasms and pertussis vaccination.

Park, in the U.S.A., has described a 2-month-old boy with a history of *paroxysmal supraventricular tachycardia* which occurred after administration of DTP and trivalent oral poliovirus (TOP) vaccines; following recovery, selective rechallenge was attempted. It was positive with DTP and TOP together, again positive with DTP alone, but negative with TOP and DT separately – an elegant piece of evidence that the tachycardia must have been precipitated by pertussis vaccine (43[C]).

Pneumococcus vaccine

Citron (38[C]) has provided a new case report of pneumococcal vaccine-induced *thrombocytopenia* in a patient with splenectomy.

Poliomyelitis

A recent review of the relationship between acute persisting spinal paralysis (APSP) and poliomyelitis vaccine, covering 13 countries, presents a good assessment of the risks associated with oral poliovaccines. Apart from many interesting details, it may be concluded that for the majority of the subjects covered by this study the risk of acquiring APSP is very low. The total number of cases in the 10 year study period 1970–1979 was 281 in 403 million patients in 6 of the 13 countries. 52 occurred in recipients of the vaccine and 70 in contacts. The remaining 159 cases were in persons without any evidence of contact. This means a risk of 0.02 per million per annum in contacts and 0.01 per million per annum in recipients. Type 3 was the most common in the recipients, whereas type 2 together with type 3 was responsible for almost all contact cases. The cases in the third group, consisting of persons without any evidence of contact, were mostly due to type 1, and these isolates were virtually never vaccine-associated. To reduce the very small risk for contact cases it is important to vaccinate young parents together with their children (39[R]).

Rabies

A case of *transverse myelitis* developing in a 50-year-old man 11 days after positive and active rabies immunization has been described in extenso. He was treated with prednisone and recovered neurologically. The vaccine used was duck embryo rabies vaccine (DEV). In an accompanying table a survey is given of 23 hitherto known neurological complications after administration of DEV; 6 of these were diagnosed as transverse myelitis (27[C]).

Rift valley fever

Rift valley fever vaccines are still in a more or less experimental stage. Recently they have been used in the Middle East, and a report from Israel, relates to 107 men aged 19–24 years who were vaccinated with a formalin inactivated virus cultivated in diploid fetal rhesus monkey cells. They received 3 injections of 0.1 to 1.0 ml vaccine. Mild and transient local reactions ranged from 5% at the lowest dose to 43% at the highest. 3 of 107 vaccinees showed *hypersensitivity reactions* and one had a suspected diagnosis of meningitis (28[c]). The findings suggested that persons with a history of hypersensitivity states should be observed carefully for allergic side effects.

A second study concerned 973 men belonging to Swedish troops serving in the Sinai desert. They received a vaccine prepared in the U.S. Army Medical Research Institute of Infectious Diseases from formalin inactivated virus grown on primary African green monkey cells. Slight local and general side effects were recorded in 6% of the vaccinees. A few moderate or severe events, including one case of *cardiac arrhythmia* and one of *Guillain-Barré syndrome,* were encountered, but these could not be attributed with any certainty to the vaccination (29[c]).

Tetanus

Case reports of *hypersensitivity reactions* after reimmunization to tetanus have been published by Lan (40[C]) and by Zaloga (41[c]).

Tuberculosis

Katznelson et al have described a polyneuritis after BCG revaccination in a tuberculin negative boy; they suspect this to be due to hypersensitivity (10[c]).

In Tashkent a frequency of 0.05 of *subcutaneous abscesses* and of 0.02 of *lymphadenitis* was found after BCG vaccination in infants by Agzamov et al (11[c]).

A boy, described by Künzel et al (12[c]), who had been vaccinated shortly after birth developed ipsilateral *axillary lymphoma* at the age of 6 months. Microscopically the picture was typical of BCG *histiocytosis.* The child survived. The underlying immunological disturbance was considered to be a temporary derangement of T-lymphocyte function.

In a series of 830 autopsies at the Children Hospital, Winnipeg, 26 of the 36 cases which had been given BCG shortly after birth showed *tuberculoid granulomas* at various sites. None of the infants had histological evidence of an immune deficiency (13[r]). According to Beyer et al (18[c]) *chronic granulomatous disease* may underlie prolonged and relapsing local complications of vaccination with BCG.

Three cases of *lupus* after BCG vaccination in India have been described by Pandhi et al (14[c]), whilst cases of *osteitis* and *osteomyelitis* have been reported by Kamran et al (15[c]), Schulze (16[c]) and Moëll (17[c]).

Finally, a brief paper originating from Swaziland describes 3 cases of anaphylactic reactions to BCG in young children, one (in a 3-month-old girl) being fatal (34[c]).

REFERENCES

1. Adler PA (1982) The effects and side effects of vaccines. *Virginia Med., 109,* 410.
2. Fenichel GM (1982) Neurological complications of immunization. *Ann. Neurol., 12,* 119.
3. Poser CM (1983) Postvaccinal Encephalitis. *Ann. Neurol., 13,* 341.
4. Remy G, Rouger C et al (1982) Angéite de Zeek dans les suites d'une vaccination par le TAB DT: a propos d'une observation. *Méd. Maladies Infect., 12,* 325.
5. Giroud M, Page G et al (1983) Les thrombopénies post vaccinales avec purpura. *J. Méd. Lyon, 64,* 97.
6. Slater DN, Underwood JCE et al (1982) Aluminium hydroxide granulomas: light- and electron microscopic studies and X-ray microanalysis. *Br. J. Dermatol., 107,* 103.
7. Orlans D, Verbov J (1982) Skin reactions after triple vaccine. *Practitioner, 226,* 1295.
8. Hirtz DG, Nelson KB et al (1983) Seizures following childhood immunizations. *J. Pediatr., 102,* 14.
9. Kheirbek AO, Molnar ZV et al (1982) Malignant lymphoma in a renal transplant recipient treated with antithymocyte globulin. *Transplantation, 35,* 267.
10. Katznelson D, Gross S et al (1982) Polyneuritis following BCG revaccination. *Postgrad. Med. J., 58,* 496.
11. Agzamov RA, Zakharova RI et al (1983) Vaccination with BCG vaccine in infants. *Probl. Tuberk., 3,* 1.
12. Künzel W, Frey G et al (1982) Geheilte BCG-Histiozytose bei isolierter temporärer Störung der T-lymphozyten-Funktion. *Dtsch. Gesundheitswes., 37,* 1384.
13. Trevenen CL, Pagtakhan RD (1982) Disseminated tuberculoid lesions in infants following BCG vaccination. *Can. Med. Assoc., 127,* 502.
14. Pandhi RK, Kanwar AJ et al (1982) Lupus vulgaris following BCG vaccination. *Indian J. Dermatol. Venereol. Lepr., 48,* 164.
15. Kamran D, Müller W et al (1982) Klinische und immunologische Befunde bei BCG-Osteomyelitis. *Monatsschr. Kinderheilkd., 130,* 899.
16. Schulze W (1982) Über BCG-Osteitis. *Orthop. Praxis, 5,* 368.
17. Moëll C, Wiebe T et al (1983) BCG vaccination as a cause of multifocal osteomyelitis in a 12-year-old girl. *Acta Paediatr. Scand., 72,* 153.
18. Beyer P, Talon P et al (1982) A propos d'une nouvelle observation. *Pédiatrie, 1,* 53.
19. Wstepne D (1981) Prophylactic vaccinations and seizure activity in EEG. *Neur. Neurochir. Pol., 5,* 553.
20. Skinner GRB, Woodman CBJ et al (1982) Preparation and immunogenicity of vaccine Ac NFU (S^-) MRC towards the prevention of herpes genitalis. *Br. J. Vener. Dis., 58,* 381.
21. Pressler K, Peukert M et al (1982) Comparison of the antigenicity and tolerance of an influenza aluminium oxide adsorbate vaccine with an aqueous vaccine. *Pharmatherapeutica, 3,* 195.
22. Gerth HJ, Mok-Hsu YC (1981) Reactogenicity and serological response to polyvalent aqueous and $Al(OH)_3$, adsorbed Tween-Ether split product influenza vaccine in young adults 1979. *Infection, 9,* 85.
23. Macoul KL (1982) Bilateral optic nerve atrophy and blindness following swine influenza vaccination. *Ann. Ophthalmol., 14,* 398.
24. Kumar R, Chandra R et al (1982) Adverse reaction after measles immunization in a rural population. *Indian Pediatr., 19,* 605.
25. Buck BE, Yang LC et al (1982) Measles virus panniculitis subsequent to vaccine administration. *J. Pediatr., 101,* 366.
26. Annunziato D, Kaplan MH et al (1982) Atypical measles syndrome: pathologic and serologic findings. *Pediatrics, 70,* 203.
27. Label LS, Batts DH (1982) Transverse myelitis caused by duck embryo rabies vaccine. *Arch. Neurol., 39,* 426.
28. Kark JD, Aynor Y et al (1982) A rift valley fever vaccine trial. *Am. J. Epidemiol., 116,* 808.

29. Niklasson B (1982) Rift valley fever virus vaccine trial: study of side-effects in humans. *Scand. J. Infect. Dis., 14,* 105.
30. Miller DL, Alderslade R et al (1982) Whooping cough and whooping cough vaccine: the risks and benefits debate. *Epidemiol. Rev., 4,* 1.
31. Cockrell JL, Richmond V (1982) Vaccine reactions: the challenge to pediatricians. *Virginia Med., 109,* 380.
32. Pollock TM, Morris J (1983) A 7-year survey of disorders attributed to vaccination in north west Thames region. *Lancet, 2,* 753.
33. Preston NW (1982) Toxicity of pertussis vaccine. *Br. Med. J., 284,* 1817.
34. Tshabalala (1983) Anaphylactic reactions to BCG in Swaziland (letter). *Lancet, 2,* 653.
35. Furesz J, Boucher DW (1983) How safe is hepatitis B virus vaccine? *Canad. Med. Ass. J., 129,* 17.
36. Bernier RH, Frank JA et al (1982) Diphtheria-tetanus toxoids pertussis vaccination and sudden infant deaths in Tennessee. *J. Pediatr., 101,* 419.
37. Torch WC (1982) Diphtheria-Pertussis-Tetanus (DPT) immunization: a potential cause of sudden infant death syndrome (SIDS). *Neurology, 32,* A169.
38. Citron ML (1982) Pneumococcal vaccine induced thrombocytopenia. *J. Am. Med. Assoc., 248,* 1178.
39. WHO Consultative Group (1982) The relation between acute persisting spinal paralysis and poliomyelitis vaccine – results of a ten-year enquiry. *Bull. World Health Org., 60,* 231.
40. Lan TA, Vandepitte J (1982) Een algemene overgevoeligheidsreaktie na tetanus vaccinatie. *Tijdschr. Geneesk., 38,* 1315.
41. Zaloga GP, Chernow B (1982) Life-threatening anaphylactic reaction to tetanus toxoid. *Ann. Allergy, 49,* 107.
42. Bellman MH, Ross EM, Miller DL (1983) Infantile spasms and pertussis immunization. *Lancet, 1,* 1031.
43. Park JM, Ledbetter EO, South MA et al (1983) Paroxysmal supraventricular tachycardia precipitated by pertussis vaccine. *J. Pediatr., 102,* 883.

J.R.B. Williams

35 Blood and blood products

Interest and anxiety about the side effects of blood products have been concerned particularly with the acquired immune deficiency syndrome, which is included in SEDA for the first time. Attention is drawn to reviews detailing the precautions advisable in laboratories and clinical units but which avoid excessive restrictions on clinical management.

This Annual also discusses the complications of granulocyte infusions and their prevention at some length, and draws further attention to the occurrence of graft-versus-host disease as a complication of blood product infusion. It is possible that this diagnosis is missed in clinical units not engaged in a transplant program, especially in the early stage of the disease when it may still be amenable to treatment. SEDA-7 is also updated with regard to hemolytic transfusion reactions and hemolytic disease of the newborn.

REACTIONS TO WHOLE BLOOD AND RED CELL TRANSFUSIONS

An antibody reacting with the high frequency antigen *Cromer* was found in a Japanese man who probably had a null phenotype in the Cromer blood group complex (1[c]). Previous examples of anti-Cr^a antibody have been found in negroes, and it appears that races of other than African origin may produce it. The antibody reacts by antiglobulin and enzyme methods and would be detected readily by routine cross-matching methods. A new variety of anti-V, which reacts in saline at room temperature, has been reported. It occurred in a multi-transfused Caucasian woman in conjunction with antiglobulin-reactive anti-CD (2[c]).

Side Effects of Drugs Annual 8
M.N.G. Dukes, editor

ISBN 0 444 90339 9
$0.80 per article per page (transactional system)
$0.20 per article per page (licensing system)

Multiple transfusions in a woman also resulted in the second example of antibody to the low-incidence antigen *Hil.* It was not possible to determine whether the antibody had been stimulated by previous transfusion or pregnancy, although the original anti-Hil was associated with hemolytic disease of the newborn (3[c]).

The distribution of the Kidd locus phenotypes varies appreciably between different ethnic groups. The Jk(a-b-) phenotype is relatively frequent in Polynesians and was present in 0.9% of this race living in New Zealand (4[C]). In this study over a period of 13 years, 9 examples of the associated antibody, *anti-Jk3*, were detected. One of these produced a delayed transfusion reaction and some others caused mild hemolytic disease of the newborn. A strange example of anti-Jk^a reacting only in the presence of methyl esters of para- and ortho-hydroxybenzoic acid was found in an individual with Jk(a+) red cells. The patient was receiving topical treatment with methyl salicylate at the time the antibody was identified, and it appears likely that immune complexes between the antibody and the chemical antigen cross-reacted with the Jk^a antigen and bound complement (5[C]). This example of anti-Jk^a was found by the indirect antiglobulin test using low-ionic-strength-solution (LISS) suspended red cells containing the preservative methyl paraben.

The use of LISS also allowed the detection of an *auto-anti-P* which was causing hemolytic anemia. The anti-P and anti-P1 were IgM in nature and the Donath-Landsteiner reaction was negative (6[c]).

Problems with polyagglutination associated with *T-activation* and severe bacterial infections have been reported again (SEDA-7, 329). Polyagglutination with features of Th and Tk activation with an acquired B antigen occurred in a 47-year-old woman with peritonitis and respiratory tract infection of mixed bacterial type. The problem was noticed by the discrepancy between the red cell and serum ABO grouping and at that stage the presence of an acquired B antigen was considered (7[C]). Fatal intravascular hemolysis associated with T-polyagglutination also occurred in a Korean man with liver abscess containing *Escherichia coli, Aspergillus niger* and probably *Clostridium perfringens* (8[c]). The authors comment on the need to consider microbial infection, especially clostridial sepsis, in patients with sudden massive hemolysis, and the development of an acquired ABO antigen or polyagglutination of red cells may also indicate severe bacterial infection requiring rapid treatment.

Difficulties in cross-matching blood may also arise in patients who have been treated with equine antilymphocyte serum (9[c]). Both direct and indirect antiglobulin tests with reactive eluates may occur in patients treated with this immunosuppressive agent and are specific to anti-IgG1.

The reverse problem of *reduced or absent laboratory evidence of red cell incompatibility* may be due to genetic factors affecting the red cell antigen or choice of the cross-matching techniques. An inherited depression of red cell antigens may affect a wide range of blood group series including H, I, i, Diego and others (10[c]). Some antibodies, however, may react only by techniques which are not in routine use for cross-matching in most hospital transfusion laboratories. Investigation of 17 patients with hemolytic transfusion reactions, associated with antibodies not detected by routine procedures, included anti-C demonstrated by ficin-capillary and Polybrene, and anti-E and anti-Jk^a shown only by Polybrene (11[C]). Pretransfusion antibody screening may allow a reduction of cross-matching to an immediate spin and room temperature incubation if blood is unlikely to be used in cold surgery. If these methods are used when transfusion is certain or probable, then occasional incompatibilities will be missed, usually due to the lack of certain specificities in the red cell screening panel (12[C]). The inclusion of a LISS technique and an antiglobulin method for both screening and cross-matching is important (13[C]). Red cell survival studies using ^{51}Cr may confirm that a hemolytic reaction was due to red cell incompatibility during transfusion. Subsequent testing with patient's serum concentrated to one-fourth its volume may allow demonstration of the incompatibility and identification of the specificity (14[c]). Whatever techniques are chosen, it may be impossible to prove the incompatibility in vitro, and repeated ^{51}Cr studies may be necessary. For example, after 4 such tests, it seemed likely that a blood group O R_2R_2 patient destroyed E negative cells in spite of compatible serological testing (15[C]).

Rare or unknown antibodies occasionally cause severe transfusion reactions, and incompatible cross-matches must always be taken seriously. A group O Rhesus positive man was found to carry anti-E and anti-c with an additional antibody shown to be anti-Co^b. He was inadvertently transfused with red cells containing this antigen which appeared to be responsible for the hemolytic reaction which followed (16[C]). A severe transfusion reaction due to anti-En^{a}TS occurred in a woman with an unusual pattern of red cell sialoglycoproteins who received three units of red cells compatible by the antiglobulin test, but incompatible by direct agglutination at 37° (17[c]). Interpretation of unusual or discrepant cross-matching tests can be difficult, as the infusion of Xg^a positive red cells into a Japanese man with anti-Xg^a caused an urticarial and febrile reaction without evidence of hemolysis (18[c]).

Delayed transfusion reactions are infrequent, a recent study recording only one in every 10,688 transfusion units (19[C]). The specificities included the usual Kidd and Rhesus antigens/antibodies and anti-S. Delayed reactions to the Kell system antigens have been reported involving anti-Js^a 23 days after transfusion (20[c]) and anti-Js^b after 15 days (21[c]). Anti-Fy^b caused a delayed reaction 2 weeks after transfusion of compatible A Rh positive cells in a woman who had been transfused twice and pregnant 4 times. The patient was transfused for excision of a ruptured spleen, and the authors suggest that this may have reduced the severity of the hemolytic reaction (22[c]). Anti-Co^a has also been reported as a cause of a delayed transfusion reaction (23[c]).

In sickle cell patients, delayed transfusion reactions may be misdiagnosed as sickle cell crises. This particularly occurs in patients with U-variants. In a 22-year-old woman with anti-U in her serum, transfusion with C positive and one U^{var} unit caused a delayed transfusion reaction 13 days later. Since delayed transfusion reactions are severe in sickle cell patients, only units confirmed as U-negative by adsorption elution should be administered to anti-U carriers (24[c]).

A primary immune response is an unusual cause for a delayed transfusion reaction but may occur with anti-C 2 months after transfusion. Serial testing for the antibody is necessary as it may not be demonstrable for a further 4 weeks (25[C]).

The *problems of massive transfusion* were reviewed in SED-9 and little new has appeared recently. A retrospective study of case records of 24 patients with severe trauma showed that red cell transfusions decreased the platelet count 2.5 times more than colloid infusions (26[C]). The authors provide equations which give the platelet requirements according to the amount of blood transfused and stress the need for fresh frozen plasma at the ratio of 2 units to 1 unit of red cells in the admission room. A review of defects in hemostasis caused by blood transfusion also comments on thrombocytopenia, which in the present author's experience is a more frequent clinical problem than abnormalities of coagulation (27[C]).

HEMOLYTIC DISEASE OF THE NEWBORN/ANTI-D PROPHYLAXIS

Since the introduction of anti-D prophylaxis, the occurrence of hemolytic disease of the newborn (HDN) from other red cell antigens has assumed proportionately greater significance. Low frequency red cell antigens may provoke HDN, and a new antigen 'Pollio' has been identified this way (28[C]). Severe HDN may occur with these antigens, especially those of the Miltenberger series such as anti-Verweyst (Vw). In puzzling cases of HDN, red cell panels in routine use may not carry the antigen involved and cross-checking the father's red cells with maternal serum at an early stage may help, together with collaboration among laboratories in different centers (29[C]). High frequency antigens may also cause HDN, although a recent report of sensitization to Lu^b with an IgG antibody was of a low level detectable by elution, but with a negative antiglobulin reaction and no clinical effects (30[C]). It is important to tailor red cell screening panels of antenatal patients to the population: HDN due to anti-Di^a occurred in an infant born to Japanese parents in Brazil, highlighting the problems of increasing mixed populations throughout the world (31[C]). A major historical review of Rhesus hemolytic disease of the newborn provides an account of the development of understanding of the disease and its treatment and prophylaxis (32[R]). In spite of prophylaxis, Rhesus HDN is still a problem. The outcome of an affected pregnancy is related to the maternal anti-D concentration. In a study using the British working standard, it was found that when serial anti-D concentrations remained below 4 IU/ml, only 3 babies in 78 were significantly affected, whereas above this level, 79 babies in 106 required exchange transfusions (33[C]). Determination of the right dose of anti-D for prophylaxis is more difficult than routine practice takes into account. The standard United States dose of 330 μg anti-D should suppress the immunogenicity of 30 ml fetal blood in the maternal circulation. Two recent studies show that enzyme-linked antiglobulin tests and a rosetting technique are sensitive and allow quantitation of a fetal/maternal bleed and adjustment of anti-D dose (34[C], 35[C]). This may be even more important in countries using lower doses of anti-D as a routine.

The formation of anti-D in male volunteers may be facilitated by the simultaneous injection of 1 μg anti-D. The degree of immunization was not augmented, but it is probable that a higher proportion of subjects was sensitized (36[C]).

REACTIONS TO WHITE CELLS

The survival of neutropenic patients with gram-negative sepsis is related to the compatibility of the granulocytes as shown by the granulocyte indirect immunofluorescence tests. This test is a measure of granulocyte-specific antibodies. There is no relation between patient outcome and a lymphocytotoxicity assay, showing that HLA compatibility is less important in this respect than specific anti-leucocyte antibody (37[C]). A study of granulocyte cytotoxins in multi-transfused patients and multiparous identified 3 granulocyte specificities (38[C]) which may well relate to the incompatibility responsible for the failure of leucocyte infusion therapy in cytotoxic-induced neutropenia.

Combined prophylactic granulocyte and platelet infusions in 23 patients with acute myelogenous leukemia resulted in frequent transfusion reactions in 10 of them. Recovery of granulocytes in all these 10 was less than

5% on at least one occasion, probably due to rapid alloimmunization (39[C]). The accompanying diminished platelet recovery was also probably due to alloimmunization and although an 'innocent bystander' effect from anti-leucocyte reaction was not excluded. In this study, at least, granulocyte infusion appeared to be effective for only 2 to 3 weeks. This raises problems in the management of induction therapy in acute leukemia of all types and with the effect of induction cytotoxic protocols on immunosuppression. Further doubt on the value of prophylactic granulocyte transfusions was cast by a prospective randomized trial, also on patients with acute myelogenous leukemia, in which there was no difference in deaths or frequency of infection, or in the frequency or duration of fever (40[C]). In another trial, no effect on response rate or survival was found, but data on infection rate and the incidence of septicemia are not yet complete (41[c]). Comparison between the groups is difficult to make because of the many clinical variables, including the nature and site of infection and choice of antibiotics (42[c]). The immune response to leucocyte antigens appears to be genetically determined. In highly transfused thalassemia patients, an increased incidence of anti-leucocyte antibodies occurred in HLA-DR2 carriers and a reduced incidence in Bw35 and DR7 individuals. (43[C]). It seems likely that immunosuppressive factors related to these HLA groups play a role in the reduced immune response.

The preparation, indications, use and side effects of granulocyte infusions have been reviewed, the author commenting on the incidence and nature of the adult respiratory distress syndrome and its relation to anti-leucocyte antigen-antibody reaction (44[r]). Whether microaggregates of leucocytes in banked blood can cause respiratory failure is still uncertain, and the evidence largely suggests that they do not do so to a significant degree (45[r]). In massive transfusions, the extent of trauma, shock and pulmonary involvement are probably more important. In a prospective study of pulmonary function in patients having elective coronary bypass surgery, there was no difference between patients receiving blood through a 20-micron filter or a 170-micron one (46[C]). Some of the patients studied had some degree of pulmonary dysfunction before transfusion and even in these there was no evidence that the use of microaggregate filters provides clinical benefit.

Microaggregate blood filtration may, however, reduce the incidence of febrile transfusion reactions by 77% and units centrifuged before filtration rarely caused reactions (reduction of 98%). The study also showed that febrile reactions are less frequent in units within 2 weeks of their shelf life due to the reduced granulocyte content (47[C]). At present, it seems that microaggregate filtration is most useful in patients who are likely to be transfused repeatedly, to reduce the onset and frequency of febrile reactions (48[r]). The removal of microaggregates from granulocyte concentrates is best done by screen filters, as depth filters remove a substantial proportion (20-60%) of neutrophils (49[c]). The best filters for the removal of leucocytes from whole blood appear to be the Imugard IG500 and Erypur, which can be relied on to reduce the absolute numbers by 98% (50[c]), although other methods such as freezing-and-thawing or centrifugation will remove appreciable numbers (51[R]). The authors of this detailed review suggest that most nonhemolytic febrile transfusion reactions will be abolished by microaggregate filtration at the bedside and should be tried before more complicated and expensive methods of leucocyte depletion are initiated.

The collection of granulocytes from donors is a fairly safe procedure, analysis of data from 190 establishments showing that adverse reactions occurred 54.9 times per 1000 procedures and that 94 per cent were mild. Moderate reactions occurred in 5.9% and severe ones in 0.4% (52[C]).

Leucocyte infusions may induce consumption coagulation changes. Fibrin degradation products may increase in association with a reduction in factor VIII and antithrombin levels (53[c]). The clinical significance of these changes is not clear.

REACTIONS TO PLATELETS

In spite of previous reports, posttransfusion purpura may respond to high-dose steroid treatment, hydrocortisone 500 mg intravenously 6-hourly producing a sharp rise in the platelet count on the 5th day after the onset of purpura (54[c]). An unusual case of posttransfusion purpura concerned a female patient with platelets negative for group PlA^1 (Zw^a) with antibody to this antigen who was treated with methylprednisolone 2 mg/kg/day. The platelet count rose 2 days later, and she was then treated by plasma exchange. Immunological studies showed that the patient's platelets did not react with the circulating antibody in vitro, but platelet survival was reduced and turnover increased. In addition to the unusual platelet antigen/antibody reaction, the patient had a delayed transfusion reaction in association with anti-E and anti-c and developed lymphocytotoxic antibodies of wide specificity (55[C]).

Further transfusions after the development of lymphocytotoxic antibodies may be possible for a time, using leucocyte poor blood and platelet concentrates, but ultimately only HLA-compatible blood may be tolerated (56[c]).

REACTIONS TO HUMAN ALBUMIN PREPARATIONS

Properly prepared human albumin should not elicit any adverse reaction, and when, from time to time, such reactions are reported, they may be attributable to impurities in a particular batch. From outside Europe, reports of such reactions do occasionally appear, and one is bound to question the conditions under which the preparations have been stored and handled when this happens. Two cases reported from Kuwait (110[c]) provide an example.

A 48-year-old man was given 100 ml of human albumin 25% (Behringwerke) for micronodular liver cirrhosis. Simultaneously, the patient was taking furosemide, spironolactone and vitamin B complex. He developed rigors, pyrexia and dyspnea on two occasions after the albumin had been administered intravenously.

A boy aged 15 received the same human albumin preparation for hypoalbuminemia, as well as receiving digoxin, furosemide and ampicillin for cardiac disease and chest infection. The patient experienced the same reaction.

In both patients, symptoms subsided on withdrawal of the infusion.

REACTIONS TO PLASMA PROTEIN FRACTIONS

Developments in the use of immunoglobulin preparations for specific therapeutic purposes require comment in this Annual. A review of their uses describes the common side effects, mentioning the possible etiology from IgA antibody reactions or the effect of contaminating proteins such as prekallikrein activator (57[r]). The new intravenous preparations cause minor side effects in some patients, but severe symptoms or anaphylaxis are only likely in known susceptible individuals. Preparations containing maltose seem to be less toxic than those in glycine alone (58[c], 59[r]).

The use of *anti-thymocyte globulin* is usually associated with adverse reactions, fever, rigor and skin rashes being frequent (60[C], 61[C]). The major dose-limiting toxicity is thrombocytopenia, especially if the bone marrow reserve is already reduced by disease and previous cytotoxic treatment.

Specific antibodies of animal origin are well known to be toxic, but an unusual effect of *tetanus antitoxin* is reported from India and is probably misdiagnosed even in countries where tetanus neonatorum is common. 14 children between the ages of 3.5 and 13 years were treated surgically for fibrosis of the quadriceps muscles. This had been noticed as painless limitation of knee flexion following repeated intramuscular injections of antitoxin in this site. The authors advise that every available intramuscular injection site is used and that consideration is given to the use of oral and intravenous routes (62[c]).

Murine monoclonal antibody T101 has been used in 2 patients with chronic lymphocytic leukemia. The first patient received 2 doses without complications but developed an anaphylactoid reaction 20 min after completing the third. The other patient became hypotensive and dyspneic 15 min after the first dose and then experienced rigors and fever (63[C]).

Rabbit-derived anti-human ovarian tumor serum has been used in women with stage-III or stage-IV epithelial ovarian cancer in addition to standard combination chemotherapy. Out of 9 patients, 3 developed low-grade fever and 2 skin rash. There was no increase in bone marrow toxicity (64[C]).

A further attempt at immunotherapy in cancer patients has been the administration of *autologous lymphocytes* stimulated by previous incubation with phytohemagglutinin and human AB serum. All 8 patients treated developed fever and some complained of headache, nausea and vomiting. There was also a temporary reduction in pulmonary diffusion capacity (65[c]).

Animal protein fractions other than immunoglobulin preparations may produce side effects presumably related to their antigenicity. *Bovine fibrin* used during ear, nose and throat operations may induce delayed hypersensitivity with cutaneous erythema and edema (66[c]).

Highly purified animal material such as *porcine factor VIII* may also cause severe allergic reactions, but its lack of cross-reaction with factor VIII inhibitors in hemophiliac patients makes it a valuable agent for treatment (67[C]). Severe reactions may also occur with human material as shown by the death in status asthmaticus of a hemophiliac who developed epileptiform fits after self-administration of *factor VIII concentrate* (68[c]).

Treatment of hemophilia with *activated prothrombin complex* is known to cause thrombotic episodes sometimes, and there are 2 further reports of myocardial infarction induced by this agent (69[c], 70[c]).

Whole plasma preparations only occasionally cause side effects (SEDA-7,331) and a recent review of adverse reactions to plasma substitutes shows that plasma protein fraction and human serum albumin have a lower incidence than any other studied except dextran 40 (71[r]).

TRANSMISSION OF DISEASE BY BLOOD PRODUCTS

Hepatitis The transmission of *hepatitis A* by blood transfusion was reviewed last year (SEDA-7, 332), and another case has been reported. 2 weeks after blood donation, the donor became ill with symptoms of hepatitis, and hepatitis-A-specific IgM was demonstrated in her serum. The blood, meanwhile, had been transfused and the recipient developed serologically confirmed hepatitis A 3 weeks later (72[c]).

The exclusion of *hepatitis B* antigen carriers from donating blood requires a sensitive test such as a radioimmunoassay system. The usual systems detect hepatitis B surface antigen (HBsAg). Testing for e antigen and its related antibody (HBeAg and anti-HBe) may help selection of those donors who carry hepatitis B antigen but who are already producing an immune response not detectable by routine tests and whose clinical management with possible treatment with hepatitis B immune serum may be modified (73[C]). Unfortunately, the commercial radioimmunoassay kits for HBsAg are not entirely specific and give a 4 per cent nonspecific reaction when tested by neutralization with pooled surface antigen (74[c]).

The incidence of markers of hepatitis B in volunteer donors is 6.3% in the United States (0.2% HBsAg), providing that they have not been transfused previously or been jaundiced (75[C]).

In spite of this relatively high incidence before exclusion of antigen carrying donors in a small survey of 164 recipients receiving 689 units of blood products, there were no cases of posttransfusion hepatitis. The donor population in this instance were US Army personnel in training who appear to be a safe source of blood for transfusion (76[c]).

The risk attached to plasma products can be reduced by manufacturing techniques or by the addition of antihepatitis B antibody (77[R]). Albumin and plasma protein fraction are heated to 60°C for 10 hours and are low-risk. A reduction in risk of antihemophilic factor, factor IX as well as antithrombin III, α-1-antitrypsin, fibronectin, C-1 inactivator and factor XIII may be obtained by a combination of chemical stabilization and heating, or by the addition of anti-HB immunoglobulin.

A recent analysis of treatment of hemophilia in the United Kingdom based on the annual reports of the directors of hemophilia centers includes data for 1980 (78[C]). The incidence of hepatitis is given in Table 1.

The annual clinical attack rate has dropped since 1974 when it was 5.2% and has remained about 3% since. This rate is relatively low, but includes all cases treated in the centers including mild ones only requiring occasional treatment. Higher infection rates as determined by serological testing for HBsAg, anti-HBs and anti-HBc were

Table 1

Coagulation defect	No. of patients treated	Cases of hepatitis	
		No.	%
Hemophilia A	2107	52	2.5
Hemophilia B	355	2	0.6
Von Willebrand's disease	235	9	3.8
Total	2697	63	2.3

found in Edinburgh being 7% and 9.5% for the two periods 1971-1975 and 1975-1979. Of the 16 patients who showed seroconversion only one developed clinically evident hepatitis (79[C]). The patients were treated predominantly with cryoprecipitate, but large-pool factor VIII concentrate was also used. Commercial factor VIII preparations now carry the same hepatitis risk as products prepared from voluntary donors (80[C]), but it still appears that the safest source of factor VIII supplements for new and mild hemophiliacs is cryoprecipitate (81[c]).

Pooled preparations of prothrombin complex still carry a high risk of hepatitis: 56% of patients undergoing cardiac surgery and receiving this material developed non-A, non-B hepatitis. In this study, only 5% of patients receiving blood transfusion without prothrombin complex developed hepatitis (82[c]), and it is evident that the use of pooled clotting factor concentrates should be avoided if at all possible. Cardiac surgery also carries a high risk of posttransfusion hepatitis in Spain, where 40 of 230 patients developed clinical or laboratory evidence of it. Of these, a quarter were due to hepatitis B, in one patient to CMV infection and the rest to non A, non B (83[C]). In the United States, a history of viral hepatitis excludes a person from blood donation, but this regulation was reduced in 1975 in the United Kingdom to a history of 12 months hepatitis or jaundice. With the modern sensitive tests, the majority of carriers of hepatitis B are identified, and in spite of the occasional occurrence of posttransfusion hepatitis B with volunteer donors, this practice seems reasonable (84[r]). A history of previous transfusion or contact with patients with hepatitis has no influence on the incidence of anti-HBc in the absence of other HBV markers strongly suggesting that these 2 factors may be ignored in the selection of donors.

The value of testing donors for abnormal serum alanine aminotransferase (ALT) is still unknown but a Special Report from the United States advises against the routine adoption of the procedure (85[R]). There is a need for more information on the significance of raised ALT levels with regard to the transmission of non-A, non-B hepatitis and the development of chronic hepatitis. The incidence of chronic hepatitis following acute non-A, non-B infection is not known, but in Italy, of 21 patients developing the acute illness, 13 progressed with histologically confirmed changes. Chronic persistent hepatitis occurred in one, chronic lobular hepatitis in 2, and chronic active hepatitis in 10. 5 of these progressed to cirrhosis and one died (86[C]).

Other infections. Post-transfusion hepatitis rarely occurs as a result of *cytomegalovirus (CMV) infection, Epstein-Barr virus* infection and extremely rarely from *toxoplasma* infection (87[R]). CMV infection without jaundice as a side effect of transfusion is frequent, especially so in neonates and neutropenic or immunologically suppressed adults. Glandular fever following transfusion of blood donated during the incubation period in the donor tends to be severe, but of the 2 seen by the present author, only one was jaundiced.

A review from Papua, New Guinea, includes discussion of the need for treating all patients with *anti-malarials* in endemic areas. *Syphilis* is still prevalent in some areas of New Guinea and as serological testing is not a complete safeguard, it is advisable to store blood for 72 hours when possible (88[r]).

Recent unusual infections transmitted by transfusion include *Babesiosis* surviving in frozen-thawed blood given to a splenectomised woman with thalassemia major. Treatment with pentamidine was successful (89[c]).

Yersinia enterocolitica contaminating blood packs was responsible for 2 severe infections, one fatal. This organism multiplies rapidly in whole blood or red cells at 4–8°C and appears to be widely distributed among the negro population in South Africa (90[C]).

Acquired immune deficiency syndrome (AIDS)

AIDS is a relatively new clinical entity, which is poorly understood. It is not, so far as is known, an adverse reaction, but it almost certainly can be transmitted via blood products. The clinical picture of malaise, fever, weight loss, lymphadenopathy and diarrhea should raise suspicion, supported further by lymph node histology of nonspecific reactive hyperplasia and the development of Kaposi's sarcoma in some cases. There is lymphopenia, defective cellular immune response with reversion of

T-helper cell/T-suppressor cell ratio but increased immunoglobulin levels.

Most cases have occurred in promiscuous male homosexuals, intravenous drug abusers and Haitian immigrants, but some have occurred in hemophiliacs, presumably in relation to the blood products they have received.

The distribution of the disease is predominantly in North America and the Caribbean, but it is also present in Europe. A report from the United Kingdom lists 14 cases of either Kaposi's sarcoma and/or AIDS between August 1982 and March 1983, and surveillance is continuing (91[c]).

In hemophiliacs, the disease may be symptom-free but associated with painless lymphadenopathy and not necessarily progressive (92[C]). Infection with micro-organisms associated with reduced immunity states may occur, and Pneumocystis carinii, Candida albicans and Herpes virus are the best known but others, including mixed infections with the preceding and Mycobacterium avium intracellulare, have been reported (93[C], 94[R]). The abnormal T-cell and increased B-cell response may be associated with clinically and hematologically typical immune thrombocytopenia occurring as a complication of severe hemophilia with high-dose factor VIII supplements, but the clinical extent of AIDS involvement varies and may be minimal (95[C]).

The etiology is at present unknown, but the disease-affected patients often have serological evidence of previous infection with hepatitis B, Epstein-Barr virus and CMV, and the altered T-cell function may perhaps be related to the complex antigen load and immune response to these combined infections (94[R]). It is also possible that human T-cell leukemia virus is involved in the pathogenesis and laboratory methods for determination for markers of this agent are becoming available (96[c]).

The precautions that seem advisable in the handling of whole blood and blood products are largely those usual in the handling of material known or suspected to be infected with hepatitis B antigen. They should provide safe conditions for work by clinical, laboratory and nursing staff and are given with some general advice on the problem in the following references (97[C], 98[R], 99[R], 100[r]).

HOST-vs-GRAFT, AND GRAFT-vs-HOST INTERACTIONS

Cytotoxic antibodies developed in 33 (14.6%) of 226 patients awaiting renal transplantation. This frequency was no different whether the transfusions were random or deliberate in timing, but the production of the cytotoxic antibodies and their anamnestic response showed that it is important to preserve all reactive patients' sera for cross-matching against possible donors later (101[C]). Alloimmunization following cardiopulmonary bypass surgery with its associated transfusions occurred in 33.6% of males and 64.3% of females, these presumably sensitized by previous pregnancies (102[C]). This alloimmunization carries implications for future transfusions and pregnancies.

The incidence of graft-versus-host disease following bone marrow transplantation is falling and depends on the careful use and timing of immunosuppressive drugs, especially methotrexate, antithymocyte globulin and prednisone (103[R]).

The use of cyclosporin A instead of methotrexate may help in the prevention of graft-versus-host disease with less bone marrow suppression, but toxic effects, especially renal, may limit dosage (104[C], 105[C]).

Granulocyte infusions may provoke graft-versus-host disease. A 5-year-old boy with Hodgkin's disease developed it after receiving nonirradiated granulocytes from his mother, and clinical and histological evidence of it followed fresh buffy coat infusions in a 59-year-old woman (106[c]).

Similar clinical and pathological changes followed syngeneic engraftment with cryopreserved buffy coat in chronic granulocytic leukemia. In the 2 cases reported, there was no reduction in suppressor T-cell numbers, and it seems possible that there was in fact an allograft derived from blood products causing the graft-versus-host disease (107[C]). This complication of cellular blood product infusion is now well recognized as occurring in immunosuppressed adults and in neonates, and requires the administration of at least 107 lymphocytes/kg. The simplest precaution to take is irradiation with a commercially available cesium source at a dose of at least 15 Gy (108[R], 109[R]).

REFERENCES

1. Daniels GL, Tohyama H, Uchikawa M (1982) A possible null phenotype in the Cromer blood group complex. *Transfusion, 22*, 362.
2. Cheng MS (1982) Saline-reactive anti-V. *Transfusion, 22*, 401.
3. Ellisor SS, Zelski D, Sugasawara E et al (1982) A second example of anti-Hil. *Transfusion, 22*, 402.
4. Woodfield DG, Douglas R, Smith J et al (1982) The Jk(a-b-) phenotype in New Zealand Polynesians. *Transfusion, 22*, 276.
5. Halima D, Garratty G, Bueno R (1982) An apparent anti-Jk^a reacting only in the presence of methylesters of hydroxybenzoic acid. *Transfusion, 22*, 521.
6. Cohen DW, Nelson L (1983) Auto-anti-P reacting only by low-ionic-strength-solutions in a patient with hemolysis. *Transfusion, 23*, 79.
7. Klarkowski DB, Ford DS (1983) A case of polyagglutination with features of Th and Tk activation associated with an acquired B antigen. *Transfusion, 23*, 59.
8. Judd WJ, Oberman HA, Flynn S (1982) Fatal intravascular hemolysis associated with T-polyagglutination. *Transfusion, 22*, 345.
9. Draper EK, Dignam CM, Yang S, Ballas SK (1982) Anti-lymphocyte globulin – a transfusion problem. *Transfusion, 22*, 345.
10. Biro V, Garratty G, Johnson CL, Marsh WL (1983) Depressed blood group antigens on red cells from a Mexican donor. *Transfusion, 23*, 65.
11. Garratty G, Vengelen-Tyler V, Postoway N et al (1982) Hemolytic transfusion reactions (HTR) associated with antibodies not detectable by routine methods. *Transfusion, 22*, 429.
12. Mintz PD, Haines AL, Sullivan MF (1982) Incompatible crossmatch following nonreactive antibody test. *Transfusion, 22*, 107.
13. Oberman HA, Barnes BA, Steiner EA (1982) Role of the crossmatch in testing for serologic incompatibility. *Transfusion, 22*, 12.
14. Whitsett CF, Daffin LE, Heffner LT et al (1982) ^{51}Cr studies verify anti-P P_1 P^k not detectable by in vitro crossmatch as cause of immediate hemolytic transfusion reaction. *Transfusion, 22*, 407.
15. Baldwin ML, Barrasso C, Ness PM, Garratty G (1983) A clinically significant erythrocyte antibody detectable only by ^{51}Cr survival studies. *Transfusion, 23*, 40.
16. Lee EL, Bennett C (1982) Anti-Co^b causing acute hemolytic transfusion reaction. *Transfusion, 22*, 159.
17. Postoway N, Anstee D, Wortman M et al (1982) A severe transfusion reaction due to anti-En^aTS in a patient with an unusual pattern of red cell sialoglycoproteins (SGP). *Transfusion, 22*, 412.
18. Azar PM, Saji H, Yamanaka R, Hosoi T (1982) Anti-Xg^a suspected of causing a transfusion reaction. *Transfusion, 22*, 340.
19. Argelagués E, Madoz P, Lluch A (1982) Reacción transfusional hemolitica retardada: a proposito de tres casos. *Biol. Clin. Hematol., 4*, 197.
20. Taddie SJ, Barrasso C, Ness PM (1982) A delayed transfusion reaction caused by anti-K6. *Transfusion, 22*, 68.
21. Waheed A, Kennedy MS (1982) Delayed hemolytic transfusion reaction caused by anti-Js^b in a Js(a+b+) patient. *Transfusion, 22*, 161.
22. Boyland IP, Mufti GJ, Hamblin TJ (1982) Delayed hemolytic transfusion reaction caused by anti-Fy^b in a splenectomised patient. *Transfusion, 22*, 402.
23. Kitzke HM, Julius H, DeLaney M et al (1982) Anti-Co^a implicated in delayed hemolytic transfusion reaction. *Transfusion, 22*, 407.
24. Beattie KM, Sigmund KE, McGraw J, Shurafa M (1982) U-variant blood in sickle cell patients. *Transfusion, 22*, 257.
25. Patten E, Reddi CR, Riglin H, Edwards J (1982) Delayed hemolytic transfusion reaction caused by a primary immune response. *Transfusion, 22*, 248.
26. Hoe DA, Graham SM, Luff R, Sohmer P (1982) Platelet counts during rapid massive transfusion. *Transfusion, 22*, 392.
27. Heinrichs C (1982) Hämostasedefekte nach Transfusionen. *Anaesthesiol. Reanimat., 7*, 245.
28. McClelland WM, McLaughlin KG, Poole J, Giles CM (1982) Haemolytic disease of the newborn due to a new red cell antigen 'Pollio'. *Clin. Lab. Haematol., 4*, 201.
29. Taylor AM, Knighton GJ (1982) A case of severe hemolytic disease of the newborn due to anti-Verweyst (Vw). *Transfusion, 22*, 165.
30. Dube VE, Zoes CS (1982) Subclinical hemolytic disease of the newborn associated with IgG anti-Lu^b. *Transfusion, 22*, 251.
31. Alves de Lima LM, Berthier ME, Sad WE, et al (1982) Characterisation of an anti-Di^a antibody causing hemolytic disease in a newborn infant. *Transfusion, 22*, 246.
32. Clarke C (1982) Historical annotation: rhesus haemolytic disease of the newborn and its prevention. *Br. J. Haematol., 52*, 525.
33. Bowell P, Wainscoat JS, Peto TEA, Gunson HH (1982) Maternal anti-D concentrations and outcome in rhesus haemolytic disease of the newborn. *Br. Med. J., 285*, 327.
34. Riley JZ, Ness PM, Taddie SJ et al (1982) Detection and quantitation of fetal maternal hemorrhage utilising an enzyme-linked antiglobulin test. *Transfusion, 22*, 472.
35. Sebring ES, Polesky HF (1982) Detection of fetal maternal hemorrhage in Rh immune globulin candidates. *Transfusion, 22*, 468.
36. Contreras M, Mollison PL (1983) Rh immunization facilitated by passively-administered

anti-Rh. *Br. J. Haematol.*, *53*, 153.
37. Dahlke MB, Keashen M, Alavi JB et al (1982) Granulocyte transfusions and outcome of alloimmunised patients with gram-negative sepsis. *Transfusion*, *22*, 374.
38. Kořinková P, Vorlíček J, Májský A (1982) A study of granulocyte cytotoxins and detection of granulocyte allospecific antigens. *Transfusion*, *22*, 379.
39. Ford JM, Brown LM, Cullen MH et al (1982) Combined granulocyte and platelet transfusions; development of alloimmunization as reflected by decreasing cell recovery values. *Transfusion*, *22*, 498.
40. Ford JM, Cullen MH, Roberts MM et al (1982) Prophylactic granulocyte transfusions: results of a randomized controlled trial in patients with acute myelogenous leukaemia. *Transfusion*, *22*, 311.
41. Sutton DMC, Shumak KH, Baker MA (1982) Prophylactic granulocyte transfusion during chemotherapy for acute myelogenous leukemia. *N. Engl. J. Med.*, *306*, 46.
42. Colombat Ph, Couret W, Garnier C et al (1982) Une année d'utilisation des unités leucocytaires et plaquettaires dans la région centre. *Rev. Méd. Tours*, *16*, 765.
43. Pollack MS, Levine LS, Oberfield SE, Markenson AL (1982) HLA-A, B, C, and DR antigen frequencies in relation to development of diabetes and variations in white cell antibody formation in highly transfused thalassemia patients. *Transfusion*, *22*, 279.
44. Neppert J (1983) Die Granulozytentransfusion. *Dtsch. Med. Wochenschr.*, *108*, 3.
45. Linko K (1982) Does blood transfusion cause respiratory failure? *Ann. Chir. Gynaecol.*, *71*, *Suppl. 196*, 37.
46. Snyder EL, Hezzey A, Barasch PG, Palerma G (1982) Microaggregate blood filtration in patients with compromised pulmonary function. *Transfusion*, *22*, 21.
47. Wenz B (1983) Microaggregate blood filtration and the febrile transfusion reaction. *Transfusion*, *23*, 95.
48. Editorial (1983) Microaggregate filtration. *Transfusion*, *23*, 89.
49. Snyder EL, Root RK, Hezzey A et al (1983) Effect of microaggregate blood filtration on granulocyte concentrates in vitro. *Transfusion*, *23*, 25.
50. Mijović V, Brozović B, Hughes ASB, Davies TD (1983) Leukocyte-depleted blood; a comparison of filtration techniques. *Transfusion*, *23*, 30.
51. Hughes ASB, Brozović B (1982) Leucocyte depleted blood; an appraisal of available techniques. *Br. J. Haematol.*, *50*, 381.
52. French JE, Solomon JM, Fratantoni JC (1982) Survey on the current use of leukapheresis and the collection of granulocyte concentrates. *Transfusion*, *22*, 220.
53. Seifried E, Pflieger H, Wiesneth M et al (1982) Haemostaseological investigations in neutropenic patients receiving granulocyte transfusion. Congress Austrian and German Soc. Hematol. Oncol., *45*, 201.
54. Moffat EH, Gerrish P, Mir MA, Darke C (1982) Remission of post-transfusion thrombocytopenic purpura with high dose intravenous corticosteroids. *Clin. Lab. Haematol.*, *4*, 333.
55. Slichter SJ (1982) Post-transfusion purpura: response to steroids and association with red blood cell and lymphocytotoxic antibodies. *Br. J. Haematol.*, *50*, 599.
56. Sorensen PG, Mickley H (1982) Problemer ved terapi med trombocytoprodukter. *Ugeskr. Laeg.*, *144*, 2345.
57. Memorandum by the Clinical Immunology Committee of the International Union of Immunological Societies and WHO (1982) Appropriate uses of human immunoglobulin in clinical practice. *Bull. WHO*, *60*, 43.
58. Editorial (1982) New formulation: immunoglobulin-intravenous drugs. *Drugs Today*, *18*, 538.
59. Bergmann H, Blauhut B (1982) Problems bei der Anwendung von Plasmafraktionen. *Hämostaseologie*, *3*, 83.
60. Fisher RI, Silver BA, Vanhaelen CP et al (1982) Objective regressions of T- and B-cell lymphomas in patients following treatment with anti-thymocyte globulin. *Cancer Res.*, *42*, 2465.
61. Wong KK, Sweet DL, Variakojis D (1982) The treatment of lymphoblastic lymphoma with anti-thymocyte globulin. *Cancer*, *50*, 57.
62. Singh KP, Sinha KI, Ganguly RR (1982) Injection fibrosis of quadriceps muscle in children. *J. Indian Med. Ass.*, *78*, 40.
63. Dillman RO, Shawler DL, Sobol RE et al (1982) Murine monoclonal antibody therapy in two patients with chronic lymphocytic leukaemia. *Blood*, *59*, 1036.
64. Hernandez D, Rosenshein NB, Pino y Torres J et al (1982) Ip immunotherapy and chemotherapy in advanced epithelial ovarian cancer. *Cancer Treatm. Rep.*, *66*, 1981.
65. Mazumder A, Grimm EA, Eberlein T et al (1982) Phase I trial of infusion into cancer patients of autologous lymphocytes activated *in vitro* with lectins. *Am. Assoc. Clin. Oncol. Abstr.*, *1*, 40.
66. Enzmann H (1982) Sensibilisierung bei der Verwendung von Fibrinkleber. *Laryng. Rhinol. Otol.*, *61*, 302.
67. Colvin BT, Ainsworth M, Buckley C (1983) Experience with highly purified porcine factor VIII in a patient with haemophilia A and a factor VIII inhibitor. *Clin. Lab. Haematol.*, *5*, 55.
68. Small M, Durward WF, Forbes CD (1983) Seizures after infusion of factor VIII. *Br. Med. J.*, *286*, 1106.
69. Schimpf K (1982) Herzinfarkt bei Hemmkörperhämophilie A nach einer Substitution mit aktiviertem Prothrombinkomplexkonzentrat. *Inn. Med.*, *9*, 424.

70. Editorial (1982) Myokardinfarkt als Therapiekonsequenz. *Münch. Med. Wochenschr.*, *124*, 21.
71. Ring J, Laubenthal H, Messmer K (1982) Incidence and classification of adverse reactions to plasma substitutes. *Klin. Wochenschr.*, *60*, 997.
72. Skidmore SJ, Boxall EH, Ala F (1982) A case report of post-transfusion hepatitis A. *J. Med. Virol.*, *10*, 223.
73. Dow BC, MacVarish I, Barr A et al (1980) Significance of tests for HBe Ag and anti-HBe in HBsAg positive blood donors. *J. Clin. Pathol.*, *33*, 1106.
74. Nath N, Fang CT, Dodd RY (1982) Specificity of and assay for antibodies to hepatitis B surface antigen. *Transfusion*, *22*, 300.
75. Tabor E, Hoofnagle JH, Barker LF et al (1981) Antibody to hepatitis B core antigen in blood donors with a history of hepatitis. *Transfusion*, *21*, 366.
76. Wozniak A, Hawksley VC (1982) Post-transfusion hepatitis: a retrospective study. *Military Med.*, *147*, 672.
77. Gerety RJ, Aronson DL (1982) Plasma derivatives and viral hepatitis. *Transfusion*, *22*, 347.
78. Rizza CR, Spooner RJD (1983) Treatment of haemophilia and related disorders in Britain and Northern Ireland during 1976–1980: report on behalf of the directors of haemophilia centres in the United Kingdom. *Br. Med. J.*, *286*, 929.
79. Stirling ML, Murray JA, MacKay P (1983) Incidence of infection with hepatitis B virus in 56 patients with haemophilia A 1971–1979. *J. Clin. Pathol.*, *36*, 577.
80. Rickard KA, Batey RG, Dority P et al (1982) Hepatitis and haemophilia therapy in Australia. *Lancet*, *2*, 146.
81. Gabra GS, Crawford RJ, Mitchell R (1982) Factor VIII cryoprecipitate and hepatitis risk. *Lancet*, *2*, 1220.
82. Hoppe K, Maass H (1982) Hepatitisrisiko von konventionellen PPSB-Poolpräparaten. *Dtsch. Med. Wochenschr.*, *107*, 1966.
83. Hernández JM, Piqueras J, Carrera A, Triginer J (1983) Posttransfusion hepatitis in Spain: a prospective study. *Vox Sang.*, *44*, 231.
84. Jones PM (1982) Blood donors with a history of jaundice. *Br. Med. J.*, *285*, 834.
85. Special Report. Report of the ad hoc committee on ALT testing (1982) *Transfusion*, *22*, 4.
86. Realdi G, Alberti A, Rugge M et al (1982) Long-term follow-up of acute and chronic non-A, non-B post-transfusion hepatitis: evidence of progression to liver cirrhosis. *Gut*, *23*, 270.
87. Tegtmeier GE, Bayer WL (1981) Those 'other agents' in the differential diagnosis of post-transfusion hepatitis. *Hepatitis, a Technical Workshop*, Amer. Ass. Blood Banks, p. 67.
88. Woodfield DG (1982) Infectious complications of blood transfusion. *Papua-New Guinea Med. J.*, *25*, 138.
89. Grabowski EF, Giardina PJV, Goldberg D et al (1982) Babesiosis transmitted by a transfusion of frozen-thawed blood. *Ann. Intern. Med.*, *96*, 466.
90. Stenhouse MAE, Milner LV (1982) Yersinia enterocolitica: a hazard in blood transfusion. *Transfusion*, *22*, 396.
91. O'Connor BH, McEvoy MB, Galbraith NS (1983) Acquired immune deficiency syndrome. *Br. Med. J.*, *286*, 1354.
92. Ragni MV, Lewis JH, Spero JA, Botempo FA (1983) Acquired-immunodeficiency-like syndrome in two haemophiliacs. *Lancet*, *1*, 213.
93. Elliott JL, Hoppes WL, Platt MS et al (1983) The acquired immunodeficiency syndrome and Mycobacterium avium-intracellulare bacteremia in a patient with hemophilia. *Ann. Int. Med.*, *98*, 290.
94. Waterson AP (1983) Acquired immune deficiency syndrome. *Br. Med. J.*, *286*, 743.
95. Ratnoff OD, Menitove JE, Aster RH, Lederman MM (1983) Coincident classical hemophilia and 'idiopathic' thrombocytopenic purpura in patients under treatment with concentrates of antihemophilic factor (factor VIII). *N. Engl. J. Med.*, *308*, 439.
96. Saxinger WC, Gallo RC (1982) Possible risk to recipients of blood from donors carrying serum markers of human T-cell leukaemia virus. *Lancet*, *1*, 1074.
97. Editorial (1983) Joint statement on acquired immune deficiency syndrome (AIDS) related to transfusion. *Transfusion*, *23*, 87.
98. Centers for Disease Control (1982) Acquired immune deficiency syndrome (AIDS): precautions for clinical and laboratory staffs. *MMWR*, *31*, 1.
99. Centers for Disease Control (1983) Prevention of acquired immune deficiency syndrome (AIDS): report of inter-agency recommendations. *MMWR*, *32*, 3.
100. Editorial (1983) Precautions against acquired immunodeficiency syndrome. *Lancet*, *1*, 164.
101. Larsen AE (1982) Selection of compatible kidney donors for recipients with multiple cytotoxic antibodies. *Transfusion*, *22*, 317.
102. Fauchet R, Genetet B, Gueguen M et al (1982) Transfusion therapy and HLA antibody response in patients undergoing open heart surgery. *Transfusion*, *22*, 320.
103. Denman AM (1982) Graft-versus-host disease. *Br. Med. J.*, *285*, 1226.
104. Barrett AJ, Kendra JR, Lucas CF et al (1982) Cyclosporin A as prophylaxis against graft-versus-host disease in 36 patients. *Br. Med. J.*, *285*, 162.
105. Atkinson K, Biggs JC, Ting A et al (1983) Cyclosporin A is associated with faster engraftment and less mucositis than methotrexate after allogeneic bone marrow transplantation. *Br. J. Haematol.*, *53*, 265.
106. Schmidmeier W, Feil W, Gebhart W et al

(1982) Fatal graft-versus-host reaction following granulocyte transfusions. *Blut, 45*, 115.

107. Starke ID, Thein SL, Goldman JM, Galton DAG (1982) Graft-versus-host disease after treatment for chronic granulocytic leukaemia in transformation. *Br. J. Haematol., 52*, 383.

108. Von Fliedner V, Higby DJ, Kim U (1982) Graft-versus-host reaction following blood product transfusion. *Am. J. Med., 72*, 951.

109. Pflieger H (1983) Graft-versus-host disease following blood transfusions. *Blut, 46*, 61.

110. Anon (1982) Reactions to normal human serum albumin, Amiri Hospital. *Kuwait Univ. Drug Adverse Reactions Series, 1*, 1.

Peter I. Folb

36 Intravenous infusions — solutions and emulsions

PROBLEMS OF TOTAL INTRAVENOUS NUTRITION

Why may total intravenous nutrition cause cholestasis?

In a recent study by Hughes et al (1[C]), conjugated hyperbilirubinemia was demonstrated in a biochemical, histological and electron microscopic investigation of 7 preterm infants who became jaundiced after prolonged total parenteral nutrition (TPN). This was apparently due to cholestasis, without significant liver cell injury. The absence of evidence of a direct toxic effect, and the analogy with the effects of total parenteral nutrition in experimental animals, suggested to the authors that this cholestasis may be the result of suppression of a trophic and/or secretion-stimulating hormone (or hormones) which is normally produced by the gut.

The clinical picture in such cases is not always the same. Other authors have described a case of cholestastic jaundice developing during TPN which mimicked the picture of large bile duct obstruction clinically and histopathologically. At post mortem examination the portal inflammatory infiltrate which had previously been demonstrated had cleared and was replaced by fibrosis (6[c]). The authors also suggest that alterations in bile chemistry could be responsible for a common pathogenetic mechanism between the lesions induced by parenteral feeding and mechanical large bile duct obstruction. The role of bile acid in the genesis of bile duct obstruction is presently under review.

Side Effects of Drugs Annual 8
M.N.G. Dukes, editor

ISBN 0 444 90339 9
$0.80 per article per page (transactional system)
$0.20 per article per page (licensing system)

The jaundice which occurs in association with total parenteral nutrition (SEDA-6, 301; SEDA-7, 338) may be due to a failure of bile secretion or excretion rather than to primary hepatocellular injury. Hughes et al (1[C]) were not able to identify any particular organelle damage. Ultrastructural changes were nonspecific, consistent with those described in association with cholestasis due to a variety of causes. A rise in plasma enzyme activity which developed shortly after the initiation of parenteral nutrition suggested that damage to hepatocytes may result from the resumption of bile flow. It is speculative whether this is due to a loss of integrity of pericanalicular tight junctions between hepatocytes which may have atrophied after total parenteral nutrition, allowing regurgitation of bile from canaliculi between the damaged hepatocytes.

This cholestasis does not appear to be related to any particular lipid, amino acid or protein hydrolysate constituents of the fluid given intravenously. Such a picture has been observed in infants not given any of these, who have not taken food by mouth in the course of a variety of gastrointestinal disorders. Cholestasis complicates TPN in 30% of cases. It develops characteristically within 2 to 4 weeks of the commencement of therapy, and clinically it mimics mechanical bile duct obstruction. It is usually transient in nature. In a report of 9 cases (8 of which had a fatal outcome) of progressive liver failure in surgical neonates maintained on prolonged TPN (for periods of 6 weeks to 15 months), several aspects of this complication emerged. It was associated with serious intra-abdominal surgical conditions, such as gastroschisis, bowel atresia with peritonitis, ante-natal peritonitis, and total colonic and ileal aganglionosis. The mean gestational age of the infants was 35 weeks with the sexes equally affected. The fatal cases had persistent cholestasis which failed to respond to alterations in parenteral protein or glucose concentrations. Enteral feeding was not tolerated. Clinical deterioration manifested by an increasing serum bilirubin, blood clotting dysfunction, hepatic enzyme elevations, and hepatomegaly. Histological examination showed significant distortion of hepatic architecture, with hepatocytes arranged in pseudoacini trapped by fibrous tissue. Bile duct proliferation was noted, but the ducts contained no bile. Bile plugs were seen in canaliculi only. Hepatocytes showed diffuse vacuolisation and stained positive for fat and iron. The portal triads were free of inflammation. Prematurity, immature liver function, dehydration, erythroblastosis fetalis, and amino acid imbalance with formation of a toxic bile salt were implicated in these findings. Sepsis and an inability to tolerate enteral feedings may have played a role (2[c]). The cause of the severe hepatic dysfunction in these patients was probably multifactorial, but TPN was certainly implicated. In many cases biochemical evidence of hepatic dysfunction disappeared when TPN was discontinued. However, even in survivors there is a risk of chronic liver disease.

Taurine may be an essential amino acid in pre-term and small neonates due to hepatic enzyme immaturity or deficiency. In premature infants adequate levels of cystine-sulfonic acid decarboxylase are required to convert methionine and cystine to taurine. A deficiency may result in decreased taurine concentrations in the bile and a fall in taurocholate. Taurolithocholate, the conjugated secondary bile salt, has been shown to cause cholestasis and consequent damage to the canalicular membrane in experimental animals. Taurocholate exerts a protective effect on taurolithocholate-induced cholestasis. Total parenteral nutrition has been linked with both acalculous cholecystitis and cholelithiasis. In a study of patients 15 years of age and older who had received TPN for a minimum of 3 months and a mean period of 13.5 months, 128 subjects were reviewed. 19 had gall bladder disease before receiving TPN. Of the 109 remaining 25 (23%) developed gall bladder disease. Patients with ileal disorders (Crohn's disease) or ileal resection, or both, were considered separately because of their known propensity for cholelithiasis. The incidence of 40% of gall bladder disease in 94 patients with ileal pathology was significantly higher than that which might be expected from a comparable group of patients not receiving TPN. On grounds of these findings the authors proposed that there is a decidedly greater risk of gall bladder disease among such patients, as a result of multiple factors working in concert to cause gall bladder stasis. Such individuals are already at risk of calculous and acalculous cholecystitis (3[c]).

The limitation of this study is that it was retrospective. The extent of ileal disease or resection was not controlled. In each case patients had undergone an ileal resection of at least 30 cm. The patients requiring TPN may have had more widespread Crohn's disease or have undergone more extensive resections than those with whom they were compared. This may explain the higher incidence of gall bladder disease observed in the TPN patients.

Stasis has been shown to be an important etiological factor in gallstone formation. A stagnant collection of bile provides an excellent milieu for cholesterol stones. Gall bladder 'sludge' developing as a result of stasis is calcium bilirubinate and contains little cholesterol. It has been demonstrated experimentally that the cholesterol saturation index does not increase as a result of gall bladder stasis during TPN. The same workers (3[c]) found an increased incidence of gall bladder disease among TPN patients treated repeatedly with narcotic or anticholinergic agents. Both of these classes of drugs have inhibitory effects on hepatic and cystic duct motility. Narcotics reduce bile flow through the sphincter of Oddi. Anticholinergics have been shown experimentally to reverse the protective effects of sphincteroplasty on gall stone formation. Whilst it is recognized that chronic administration of these medications may reflect more severe ileal or large bowel disease, their known effect on biliary function strongly suggests that they may be an important contributory factor in TPN-related gall bladder disease. It is still not known whether any particular element of the TPN solution is cholelithogenic (SEDA-7, 338; 3[c]). In a closely linked paper by the same authors (4[C]), it was suggested that hyperalimentation for an underlying intestinal disorder which does not permit oral feeding does not activate food-stimulated intestinal hormone secretion. This might be expected to influence the normal enterohepatic circulation of bile salt, alter bile composition, and result in stasis of bile within the gall bladder. These effects might in turn predispose to cholecystitis. It may be possible in the future to reduce the formation of gall stones by eliminating biliary stasis.

In an alternative approach, the effect of metronidazole on liver function tests was studied in 16 patients given total parenteral nutrition for an acute attack of Crohn's disease. In those patients receiving TPN and metronidazole concurrently, serum activities of alkaline phosphatase and γ-glutamyl transferase decreased or remained normal after 30 days of treatment. In contrast, serum enzyme activities increased sharply after prolonged TPN alone (5[C]). These findings were interpreted as indicating that TPN-associated intrahepatic cholestasis is caused by intestinal overgrowth of anaerobic bacteria. The latter may elevate biliary lithocholic acid concentrations, which have been shown to be higher in patients whose liver function tests have become abnormal during TPN than in patients whose liver function has remained normal. Intestinal overgrowth of anaerobic organisms may lead to production of hepatotoxic substances such as endotoxins and/or abnormal bile salts. In neonates and infants particularly, endotoxins may induce canalicular cholestasis as a result of inhibition of bile salt-independent biliary flow. Lithocholic acid, a secondary bile acid normally formed by bacterial 7-α-dehydroxylation of chenodeoxycholic acid, produces severe liver damage with cholestasis in several animal species. The histological changes (portal and periportal inflammation and fibrosis, and ductular proliferation) observed in animals given lithocholic acid and in patients receiving TPN are very similar. The demonstrated efficacy of metronidazole in reducing abnormalities of hepatic function associated with TPN suggests that anaerobic organisms may be involved in the pathogenesis of these changes.

Micronutrient deficiencies

Two adult patients receiving TPN long-term at home presented with extensive *loss of hair.* Both had had gut resections and had received no *biotin* orally or parenterally. Supplementation with biotin 200 mg daily resulted in gradual regrowth of healthy hair. Treatment was subsequently recommenced with a parenteral solution containing biotin, and the patients showed no recurrence of alopecia (7[c]). Unfortunately, no definitive assessment of the biotin status was obtained in these patients before supplementation was initiated.

Body biotin is obtained from both dietary sources and from enteric biosynthesis. The contribution from the latter source appears to be considerable. Biotin absorption is believed to take place in the proximal intestine by passive diffusion rather than active transport, and it would thus be dependent, at least to an extent, on intraluminal biotin concentration. The authors suggest that biotin deficiency may develop in an adult when no preformed biotin is provided and when in addition the contribution of this vitamin by intestinal microbial biosynthesis is compromised. They recommend, on the basis of their limited experience, that biotin should be added routinely to the micronutrient supplementation of all patients receiving TPN. This may be most critical in the case of patients in whom intestinal microbial synthesis is suppressed by antibiotic treatment, and in patients with a markedly shortened gut.

A child receiving TPN for approximately 1½ years developed intermittent *muscle pain and tenderness* in her legs with *elevations in serum enzymes* (glutamic oxaloacetic transaminase, glutamic pyruvic transaminase and creatine kinase). 6 months later her finger nails became whitened. Detailed cardiological evidence revealed no evidence of cardiac muscle cell damage, despite markedly elevated serum activities of the MB isoenzyme of creatine kinase. The entire picture was typical of selenium deficiency (SEDA-6, 299). Retrospective analyses during this period demonstrated very low serum selenium concentration and urine excretion of selenium. Intravenous supplementation of selenium 42 mg daily as elemental selenium (H_2SeO_3) and a prospective study of biochemical selenium status were begun 33.5 months after initiation of TPN. Both serum selenium concentration and whole blood glutathione peroxidase activity improved after selenium therapy. The finger nail bed abnormalities resolved (8[c]).

The authors suggest, on the basis of their own experience, that biochemical selenium deficiency is likely to develop within 6 months of commencing selenium-free TPN.

Since standard TPN preparations containing crystalline amino acids are unlikely to provide more than trivial amounts of selenium, they recommend that selenium supplementation should be administered to all patients receiving prolonged TPN. Implied in this is the necessity to monitor blood selenium levels and blood glutathione peroxidase activity as indicators of the need for continued selenium supplementation. Intracellular selenium deficiency is likely to develop after the serum selenium has been depleted. Reduction of serum selenium and fall in urine selenium excretion may be early indicators of total body depletion, but they are not sensitive indices of prolonged and clinically significant selenium deficiency. Patients with comparably reduced levels of serum selenium may differ considerably in the extent of cellular depletion.

The clinical significance of selenium deficiency remains unclear. The limitation of the aforementioned study, and the difficulty in evaluating it, is that, besides having selenium and possible magnesium deficiency, the patient had been receiving a fat emulsion that had low concentrations of chromium and linolenic acid. Both chromium and linolenic acid deficiencies could have contributed to the symptoms and to the peripheral neuropathy which developed late in the disease.

A possible case of human *linolenic acid* deficiency associated with *neurological abnormalities* has been described (9[c]). The association was mooted when the deficiency was corrected, with relief of the symptoms, suggesting that linolenic acid and its metabolites may have a physiological function in the nervous system. The authors are careful not to link the neuropathy categorically with linolenic acid deficiency. An alternative possibility for peripheral neuropathy in a patient of this kind is chromium deficiency, with which long-term TPN has been associated. In the case concerned serum chromium was not measured.

Metabolic bone disease

Although hypercalciuria and osteopenic bone disease have been identified in many patients maintained on long-term parenteral nutrition, and have been widely debated (SEDA-6; SEDA-7), the causes of the disturbance in calcium balance have not yet been clarified. On the basis of a study of the contents of a commercially available amino acid solution, Cole and Zlotkin (10[c]) suggest that the increased sulfate burden experienced with TPN may disturb calcium balance. They found increased sulfur-amino acid and inorganic sulfate content in the amino acid solution container. Its administration to a group of premature newborns resulted in an elevation of serum sulfate and increased calcium excretion. Supplemental cysteine resulted in a further increase in serum sulfate and urinary calcium excretion. In a group of 8 infants receiving either TPN or TPN plus cysteine, the sulfate levels in serum and the urinary calcium loss increased substantially. An association of hypersulfatemia, hypercalciuria and TPN-associated bone disease was suggested on grounds of these observations. The sulfate molecule is a polyanionic ligand capable of forming ion-pair complexes with calcium. As an excreted metabolite it inhibits reabsorption of calcium by the kidneys. The oxidation of sulfur amino acids produces two equivalents of hydrogen ion for every mole of sulfate formed. In this study metabolic acidosis was not detected, although modest changes in acid-base status may not have been apparent in the premature and full term infants that were studied (28 subjects).

The suggestion that increased sulfate may have a direct deleterious effect on bone is of interest. There is experimental evidence in rats and dogs that supplemental administration of sulfate or methionine results in an increased release of minerals from bone and subsequent osteopenia. Studies have shown that sulfate may substitute for phosphate in the apatite matrix (10[c]). However, it seems more likely that elevated sulfate is one of several etiological factors contributing to increased calcium loss from bone which develops with TPN given for prolonged periods, and its relative contribution has still to be determined.

Respiratory problems

A report of *hypophosphatemic respiratory failure* developing in an elderly woman with multiple intestinal fistulae who was treated with TPN serves to draw attention to the fact that the formulae for TPN either may not contain or may be deficient in their *phosphate* concentration. In such instances absence of exogenous phosphate supplementation can, with prolonged treatment, lead to hypophosphatemia, serious neurological and muscular disorders, and eventually hypophosphatemic respiratory failure (11[c]).

Patients treated with TPN for prolonged periods have been demonstrated to have *increased carbon dioxide production* (12[c]). This may be ascribed to the calorigenic action of the infused substances (specific dynamic action) and/or a metabolic stimulus as a result of reduced energy intake, counteracting the fall in basal metabolic rate induced by fasting. In a comparison of oxygen intake ($\dot{V}O_2$) during TPN with 100% glucose and with 62% glucose plus 38% fat respectively, $\dot{V}O_2$ was 21% less in the former case than in the latter. The $\dot{V}CO_2$ (carbon dioxide output) was 27% higher, and minute ventilation 26% higher in response to the change in $\dot{V}CO_2$. The diminished oxygen consumption which was found after substituting the mixture of glucose and fat with glucose alone may be attributed to (a) the known lower oxygen consumption involved in the combustion of glucose as opposed to fat; and/or (b) oxygen released by glucose-based lipogenesis. Glucose is much richer in oxygen than is fat. The authors are of the opinion that variations in $\dot{V}O_2$ and $\dot{V}CO_2$ developing during TPN may be clinically important in patients with impaired cardiovascular function (12[c]).

Miscellaneous complications

A case has recently been reported of *cortical venous thrombosis* developing as a result of administration of hyperosmolar parenteral nutrition fluid through a misplaced central venous catheter. The catheter had accidentally been placed in the internal jugular vein. It was suggested that central venous thrombosis developed in this patient as a result of retrograde perfusion of TPN fluid (13[c]). This stresses the importance of correct placing of the central catheter in the superior vena cava, and of confirming its position radiologically before any solution other than isotonic electrolytes is given.

A patient has been described who developed *hydrothorax* due to an extrapleural collection of parenteral nutrition fluid delivered via a centrally placed catheter. The tip of the catheter was in the right innominate vein or at the origin of the superior vena cava. The complication suddenly became apparent on the 5th day of treatment and probably resulted from the catheter finding its way into a small vein which had become thrombosed and eroded by the irritant fluid (14[c]).

Fat emulsions

The serum of over half of a group of 26 acutely ill patients *agglutinated Intralipid*, a fat emulsion based on soya bean oil, designed for intravenous infusion. The reaction was thought to be precipitated by C-reactive protein in the presence of calcium ions. Post mortem examination of the patients who had died showed evidence of lipid micro-embolism which could have been caused by agglutination of Intralipid. The study suggested that creaming of Intralipid may be a property of acute phase sera. This would explain the high proportion of 'creamers' in intensive care and coronary care units. The authors found a strong correlation between acute-phase serum C-reactive protein and ability to cream Intralipid (15[c]). C-Reactive protein is known to agglutinate lipid suspensions in vitro in the presence of calcium ions, and it seems possible that creaming of Intralipid and other intravenous fat emulsions occurs by the same mechanism.

Agglutination of Intralipid in vivo is only important if it occurs to a large extent. If agglutination in the blood stream takes place only to a minor degree, it will probably be cleared rapidly by the reticulo-endothelial system. Large-scale agglutination may result in lipid micro-embolization. Patients who have received Intralipid immediately before death have had lipid deposition demonstrated post mortem in the lungs and other tissues, including brain, kidney and spleen. Perhaps Intralipid should not be administered to certain acutely ill patients.

PLASMA SUBSTITUTES

Dextrans

Dextran-induced anaphylactic or anaphylactoid reactions were recorded in 1.99% of patients in whom dextran was used prophylactically against postoperative thromboembolism at the Central Hospital of Sogn og Fjordane, Norway. Of these 0.83% were serious. This represents a high incidence of dextran-induced reactions compared with data from other investigators (16[r]).

Using the red cell-linked antigen-antiglobulin reaction (RCLAAR) with stearoyl-dextran-coated erythrocytes, the immunoglobulin classes and IgG sub-classes of dextran reactive antibodies (DRA) were compared in 27 dextran-reactors and 96 non-reactors. High titres of dextran-reactive IgG were regularly found prior to the infusion in sera of patients who subsequently developed severe dextran-induced anaphylactoid or anaphylactic reactions. In 4 lethal cases IgG antibodies were found in high titre. Furthermore, high titres of IgA and IgM have been found in severe dextran-induced anaphylactoid reactions. Dextran non-reactors tend to have considerably lower titres of dextran reactive antibodies of the IgG, IgM and IgA classes. Immunoglobulin D antibody was absent in the serum of both groups. Dextran-reactive IgE antibodies were not demonstrable in dextran reactors. Dextran-reactive IgG1, IgG2, IgG3 and IgG4 were demonstrated (by indirect measurement) in both reactors and nonreactors. Dextran infusion caused variable neutralization of all IgG subclasses, but the contribution of IgG2 was considered most important because of its high titres and most pronounced neutralization in severe dextran reactions (17[C]).

The conclusions of these workers are that dextran reactive antibodies, mainly of the IgG class, play a critical role in the induction of severe dextran-induced anaphylactic reactions. The RCLAAR method facilitates definition of a patient risk group. It appears that predisposition to severe dextran-induced reactions of this nature may reside in a small number of individuals with high titres of dextran-reactive antibodies. Infusion of dextran in such patients generates immune complexes which produce symptoms as a result of a Type 3 immune response associated with complement activation and release of mediators.

Hetastarch

Hetastarch is a plasma volume expander used in adults for the treatment of shock caused by hemorrhage, burns, surgery, sepsis or trauma. It is a heterogenous macromolecular agent derived from starch and is composed primarily of amylopectin. Its major route of elimination is in the urine, and accumulation may occur in patients with severe renal impairment unless the dosage is adjusted. Adverse reactions associated with its use include minor defects in coagulation, and dose-related hematological abnormalities with high dose infusions (in excess of 1,500 ml). Elevations in serum α-amylase and indirect bilirubin have been reported. The incidence of allergic reactions was less than 0.01% of 16,405 infusions of hetastarch (18[r]). The majority of reactions were mild or moderate in severity. The incidence of severe allergic reactions involving shock, life-threatening spasm of smooth muscle, or cardiac or respiratory arrest is reported as 0.006% (18[r]).

Hetastarch should be used with caution in patients at risk of pulmonary edema or congestive heart failure. Circulatory overload may be induced. Large volumes of hetastarch may cause transient prolongation of prothrombin time, partial thromboplastin time, clotting time and bleeding time. It is contraindicated in patients with severe bleeding disorders.

More data are required to evaluate the acute and chronic effects of hetastarch compared with other plasma volume expanders, and to characterize its hematological effects. It is cheaper than albumin and appears to be equally effective as a volume expander.

Infectious complications of intravenous therapy

Over recent years nosocomial bacteremia and septicemia caused by contaminated intravenous products, and the development of sepsis as a hazard of the intravenous access line, have reached epidemic proportions (SED-9, 578). A study of 378 patients in 25 different American hospitals who developed Enterobacter cloacae or Enterobacter agglomerans septicemia (the latter was better known as a plant pathogen and had only been partly recognized as a human pathogen in the past) served to underline the high morbidity and mortality (13.4% mortality) of such a complication, and it focused attention on infusion fluid as a vehicle of infection. Furthermore, the point was highlighted that a high index of suspicion is required for the correct diagnosis to be made (19[CR]). The signs and symptoms of septicemia caused by con-

taminated intravenous fluid are similar to those of gram-negative septicemia of other etiologies. Nonspecific respiratory, gastrointestinal and neurological effects may divert attention from the primary etiology. There may be only mild and transient illness; most patients develop severe and debilitating disease. Patients with serious underlying diseases succumbed to infection more frequently (44.2%) than patients without underlying illness (7.4% incidence) (20[CR]). Although the organisms which were isolated were sensitive in vitro to nearly all antibiotics tested, it was characteristic of these infections that there was an inadequate response to therapy when the offending intravenous system had not been removed (20[CR]). Members of the tribe Klebsielleae, Enterobacterium, Pseudomonas, and Serratia, which are able to multiply at room temperature in intravenous solutions, predominated in these infections. In any case of septicemia that may be attributable to contaminated infusion fluid, members of the tribe Klebsielleae are likely to be predominant pathogens.

Infusion systems in continuous use are more vulnerable to introduction of organisms during manipulation or interference (e.g. injections, introduction of additives, cannula changes). The longer the device is left in place the higher the risk of related bacteremia. Routine replacement of the delivery system every 24–48 hours appears to reduce the likelihood of infections due to contaminated intravenous fluid, regardless of the source of contamination (19[CR]). This would not prevent clinical illness from intravenous fluid contaminated bacteriologically at the time of infusion.

Of the large number of epidemics of hospital-acquired bacteremia reported between 1965 and 1978 fully one-third were attributed to intravenous therapy. From a consideration of the documented epidemics of nosocomial infections related to contamination of large volume parenterals for intravenous administration or of intravenous access lines (19[CR], 20[CR]) the following general principles emerge:

1. *No infusion fluid can be assumed to be sterile at the time of use. Turbidity is not a reliable indicator of contamination.*
2. *When bacteremia is suspected, the entire infusion set should be immediately removed and cultured. This includes the fluid and cannula.*
3. *Identification, at least of genus, of all isolates is essential to programs of infection control.*
4. *Cannula-related septicemia most commonly begins as local infection of the dermal cannula wound.*
5. *Isolation of aerobic gram-negative organisms from the blood of a patient receiving infusion therapy raises suspicion of a contaminated infusate and may signal an epidemic.*
6. *The risk of fluid becoming contaminated during use is linked to the duration of uninterrupted infusion through the same administration set.*
7. *Immunocompromized patients are more susceptible to hospital-related infections of all types, including infusion-related bacteremia, but nosocomial bacteremia may also occur in patients whose immune responses are not suppressed.*

In two prospective clinical studies (21[c], 22[c]), one of which was randomized and controlled (22[c]), the conclusion was reached that routine replacement of the delivery system every 48 hours should normally control intravenous-associated bacteremia, in-use intravenous fluid contamination, and phlebitis, and that little benefit is likely to accrue from changing the administration sets more frequently.

Newborn infants are at special risk of infection caused by coagulase-negative staphylococci when a foreign body such as a vascular catheter is present in a large vessel (23[c]). The risk appears to be greater when parenteral nutrition is administered by a central venous catheter. Removal of the catheter and appropriate antimicrobial therapy results in resolution of the infection.

In a prospective study in adult patients of total parenteral nutrition-related infections 12 of 100 courses (12%) in 69 patients resulted in infections – 5 had sepsis, and 7 local infection. S. epidermidis, Candida species, S. aureus, Serratia marcescens, and mixed bacterial pathogens were most commonly identified. No differences were found among patients with and without infection with regard to age, underlying disease, surgery, systemic antibiotic usage, or the presence of other infections. A significant association was found between infection and violation of the access line by procedures such as extraction of a clot, using the line for central venous pressure readings, administering medications, and allowing the line to fall apart into a non-sterile field and then reconnecting it (24[C]).

The origins of bacteria responsible for catheter-related sepsis developing during total parenteral nutrition are unclear. Of 53 patients, in whom 74 catheters were used to administer TPN, bacteria and/or fungi were recovered from 19 catheters, and in 13 of the patients organisms were isolated in significant numbers concurrently from the insertion site. The results of this investigation were interpreted as demonstrating that skin colonization is a more frequent source of bacterial colonization of catheters than the hematogenous route (25[C]). A similar conclusion was reached in another study of 54 patients who received 59 courses of total parenteral nutrition, in whom a positive skin culture was found to have a positive predictive value of 61% for the development of infection (26[C]). The same authors argue that negative skin-entry-site cultures indicate strongly against the cannula as a source of infection in a patient receiving TPN. The study further emphasizes the importance of S. epidermidis as a pathogen in the septicemia complicating TPN, and as a common false-positive isolate. The conclusion that most cases of catheter related sepsis stem from skin colonization is contested by Sitges-Serra and colleagues (27[r]), who regard it as unproven and point out that concomitant culture from skin and catheter does not necessarily implicate the skin as the origin of microorganisms causing catheter related sepsis because contiguous seeding cannot be ruled out.

In a comparative investigation of four different brands of intravenous cannulae in patients undergoing elective surgery in Australia it was found that the dorsum of the hand was the anatomical site which developed the least number of complications, and that gauge of cannula had no influence on the incidence of complications. Phlebitis, thrombophlebitis, extravasation and blockage were more common with blood transfusion or when potassium or antibiotics were added to the infusion, and with prolonged duration of infusion (28[c]).

DRUG INCOMPATIBILITIES WITH INTRAVENOUS FLUIDS

The drugs added to intravenous fluids are mainly antibiotics, electrolytes, vitamins, aminophylline and heparin. The hazards of introducing an additive into an intravenous drip include breakdown of sterility, drug incompatibility, risk of thrombophlebitis, introduction of particulate matter, and an increased incidence of dose-related and idiosyncratic drug reactions.

A practical approach to antibiotic incompatibilities is indicated in Table 1. These are the drug incompatibilities with intravenous fluids that are best documented (29[R], 30[R], 31[R]).

Guidelines for the addition of drugs to intravenous fluids, aimed at maximum safety, include the following:

1. the addition of drugs to intravenous fluids should be discouraged, except in cases of emergency and for treatment of infants;
2. where addition of drugs to an intravenous fluid unit is indicated only one should be added;
3. the only intravenous fluids which should be used for this purpose are isotonic saline and 5% dextrose. More complicated electrolyte solutions and other fluids which contain amino acids and emulsions are not suitable.

An investigation of concentrations of active agents in common carrier media for intravenous infusion revealed that potassium chloride tends to form a pool when it is added without mixing in glass or polyvinyl chloride (PVC) containers which are already suspended in their functional position pointing downwards. Heparin behaves in a similar fashion when added without mixing to carrier media in PVC containers. Such uneven distribution may expose a patient to potentially dangerous, possibly lethal, concentrations of a drug, even when a relatively small amount of it is used. Insulin floats to the top of a hemacell container if its contents are not adequately mixed after addition. The irregularity of dosage that may result may make the management of diabetic ketoacidosis very difficult (32[R]).

Table 1. *Intravenous antibiotic admixture incompatibilities*[1,2] *(Based on references 29R, 30R, and 31R)*

	Amino acids	Aminophylline	Amphotericin B	Ampicillin	Calcium chloride	Carbenicillin	Chloramphenicol	Cimetidine	Erythromycin	Heparin Na^-	Hydrocortisone	Methylprednisolone	Sodium bicarbonate	Tetracyclines	Vitamin infusions	Vancomycin
Ampicillin[3,4]								+						+		
Carbenicillin			+				+	+	+					+	+	
Chloramphenicol						+		+	+		+	+	+	+	+	+
Clindamycin								+							+	
Erythromycin[4]						+	+	+		+				+	+	
Methicillin[4]								+			+		+	+	+	
Penicillin[5]	+		+					+		+			+	+	+	+
Tetracyclines[4,6]		+		+	+	+	+	+	+	+	+	+	+		+	

1. No antibiotics can safely be added to the following:
   Blood and blood components (human)
   Fat emulsion 10%
   Amino acid solutions
2. The following antibiotics are incompatible with all other drugs in admixture:
   cefazolin sodium — lincomycin hydrochloride
   gentamicin — minocycline hydrochloride
   kanamycin sulfate — oxacillin sodium
3. Sodium ampicillin is an alkaline antibiotic, and it may raise the pH of the intravenous fluid to 8.0 or higher, at which level ampicillin is slowly inactivated. In more acid solutions, such as 5% dextrose in water (pH about 4.7), ampicillin is more stable, but the pH of individual bottles may vary. For these reasons it is advisable to avoid adding ampicillin to intravenous solutions if possible.
4. The following indicates the stability of some antibiotics in intravenous fluids:

drug	intravenous fluid	% drug activity lost	time (hr)
erythromycin	dextrose/saline	21	12
nafcillin Na^+	dextrose 10%	47	24
oxytetracycline	dextrose 5%	25	24
ampicillin	dextrose 5%	24	8
methicillin Na^+	dextrose/saline	50	0.5
methicillin Na^+	dextrose	50	4.6

5. Penicillin G and semisynthetic penicillins are almost completely inactivated within a few hours in carbohydrate solutions containing sufficient bicarbonate to elevate the pH above 8.0. Penicilloic acid, which appears to play a role in some allergic reactions, is a major product of such inactivation.
6. Tetracyclines form stable insoluble chelates with polyvalent metal cations, eg Al^{+++}, Ca^{++}, Fe^{++}, Mg^{++}, that may be present in infusion fluids or in other medicines administered simultaneously.

Particulate contamination

The term particulate matter describes the suspended undissolved substances which may unintentionally be present in solutions for parenteral administration. Such substances can be detected and quantified by light and scanning electron microscopy, and energy dispersive X-ray analysis can be used to identify the inorganic element content (33[C]).

The particles may range in size from less than 0.5 μ to 450 μ, and contain elements such as chromium, copper, iron, zinc, silicon, manganese, calcium, sodium, potassium and chlorine. Organic particles including fibres of plastic, cellulose, cotton and other material, and rubber and similar substances from vial stoppers have been identified.

The shape and size of the particles may determine where in the body such particles will become lodged.

Particles introduced by injection or infusion may give rise to thromboembolic complications or foreign body reactions. The nature and extent of the pathological response may depend on

1. the site of injection (vein or artery, systemic or selective);
2. the site of lodgement of the particles;
3. the physical, chemical and biological properties of the particles;
4. the number of particles, their size and spatial configuration (34[C]).

In certain cases it has been recommended that parenteral solutions should be filtered, using a micropore filter with a pore size of 5 μ or less. It is important that such filters should not themselves shed particles into the solutions (35[c]).

The infusion into rabbits of particulate matter found in intravenous infusion solutions has produced disseminated vascular granulomas. Foreign body granulomas have been demonstrated post mortem in the lungs of patients as a result of infusion of 500 ml of solution. In post mortem examinations of patients who had received long-term intravenous therapy whilst terminally ill, vascular granulomas and evidence of chronic fibrosing pneumonitis have been found in which cellulose fibres and crystals were identified. Infusion phlebitis developing as a common consequence of intravenous therapy may be the result of infused particulate matter. Catheter-associated phlebitis of whatever cause is associated with an increased risk of septicemia. In extracorporeal infusion it has been suggested that plastic particles may be responsible for much of the cardiac, cerebral and other organ damage that may develop. Particles of silicone have been identified in kidney, heart, and in areas of cerebral softening after clinical and experimental heart surgery employing a bubble oxygenator which was coated with silicone to retard coagulation (36[R]).

The leaching of plasticizers from plastic containers and blood lines has been a major concern. A viral hepatitis-like syndrome developing in 6 patients after exposure to new PVC tubing during hemodialysis was attributed to high levels of plasticizer found in the blood, although in a subsequent paper the same authors express reservations over the association. The infusion of the plasticizer di-2-ethyl-phanthalate (DEHP) into subhuman primates has produced definite biochemical as well as morphological abnormalities in the liver. It is essential that physicians should ensure that all equipment and products related to intravenous therapy and extracorporeal circulation are adequately tested for particulate contamination before clinical use (36[R]).

Hazards of the intravascular catheter

Besides the potential thrombogenic effects and chemical irritation caused by catheters and guide-wires, there is always a risk, regardless of the material used, of fragmentation and embolism of such fragments (37[c]).

Particles shed by catheters may consist of fibres, carbon, or other unidentified material from the environment, manufacturing procedure or packing material. Plastic, bismuth, and unidentified grains of dyes and fillers may be released by shedding of catheter material as a result of irrigation or scraping by the guide-wire. Particles up to several centimeters in size have been found. The insertion of a guide-wire is likely to increase the number of particles measuring 5–10 μ in size released from a catheter up to 16-fold (37[C]).

ACKNOWLEDGEMENTS

The sections on particulate contamination and hazards of the intravascular catheter were contributed in large part by Dr. O. Winding, Institute of Hygiene, Faculty of Medicine, University of Copenhagen.

The section on Drug Incompatibilities with Intravenous Fluids is reproduced from Folb, P.I., Drug Safety in Clinical Practice. Springer-Verlag, Berlin, Heidelberg, New York, Tokyo, 1984, by permission of the publishers.

REFERENCES

1. Hughes CA, Talbot IC, Ducker DA et al (1983) Total parenteral nutrition in infants: effect on the liver and suggested pathogenesis. *Gut, 24*, 241.
2. Hodes JE, Grosfeld JL, Weber TR et al (1982) Hepatic failure in infants on total parenteral nutrition (TPN): clinical and histopathologic observations. *J. Ped. Surg., 17*, 463.
3. Roslyn JJ, Pitt HA, Mann LL et al (1983) Gallbladder disease in patients on long-term parenteral nutrition. *Gastroenterology, 84*, 148.
4. Pitt HA, King W, Mann LL et al (1983) Increased risk of cholelithiasis with prolonged total parenteral nutrition. *Am. J. Surg., 145*, 106.
5. Capron J-P, Gineston J-L, Herve M-A et al (1983) Metronidazole in prevention of cholestasis associated with total parenteral nutrition. *Lancet, 1*, 446.
6. Body JJ, Bleiberg H, Bron D et al (1982) Total parenteral nutrition-induced cholestasis mimicking large bile duct obstruction. *Histopathology, 6*, 787.
7. Innis SM, Allardyce DB (1983) Possible biotin deficiency in adults receiving long-term total parenteral nutrition. *Am. J. Clin. Nutrit., 37*, 185.
8. Kien CL, Ganther HE (1983) Manifestations of chronic selenium deficiency in a child receiving total parenteral nutrition. *Am. J. Clin. Nutrit., 37*, 319.
9. Meng HC (1983) A case of human linolenic acid deficiency involving neurological abnormalities. *Am. J. Clin. Nutrit., 37*, 157.
10. Cole DEC, Zlotkin SH (1983) Increased sulfate as an etiological factor in the hypercalciuria associated with total parenteral nutrition. *Am. J. Clin. Nutrit., 37*, 108.
11. Youssef HAE (1982) Hypophosphatemic respiratory failure complicating total parenteral nutrition – an iatrogenic potentially lethal hazard. *Anesthesiology, 57*, 246.
12. Mondejar EF, Lombardo MD, De la Cruz AJP et al (1982) Variations in oxygen consumption and carbon dioxide production during parenteral nutrition. *Intens. Care Med., 8*, 169.
13. Souter RG, Mitchell A (1982) Spreading cortical venous thrombosis due to infusion of hyperosmolar solution into the internal jugular vein. *Br. Med. J., 285*, 935.
14. Wright JE (1982) Hydrothorax: a delayed complication of parenteral nutrition via a central venous catheter. *Austr. Paediatr. J., 18*, 216.
15. Hulman G, Fraser I, Pearson HJ et al (1982) Agglutination of Intralipid by sera of acutely ill patients. *Lancet, 2*, 1426.
16. Flaatten H (1982) Dextran-induced anaphylactic reactions. *Tidsskr. Nor. Laegeforen, 11*, 102.
17. Kraft D, Hedin H, Richter W et al (1982) Immunoglobulin class and subclass distribution of dextran-reactive antibodies in human reactors and non reactors to clinical dextran. *Allergy, 37*, 481.
18. Nakasato SK (1982) Evaluation of hetastarch. *Clin. Pharmacol., 1*, 509.
19. Maki DG, Rhame FS, Mackel DC et al (1976) Nationwide epidemic of septicemia caused by contaminated intravenous products. *Am. J. Med., 60*, 471.
20. Maki DG (1981) Nosocomial bacteremia: an epidemiologic overview. *Am. J. Med., 70*, 719.
21. Buxton AE, Highsmith AK, Garner JS et al (1979) Contamination of intravenous infusion fluid: effects of changing administration sets. *Ann. Intern. Med., 90*, 764.
22. Band JD, Maki DG (1979) Safety of changing intravenous delivery systems at longer than 24-hour intervals. *Ann. Intern. Med., 91*, 173.
23. Munson DP, Thompson TR, Johnson DE et al (1982) Coagulase-negative staphylococcal septicemia: Experience in a newborn intensive care unit. *J. Pediatr., 101*, 602.
24. Snydman DR, Murray SA, Kornfeld SJ et al (1982) Total parenteral nutrition-related infections: prospective epidemiologic study using semiquantitative methods. *Am. J. Med., 73*, 695.
25. Bjornson HS, Colley R, Bower RH et al (1982) Association between microorganism growth at the catheter insertion site and colonization of the catheter in patients receiving total parenteral nutrition. *Surgery, 92*, 720.
26. Snydman DR, Gorbea HF, Pober B et al (1982) Predictive value of surveillance skin cultures in total-parenteral-nutrition-related infection. *Lancet, 2*, 1385.
27. Sitges-Serra A, Jaurrieta E, Liñares J et al (1983) Bacteria in total parenteral nutrition catheters: where do they come from? *Lancet, 1*, 531.
28. Holland RB, Levitt MWD, Steffen CM et al (1982) Intravenous cannulas: survey of their use in patients undergoing elective surgery. *Med. J. Austr., 2*, 86.
29. Engel G (1971) Addition of drugs to intravenous fluids. *Med. J. Aust., 2*, 962.
30. Newton DW (1978) Physicochemical determinants of incompatibility and instability in

injectable drug solutions and admixtures. *Am. J. Hosp. Pharm.*, *35*, 1213.

31. Medical Economics Company (by arrangement with New England Deaconess Hospital, Boston, Massachussets) (1980) *A Guide to I.V. Admixture Compatibility*. Oradell, New Jersey.
32. Bergman N, Vellar ID (1982) Potential life-threatening variations of drug concentrations in intravenous infusion systems: potassium chloride, insulin, and heparin. *Med. J. Aust.*, *2*, 270.
33. Winding O, Holma B (1976) Method for determination and element analysis of particulate contamination in injectable solutions. *Am. J. Hosp. Pharm.*, *33*, 1154.
34. Winding O (1981) Foreign-body contamination at angiography. Thesis FADL's Forlag.
35. Winding O (1980) Intrinsic particles in angiographic contrast media. *Radiology*, *134*, 317.
36. Leading Article (1982) Particulate contamination in intravenous therapy and extracorpoeal systems. *Med. J. Aust.*, *2*, 309.
37. Winding O (1981) Particle release from angiographic utensils. *Eur. J. Radiol.*, *1*, 114.

E.A. Loeliger

37 Drugs affecting blood clotting and hemostasis

HEMORRHAGIC COMPLICATIONS

Quantitative assessment of the bleeding risk

Hospitalized patients with proximal vein thrombosis, initially treated intensively for 14 days with continuous intravenous heparin combined during the last 4 days with a standard regimen of warfarin, were randomly allocated to 2 groups for a further 3 months of prophylaxis using either conventional oral anticoagulation (to prolong the prothrombin time up to more than 5 times normal in terms of International Normalized Ratio) or low-dose oral anticoagulation (with target values close to 2 INR). The less intensive anticoagulant therapy was apparently associated with the same low frequency of recurrent venous thromboembolic complications as was the highly intensive treatment, but with a much reduced risk of hemorrhage (22[C]).

Both spinal and epidural anesthesia could be administered without any signs of local bleeding in 187 patients given prophylaxis with dihydroergotamine (0.5 mg) combined with heparin (5,000 IU) 2 hours preoperatively and continued at 12-hour intervals for at least 7 days post-operatively (4[C]).

The results of a prospective randomized double-blind clinical trial to compare venous prophylaxis by means of 5,000 IU heparin s.c., administered every 12 hours, with an alternative regimen employing 2,500 IU heparin combined with 0.5 mg dihydroergotamine (DHE) given at the same intervals, have shown convincingly that the risk of wound hematomata and reinterventions due to local hemorrhagic complications is significantly lower in the patients given the combination of heparin and DHE (5[C]).

The extensive experience acquired by the European cooperative study group with a glucose-controlled *one-day systemic infusion of streptokinase* (250,000 IU over 20 min, followed by 100,000 IU over the next 24 hours) in 156 patients included 2 *intracerebral hemorrhages*, one small and subsiding within some weeks, the other of unknown clinical severity, the patient having died of cardiac rupture 24 hours after the onset. In 5 patients the infusion had to be stopped because of severe bleeding at the puncture sites. All other bleedings were minor. The only patient requiring blood transfusion was in the control group. Chills and rigors were observed in roughly 1 in 10 patients. The mean hematocrit decrease was 3.4% in the streptokinase group and 1.8% in the glucose group, a significant though clinically irrelevant difference (43[CR]).

Fatal transmural hemorrhagic infarcts developed in 4 out of 101 patients with acute myocardial infarction whose coronary arteries were successfully recanalized by *local application of intracoronary streptokinase.* Unfortunately, no data were given on the pretreatment hemostasis profile or on the posttreatment heparin dosage, both of which could have been of decisive importance in the development of severe hemorrhagic imbibition of the myocardium after thrombolysis (26[C]). The safety data on 209 US cases in the Hoechst-Roussel intracoronary streptokinase registry also underscore the danger of excessive bleeding when thrombolysis is associated with general heparinization (50[C]).

The *combined streptokinase/plasminogen infusion* to induce permanent plasminemia was again shown to be accompanied by a high (about 30%) incidence of macro-hematuria and other major hemorrhages (46[C]).

Side Effects of Drugs Annual 8
M.N.G. Dukes, editor

ISBN 0 444 90339 9
$0.80 per article per page (transactional system)
$0.20 per article per page (licensing system)

Specific bleeding complications

For the first time, *mono-articular joint destruction* due to recurrent hemarthrosis and resembling hemophilic arthropathy has been described; this case concerned a 56-year-old patient who had been on long-term prophylaxis with warfarin for 10 years after receiving a Starr-Edwards aortic valve prosthesis (6^C).

4 cases of *calf hematoma* after treatment with heparin prescribed on the basis of an incorrect diagnosis, i.e. deep venous thrombosis, have been reported in patients suffering from synovial rupture of the knee (Baker's cysts) (51^{CR}).

Rare bleeding complications

In the French literature there is the report of a case of an endoscopically confirmed *hematoma of the oesophagus* in a patient treated with acenocoumarin combined with ticlopidine (!). The laboratory data point to over-treatment with oral anticoagulants. The symptoms mimicked acute myocardial infarction or dissection of the aorta (18^C).

Equally rare is the *intramural duodenal hematoma*, of which only 14 cases have thus far been reported in the world literature (15^{CR}).

The case of an *anterior mediastinal hematoma* and left hemothorax occurring during well-controlled oral anticoagulation may well be an example of a severe hemorrhagic complication in a patient with an additional disturbance of the intrinsic coagulation mechanism, since the partial thromboplastin time appeared to be disproportionately prolonged (1^C).

A 22-year-old man with obstructive uropathy and renal failure who was given pre-operative hemodialysis collapsed and died 5 hours later. Autopsy revealed massive *intrarenal hemorrhage and intraperitoneal rupture* of a dilated superior calix. Anticoagulation with heparin employed during hemodialysis was, although apparently well controlled, assumed to have been responsible for the calamity (35^C).

PROBLEM SITUATIONS IN ANTI-COAGULATION

Toxicity

Vitamin K_1 epoxide accumulation in the plasma, reaching a maximum 3–4 hours after intravenous application of 10 mg vitamin K_1, and specifically assessed by means of a gas-liquid chromatographic method, is claimed to be the best method for rapid assessment or confirmation of *surreptitious or accidental ingestion/overdosage* of an oral anticoagulant (8).

Transcutaneous uptake of warfarin present in talcum powder used for infant hygiene caused severe hypoprothrombinemia leading to death in 177 of 741 children (25).

Skin necrosis

Cases of coumarin necrosis in patients with obvious initial overshooting hypoprothrombinemia continue to be reported (19^C, 20^C, 44^C). The classic picture of skin necrosis was observed on repeated occasions, not only after intake of coumarin, but for the first time also (once) during an episode of cholestasis associated with the development of hypoprothrombinemia (19^C). This case gave occasion for further investigation, which incriminated hereditary protein-C deficiency as one of the predisposing conditions for the development of coumarin necrosis (10). Severe shortage of protein C, developing immediately after an initial loading dose of coumarin, is probably responsible for diffuse thrombosis of small venules in the affected skin areas. It is obvious that protein-C deficiency will be especially pronounced in patients with low baseline values, as in, for example, heterozygotes (having the severe defect) or in cases with a mild (homozygotic?) protein-C deficiency (about 20% of normal), the latter having been the case in the patient with a coumarin-type necrosis (10).

HEPARIN *(SED-9, 599; SEDA-6, 304; SEDA-7, 344)*

Calcium versus sodium heparin

The relative efficacy and side effects of subcutaneously administered sodium and calcium heparin have been studied in another randomized double-blind placebo-controlled trial. The two preparations were products of the same manufacturer (Allen & Hanburys). While calcium heparin tended to be more effective, this preparation led to significantly more local hematoma and pain (12), a conclusion which is at variance with earlier reports (2, 45).

Osteoporosis *(SED-9, 601)*

The Swedish Adverse Drug Reactions Advisory Committee (57[Cr]) had up to 1982 received reports of 4 cases of osteoporosis and multiple vertebral compression where a connection with heparin therapy was suspected; 3 of the patients were young (27–33 years of age). All these 3 had developed the complication during or shortly after pregnancy. The shortest period of treatment prior to symptoms was about 10 weeks, and the lowest heparin dose was 10,000 IU/day. One of the pregnant women had been treated concurrently with phenemal and phenytoin, which in rare cases may elicit osteomalacia.

Vasospastic reactions

Cases of suspected serious vasospastic reactions observed during routine thrombosis prophylaxis with heparin-dihydroergotamine continue to be published (5[C], 47[C], 48[C]); at least some of these may have been due to overdosage (36[C]). Some of the cases of supposed ergotism may be caused by undesirably severe vasoconstriction in areas of diminished sympathic innervation, known for instance in paraplegia patients, patients with epidural anesthesia after sympathectomy, or in cases where the extremities have been compromized by surgical or accidental trauma (38[CR], 40[C]).

Thrombocytopenia, thrombosis and skin necrosis

IgG has once again been shown to be responsible for the heparin-dependent severe type thrombocytopenia which is often complicated by thromboembolism (14[C], 21[C], 32[CR], 54[C]), one Australian paper reporting as many as 12 delayed-onset cases, 7 of them with thromboembolic complications (54[C]). Cipolle et al (56[C]) found that of a series of 211 patients treated with i.v. heparin for thromboembolic disease 11 (5.2%) developed thrombocytopenia between days 2 and 10 of therapy; of these, 10 were receiving beef lung heparin and only 1 porcine intestinal mucosal heparin, although the 2 products had been employed in similar numbers of patients. The platelet-aggregating property of heparin was found to be associated with its high molecular weight fractions (21[C]).

For the first time, a necrotizing leucocytoclastic vasculitis was identified as the pathological mechanism underlying heparin necrosis at the sites of subcutaneous heparin injections (23[C]). The reaction is independent of the type and brand of heparin used, as demonstrated by positive intradermal skin tests of 5 brands of heparin (4 originating from a porcine source and 1 from a bovine source); these tests were performed in a patient with the classical picture of large tender erythematous plaques developing from the second week of treatment onwards in the skin overlying the sites of subcutaneous heparin injection (41[CR]).

A review of the world literature on heparin-induced thrombocytopenia, written in French, is worth consultation (39[CR]).

Interferences with laboratory tests

The artefactual increases of as much as 50% in total thyroxine (T4), estimated by a competitive protein-binding assay, and of as much as 30% in tri-iodothyroxine (T3) resin uptake are in all probability the results of rapid and continuing lipolytic hydrolysis of triglycerides after blood has been drawn. The equilibrium between bound and free hormones is disturbed by in vitro generated nonesterified fatty acids, which compete strongly with T4 (and T3) for binding sites on serum albumin. Thyroid function tests should therefore always be performed on blood samples taken before (or a sufficient time after) heparin treatment (52).

WARFARIN AND OTHER COUMARIN CONGENERS *(SED-9, 601; SEDA-7, 348)*

Risk factors

The observation of an unusually long elimination half-life of warfarin (78 h instead of the normal 37 ± 2.1 h) in a patient with profound iron deficiency points to the possibility of alteration of warfarin metabolism, under conditions of severe iron deficiency, at the level of the hepatic microsomal cytochrome P-450 drug-metabolizing system (31).

Drug interactions

Sulphinpyrazone, in sharp contrast to phenylbutazone, did not significantly influence the reaction to a single dose of racemic phenprocoumon (0.6 mg/kg) in 6 volunteers. The slight prolongation of the prothrombin time was not significant, nor was the slightly slower disappearance from plasma (34). This apparent lack of interaction is in contrast with the highly significant augmentation by sulphinpyrazone of the hypoprothrombinemia induced by acenocoumarol and warfarin reported earlier (29, 33).

It is now claimed that the anti-arrhythmic compounds *quinidine* and *disopyramide* do not interfere with oral anticoagulants. The slight (10–20%) though significant decrease in the anticoagulant effect of dicoumarol or warfarin is attributed to improved liver blood flow after DC conversion (42[C]).

Husserl (55[c]) has described the case of a man of 69 on peritoneal dialysis taking various drugs including warfarin. Prothrombin time increased (31.3 sec; control 11 sec) when erythromycin was added to the therapeutic regimen; both warfarin and erythromycin were withdrawn and there was recovery; one cannot of course know what would have happened had only erythromycin been withdrawn, but the possibility of an interaction in this case must be borne in mind.

THROMBOLYTIC AGENTS

The case of a 63-year-old female patient with massive pulmonary embolism who developed the *adult respiratory distress syndrome* (ARDS) shortly after a course of streptokinase therapy has been reported. The possible association between streptokinase therapy for pulmonary embolism and ARDS should be kept in mind now that streptokinase is gaining wider clinical application. A full discussion of the possible pathogenic mechanism is presented in this report (24[C]).

The report of a case of transient leukemoid plasmocytosis with up to 7×10^9 plasma cells per liter and an increase of IgM and IgG up to 9.3 and 22 g/l respectively, is a good example of the well-known *immune complex syndrome* developing after thrombolysis induced by streptokinase (27[C]).

Streptokinase induced a severe, though nonfatal *shock reaction* when it was injected for the second time 4 weeks after successful clearance of a thrombosed Scribner shunt (7[C]).

Pick et al from San Diego (53[C]) have described the occurrence of acute renal failure in a 38-year-old man treated with streptokinase for pulmonary embolism; he had received streptokinase before. The serum creatinine rose to 4.8 mg/dl, and urea nitrogen to 57 mg/dl; there was recovery on withdrawal of the treatment.

ANTI-PLATELET DRUGS

Ticlopidine

7 additional cases of complete *agranulocytosis*, observed within 1–7 weeks after the start of ticlopidine (co-)medication and disappearing rapidly after withdrawal of the drug, and 1 case of *cholostatic hepatopathia* developing 3 months after the start of ticlopidine (co-)medication and subsiding after discontinuation of the drug, have been reported (9[C], 13[C], 16[C], 28[C]). Causality has been challenged, because treatment with ticlopidine often coincides with treatment with vasodilating agents and the latter can also cause agranulocytosis or may enhance ticlopidine toxicity (17).

ANTIDOTES

Vitamin K_1

On the basis of the report of 2 more cases of serious complications, one of them fatal, it is recommended that intravenous infusion of phytonadione be given at a rate considerably slower than 1 mg/min (37[C]).

EACA (ϵ-aminocaproic acid) and AMCHA (tranexamic acid)

A large *cerebral infarction* detected by a CT scan which became fatal within 6 weeks occurred in a 26-year-old female patient who had been given 1.5 g AMCHA daily for several weeks to stop uterine bleeding after the insertion of an IUD (3[C]). An additional case and an exhaustive review of the world literature concerning myopathy secondary to EACA administration have been presented (11[CR]).

Protamine sulfate

A severely debilitating anaphylactic reaction in a diabetic woman given about 10 mg of protamine sulfate to reverse the anticoagulant effect of heparin, points once again to the risk of inducing immunological reactions in patients previously exposed to protamine contained in neutral protein Hagedorn insulin (49[C]), the response resembling that of patients treated with protamine zinc insulin (30[C]).

REFERENCES

1. Abaskaron M, Peterson G, Huang TY (1983) Anterior mediastinal haematoma and left haemothorax on well-controlled oral anticoagulant therapy. *Postgrad. Med. J., 59*, 95.
2. Abou-Abdallah E, Rausis C, Loup P, Mosimann R (1975) Etude comparative héparinate de sodium et de calcium dans la prophylaxie des maladies thrombo-emboliques en chirurgie. *Helv. Chir. Acta, 42*, 691.
3. Agnelli G, Gresele P, De Cunto M et al (1982) Tranexamic acid, intrauterine contraceptive devices and fatal cerebral arterial thrombosis. Case report. *Br. J. Obstet. Gynaecol., 89*, 681.
4. Allemann BH, Gerber H, Gruber UF (1983) Rückenmarksnahe Anaesthesie und subkutan verabreichtes low-dose Heparin-Dihydergot zur Thromboembolieprophylaxe. *Anaesthesist, 32*, 80.
5. Amman JF, Aebi B (1983) Das Blutungsrisiko der Thromboembolie-Prophylaxe in der Allgemeinchirurgie: Vergleich von low-dose-Heparin mit Heparin-Dihydergot 2500. *Chirurg, 54*, 29.
6. Andes WA, Edmunds JO (1983) Hemarthroses and warfarin: joint destruction with anticoagulation. *Thromb. Haemostas., 49*, 187.
7. Baumgartner TG, Davis RG (1982) Streptokinase-induced anaphylactic reaction. *Clin. Pharm., 1*, 470.
8. Bechtold H, Trenk D, Jähnchen E, Meinertz T (1983) Plasma vitamin K_1-2,3-epoxide as diagnostic aid to detect surreptitious ingestion of oral anticoagulant drugs. *Lancet, 1*, 596.
9. Biour M, Toussaint P, Duhamel G et al (1982) Ticlopidine: atteintes sanguines et hépatiques? (letter). *Thérapie, 37*, 222.
10. Broekmans AW, Bertina RM, Loeliger EA et al (1983) Protein C and the development of skin necrosis during anticoagulant therapy. *Thromb. Haemostas., 49*, 251.
11. Brown JA, Wollmann RL, Mullan S (1982) Myopathy induced by epsilon-aminocaproic acid. *J. Neurosurg., 57*, 130.
12. Cade JF, Andrews JT, Stubbs AE (1982) Comparison of sodium and calcium heparin in prevention of venous thromboembolism. *Aust. N. Z. J. Med., 12*, 501.
13. Chomienne C, Baumelou E, Rio B et al (1983) Deux observations d'agranulocytose aiguë au cours d'un traitement antiagrégant par la ticlopidine. *Rev. Méd. Thérapeutique, 13*, 589.
14. Chong BH, Pitney WR, Castaldi PA (1982) Heparin-induced thrombocytopenia: association of thrombotic complications with heparin-dependent IgG antibody that induces thromboxane synthesis and platelet aggregation. *Lancet, 2*, 1246.
15. D'Amato A, Ferrara A, Fuortes M et al (1982) Intramural duodenal hematoma. A case occurred during anticoagulant therapy with vitamin K antagonists. *Ital. J. Surg. Sci., 12*, 303.
16. De Gramont A, Canuel C, Krulik M et al (1982) Toxicité hématologique de la Ticlopidine? *Nouv. Rev. Fr. Hématol., 24*, 35.
17. Desablens B, Messerschmitt J (1982) Toxicité hématologique des vasodilatateurs? *Nouv. Rev. Fr. Hématol., 24*, 313.
18. Dumas D, Faux N, Levillain Cl et al (1983) L'hématome intra-mural spontané de l'oesophage. *Méd. Chir. Dig., 12*, 47.
19. Hofmann V, Frick PG (1982) Repeated occurrence of skin necrosis twice following coumarin intake and subsequently during decrease of vitamin K dependent coagulation factors associated with cholestasis. *Thromb. Haemostas., 48*, 245.
20. Howitt AJ, Williams AJ, Skinner C (1982) Warfarin-induced vasculitis: A dose-related phenomenon in susceptible individuals? *Postgrad. Med. J., 58*, 233.
21. Huisse M-G, Guillin M-C, Bezeaud A et al (1982) Heparin-associated thrombocytopenia. In vitro effects of different molecular weight heparin fractions. *Thromb. Res., 27*, 485.
22. Hull R, Hirsh J, Jay R et al (1982) Different intensities of oral anticoagulant therapy in the treatment of proximal vein thrombosis. *N. Engl. J. Med., 307*, 1676.
23. Kearsley JH, Jeremy RW, Coates AS (1982) Leucocytoclastic vasculitis and skin necrosis following subcutaneous heparin calcium. *Aust. N. Z. J. Med., 12*, 288.

24. Martin TB, Sandblom RL, Johnson RJ (1983) Adult respiratory distress syndrome following thrombolytic therapy for pulmonary embolism. *Chest, 83*, 151.
25. Martin-Bouyer G, Linh PD, Tuan LC et al (1983) Epidemic of haemorrhagic disease in vietnamese infants caused by warfarin-contaminated talcs. *Lancet, 1*, 230.
26. Mathey DG, Shofer J, Kuck K-H et al (1982) Transmural, haemorrhagic myocardial infarction after intracoronary streptokinase. Clinical, angiographic, and necropsy findings. *Br. Heart J., 48*, 546.
27. Maubach PA, Emmerich B, Theiss W et al (1983) Reaktive leukämoide Plasmozytose mit polyklonaler Gammaglobulinvermehrung unter Streptokinasetherapie. *Dtsch. Med. Wochenschr., 108*, 383.
28. Meyer C, Chassagnon Ch, Prignet JM (1982) Agranulocytose en relation avec un traitement de ticlopidine (letter). *Lyon Méd., 248*, 407.
29. Michot F, Holt NF, Fontanilles F (1981) Über die Beeinflussung der gerinnungshemmenden Wirkung von Acenocoumarol durch Sulfinpyrazon. *Schweiz. Med. Wochenschr., 111*, 255.
30. Moorthly SS, Pond W, Rowland RG et al (1980) Severe circulatory shock following protamine (an anaphylactic reaction). *Anesth. Analgetica, 595*, 77.
31. Nicholls DP, Shepherd AM (1978) Altered warfarin metabolism in iron-deficient patient (letter). *Lancet, 2*, 215.
32. Olin JW, DeWolfe VG (1981) Paradoxical thromboembolism associated with heparin therapy. *Cleveland Clin. Q., 48*, 379.
33. O'Reilly RA, Goulart DA (1981) Comparative interaction of sulfinpyrazone and phenylbutazone with racemic warfarin: alteration in vivo of free fraction of plasma warfarin. *J. Pharmacol. Exp. Ther., 219*, 691.
34. O'Reilly RA (1982) Phenylbutazone and sulfinpyrazone interaction with oral anticoagulant phenprocoumon. *Arch. Intern. Med., 142*, 1634.
35. Palaniswamy R, Singhal PC, Rao MS et al (1983) Fatal renal haemorrhage following haemodialysis in a patient with obstructive uropathy. *Postgrad. Med. J., 59*, 57.
36. Paquet K-J (1982) Vasospastische Reaktionen nach Heparin-Dihydroergotamin (letter). *Dtsch. Med. Wochenschr., 107*, 1333.
37. Rich EC, Drage CW (1982) Severe complications of intravenous phytonadione therapy. Two cases with one fatality. *Postgrad. Med., 72*, 303.
38. Rummel W (1982) Komplikationsgefahr bei Heparin-Dihydergot. *Dtsch. Ärztebl., 79*, 32.
39. Samama M, Kher A, Horellou MH et al (1982) Thrombopénies à l'héparine. *J. Mal. Vasc., 7*, 237.
40. Schneck HJ, Tempel G (1983) Ergotismus bei Heparin-Dihydroergotamin-Medikation. *Dtsch. Med. Wochenschr., 108*, 397.
41. Shelley WB, Saÿen JJ (1982) Heparin necrosis: an anticoagulant-induced cutaneous infarct. *J. Am. Acad. Dermatol., 7*, 674.
42. Sylvén C, Anderson P (1983) Evidence that disopyramide does not interact with warfarin. *Br. Med. J., 286*, 1181.
43. The European Cooperative Study Group (1981) Streptokinase in acute myocardial infarction. Extended report of the European cooperative trial. *Acta Med. Scand., Suppl. 648*, 7.
44. Törngren S, Somell A (1982) Warfarin skin necrosis of the breast. *Acta Chir. Scand., 148*, 471.
45. Toulemonde F, Khier A, Bertrand H (1974) Tolerance locale et générale de l'héparinate de calcium administré par voie sous-cutanée. *Cahiers Méd. Lyon. d'Enseignement Postuniversitaire, 50*, 1983.
46. Trübestein G, Ludwig M, Etzel F (1983) Ergebnisse einer Streptokinase-Plasminogen-Therapie bei tiefer Venenthrombose. *Med. Welt, 34*, 448.
47. Van den Berg E, Rumpf K-D, Fröhlich H et al (1982) Vascular spasm during thromboembolism prophylaxis with heparin-dihydroergotamine. *Lancet, 2*, 268.
48. Van den Berg E, Walterbusch G, Gotzen L et al (1983) Ergotismus – eine ernste Komplikation der medikamentösen Thromboemboliephrophylaxe mit Heparin-DHE. *VASA, 12*, 64.
49. Vontz FK, Puestow EC, Cahill Jr DJ (1982) Anaphylactic shock following protamine administration. *Am. Surg., 48*, 549.
50. Weinstein J (1982) Treatment of myocardial infarction with intracoronary streptokinase: Efficacy and safety data from 209 United States cases in the Hoechst-Russel registry. *Am. Heart J., 104*, 894.
51. Wigley RAD, Paterson DE (1982) Calf haematoma following anticoagulants in synovial rupture. *N.Z. Med. J., 95*, 630.
52. Wilkins TA, Midgley JEM, Giles AF (1982) Treatment with heparin and results for free thyroxin. An in vivo or an in vitro effect? *Clin. Chem., 28*, 2441.
53. Pick RA, Joswig BC (1983) Acute renal failure following repeated streptokinase therapy for pulmonary embolism. *West. J. Med., 138*, 878.
54. Van der Weyden MB et al (1983) Delayed-onset thrombocytopenia. *Med. J. Aust., 2*, 132.
55. Husserl F (1983) Erythromycin-warfarin interaction. *Arch. Int. Med., 143*, 1831.
56. Cipolle RJ, Rodvold KA, Seifert R et al (1983) Heparin-associated thrombocytopenia: a prospective evaluation of 211 patients. *Ther. Drug Monit., 5*, 205.
57. Anon (undated, 1982) Osteoporosis during heparin therapy. *Bull. Swedish Adverse Drug Reactions Advisory Committee, 38*, 5.
58. Weinberg AC, Lieskovsky G, McGehee WG et al (1983) Warfarin necrosis of the skin and subcutaneous tissue of the male external genitalia. *J. Urol., 130*, 352.

M.J.S. Langman

38 Gastrointestinal drugs

ANTISECRETORY DRUGS AND ANTIULCER AGENTS

Histamine H_2 antagonists *(SED-9, 268; SEDA-4, 111; SEDA-5, 156; SEDA-6, 157; SEDA-7, 174)*

Cimetidine Cimetidine can now be regarded as the classic H_2 antagonist, but as time progresses others may prove to differ from it to a greater or lesser degree. Analyses of morbidity patterns in some 10,000 cimetidine takers and 10,000 controls showed that takers were about twice as likely to die in the year succeeding treatment as were controls (1[R]). However the excess deaths amongst the takers arose from a wide variety of causes including lung cancer, vascular disease and chronic lung disease, and none of the excess seemed likely to be drug related.

Drug interactions *(2[R], 3[R])* A large number of interactions have by now been described. In general terms they stem from interference with the cytochrome P450 mediated phase I of drug metabolism, whilst phase II (conjugative) is unaltered. Reactions receiving attention in the last year include the following.

Beta blocking agents Metoprolol and propranolol metabolism have been retarded, but atenolol handling seems to be unaffected (4[C]).

Chlorpromazine Raised steady state levels have been detected in cimetidine takers (5[C]).

Digoxin Raised steady state levels have been found (6[C]).

Imipramine Undesirable anticholinergic effects have been noted as a result of retarded drug degradation (7[C]).

Indomethacin Metabolism is retarded (5[C]).

Lignocaine Toxic levels have been reached in studies of normal volunteers with associated transient confusion (8[C], 9[C]).

Theophylline Toxic levels have been reached (10[C]–14[C]), associated with the induction of seizures (13[C]).

In addition cimetidine treatment has been shown to retard modestly the elimination of *alcohol* (15[C], 16[C]), an unexpected result given that metabolism predominantly takes place outside the microsomal cytochrome system.

Antiandrogenic properties These are already well documented. A recent study emphasized the high frequency of impotence when large doses of cimetidine were used to control the hypersecretion of the Zollinger-Ellison syndrome, 9 of 22 patients so treated being affected (17[C]). Weak antiandrogenic properties associated with disturbed hormone levels and diminished sperm counts have again been reported (18[C]).

Central nervous disturbances Respiratory depression has been noted in an elderly patient given intravenous treatment, and possible extrapyramidal and cerebellar disturbances have also been described (19[C], 20[C]). The respiratory depression was reversed by physostigmine treatment, whilst the neurological disturbances righted themselves spontaneously when cimetidine treatment was stopped. Exacerbation of mania has been described in a single case (89[c]).

Hematological changes Thrombocytopenia, with recurrence on rechallenge with cimetidine, has been noted on two occasions (21, 22), and experimental treatment in vitro has been shown to reduce granulocyte-macrophage colony formation (23[C], 24[C]).

Intravenous bolus dosage with cimetidine has also been found to *retard thrombin formation* (25[C]), but the same effect has not been noted during infusion treatment, nor

Side Effects of Drugs Annual 8
M.N.G. Dukes, editor

ISBN 0 444 90339 9
$0.80 per article per page (transactional system)
$0.20 per article per page (licensing system)

when amounts of ranitidine which were equipotent in hyposecretory effect were used instead.

Cardiovascular effects Isolated instances where cimetidine treatment seemed to induce arrhythmias have again been reported (26[C]–29[C]). These have usually been bradycardias, often with some degree of sinu-atrial or atrio-ventricular block. Experimental attempts to reproduce these abnormalities in man with cimetidine, or ranitidine, have been unsuccessful (30[C], 31[C]).

Renal abnormalities Transiently raised serum creatinine levels have been noted, as in the past, during cimetidine treatment (32[C]), the same effect being detectable during oxmetidine treatment. Acute interstitial nephritis (33[C], 34[C]), with recurrence on rechallenge (33[C]) has been described, the immunological abnormalities suggested to the authors that there was activation of cell mediated immunity; polymyositis was also associated (34[C]).

Other possible actions Raised serum high density lipoprotein levels (35[c]), xerosis and asteatotic dermatitis (possibly antiandrogenic origin) (36[C]) and anaphylaxis, with recurrence on rechallenge (37[C]) have all been reported.

Two reports from Kuwait (84[c]) merit attention, though their significance is not yet clear.

Cimetidine was given to a patient for the treatment of duodenal ulcer disease in a dose of 200 mg 3 times daily and 400 mg at night. He was concurrently using 'Librax' (chlordiazepoxide with clidinium) and magnesium trisilicate. Four weeks after treatment started, the patient developed signs of *optic neuritis.* The condition resolved after withdrawal of cimetidine leaving a slight residual visual impairment.

Another adult patient received cimetidine 200 mg 3 times daily for 2 weeks. Within one day of commencing therapy the patient developed *nummular eczema,* the areas affected were coin-shaped and it was considered that a *neurodermatitis* might be present.

A report by Watson et al that cimetidine might cause *polymyositis* appears to have been discredited by follow-up of the case in question by the same authors (88[r]).

Ranitidine

The general properties of this newer more potent histamine H_2 antagonist have been reviewed (38[R]). General experience has been reassuring, but several reports (usually isolated) deserve attention.

In the first report of the University of Southampton's new Drug Surveillance Research Unit, issued in 1983, an account is presented of a pilot experiment to learn more about the population of patients receiving ranitidine ('Zantac'). Data on 9,600 cases were collected, treatment covering an average of 12.5 months. A total of 3,822 events were recorded during treatment, though many of these were clearly coincidental, many events also being recorded in patients who had stopped treatment. It is interesting that *herpes* was reported in 28 patients on treatment and in only 13 off treatment. Manufacturer's data also noted 5 reports of herpes in 1,108 patients treated with ranitidine and none in a similar group receiving placebo.

There were 453 musculoskeletal events during treatment compared with 372 after treatment had ceased. 86 reported *headache* and 90 *dizziness* or vertigo on treatment, compared with 45 and 41 respectively after treatment had ceased. Depression and anxiety were not recorded more often during treatment than thereafter. No cases of liver disorders were attributed to ranitidine, but it was noted that 26 cases of *gall bladder disease* were diagnosed during the treatment period compared with only 11 after treatment. The author remarks that 'it seems likely that the underlying cause of the symptoms for which 'Zantac' had been prescribed (gall stones) was only revealed for the first time after the drug had been started. The general impression from this pilot study is that ranitidine has a very low incidence of side effects (90[C]).

Drug interactions Metoprolol metabolism, but not atenolol or propranolol metabolism (39[C], 40[C]) seem to be retarded. Experiments in man with the model drugs amino- and antipyrine and with theophylline suggest that in contrast with cimetidine, interference with metabolism does not occur (41[C], 42[C]).

Antiandrogenic properties These have not been generally described, though minor elevation of serum prolactin levels has been suggested following intravenous bolus dosage (43[C]).

Cardiovascular effects Ranitidine has been suggested to cause bradycardia (44[C]) and the proposed action has also been claimed to be unlikely (45[r]).

Miscellaneous effects Inhibition of cholinesterases has been proposed to explain a possible cholinergic action (46[c]), the extent and nature of which is doubtful.

Oxmetidine

This H_2 antagonist is more powerful than cimetidine; it also possesses an imidazole ring, but preliminary studies suggest that despite this it does not interfere with hepatic drug metabolism (3[C]). Initial clinical experience is limited but generally reassuring (32[C], 47[R]).

Histamine H_2 antagonists today

Exposure, particularly to cimetidine since its introduction some 7 years ago, has been extensive, and studies of the properties and possible adverse effects have been as intensive and perhaps more intensive than any other group of drugs. In general terms cimetidine has proved to be a safe and effective antisecretory agent in short-term use. Such a conclusion may initially seem unreasonable, given the variety and number of reports of possible adverse effects. These can be considered under the following headings.

Effects which are well proven with a plausible basis

Interference with phase I of hepatic drug metabolism *This is now well described for cimetidine, and a clear mechanism is available in the tendency of the drug to bind to cytochrome P450. This is probably the major mechanism rather than altered drug absorption or slowed hepatic blood flow. The result is a slowing, by about a third, of the metabolism of other agents which is rapidly reversed when treatment is stopped. Such interference is likely to be important where the other agents have to be maintained within a narrow therapeutic range, and these include theophylline, lignocaine, oral anticoagulants and phenytoin. Adverse effects due to increased drug potency with slowed metabolism could occur with other drugs, such as beta blocking agents and benzodiazepines handled, as they largely are, by a phase I mechanism; but are generally likely to be inapparent. Ranitidine largely, but perhaps not completely, is free of such effects.*

Antiandrogenic properties *Cimetidine is mildly antiandrogenic and can cause gynecomastia, impotence, and with bolus doses a transient rise in serum prolactin levels. Clinically such actions are uncommon, except when high doses are used in treating the Zollinger-Ellison syndrome. Ranitidine is probably largely, if not completely, free of such effects; oxmetidine has been too little studied for any certainty to be possible.*

Central nervous effects *There are H_2 receptors in the brain and cimetidine enters the cerebrospinal fluid. Abnormalities, usually mental confusion, occur with intravenous dosage in elderly people or those with hepatic or renal impairment, and are uncommon.*

Rare effects which are reasonably well proven and which are mainly idiosyncratic

These include interstitial nephritis, thrombocytopenia and agranulocytosis.

Postulated adverse effects which are ill proven

Claims have been made that treatment might increase liability to cancer, particularly gastric cancer, predispose to ulcer perforation on stopping treatment, induce pancreatitis, cause joint pains and interfere with immunological function.

The most important claim has been that cimetidine treatment might predispose to gastric cancer either because the drug itself could form a carcinogenic metabolite, nitrosocimetidine, or because suppression of gastric acid production could allow nitrate-reducing bacteria to proliferate in the stomach and so predispose to the formation of nitrosamines from nitrites and amines in the stomach. The experimental evidence is complex, and a body of material which suggests that treatment can predispose to nitrosamine formation is counterbalanced by another set which denies that such an effect is likely (48[C], 49[C]). The critical evidence must derive from clinical studies, and the anecdotal case reports are unconvincing, with apparently short incubation periods before the detection of gastric cancer where biological likelihood would lead one to expect long incubation periods. The results of surveillance studies have not so far helped to clarify matters. A larger study in progress in the United Kingdom has shown that though many people with gastric cancer have received cimetidine treatment, in most patients, and perhaps all, the symptoms associated with the tumour were the underlying reason for treatment (81[C]). A second report from the same survey (1[C]) has also emphasized the difficulties of interpretation, even when controlled data are collected; the results showing a large number of excess deaths in cimetidine recipients are best explained by the hypothesis that recipients differ in many ways, including a greater likelihood of having a second associated disease ab initio, from controls.

Experience with oxmetidine is too limited for any useful comparison with cimetidine to be possible. Ranitidine has now been available, particularly in the United Kingdom for several years, but comparisons with cimetidine are difficult because much of the side effect experience with cimetidine only became apparent after an interval of several years. It would seem that ranitidine is largely if not completely free of a tendency to slow the metabolism of other drugs, to cause confusion and to produce antiandrogenic effects. The profile of idiosyncratic adverse effects is less clear; so far the drug seems remarkably free of harmful properties but more time is needed to be sure.

For ordinary purposes it seems clear that there is little to choose between ranitidine and cimetidine, but in the elderly, in those receiving other drugs, and where high dosage is needed, ranitidine may have advantages.

Other antiulcer agents

Antacids *(SED-9, 618; SEDA-5, 333; SEDA-6, 315; SEDA-7, 353)* Metabolic alkalosis has been described as a result of taking a non-absorbable antacid mixture of aluminium and magnesium hydroxides (50[C]). The absorption of phenytoin was retarded by an antacid-dimethicone mixture, the dimethicone alone being devoid of this property (51[C]). Severe copper deficiency has also been described in a woman taking a gel of bismuth, aluminium, silica, magnesium and sodium (52[C]).

Scopolamine Given transdermally this has precipitated glaucoma (53[C]); perhaps to be expected if pharmacologically effective antisecretory doses are to be absorbed.

Sucralfate The concurrent use of sucralfate, a polyaluminium sucrose preparation with probable binding properties to the damaged mucosa has resulted in a decreased bioavailability of warfarin (54[c]), presumably because of warfarin binding in the stomach by ingested sucralfate. A further report that sucralfate treatment precipitated ulcer perforation (55[c]) seems more likely to be coincidence than cause and effect. A sucralfate *bezoar* has been described in an elderly man (85[c]).

Trithiozine *(SEDA-6, 318)* A single case in which treatment may have precipitated acute hepatitis has recently been described (56[c]).

ANTIEMETICS

Bendectin *(SEDA-5, 334; SEDA-6, 316; SEDA-7, 313; 86[R])*

In a general review of congenital malformations no risk was attached to treatment with bendectin (57[R]), but in another study takers of the drug were about 4 times more likely than expected to have a child with pyloric stenosis (58[C]). It should be noted, however, that the confidence limits were wide and that 15 other factors, none with a significantly increased risk, were examined. One plausible possibility is that the pyloric stenosis result is a normal outlier.

Cannabinoids

These have been reviewed (59[R]). Side effects of sedation, dry mouth, decreased coordination, lowered blood pressure and blurred vision were occasionally recorded with both delta- and tetrahydrocannabinol and nabilone. Dysphoria seemed to be a prominent side effect of levonantradol (59[C]) and major affective problems and pain at the injection site were commonly noted in another study (60[C]). Another study suggested, however, that dysphoria is not uncommon with nabilone treatment (61[C]), and a diminished rate of alcohol metabolism, diminished mixed function oxidase activity and hyperalgesia to thermal pain have been suggested as undesirable effects of tetrahydrocannabinol (62[C]).

Domperidone

Its properties have been generally reviewed (53[R]). Although a generally satisfactory safety profile is evident, there has been a recent disturbing report of sudden death with ventricular fibrillation following intravenous treatment (64[C]). Two cases of extrapyramidal disturbance in an adolescent and a young adult given ordinary doses have been described (82[C]), and gynecomastia, raised serum prolactin levels and galactorrhea have been noted in a male infant given the drug (83[C]).

Metoclopramide

The most prominent and consistent adverse effects are sedation, diarrhea and extrapyramidal disturbances (65[R]). It has also been suggested recently that it can cause transient hypertension (66[C]) and edema (67[c]), effects which sound aldosterone-like, as well as depression (87[r]).

Emetics

An unusual case report has described massive gastroduodenojejunal mucosal necrosis after the ingestion of 1 kg of salt in 600 ml of water following self poisoning with Distalgesic, chlordiazepoxide and alcohol (68[C]).

ANTIDIARRHEAL AGENTS *(SED-9, 621; SEDA-5, 335; SEDA-6, 318; SEDA-7, 355)*

Oxyquinolines

The gradual withdrawal of clioquinol is to be welcomed; there is no therapeutic place for this drug in managing or preventing diarrheal illness. Typical quinoline neurotoxicity has been described recently in a taker of tilbroquinol and tiliquinol (69[C]). Gross hematuria has also been reported in neonates and infants given quinone and 8-quinolinol (Mexaform) (70[C]).

Sulfasalazine *(SED-9, 621; SEDA-5, 336; SEDA-6, 319; SEDA-7, 354)*

Recently reported adverse effects include single cases with exacerbation of ulcerative colitis (71[C]), with interstitial pneumonia (recurring after rechallenge) (72[C]), lupus syndrome (73[C]) and glandular fever-like illness (74[C]). All have parallels in earlier literature. In a further study desensitization to sulfasalazine is reported as successfully undertaken; however on this occasion only 2 of those described had skin rashes, and in the remainder with a variety of complaints often generally associated with high dosage (75[C]) clinical improvement may have been more likely due to dosage reduction than to true desensitization.

LAXATIVES *(SED-9, 622; SEDA-5, 337; SEDA-6, 318; SEDA-7, 355)*

Oxyphenisatin-induced liver damage has once again been described (76[c]). There is little reason for continuing to market this drug.

Bisacodyl treatment has been shown to reduce steady state levels of digoxin (77[C]); the same might be true for other drugs.

DRUGS USED IN MANAGING GALLSTONES

Mono-octanoin *(SED-9, 637; SEDA-5, 340; SEDA-6, 323; SEDA-7, 358)*

The drug may not be entirely safe. Necrotizing choledochomalacia has been ascribed to the use of this glycerol derivative to dissolve common duct stones (78[C]).

Glucagon

In a trial of treatment for symptomatic biliary tract disease no serious side effects occurred, but vomiting seemed to be about twice as common in treated as in control individuals (79[C]).

Bile acid therapy

Ursodeoxycholic acid. A recent review has stressed again the general absence of side effects with much less diarrhea than in takers of chenodeoxycholic acid, and no evidence of liver injury (80[R]).

REFERENCES

1. Colin-Jones D, Langman MJS, Lawson DH, Vessey MP (1983) Post-marketing surveillance of the safety of cimetidine: 12 month mortality report. *Br. Med. J., 286,* 1713.
2. Mangini RJ (1982) Clinically important cimetidine drug interactions. *Clin. Pharm., 1,* 433.
3. Henry D, Kitchingman G, Langman M (1982) H_2-Receptor antagonists: the problem of hepatic drug interaction. In: Misiewicz JJ, Wormsley KG (Eds), *The Clinical Use of Ranitidine.* Medicine Publishing Corporation, Oxford.
4. Kirch W, Spahn H, Köhler H et al (1982) Interaction of metoprolol, propranolol and atenolol with concurrent administration of cimetidine. *Klin. Wochenschr., 60,* 1401.
5. Howes CA, Pullar T, Sourindhrin I et al (1983) Reduced steady-state plasma concentrations of chlorpromazine and indomethacin in patients receiving cimetidine. *Eur. J. Clin. Pharmacol., 24,* 99.
6. Fraley DS, Britton LH, Schwinghammer TL, Kalla R (1983) Effect of cimetidine on steady-state serum digoxin concentrations. *Clin. Pharm., 2,* 163.
7. Miller DD, Macklin M (1983) Cimetidine-imipramine interaction: a case report. *Am. J. Psychiatr., 140,* 351.
8. Feely J, Wilkinson GR, McAllister CB, Wood AJJ (1982) Increased toxicity and reduced clearance of lidocaine by cimetidine. *Ann. Intern. Med., 96,* 592.
9. Knapp AB, Maguire W, Keren G et al (1983) The cimetidine-lidocaine interaction. *Ann. Intern. Med., 98,* 174.
10. Fenje PC, Isles AF, Baltodano A et al (1982) Interaction of cimetidine and theophylline in two infants. *Can. Med. J., 126,* 118.
11. Vestal RE, Thummel KE, Musser B, Mercer GD (1983) Cimetidine inhibits theophylline clearance in patients with chronic obstructive pulmonary disease: a study using stable isotope methodology during multiple oral dose administration. *Br. J. Clin. Pharmacol., 15,* 411.
12. Lalonde RL, Koob RA, McLean WM, Balsys AJ (1983) The effect of cimetidine on theophylline pharmacokinetics at steady state. *Chest, 83,* 221.
13. Bauman JH, Kimelblatt BJ, Caraccio TR et al (1982) Cimetidine-theophylline interaction. Report of four patients. *Ann. Allergy, 48,* 100.
14. Schwartz JI, Bachmann KA, Bond LW, Mahajan VK (1982) Impact of cimetidine on the pharmacokinetics of theophylline. *Clin. Pharm., 1,* 534.
15. Seitz HK, Bösche J, Czygan P et al (1983) Increased blood ethanol levels following cimetidine but not ranitidine. *Lancet, 1,* 760.
16. Feely J, Wood JJ (1982) Effects of cimetidine on the elimination and action of ethanol. *J. Am. Med. Assoc., 247,* 2819.
17. Jensen RT, Collen MJ, Pandol SJ et al (1983) Cimetidine-induced impotence and breast changes in patients with gastric hypersecretory states. *N. Engl. J. Med., 308,* 883.
18. Wang C, Lai CL, Lam KC, Yeung KK (1982) Effect of cimetidine on gonadal function in man. *Br. J. Clin. Pharm., 13,* 791.
19. Bostrom R, Holmgren E, Lundberg D (1982) Respiratory depression after cimetidine reversed by physostigmine. *Intensive Care Med., 8,* 153.
20. Handler CE, Bessa CP, Wilson AO (1982) Extrapyramidal and cerebellar syndrome with encephalopathy associated with cimetidine. *Postgrad. Med. J., 58,* 527.
21. Glotzbach R (1982) Cimetidine-induced thrombocytopenia. *South. Med. J., 75,* 232.
22. Mann HJ, Schneider JR, Miller JB, Delaney JP (1983) Cimetidine-associated thrombocytopenia. *Drug Intell. Clin. Pharm., 17,* 126.
23. Aymard JP, Herbeuval M, Herbeuval R et al (1982) Action de la cimétidine sur les cellules souches de la granulopoièse humains. *Path. Biol., 30,* 855.
24. Eridani S, Johnston IDA, Villa S (1982) Cimetidine and granulopoiesis. *Ann. Intern. Med., 97,* 620.
25. Lubcke P, Herrmann W (1982) Auswirkungen von Cimetidin und Ranitidin auf die plasmatische Gerinnungsfähigkeit des Blutes. *Dtsch. Med. Wochenschr., 107,* 1671.
26. Watson AJS, Watson R, Keogr JAB (1982) Cimetidine induced arrhythmias. *Ir. J. Med. Sci., 151,* 348.
27. Hiss J, Hepler BQ, Falkowski AJ, Sunshine I (1982) Fatal bradycardia after intentional overdose of cimetidine and diazepam. *Lancet, 2,* 982.
28. Nikolic G, Singh JB (1982) Cimetidine, vasopressin and chronotropic incompetence. *Med. J. Aust., 2,* 435.
29. Matthews SJ, Michelson PA, Cersosimo RJ (1982) Cimetidine-induced sinus bradycardia. *Clin. Pharm., 1,* 556.
30. Jackson G, Upward JW (1982) Cimetidine,

ranitidine and heart rate. *Lancet, 2,* 265.

31. Liedberg G, Fletcher E, Davies J (1982) Cimetidine, ranitidine and heart rate. *Lancet, 2,* 265.
32. Paoluzi P, Fave GD, Proietti F et al (1982) Oxmetidine and cimetidine in the treatment of duodenal ulcer: results of a double-blind study. *Ital. J. Gastroenterol., 14,* 176.
33. Pitone JM, Santoro JJ, Biondi RJ et al (1982) Cimetidine-induced acute interstitial nephritis. *Am. J. Gastroenterol., 77,* 169.
34. Watson AJS, Dalbow MH, Stachura I et al (1983) Immunologic studies in cimetidine-induced nephropathy and polymyositis. *N. Engl. J. Med., 308,* 142.
35. Miller NG, Lewis B (1983) Cimetidine and HDL cholesterol. *Lancet, 1,* 524.
36. Greist MC, Epinette WW (1982) Cimetidine-induced xerosis and asteatotic dermatitis. *Arch. Dermatol., 110,* 253.
37. Knapp AB, Grimshaw RS, Goldfarb JP et al (1982) Cimetidine-induced anaphylaxis. *Ann. Intern. Med., 97,* 374.
38. Brogden RN, Carmine AA, Heel RC et al (1982) Ranitidine: a review of its pharmacology and therapeutic use in peptic ulcer disease and other allied diseases. *Drugs, 24,* 267.
39. Spahn H, Mutschler E, Kirch W et al (1983) Influence of ranitidine on plasma metoprolol and atenolol concentrations. *Br. Med. J., 1,* 1546.
40. Hegarty AM, Casteleden CM, Patel L (1982) Failure of ranitidine to interact with propranolol. *Br. Med. J., 284,* 1304.
41. Henry DA, MacDonald IA, Kitchingman G et al (1980) Cimetidine and ranitidine – comparison of effects on hepatic drug metabolism. *Br. Med. J., 281,* 775.
42. Breen KJ, Bury R, Desmond PV et al (1982) Effects of cimetidine and ranitidine in hepatic drug metabolism. *Clin. Pharm. Therap., 31,* 297.
43. Francavilla A, Panella C, Ieradi E et al (1983) Effects of ranitidine, a short term clinical trial for duodenal ulcer treatment using two different types of oral administration. *Ital. J. Gastroenterol., 15,* 39.
44. Camarri E, Chirone E, Fanteria G, Zocchi M (1982) Ranitidine induced bradycardia. *Lancet, 2,* 160.
45. Jack D, Richards DA, Grenats F (1982) Side effects of ranitidine. *Lancet, 2,* 264.
46. Hansen WE, Bertl S (1983) Inhibition of cholinesterases by ranitidine. *Lancet, 1,* 235.
47. Somerville KW, Langman MJS (1983) Newer antisecretory agents for peptic ulcer. *Drugs, 25,* 315.
48. Reed PI, Smith PLR, Haines K et al (1981) Effect of cimetidine on gastric juice N-nitrosamine concentrations. *Lancet, 2,* 553.
49. Muscroft TJ, Youngs DJ, Bardon DW et al (1981) Cimetidine is unlikely to increase formation of intra-gastric N-nitroso-compounds in patients taking a normal diet. *Lancet, 1,* 408.
50. Medias NE, Levey AS (1983) Metabolic alkalosis due to absorption of 'nonabsorbable' antacid. *Am. J. Med., 74,* 155.
51. McElney JC, Uprichard G, Collier PS (1982) The effect of activated dimethicone and a proprietary antacid preparation containing this agent on the absorption of phenytoin. *Br. J. Clin. Pharm., 13,* 501.
52. Kalmthont PMV, Engels LGJ, Baker HH, Burghouts JTM (1982) Severe copper deficiency due to excessive use of an antacid combined with pyloric stenosis. *Dig. Dis. Sci., 27,* 859.
53. Frauenfelder FT (1982) Transdermal scopolamine precipitating narrow-angle glaucoma. *New Engl. J. Med., 307,* 1079.
54. Mungall D, Talbert RL, Phillips C et al (1982) Sucralfate and warfarin. *Ann. Intern. Med., 97,* 557.
55. Bitran JD, Sweet DL, Vardiman J et al (1982) Sucralfate and ulcer perforation. *Ann. Intern. Med., 97,* 619.
56. Cruz DJV, Calvet MN, Galipienzo JMR et al (1983) Hepatitis aguda tras la administracion de tritiozine. *Rev. Esp. Enf. Ap. Digest., 63,* 188.
57. Kalter H, Warkany J (1983) Congenital malformation. *N. Engl. J. Med., 308,* 491.
58. Eskenazi B, Bracken MB (1982) Bendectin (Debendox) as a risk factor for pyloric stenosis. *Am. J. Obstet. Gynecol., 144,* 919.
59. Vincent BJ, McQuiston DJ, Einhorn LH et al (1983) Review of cannabinoids and their antiemetic effectiveness. *Drugs, 25, Suppl. 1,* 52.
60. Joss RA, Galeazzi RL, Bischoff A et al (1982) Levonantradol, a new antiemetic with a high rate of side effects for the prevention of nausea and vomiting in patients receiving cancer chemotherapy. *Cancer Chemother. Pharm., 9,* 61.
61. Cone LA, Greene DS, Helm NA (1982) Use of nabilone in the treatment of chemotherapy-induced vomiting in an outpatient setting. *Cancer Treat. Rev., 9, Suppl. B,* 63.
62. Robinson CP (1982) Tetrahydrocannabinol – a minireview. *Drugs Today, 18,* 669.
63. Brogden RN, Carmine AA, Heel RC et al (1982) Domperidone. A review of its pharmacological activity, pharmacokinetics and therapeutic efficacy in the symptomatic treatment of chronic dyspepsia and as an emetic. *Drugs, 24,* 360.
64. Joss RA, Goldhirsch A, Brunner KW, Galeazzi RL (1982) Sudden death in cancer patient on high-dose domperidone. *Lancet, 1,* 1019.
65. Gralla RJ (1983) Metoclopramide. A review of anti-emetic trials. *Drugs, 25,* 63.
66. Sheriden C, Chandra P, Jacinto M, Greenwald ES (1982) Transient hypertension after high doses of metoclopramide. *N. Engl. J. Med., 307,* 1346.
67. Zumoff B (1982) Metoclopramide and edema. *Ann. Intern. Med., 97,* 557.
68. Calam J, Krasner N, Haqqani M (1982) Extensive gastrointestinal damage following a

saline emetic. *Dig. Dis. Sci.*, *27*, 936.
69. Soffer M, Basdevant A, Sarragoussi JJ et al (1983) Oxyquinoline toxicity. *Lancet*, *1*, 709.
70. Bajoghli M (1982) Gross hematuria of newborns and infants induced by quinone and 8-quinolinol (Mexaform). *Eur. J. Pediatr.*, *138*, 359.
71. Schwartz AG, Targan SR, Saxon A, Weinstein WM (1982) Sulfasalazine-induced exacerbation of ulcerative colitis. *N. Engl. J. Med.*, *306*, 409.
72. Sigvaldason A, Sörenson S (1983) Interstitial pneumonia due to sulfasalazine. *Eur. J. Respir. Dis.*, *64*, 229.
73. Carr Locke DL (1982) Sulfasalazine-induced lupus syndrome in a patient with Crohn's disease. *Am. J. Gastroenterol.*, *77*, 614.
74. Carr Locke DL, Ali M (1982) Glandular fever-like illness associated with sulphasalazine. *Postgrad. Med. J.*, *58*, 665.
75. Taffet SL, Das KM (1982) Desensitization of patients with imflammatory bowel disease to sulphasalazine. *Am. J. Med.*, *73*, 520.
76. Schmitz D, Walster B, Becker JM et al (1982) Hépatopathies et oxyphénisatine. *J. Méd. Strasbourg*, *14*, 155.
77. Botzler R, Ritter U (1982) Einfluss von Abfürmassnahmen auf die Serumkonzentration von Digoxin beim Menschen. *Leber Magendarm.*, *12*, 255.
78. Crabtree TS, Dystra R, Kelly J, Preshaw RM (1982) Necrotising choledochomalacia after use of monoactanoin to dissolve bile-duct stones. *Can. J. Surg.*, *25*, 644.
79. Stower MJ, Foster GE, Hardcastle JD (1982) A trial of glucagon in the treatment of painful biliary tract disease. *Br. J. Surg.*, *69*, 591.
80. Bachrach WH, Hofman AF (1982) Ursodeoxycholic acid in the treatment of cholesterol cholelithiasis. *Dig. Dis. Sci.*, *27*, 833.
81. Colin-Jones DG, Langman MJS, Lawson DH, Vessey MP (1982) Cimetidine and gastric cancer: preliminary report from post-marketing surveillance study. *Br. Med. J.*, *285*, 1311.
82. Gonce M, Bury J, Burton L, Delwaide PJ (1982) Syndrome neurodysleptique induit par le dompéridone. *Nouv. Presse Méd.*, *11*, 2298.
83. Van der Steen M, Du Caju MVL, Van Acker KJ (1982) Gynaecomastia in a male infant given domperidone. *Lancet*, *2*, 884.
84. Anon (1983) Cimetidine. *Kuwait Drug Adverse Reactions Series*, *2*, 12.
85. Algozzine GJ, Hill G, Scoggins WG et al (1983) Sucralfate bezoar. *N. Engl. J. Med.*, *309*, 1387.
86. Holmes LB (1983) Is benedictin dysmorphogenic? *Teratology*, *27*, 277.
87. Anon (1983) Metoclopramide and depression ADR. *Scrip*, *830*, 21.
88. Hawkins RA et al (1983) Does cimetidine cause polymyositis? *N. Engl. J. Med.*, *309*, 187.
89. Titus JP (1983) Exacerbation of mania. *J. Clin. Psychiatr.*, *44*, 267.
90. Inman W (1983) Zantac. *PEM News*, *1*, 9. University of Southampton Drug Surveillance Research Unit.

J. Descotes and J.Cl. Evreux

39 Immunomodulating agents

Although immunomodulating agents are progressively emerging as valuable therapeutic tools in the light of encouraging clinical results, particularly in the field of cancer immunotherapy as recently reviewed by Baker and Taub (1[R]) and Shapiro et al (2[R]), specific data bearing on their side effects are still sparse.

DRUG INTERACTIONS

Immunostimulants of both bacterial and synthetic origin may inhibit the cytochrome P 450-dependent drug oxydizing system (SED-10). Recent experimental work provides additional evidence that interferon preparations and interferon-inducing agents are the most likely candidates for causing such inhibition, the main consequence of which is increased pharmacological activity, hence toxicity, of any drug given at the same time, e.g. hexabarbital, zoxazolamine, phenytoin or acetaminophen (3, 4, 5). However, not all interferon preparations were found to behave similarly, at least in mice (5). It should again be stressed that most data have been obtained in laboratory animals and that there is an urgent need for confirmation of their clinical relevance inasmuch as negative results with immunomodulating agents, e.g. synthetic muramyl-dipeptide in rats (6), have also been reported.

EFFECTS RELATED TO INDIVIDUAL COMPOUNDS

C 1740

C 1740 (Biostim) is a glycoproteinic extract from *Klebsiella pneumoniae* serotype 2. No side effects were noted in a phase-I short-term open trial involving 21 adult patients (7[C]). In a double-blind investigation Viallat et al (8[C]) studied Biostim versus placebo as a preventive measure against acute infectious episodes in chronic bronchitis. None of the 38 patients who received Biostim 4 mg per day orally for 6 days, then 1 mg per day for 8 days every 2 months, developed side effects, increased IgE levels or anti-Biostim antibodies.

Diethyldithiocarbamate (DTC)

A comprehensive review of 182 references devoted to the immunopharmacology and general pharmacology of diethyldithiocarbamate can be warmly recommended (9[R]). Slow intravenous infusion is usually well tolerated. By contrast, patients who were rapidly administered i.v. DTC complained of malaise, dyspnea or transient cyanosis. The oral, intrathecal and aerosol routes of administration have so far not been associated with side effects.

Lentinan

Lentinan is a neutral polysaccharide isolated from a Japanese fruit, *Lentinus edodes,* the application of which in cancer treatment has been reviewed by Chihara and Taguchi (10[R]). During phase-I study, 3 out of 50 patients developed side effects. They comprised 1 case of slight liver dysfunction detected by GOT and GPT analysis at a dose of 0.5 mg/day, 1 case of mild oppressive sensations in the chest at a dose of 5 mg/day, and 1 case of petechiae in the legs at a dose of 50 mg/day. These side effects were all transient. In a phase-III trial of nearly 300 patients, untoward reactions were seldom noted: only 10 treated patients complained of transient nausea and vomiting, heaviness on the chest, skin rash or sweating, or showed an increase of blood pressure.

Levamisole

The side effects of levamisole are reviewed primarily in Chapter 32.

Side Effects of Drugs Annual 8
M.N.G. Dukes, editor

ISBN 0 444 90339 9
$0.80 per article per page (transactional system)
$0.20 per article per page (licensing system)

Despite its frequent and potentially serious side effects, levamisole is indeed regarded by some workers, e.g. Veys et al (11[C]), as a valuable treatment for rheumatoid arthritis. In their experience, discontinuation of drug administration due to serious side effects was nevertheless required in 37 out of 142 patients (26%), leukotoxicity being the commonest problem (16%). Chahinian et al (12[C]) confirmed the hematological safety of levamisole in patients with advanced lung cancer, a finding unhappily devoid of practical importance owing to levamisole's lack of therapeutic efficacy.

The dosage regimen is probably the critical factor with respect to levamisole's efficacy and safety in cancer patients. A comprehensive survey of 2635 patients in 46 controlled studies concluded that 2.5 mg/kg levamisole given for 3 consecutive days every fortnight provided optimal therapeutic efficacy and safety (13[R]). The same may possibly apply in rheumatoid arthritis; Bussière et al (14[C]) noted less frequent and less severe side effects, particularly hematological, in patients given levamisole 150 mg once a week. These findings are in keeping with those of Veys et al (11[C]), who reported less leukotoxicity in patients receiving levamisole once a week. However, flu-like reactions, possibly indicating an immunostimulation, tended to be more pronounced in these patients.

Interindividual variability in the pharmacokinetics of levamisole is another factor to be taken into account (15[C]): low doses are required to reach the minimal effective plasma concentrations necessary to trigger an immunostimulatory response, while high plasma concentrations may be associated with immunodepression.

NPT 15392

NPT 15392 is structurally related to isoprinosine and has immunomodulating properties of potentially therapeutic interest (16[R]). Mild and reversible hair loss without true alopecia was the only toxic effect so far reported during tolerance studies in humans.

OK 432

OK 432 is an immunomodulating agent initially extracted from Group A streptococcus. Systemic fever, local pain and induration of no clinical importance have been described in patients with gestational choriocarcinoma (17[C]).

Poly(ICLC)

Poly(ICLC) is a potent interferon-inducing agent, currently under phase-II trial study. Nakamura et al (18[C]) treated 7 patients with intravenous doses ranging from 0.05 and 0.2 mg/kg every week. A febrile reaction up to 39.0°C was noted in every patient. Modest hypotension occurred once, transient elevation of liver enzyme levels and leukopenia twice. However, doses well tolerated in adults are likely to be toxic in children; Lampkin et al (19[C]) described 3 cases of severe hypotension, 8 cases of serious myalgia, arthritis or arthralgia, and 2 cases of coma among 30 children given 12 mg/m^2 of poly(ICLC) intravenously. No correlation between drug toxicity and interferon levels could be detected in these patients.

Thymic hormones

Of a series of patients receiving thymopoietin pentapeptide for the treatment of rheumatoid arthritis, 1 experienced fever after 1 mg intramuscularly once a week, while 2 reported skin rash, 1 herpes zoster and 1 diarrhea after 50 mg intravenously once a week (20[C]).

REFERENCES

1. Baker MA, Taub RN (1982) Immunotherapy of cancer. In: Greenspan EM (Ed), *Clinical Interpretation and Practice of Cancer Chemotherapy*, p 633. Raven Press, New York.
2. Shapiro A, Kadman D, Catalona WJ, Ratliff TL (1982) Immunotherapy of superficial bladder cancer. *J. Urol., 128*, 892.
3. Parkinson A, Lasker J, Kramer MJ et al (1982) Effects of three recombinant human leukocyte interferons on drug metabolism in mice. *Drug Metab. Dispos., 10*, 579.
4. Harned CL, Nerland DE, Sonnenfeld G (1982) Effects of passive transfer and induction of gamma (type II immune) interferon preparations on the metabolism of diphenylhydantoin by murine cytochrome P-450. *J. Interferon Res.,*

2, 5.
5. Moore JA, Marafino BJ, Stebbing N (1983) Influence of various purified interferons on effects of drugs in mice. *Res. Commun. Chem. Pathol. Pharmacol.*, *39*, 113.
6. Zidek Z, Kamenikova, Buchar E, Janku I, Mazk K (1983) Biotransformation of drugs in rats treated with a synthetic muramyldipeptide, N-acetylmuramyl-L-alanyl-D-isoglutamine. *Int. J. Immunopharmacol.*, *5*, 151.
7. Lang JM, Giron C, Zalicz R et al (1982) C 1740 (Biostim®): an overview of preclinical studies. In: Serrou B, Rosenfield C, Wybran J, Meyer G (Eds), *New Immunomodulating Agents and Biological Response Modifiers*, p 133. Elsevier Biomedical Press, Amsterdam, New York.
8. Viallat JR, Constantini D, Boutin C, Fournier P (1983) Etude en double-aveugle d'un immunomodulateur d'origine bactérienne (Biostim®) dans la prévention des épisodes infectieux chez le bronchitique chronique. *Poumon-Coeur, 39*, 53.
9. Renoux G (1982) Immunopharmacologie et pharmacologie du diéthyldithiocarbamate (DTC). *J. Pharmacol. (Paris), 13, Suppl. 1*, 95.
10. Chihara G, Tagushi T (1982) Lentinan: biological activities and possible clinical use. *E.O.S.*, *2*, 93.
11. Veys EM, Mielants H, Hermanns P, Verbruggen G (1981) Recent advances in the immunological monitoring and treatment of rheumatoid arthritis patients. *Acta Rheumatol.*, *5*, 267.
12. Chahinian AP, Goldberg J, Holland JF et al (1982) Chemotherapy versus chemoimmunotherapy with levamisole or Corynebacterium parvum in advanced lung cancer. *Cancer Treat. Rep.*, *66*, 1291.
13. Amery WK, Butterworth BJ (1983) The dosage regimen of levamisole in cancer: is it related to efficacy and safety? *Int. J. Immunopharmacol.*, *5*, 1.
14. Bussière JL, Ristori JM, Sauvezie B, Rampon S (1982) Traitement de la polyarthrite rhumatoïde. Tolérance du lévamisole `a dose unique (150 mg) hebdomadaire. *Nouv. Presse Méd.*, *11*, 1144.
15. Luyckx M, Rousseau F, Cazin M et al (1982) Pharmacokinetics of levamisole in healthy subjects and cancer patients. *Eur. J. Drug Metab. Pharmacokinet.*, *7*, 247.
16. Wybran J (1982) Immunological properties of NPT 15392: a review. In: Serrou B, Rosenfeld C, Wybran J, Meyer G (Eds), *New Immunomodulating Agents and Biological Response Modifiers*, p 89. Elsevier Biomedical Press, Amsterdam, New York.
17. Kanazawa K, Ohno M, Takeuchi S (1982) Immunochemotherapy using OK 432 in gestational choriocarcinoma. *J. Jpn. Soc. Cancer Ther.*, *17*, 1902.
18. Nakamura O, Shitara N, Matsutani M, Takakura K, Machida H (1982) Phase I-II trials of poly(ICLC) in malignant brain tumor patients. *J. Interferon Res.*, *2*, 1.
19. Lampkin B, Levine AS, Krivit W, Hammond D (1982) Phase II trial of poly(ICLC) (an interferon inducer) in the treatment of children with acute leukemia. *Am. Soc. Clin. Oncol. Abstracts*, *1*, 123.
20. Veys EM, Huskisson EC, Rosenthal M et al (1982) Clinical response to therapy with thymopoeitin pentapeptide in rheumatoid arthritis. *Ann. Rheum. Dis.*, *41*, 441.

H.D. Reuter

40 Vitamins

Vitamin A

The widespread availability of high-dose vitamin preparations, which are defined as food supplements, may be helping to nurture a form of vitamin intoxication. Two cases of a serious multisystem disease with the ingestion of excessive amounts of vitamins A and D have been described (1[r]). Potential lethal intoxication occurred in 2 young boys from different families whose parents administered as much as 250,000 I.U. of vitamin A and 4,000 I.U. of vitamin D daily. On examination increased calcium levels in the blood, increased sedimentation rate, fluid retention in the face and limbs, bone pain and tenderness were found. The boys recovered after hospital treatment.

According to the authors, the multi-million-dollar health food industry, the increased emphasis of physicians on more natural approaches to disease treatment, a population of consumers interested in holistic medicine and, in the USA, a court decision that vitamins are not drugs and may be marketed without control by the health authorities, might have contributed to the increased accessibility and use of high-dose vitamin preparations. This situation has a dangerous potential for abuse of megavitamins and the occurrence of new diseases (1[r]).

Hypercalcemia may occur after daily doses of as high as 200,000 I.U. of vitamin A (2[c]). In an 8-year-old girl with psoriasis, the clinical features after receiving this dose for 6 months included hypercalcemia, dehydration, bone pain and decreased renal function.

In a review of the available information on the clinical effects of retinol (vitamin A), tretinoin (retinoic acid) and isotretinoin (13-cis-retinoic acid) it is indicated that while they express similar spectra of toxicity, they also differ in the extent to which they affect various body systems (3[C]). This suggests that differential efficacy of the retinoids may be related, in part, to the cutaneous sites of maximum activity.

With vitamin A acute toxicity is said to occur within 12–24 hours after the ingestion of 30,000 I.U. by children or 1,000,000 I.U. or more by adults. The adverse effect of a very high dose of vitamin A is documented by the report on a 62-year-old man, in whom some hours after ingestion of 4,000,000 I.U. of vitamin A severe headache, transient blurring of vision accompanied by scotomas occurred (4[C]). The patient was hospitalized for 5 days. Emesis, photophobia, scotomas and headache remitted by day 3 while exfoliation of the skin of hands and face began at the same time and ceased about 12 days after the vitamin A ingestion.

Investigations in 66 patients with acne who had been treated for several months with daily doses of 300,000 and 500,000 I.U. of vitamin A revealed only minor increases of serum SGOT, SGPT, alkaline phosphatase and triglycerides in 14%, 10%, 9% and 89% of the patients treated with low dose, and in 20%, 40%, 10% and 100% of those treated with the high dose (3[C]). The rate of cheilitis, xerosis of the skin and mucous membranes, epistaxis and headache was 96%, 95%, 46% and 68% with the low dose, and 80%, 90%, 50% and 60% with the high dose.

In a 43-year-old woman only dermatological symptoms were seen after eating 100,000 I.U. of vitamin A daily every second month for approximately 15 months. Her dermatitis disappeared slowly after stopping the vitamin intake (5[C]).

Hypervitaminosis A can also result with very low levels of 10 times the daily allowance. A 16-year-old boy, after intake of daily doses of 50,000 I.U. vitamin A for 2.5 years as a form of self-treatment for acne, was admitted with bilateral mild

Side Effects of Drugs Annual 8
M.N.G. Dukes, editor

ISBN 0 444 90339 9
$0.80 per article per page (transactional system)
$0.20 per article per page (licensing system)

papilledema, a slightly stiff neck, dry skin and fissuring of the lips (6[c]). About 14 days after the last vitamin A supplement he showed increased intracranial pressure. The SGOT level was approximately twice normal. The total serum vitamin A was greatly elevated as was the serum retinol binding protein. The patient suffered from headache, nausea and vomiting, abdominal, back and joint pain. He was treated with mannitol and dexamethasone. Improvement occurred very slowly and only 2 months after discharge the patient had regained normal weight and was fully active.

In a 7.5-year-old boy hypervitaminosis A was seen after daily intake of 25,000–50,000 I.U. for 1 year. In addition he was taking an unspecified amount of multivitamins that also contained vitamin A. The serum level of vitamin A was 1,489 I.U. (normal 65–275 I.U.) (7[c]). Improvement was noted within 3 days after discontinuation of the medication and he returned to his usual state of health within 2 weeks.

Some other authors report adverse effects associated with the intake of vitamin A doses of 50,000–100,000 I.U. per day, such as marked weight loss, psychiatric disturbance, total body alopecia, liver disease and increased calcium levels in the blood (8[C]–11[C]).

From the report on a case of vitamin A intoxication in a severely atopic 6-year-old boy who suffered from protein-calorie deficiency, it can be suggested that large doses of vitamin A (about 20,000 I.U. vitamin A daily) given over a long period to children with restricted protein intake will circumvent normal metabolic processes in the liver leading to hypervitaminosis A (12[C]).

Administration of oral vitamin A and the synthetic retinoids to humans and experimental animals have been accompanied by changes in lipid metabolism (13[R]). These changes include alterations in serum, liver and skin surface lipids. While the immediate cause of the serum and liver changes remain obscure, the skin surface alterations appear to be secondary to changes in sebum production. The most marked effect seen in clinical and animal studies is that of hypertriglyceridemia (increase of the VLDL fraction) and occurs during the fasted and the fed state.

all-trans-Retinoic acid (tretinoin, retin A)

Phototoxicity by UVA and the visible spectrum in the presence of tretinoin seems to occur in about 10% of treated patients. The symptoms, however, are generally mild (14[C]).

Retinoids

In rats oral all-trans-retinoic acid, 13-cis-retinoic acid and natural vitamin A have resulted in hyperglyceridemia while in man 13-cis-retinoic acid, etretinate and natural vitamin A have been reported to elicit this response (13[R]).

For the last several years there has been growing interest in the use of retinoids in the treatment of a variety of dermatoses. Tables 1 and 2 compare the systemic and mucocutaneous side effects of retinoids taken orally (15[r]).

13-cis-Retinoic acid (isotretinoin, Accutane)

Although experience with isotretinoin is limited, the drug appears to share some of the adverse effects of other retinoids although it appears to have a greater benefit-to-risk ratio and fewer CNS effects than systemically administered vitamin A or tretinoin. The frequency and severity of adverse reactions to isotretinoin are generally dose-related with more pronounced effects occurring at dosages greater than 1 mg/kg/day. Adverse effects usually subside with a reduction in dosage and are usually reversible following discontinuance of therapy (16[R], 17[R]). Adverse mucocutaneous effects occur frequently (cheilitis, xerosis, xerostomia, dry nose, epistaxis, pruritus); conjunctivitis and irritation of the eye in about 40% of the patients; temporary thinning of the hair, palmoplantar desquamation, skin fragility, infection of the skin and photosensibility are seen in 5–10% of the patients. Rarely mucocutaneous effects are hypo- and hyperpigmentation, urticaria and bruising. Hypertriglyceridemia occurs in about 25% of treated patients, serum concentrations greater than 500 mg/100 ml have been observed in some cases, increases in VLDL and decreases in HDL in about 15% of the patients, and increases in serum cholesterol in 7%. Adverse musculoskeletal effects, bone

Table 1. *Comparison of systemic side effects of retinoids taken orally*

Side effects	Natural		Synthetic	
	Retinol (vitamin A)	all-trans-Retinoic acid (tretinoin; Retin A)	Aromatic retinoid (etrinate; Ro 10-9359)	13-cis-Retinoic acid (isotretinoin; Accutane)
CNS				
Coma		rare	0	0
Intraocular pressure	common	common	0	0
Headache	common	always	rare	rare
Psychological changes	often	often	0	rare
Other systems				
Fatigue	common	common	rare	rare
Anorexia	often	often	0	rare
Thirst	common	common	rare	often
Nausea	often	common	0	0
Dizziness/ arthralgias/ arthritis	often		rare	rare
Altered menses	common		0	0

or joint pain and generalized muscle aches occur in about 5% of the patients. In patients with disorders of keratinization, treated with isotretinoin for more than 2 years, skeletal abnormalities have been diagnosed. Hematological effects comprise: increased erythrocyte sedimentation rates (40%), decreased hemoglobin concentration and hematocrit, decreased erythrocyte and leucocyte counts and increased platelet counts. Adverse nervous system effects of isotretinoin include lethargy, fatigue and headache. Very rarely paresthesias and dizziness occur. Gastrointestinal effects of isotretinoin are anorexia, nausea, vomiting, increased appetite and thirst. No hepatic effects have been reported to date. In 10% of the patients minimal transient increases in serum concentrations of alkaline phosphatase, SGOT and SGPT occur. In addition to conjunctivitis and irritation of the eyes isotretinoin therapy has been associated with the development of corneal opacities in some patients with disorders of keratinization.

In a phase I study of 13-cis-retinoic acid in 16 patients with head and neck malignancies (18[C]) it was found that drug doses > 60 mg/m^2 induced intense headaches, urethritis, desquamative dermatitis, vertigo and ataxia. The severity of these side effects precludes the use of 13-cis-retinoic acid as a potential chemopreventive agent at doses higher than 60 mg/m^2.

Adverse effects in patients with severe

Table 2. *Comparison of mucocutaneous side effects of retinoids taken orally*

Side effects	Retinol	Tretinoin	Etrinate	13-cis-Retinoic acid
Dry skin/desquamation	always	common	common	often
Cheilitis	often	always	always	always
Conjunctivitis			often	common
Skin fragility			often	common
Pruritus	always	common	often	rare
Epistaxis	common	often	rare	common
Mucosal erosions	often	0	often	0
Edema	common (legs)	often (face)	rare (legs)	0
Alopecia	common	often	often	rare
Altered hair texture	common		often	rare
Brittle nails	common			
Paronychia	rare		rare	rare

nodulo-cystic acne treated with 40 mg/day in the course of 6–12 months were dryness of the lips, cheilitis with rhagades, facial dermatitis, increased hepatic enzymes and triglycerides occurred (19[C]).

In 6 patients with keratosis palmaris et plantaris treated for 113 days with a mean dose of 1.95 mg/kg/day isotretinoin the major recorded clinical toxicity included cheilitis, dryness of the nasal mucosa and conjunctiva, central facial desquamation, increased skin fragility, pruritus, occasional hair loss and headache (20[C]).

Similar side effects were observed in 18 patients with advanced breast cancer whose treatment began with 0.5 mg/kg and rose to 8 mg/kg over a 1-month period, unless toxicity forced dose reduction (21[C]), and in 33 patients with treatment-resistent cystic and conglobate acne treated with 0.5 mg/kg/day (22[C]).

Dose-limiting toxic effects of isotretinoin as dermatitis, emotional lability and headaches were seen in patients treated because of advanced cancers (23[C]).

Blepharoconjunctivitis has been reported as a side effect in 43% of patients receiving 13-cis-retinoic acid in doses of 2 mg/kg/day and other eye symptoms have also been described, while 20% of patients with acne treated with 1.0 mg/kg isotretinoin also experienced blepharoconjunctivitis (24[c]).

Premature epiphyseal closure of the right tibia was seen in a 10.5-year-old boy with epidermolytic hyperkeratosis who had been treated systemically for 4.5 years with 13-cis-retinoic acid (25[C]). Similar changes have been described in individuals ingesting excessive amounts of vitamin A.

Etretinate (Ro 10-9359)

The most striking side effects of etretinate (Tigason) treatment of keratinizing disorders of the skin and mucous membranes with doses of 25–100 mg were cheilitis (70%), dryness of mucous membranes (27%) and hair loss (27%) (26[C]).

Similar effects were seen in 50% of patients with pustulosis palmo-plantaris and eczema keratoticum treated for up to 24 months with 25–75 mg/24 hr etretinate (27[C]) and in patients with keratodermia punctata hereditaria (28[c]). Also 2 patients with ear ache related to 50–75 mg etretinate are reported (29[c]).

In a retrospective study of 27 patients with hyperkeratotic dermatoses the following side effects due to Ro 10-9395 were seen: dryness of the lips and mucous membranes (14), diffuse hair loss (5), epistaxis (1) and conjunctivitis (1). Abnormal liver tests were found in 7 patients, while in 2 patients liver biopsy showed changes indicative of toxic hepatitis (30[C]).

Dryness of the mouth, rhagades and fissures, as well as mild headache, increased transaminases and recurrent fever in one case, were side effects observed in patients with erythrokeratoderma who had been treated for 2.5 years with Tigason (31[C]).

In the successful treatment of extensive virus warts with 100 mg/day etretinate in a patient with sarcoidosis, mild cheilitis, skin thinning and hair loss were observed (32[c]).

Ro 13-6298

In a clinical phase I study of Ro 13-6298 in patients with cancer the following adverse effects were seen in the course of a treatment with 5–10 mg/kg/week: 10/11 patients showed skin toxicity (scaling, desquamation, dryness of the mucous membranes, cheilitis and erythema). One of the patients lost his fingernails. In 10/12 patients given 1–2 mg/kg/day skin toxicity was observed, being severe in one (localized erythema of a fistula). Mild side effects other than those mentioned in both groups consisted of dizziness, headache, loss of appetite, constipation, hair loss and pain at the site of metastases (33[c]).

REFERENCES

1. Anon (1981) Vitamin intoxication is new abuse. *Amer. Pharmacy, 821,* 91.
2. Kjaergaard J-J, Nielsen JL, Mosekilde L (1981) A case of vitamin A toxicity with hypercalcemia. *Ugeskr. Laeg., 143,* 757.
3. Windhorst DB, Nigra T (1982) General clinical toxicology of oral retinoids. *J. Am. Acad. Dermatol., 6,* 675.
4. LaMantia RS, Andrews CE (1981) Acute vitamin A intoxication. *South. Med. J., 74,* 1012.
5. Hamann K, Avnstorp C (1982) Chronische Hypervitaminose A mit Hautveränderungen. *Hautarzt, 33,* 559.
6. Farris WA, Erdman JW (1982) Protracted

hypervitaminosis A following long-term, low-level intake. *J. Am. Med. Assoc.*, *247*, 1317.

7. Wason S, Lovejoy Jr H (1982) Vitamin A toxicity. *Am. J. Dis. Child.*, *136*, 174.
8. Ragavan VV, Smith JE, Bilezikian JP (1982) *Am. J. Med. Sci.*, *283*, 161.
9. Fumich RM, Essig GW (1983) Hypervitaminosis A. Case report in an adolescent soccer player. *Am. J. Sports Med.*, *11*, 34.
10. Van de Loo W (1983) Chronische Vitamin-A-Intoxikation. *Dtsch. med. Wschr.*, *108*, 75.
11. Baxi SC, Dailey III GE (1982) Hypervitaminosis A. A cause of hypercalcemia. *West. J. Med.*, *137*, 429.
12. Silverman SH, Lecks HI (1982) Protein-calorie deficiency and vitamin indiscretion in an atopic child who developed hypervitaminosis A. *Clin. Pediatr.*, *21*, 172.
13. Gerber LE, Erdman JW (1982) Changes in lipid metabolism during retinoid administration. *J. Am. Acad. Dermatol.*, *6*, 664.
14. Béani JC, Peyron JL (1982) Antibio-Aberel®: Photo-innocuité? *Inform. Thérap.*, *18*, 5939.
15. Bayrd GT, Goltz RW (1982) Oral retinoids in dermatology. *Minnesota Med.*, *65*, 741.
16. Perry MD, McEvoy GK (1983) Isotretinoin: New therapy for severe acne. *Clin. Pharmacy*, *2*, 12.
17. Roduner J, Krebs A (1982) Die perorale Behandlung mit Retinoiden – aktueller Stand. *Ther. Umschau*, *39*, 897.
18. Band PR, Besner JG, Leclaire R et al (1982) Phase I study of 13-cis-retinoic acid toxicity. *Cancer Treatm. Rep.*, *66*, 1759.
19. Ott F, Geiger JM (1982) Traitement à long terme par l'acide rétinoïque 13-cis de l'acné sévère nodulo-kystique. *Ann. Dermatol. Vénéréol. (Paris)*, *109*, 849.
20. Bergfeld WF, Derbes VJ, Elias PM et al (1982) The treatment of keratosis palmaris et plantaris with isotretinoin. *J. Am. Acad. Dermatol.*, *6*, 727.
21. Cassidy J, Lippman M, Lacroix A, Peck G (1982) Phase II trial of 13-cis-retinoic acid in metastatic breast cancer. *Eur. J. Cancer Oncol.*, *18*, 925.
22. Peck GA, Olsen TG, Butkus D et al (1982) Effect of oral synthetic retinoids on sebaceous glands and acne. *J. Am. Acad. Dermatol.*, *6*, 735.
23. Meyskens FL, Gilmartin E, Alberts DS et al (1982) Activity of isotretinoin against squamous cell cancers and preneoplastic lesions. *Cancer Treatm. Rep.*, *66*, 1315.
24. Milson J, Jones DH, King K, Cuncliffe WJ (1982) Ophthalmological effects of 13-cis-retinoic acid therapy for acne vulgaris. *Brit. J. Dermatol.*, *107*, 491.
25. Milstone LM, McGuire J, Ablow RC (1982) Premature epiphyseal closure in a child receiving oral 13-cis-retinoic acid. *J. Am. Acad. Dermatol.*, *7*. 663.
26. Mahrle G, Meyer-Hamme S, Ippen H (1982) Oral treatment of keratinizing disorders of skin and mucous membranes with etretinate. Comparative study of 113 patients. *Arch. Dermatol.*, *118*, 97.
27. Reymann F (1982) Two years' experience with Tigason treatment of pustulosis palmoplantaris and eczema keratoticum manuum. *Dermatologica*, *164*, 209.
28. Christiansen JV (1983) Keratodermia punctata hereditaria treated with etretinate (Tigason). *Acta Dermatov. (Stockh.)*, *63*, 181.
29. Juhlin L (1983) Ear ache during etretinate treatment. *Acta Dermatov. (Stockh.)*, *63*, 181.
30. Foged EK, Jacobsen FK (1982) Side effects due to Ro 10-9359 (Tigason). A retrospective study. *Dermatologica*, *164*, 395.
31. Kantner V (1982) Tapaszatalataink hosszabb ideje kezelt erythrokeratodermás betegeinknél Tigasonnal. *Börg. Venerol. Szemle*, *58*, 266.
32. Boyle J, Dick, DC, Mackie RM (1983) Treatment of extensive virus warts with etretinate (Tigason) in a patient with sarcoidosis. *Clin. Exp. Dermatol.*, *8*, 33.
33. Hartmann D, Hofmann V, Hindermann E et al (1982) Clinical phase I study of a new retinoid (Ro 13-6298). *Am. Soc. Clin. Oncol.*, *1*, 153 (Abstr.).

W. Heyns

41 Corticotropins and corticosteroids

Before treating a patient with corticosteroids, in particular when the intended treatment involves the use of high doses of corticosteroids for a long period, the possible beneficial effects of therapy should always be evaluated versus the real risk of a number of serious complications. Some of the side effects which have received particular attention in recent literature are reviewed in the present Chapter.

SYSTEMIC SIDE EFFECTS OF CORTICOSTEROIDS

The systemic adverse effects of these compounds are due to the general impregnation of the organism with excessive levels of corticosteroids and therefore they occur most frequently after systemic administration. They may, however, also be induced by local or topical administration of these drugs, depending on their dosage, potency, and route and frequency of administration.

Corticosteroids and peptic ulcer disease *(SED-9, 650; SEDA-7, 376)*

The possibility that corticosteroids are potentially ulcerogenic continues to be the subject of considerable debate. Although there are numerous clinical reports which favor this hypothesis, it was not confirmed in certain randomized-control trials. Messer et al ([1R]) have reexamined the question by pooling data from 71 clinical trials, in which randomized control patients were compared with corticosteroid-treated patients ($n = 3064$). A significantly ($P < 0.001$) higher incidence of peptic ulcer disease (1.8%) was observed in the steroid-treated patients than in the controls (0.8%) and this incidence varied directly with the dosage of steroids. Gastrointestinal hemorrhage also occurred more frequently ($P = 0.03$) in steroid-treated patients (2.5%) than in controls (1.6%). This study thus strongly suggests that there really is an increased risk of peptic ulcer and gastrointestinal hemorrhage, which should be taken into account when prescribing corticosteroids.

Side Effects of Drugs Annual 8
M.N.G. Dukes, editor

ISBN 0 444 90339 9
$0.80 per article per page (transactional system)
$0.20 per article per page (licensing system)

Corticosteroids and pancreatitis *(SEDA-7, 316)*

The association of pancreatitis with the use of corticosteroids is based mainly on multiple case reports, and there is still insufficient statistical proof to establish it with certainty. In most of the relevant published reports, pancreatitis was observed after treatment with corticosteroids given in combination with other drugs. This is again the case in 3 new case reports, 1 of chronic pancreatitis with cyst formation ([2cr]), and 2 of fatal hemorrhagic pancreatitis ([3c], [4c]), in which prednisone (40 to 60 mg daily) was taken alongside various other drugs. For this reason, it is not clear in how far the corticosteroids, the underlying disease or the other drugs (given alone or in combination) should be considered etiological agents. Nevertheless, the possibility that corticosteroids cause or favor pancreatitis should not be overlooked.

Neurological complications

Allergic reactions to corticosteroids are occasionally reported (SED-9, 646) in spite of the antiinflammatory and immunosuppressive activity of these drugs. Behan et al ([5cr]) report on 2 patients who developed *neurological symptoms* after the local injection of methylprednisolone. In both patients antibodies against methylprednisolone could be demonstrated. In 1 patient, who also had a positive skin reaction to methylprednisolone, ataxia, diplopia and right hemiparesis gradually developed during the days following the injection. In this case the symptoms were ascribed to acute disseminated *encephalomyelitis* probably precipitated by the drug. In the case of the second patient an *epileptic grand mal seizure* was probably triggered by an anaphylactic reaction to methylprednisolone.

Epidural lipomatosis Extradural fat deposition induced by corticosteroids has been reported occasionally as a cause of myelopathy, with neurological and radiological signs of spinal cord compression (SEDA-5, 354). Additional cases of this complication have been described by Guegan et al (6[c]) and by George et al (7[cR]), who also provide a brief review of earlier cases. Most of these patients received high doses (40 mg or more) of prednisone for a prolonged period and required surgical decompression for treatment. A 14-year-old renal transplant patient, reported by George et al, was, however, treated successfully by tapering the dose of prednisolone (from 45 to 25 mg daily) and by prescribing a 1000-kcal diet high in protein and low in carbohydrate, thus also eliminating his insulin requirement which had developed during steroid therapy.

Mental changes occur frequently during corticosteroid therapy. Usually there is euphoria, but depressive reactions are also observed. Carpenter and Gruen (8[R]) have reviewed the effects of corticosteroids on human mental function and discussed the general principles for treatment of these abnormal emotional reactions. Patients with exogenous hypercortisolism may require psychiatric treatment because of a serious risk of suicide, behavioral problems related to the state of excitation, or perceptual abnormalities including hallucinations. In the presence of these symptoms, corticosteroids should be reduced to physiological levels, but this should be done gradually since an abrupt cessation can result in rebound depression and increased anxiety, or possibly lead to adrenal insufficiency (see 'Steroid withdrawal syndrome'). Furthermore, new psychological problems, such as reactive disappointment, anxiety and depression, may develop after reduction of corticosteroid therapy, in part due to the exacerbation of the original medical condition.

In patients on alternate-day therapy these mental changes may present a typical cyclic character. Sharfstein, Sack and Fauci (9[C]) have described behavioral abnormalities in 3 patients on long-term alternate-day therapy. On the day of corticosteroid intake (50–60 mg of prednisone), the patients developed serious symptoms of hyperactivity and hypomania and they had difficulty in sleeping that night. The next day (with no treatment) they became progressively depressed and lethargic. The 2-day cycle would then start again with the intake of prednisone the following morning. In 2 patients the symptoms of rapid changes of mood improved markedly when the dosage of corticosteroids was diminished.

Osteonecrosis

A frequent occurrence of this complication has been noted in renal transplant patients treated with corticosteroids for prolonged periods (SEDA-6, 333). Nevertheless, this adverse effect has occasionally been observed in other patients as well after a short period of treatment with high doses of corticosteroids (SEDA-7, 376). In 1 recently reported case, for instance, osteonecrosis of both humoral and femoral heads became clinically manifest 1 year after a 7-day course of treatment with 16 mg dexamethasone daily (10[c]).

In the meantime, Williams and Corbett (33[C]) have provided extensive case descriptions of a 33-year-old diabetic man and a 33-year-old woman with Addison's disease who both developed avascular bone necrosis after steroid replacement therapy; in both cases the complication developed about a year after the start of therapy.

Avascular bone necrosis has also been described as a complication of the treatment of malignant lymphoma with systemic chemotherapy including high-dose corticosteroids. In a retrospective study on 3500 patients, Thorne et al (11[CR]) found 12 patients in whom osteonecrosis developed during or after such treatment. The first symptoms were observed 8 to 72 months after the start of steroid therapy. The predominance of Hodgkin's disease over non-Hodgkin's lymphoma in the affected patients suggests that these patients are more at risk of this complication. This seems to be confirmed by another study in which Mould and Adam (12[C]) observed osteonecrosis in 7 out of 312 patients treated for Hodgkin's disease with combined chemotherapy including corticosteroids and radiotherapy.

The currently most widely accepted theory for the pathogenesis of steroid-induced osteonecrosis is the blockage of the bone and arteries by corticosteroid-induced lipid microemboli. Pastore and Kessler (13[cR]) have described 3 fatal cases of *pulmonary fat embolization*, occurring in immunosuppressed patients while receiving steroids. 2 of these patients had systemic lupus erythematosus, which may have been a contributing factor since these patients also display a high incidence of avascular bone necrosis during corticosteroid therapy.

Steroid-induced cataracts *(SEDA-6, 334)*

Kollarits et al (14[C]) have compared the incidence of this complication in steroid-treated renal transplant patients with that in age-matched controls. They found posterior subcapsular lens changes in 32 of 33 steroid-treated patients, but only in 1 of 33 controls. Cataract surgery was necessary in 6 of the renal transplant patients, and in 4 of these patients HLA-A1 antigen was present, suggesting that susceptibility to steroid-induced cataract might be related to the presence of this antigen.

Steroid withdrawal syndrome

The treatment of a patient with corticosteroids for a more or less prolonged period will induce an adaptation of the system to excessive steroid levels. When the treatment is interrupted or even reduced, this may lead to a number of symptoms which have been classified as 'steroid withdrawal syndrome' (15[R], 16[R], 17[CR], 18[cr]). In this relatively vague syndrome a number of elements can be distinguished which may be present alone but more often appear in combination.

1. **Recrudescence of the underlying disease** *Since many steroid-treated diseases are chronic in nature, the withdrawal or even the reduction of the steroid dose may lead to a reappearance of the disease, sometimes with marked changes in its symptomatology. This flaring-up of symptoms may be related to the time schedule of steroid administration, e.g. if a reduced single morning dose of the corticosteroid is no longer able to suppress the disease adequately over the full 24 hours (18[cr]). A similar problem may also occur during alternate-day therapy. Since the risk of a flare-up depends largely on the nature of the underlying disease, it is difficult to provide general guidelines for this aspect of steroid withdrawal. It is, however, clear that tapering should be performed very gradually, particularly after prolonged steroid treatment, and with careful monitoring of the individual patient.*

2. **Hypothalamo-pituitary adrenal hypofunction** *(SEDA-4, 270) Very often during systemic corticosteroid treatment the hypothalamo-pituitary adrenal (HPA) axis will be partially or completely suppressed. When the treatment is short (less than 1 week), even complete suppression by high doses of corticosteroids will have little permanent effect, but the effects of suppression become quite pronounced and long lasting after prolonged treatment. The nature of the steroid, its dosage and time schedule (e.g. alternate-day therapy) and the susceptibility of the individual patient play an important role in determining the degree of suppression.*

When steroid therapy is interrupted this may thus lead to a more or less pronounced degree of adrenal insufficiency with the corresponding clinical picture. The reduced cortisol output can be demonstrated by various means but the 8 A.M. plasma cortisol level and the response of plasma cortisol to ACTH-injection are probably the most useful parameters to monitor the basal cortisol impregnation and the adrenal response to ACTH. The same parameters can also be used to follow the recovery of the adrenal function in patients who have steroid-induced HPA-hypofunction and still require non-suppressive corticosteroid substitution for that reason.

Normal basal cortisol levels and a normal response to ACTH, or even a normal response to more complex tests (metapyrone, hypoglycemia) which give additional information on the hypothalamo-pituitary function, do not preclude the possibility that the patient will react inadequately to medical or surgical stress. For this reason steroid coverage of major stress should be used in a general way in these patients during, or even up to 1 year after, steroid withdrawal.

3. **Dependence upon increased corticosteroids** *After cessation of corticosteroid therapy a number of patients show symptoms reminiscent of adrenal insufficiency, although their adrenal function tests are normal. The clinical picture in these cases is rather vague and includes subjective symptoms such as anorexia, nausea, fatigue, lethargy, arthralgia and myalgia, but also objective symptoms such as fever, desquamation and weight loss. The symptoms disappear when additional corticosteroids are given. The mechanism of this increased corticosteroid requirement is not understood, but the patients appear to suffer from a kind of relative adrenal insufficiency, which is not necessarily physical. In the same context the marked mental effects of corticosteroids should be mentioned (SEDA-7, 375) which may lead occasionally to a degree of psychic dependence, so that depression and anxiety can occur when corticosteroids are withdrawn.*

It will be clear that the various elements involved in steroid withdrawal often occur simultaneously in the same patient and that symptoms cannot always be classified unambiguously in one category or another. It will also be obvious that the management of the patient during steroid withdrawal should be adapted carefully to the individual, his previous case history and his clinical evolution.

SIDE EFFECTS OF ANTENATAL GLUCOCORTICOIDS

Antenatal glucocorticoid therapy is widely used to promote fetal lung maturation in cases of premature labor, and in such cases it is often employed in combination with tocolytic drugs. 2 recent reports again describe the occurrence of *maternal pulmonary edema* in patients treated with this combination of drugs (see also SEDA-5, 354; SEDA-6, 333). In one report on 3 cases (19[cr]), a high dose of hydrocortisone (1 g every 8 hours) was combined with isoxsuprine or with ritodrine. In another report on 3 cases (20[C]) isoxsuprine, metaproterenol or ritodrine were associated with betamethasone (12 mg/l i.m.). Although the administration of intravenous fluid and the simultaneous administration or other drugs probably contributed to the development of pulmonary edema, one should be aware of the possible risks of this complication, and the patients should be monitored accordingly. Another possible side effect of this combination of drugs (betamethasone in combination with ritodrine) is a *hypertensive crisis*, which was observed in one patient under similar conditions (21[c]). It should never be forgotten that the combination may also induce *hyperglycemia* (SED-9, 224).

The maternal antenatal administration of corticosteroids also affects the neonate, and in fact fetal lung maturation is the primary goal of this treatment. A side effect of this treatment, which is primarily of diagnostical value, is a neonatal leukemoid reaction (SEDA-7, 377). Anday and Harris (22[c]) describe a similar neutrophilic leucocytosis in 5 infants (all girls) whose mothers had been treated with dexamethasone. In 3 cases the last dose of dexamethasone had been given more than 1 week before delivery. The authors stress that other causes of such a leukemoid reaction should be excluded before the leucocytosis is attributed to the administration of the steroid. The same holds true in adults, where corticoids also induce a predominantly polymorfonuclear leucocytosis, which is extremely variable in intensity and evolution (23[CR]).

SAFETY OF CORTICOSTEROID AEROSOLS

Inhaled corticosteroids. The large scale use of inhaled corticosteroids has provided further evidence for their safety. This subject has been newly reviewed by Clark (24[R]) and by Mygind (25[R]). When the dose of beclomethasone dipropionate is kept below 1 mg a day there seems to be little or no suppression of the hypothalamo-pituitary adrenal axis, and doses of 2 mg or more are required to produce marked suppression. Other systemic side effects (hyperglycemia, osteoporosis, growth retardation, etc.) are usually absent. With regard to local side effects, an increased risk of infection has not been substantiated, although there is a higher frequency of oropharyngeal candidiasis, which does, however, not lead to pulmonary infection. Histological examination of bronchial biopsy specimens reveals no pathological changes of the bronchial mucosa even after as much as 36 months of treatment.

Nasal aerosols of beclomethasone dipropionate (50 μg, 3 or 4 times daily) used for the treatment of perennial or seasonal rhinitis also produce little or no pathological change in the nasal mucosa, although the resulting local corticosteroid concentrations are much higher. About 10% of the patients have episodes of hemorrhagic secretion, but this side effect is usually of little importance. Sneezing and nasal burning have also been noted. No increased risk of candidiasis or HPA-suppression was demonstrated (26[CR], 27[CR]).

It should be noted, however, that the safe use of corticosteroid aerosols involves the use of specifically chosen corticosteroids (e.g. beclomethasone dipropionate, budenoside) under well-controlled conditions. Important side effects and even a full-blown Cushing's syndrome have been noted, for instance, with nasal sprays containing other corticosteroids, such as dexamethasone (SEDA-5, 354). In this respect we may also mention some recent reports of pseudohyperaldosteronism with hypertension (SEDA-7, 378) and of electrolyte changes, observed during the use of nasal sprays containing 9α-fluoroprednisolone acetate, a corticosteroid with relatively strong mineralocorticoid activity (28[c], 29[c]).

SIDE EFFECTS OF CORTICOTROPINS

Allergic reactions The incidence of these reactions has been reduced markedly by the use of synthetic ACTH-derivatives (notably tetracosactide). Nevertheless, very severe allergic reactions are still observed occasionally (SEDA-6, 335). Müller et al (30[cr]) report the case of a 14-year-old girl who died in anaphylactic shock after the intravenous injection of tetracosactide. The presence of ACTH-antibodies could be demonstrated in serum and ascites fluid. The patient had been treated for asthma with ACTH-injections (tetracosactide-depot, 1 mg twice monthly). From literature data the authors conclude that ACTH-antibodies can always be demonstrated by radioimmunology in cases of an anaphylactic reaction to corticotropins, but only in 30% of the patients who present only a slight reaction (urticaria, hot flush, local swelling). In fact, in some of these patients the reaction may be based on a histamine-releasing activity of ACTH and its derivatives, rather than an allergic mechanism. The authors warn against the risk of severe allergic reactions to ACTH in patients treated for a long period with this peptide, in particular in those patients who already show some symptoms of an allergic reaction (urticaria, itching) or who are positive for anti-ACTH-antibodies. Diagnostic ACTH-stimulation tests in those patients should be covered with dexamethasone.

In this connection it may be noted that the Belgian National Center for Adverse Reaction Monitoring has received a report of a 79-year-old man who died from bronchospasm due to administration of a slow-release preparation of tetracosactide (32[C]); the use of tetracosactide in Belgium has now been restricted to diagnosis of secretory activity of the adrenal cortex and (for the slow-release preparation) to certain neurological conditions and the treatment of myoclonic spasms (see, however, below).

Brain atrophy During treatment of infantile spasms with ACTH-injections, cranial computed tomography (CT) very frequently reveals radiological signs of brain atrophy (SEDA-5, 351), in fact a reversible brain shrinkage, caused by extremely high induced endogenous corticosteroid levels, probably through intracranial water and electrolyte changes. Satoh et al (31[CR]) have reported another 13 cases with this radiological finding in children treated with ACTH-treatment for intractable epilepsy. In 2 of these cases the ACTH-treatment was further complicated by a subdural diffusion. The authors suggest that the short- and long-term influence of this treatment should be reconsidered and that ACTH should not be administered as a first drug in the treatment of infantile spasms.

REFERENCES

1. Messer J, Reitman D, Sacks HS et al (1983) Association of adrenocorticosteroid therapy and peptic-ulcer disease. *N. Engl. J. Med.*, *309*, 21.
2. Weaver GA, Bordley J, Guiney WB, D'Accurzio A (1982) Chronic pancreatitis with cyst formation after prednisone and thiazide treatment. *Am. J. Gastroenterol.*, *77*, 164.
3. Bhatia R, Shankar SK, Tandon PN (1981)

Iatrogenic pancreatitis in a neurosurgical patient. *Neurology India, 29*, 199.

4. Tuder RM, Pinto RV (1982) Pancreatite necro-hemorragica pelo corticoide. *Rev. Hosp. Clin. Fac. Med. S. Paulo, 37*, 152.
5. Behan PO, Thomas M, Behan WMH (1982) Allergic reactions to steroids presenting with neurological symptoms. *Acta Neurol. Scand., 65*, 432.
6. Guegan Y, Fardoun R, Launois B, Pecker J (1982) Spinal cord compression by extradural fat after prolonged corticosteroid therapy. *J. Neurosurg., 56*, 267.
7. George Jr WE, Wilmot M, Greenhouse A, Hammeke M (1983) Medical management of steroid-induced epidural lipomatosis. *N. Engl. J. Med., 308*, 316.
8. Carpenter WT, Gruen PH (1982) Cortisol's effects on human mental functioning. *J. Clin. Psychopharmacol., 2*, 91.
9. Sharfstein SS, Sack DS, Fauci AS (1982) Relationship between alternate-day corticosteroid therapy and behavioral abnormalities. *J. Am. Med. Assoc., 248*, 2987.
10. Anderton JM, Helm R (1982) Multiple joint osteonecrosis following short-term steroid therapy. Case report. *J. Bone Joint Surg., 64*, 139.
11. Thorne JC, Evans WK, Alison RE, Fournasier V (1981) Avascular necrosis of bone complicating treatment of malignant lymphoma. *Am. J. Med., 71*, 751.
12. Mould JJ, Adam NM (1983) The problem of avascular necrosis of bone in patients treated for Hodgkin's disease. *Clin. Radiol., 34*, 231.
13. Pastore L, Kessler S (1982) Pulmonary fat embolization in the immunocompromised patient. Its relationship to steroid medication. *Am. J. Surg. Pathol., 6*, 315.
14. Kollarits C, Swann ER, Shapiro RS et al (1982) HLA-A1 and steroid-induced cataracts in renal transplant patients. *Ann. Ophthalmol., 14*, 1116.
15. Fass B (1979) Glucocorticoid therapy for nonendocrine disorders: withdrawal and 'coverage'. *Pediatr. Clin. North Am., 26*, 251.
16. Sullivan JN (1982) Saturday Conference: steroid withdrawal syndromes. *South. Med. J., 75*, 726.
17. Dixon RB, Christy NP (1980) On the various forms of corticosteroid withdrawal syndrome. *Am. J. Med., 68*, 224.
18. Studer H, Straub W (1981) Das Steroidentzug-Syndrom. Ein aktuelles Problem der ambulanten Medizin. *Schweiz. Med. Wochenschr., 111*, 1462.
19. Semchyshyn S, Zuspan FP, O'Shaughnessy R (1983) Pulmonary edema associated with the use of hydrocortisone and a tocolytic agent for management of premature labor. *J. Reprod. Med., 28*, 47.
20. Coggiola F, Scarrone G, Cabiati EG (1982) Su 3 casi di edema polmonare acuto in gravide trattate con tocolitici e betametasone. *Minerva Ginecol., 34*, 191.
21. Gonen R, Samberg I, Sharf M (1982) Hypertensive crisis associated with ritodrine infusion and betamethasone administration in premature labor. *Eur. J. Obstet. Gynecol. Reprod. Biol., 13*, 129.
22. Anday EK, Harris MC (1982) Leukemoid reaction associated with antenatal dexamethasone administration. *J. Ped., 101*, 614.
23. Shoenfeld Y, Gurewich Y, Gallant LA, Pinkhas J (1981) Prednisone-induced leukocytosis. Influence of dosage, method and duration of administration on the degree of leukocytosis. *Am. J. Med., 71*, 773.
24. Clark TJH (1982) Safety of inhaled corticosteroid. *Eur. J. Resp. Dis., 63* (122 Suppl.), 235.
25. Mygind N (1982) Mucosal changes in the airways during long-term corticosteroid treatment. *Eur. J. Resp. Dis., 63* (122 Suppl.), 229.
26. Siegel SC, Katz RM, Rachelefsky GS et al (1982) Multicentric study of beclomethasone dipropionate nasal aerosol in adults with seasonal allergic rhinitis. *J. Allergy Clin. Immunol., 69*, 345.
27. Small P, Black M, Frenkiel S (1982) Effects of treatment with beclomethasone dipropionate in subpopulations of perennial rhinitis patients. *J. Allergy Clin. Immunol., 70*, 178.
28. Russolo M, Marusi F, Bellini G et al (1982) Ipertensione arteriosa da abuso di preparato cortisonico contenuto in nebulizzatore nasale. *Oto-Rino-Laringol. Ital., 32*, 399.
29. Fogari R, Zoppi A, Clivati L et al (1982) Pseudo-iperaldosteronisimo primitivo da spray nasale contente 9-alfa-fluoro-prednisolone acetato: un caso clinico. *Prog. Med. Roma, 38*, 307.
30. Müller M, Fehm HL, Homoki J, Teller WM (1982) Tödlicher Zwischenfall nach intravenöser Injektion von synthetischem ACTH. *Dtsch. med. Wochenschr., 107*, 1353.
31. Satoh J, Takeshige H, Hara H, Fukuyama Y (1982) Brain shrinkage and subdural effusion associated with ACTH administration. *Brain Dev., 4*, 13.
32. Personal Communication to the Editor (1983).
33. Williams PL, Corbett M (1983) Avascular necrosis of bone complicating corticosteroid replacement therapy. *Ann. Rheum. Dis., 42*, 276.

P.E. Lebech and B. Ottesen

42 Sex hormones and related compounds, including oral contraceptives

PROGESTAGENS

General considerations

Until recently, it was customary to regard the estrogens as being the agents primarily responsible for various of the adverse reactions seen with the use of estrogen-progestagen preparations, such as the combined oral contraceptives. In many instances this is true, but the role of the progestagen must also be carefully examined when a problem is discussed. Typical is the debate relating to effects on serum lipids and lipoproteins; recent work has made it clear that the progestagens (largely by virtue of their antiestrogenic and androgenic effects) can influence lipid factors, and that both the nature and dose of the progestagen in a combined preparation can be of some importance in this respect.

Most known progestagens are derived from one of two groups. The first comprises the derivatives of progesterone itself, and includes 17-hydroxyprogestagens, medroxyprogesterone and megestrol acetate. The second comprises derivatives of testosterone and includes norethindrone, norgestrel and lynestrenol. Compounds in the latter group tend to be weight for weight more potent (1[R]).

Few new progestagens have been developed in the last two decades. An exception is desogestrel, currently available in various countries in combination with mestranol for oral contraception (Marvelon) (SEDA-7, 386). Structurally, desogestrel resembles lynestrenol, but there are some pharmacological differences; desogestrel has strong progestational and antiestrogenic activity, but no estrogenic properties, and it is only weakly bound to androgen receptors; it has little or no androgenic effect. Plasma levels of sex hormone-binding globulin (SHBG) were found to be higher in women using products containing desogestrel than in those taking levonorgestrel, and a decrease in free androgens was seen (2[R], 3[c], 4[C]). The hypothesis that it might be 'safer' in view of this profile still has to be proven in long-term use.

The progestational 'mini-pill'

The low-dose progestagen mini-pill has been considered as a contraceptive method which is safer but rather less effective than the combination pill (5[R]). Small doses of progestagen are here administered orally without a monthly break. Bleeding disturbances are generally the only clinical side effect experienced, spotting being common.

The low-dose progestagen mini-pill exerts its contraceptive effect largely by an action on the cervical mucus, but Detaeuf and Kuttenn (6[r]) found that in some 50% of cases alterations of the gonadotropins FSH and LH secretion occurred. A relative hyperestrogenic state ensues, which can result in uterine and mammary dystrophies. For this reason, this type of preparation should not be administered to patients with benign breast disease, to premenopausal women with endometrial or myometrial hyperplasia, or to women with a history of dysovulation or a high risk of genital cancer.

Side Effects of Drugs Annual 8
M.N.G. Dukes, editor

ISBN 0 444 90339 9
$0.80 per article per page (transactional system)
$0.20 per article per page (licensing system)

Progestagens as injectable hormonal contraceptives *(SEDA-7, 390)*

The effectiveness of some progestagens can be prolonged by incorporating them in an injectable solution or a carrier which gradually releases the hormone. Thus used, they can be effective for long periods. Three progestagens have proved highly effective as long-acting contraceptives: medroxyprogesterone-acetate, norethindrone-enanthate, and levonorgestrel. The first two are injectable preparations and the third is used in implants, vaginal rings or other carriers.

Since the review presented in SEDA-7 (p. 390) only a few papers have appeared (7[R], 8[R], 9[C], 10[C], 11[c], 12[c]) and they provide little new information. From a clinical point of view the bleeding problem is the major short-term drawback of these methods. Long-term concern has been focussed on the fact that these gestagens decrease the circulating levels of high density lipoprotein (HDL) cholesterol, which might in the long run raise the risk of cardiovascular disease. So far there are insufficient clinical data to determine whether any increase in the incidence of cardiovascular disease in fact occurs.

In the meantime, however, the heated social debate about medroxyprogesterone acetate (Depo-Provera) continues, a debate fostered as much by moral concern that injectable preparations might be used against a woman's will (e.g. in the mentally defective or asocial groups) as by concern about its possible physical risks (13[R]).

Progesterone therapy in threatened abortions *(SED-7, 389)*

Progestagens are in widespread use in many countries for supportive treatment in pregnancy. It has often been pointed out that in view of possible risks (e.g. masculinization of the fetus) the benefits of progestagen therapies need to be proven before any of these drugs can be recommended for supportive treatment in pregnancy. In a recent double-blind clinically controlled study Søndergaard et al (14[C]) investigated the effect of natural progesterone in women admitted to the hospital with threatened first trimester abortion and reduced progesterone levels. They did not find any significant effect of progesterone on the abortion rate as compared to the placebo group. They conclude that threatened abortion and low serum progesterone is no indication for routine progesterone replacement therapy.

ANDROGENS

Obstructive sleep apnea syndrome

The obstructive sleep apnea syndrome is a recently described clinical disorder that results from repetitive episodes of upper-airway occlusion during sleep (15[c]). Since the syndrome occurs much more frequently in males than in females it is reasonable to postulate that androgens may be important in its causation. Sandblom et al (16[c]) have described a man in whom the symptoms of obstructive sleep apnea syndrome developed on two occasions in association with administration of testosterone.

A 36-year-old man volunteered to participate in a study of contraceptive agents for men. His medical history and physical examination were normal except for moderate obesity. The results of routine hematological and blood-chemistry studies were normal. Total serum testosterone was 3.4 ng/ml and free serum testosterone 143 pg/ml. After a 5-month control period, the subject received 200 mg of intramuscular testosterone enanthate per week for 7 months. Thereafter, while testosterone administration was continued, human chorionic gonadotropin (5000 I.U. given intramuscularly 3 times weekly) was added for the next 3 months.

10 months after the beginning of the study, the subject reported progressive difficulty in sleeping, daytime somnolence, and mood depression. He denied having respiratory symptoms, but he did have a lifelong history of loud snoring. A complete examination of the upper airway revealed no source of obstruction, and the remainder of the examination was remarkable only for pitting pedal edema.

Sleep studies and ventilatory-drive studies were conducted to evaluate the symptoms of sleep apnea. When these studies were completed, testosterone and human chorionic gonadotropin were discontinued, and the patient was restudied 5 weeks later. At this time, he described a definite improvement in the quality of his sleep and in his mood, as well as a reduction of daytime somnolence. The results of a physical examination were similar except for the abscence of pedal edema and systemic hypertension. Testosterone enanthate injections of 200 mg weekly were then resumed, and after 5 injections the symptoms returned, as did the pedal edema. Sleep studies and ventilatory-drive studies were repeated, after which testosterone was again discontinued. After 6 months

without exogenous testosterone all the patient's symptoms had resolved.

A relation between sex steroids and sleep apnea has often been suggested. The male seems more prone to develop obstructive sleep apnea than the female, and disordered breathing during sleep is more common among normal males than premenopausal females. These observations, and the fact that progesterone is known to stimulate waking ventilatory drives (17[c]), suggest that the abnormal relaxation of the pharyngeal muscles found both in snoring and obstructive sleep apnea is effected by levels of circulating hormones.

Danazol *(SEDA-5, 375; SEDA-6, 355)*

Danazol was initially used only in the treatment of pelvic endometriosis but has also been employed in the treatment of chronic cystic mastitis, precocious puberty and congenital angioneurotic edema. It has furthermore been used as an antifertility agent in both men and women, and for the treatment of menorrhagia (18[R]).

Effects on the fetus Because danazol is capable of causing amenorrhea, a patient who becomes pregnant while taking the medication may not be diagnosed until considerable fetal exposure has occurred. Evidence is accumulating that danazol has an androgenic effect on the fetus leading to fetal genital malformations (19[R], 20[c], 21[c]). That danazol is contraindicated in early pregnancy must be emphasized. It has been suggested that therapy with danazol should begin after several days of a normal menstrual flow and at a dose greater than 200 mg/day, since lower doses may not effectively inhibit hormonal output, folliculogenesis and ovulation (19[R]).

It must never be forgotten that danazol is an androgen and that some women are very prone to develop *signs of virilization* even with weak androgens. Briefly reviewing the literature, Wardle et al (22[r]) remark that according to recent studies danazol causes acne in between 21% and 27% of patients, hirsutism in 17–21% and deepening of the voice in 7–10%. Early studies suggested that the effect on the voice was merely a deepening of pitch which would prove reversible when the drug was stopped. That this has not always proved to be so is not surprising, since it is well known that beyond a certain point – and sometimes quite quickly – androgens can induce permanent changes in the vocal cords. Wardle et al themselves (22[C]) report on a 27-year-old woman treated for endometriosis with 600 mg danazol daily who began to complain of voice changes within 7 months, after which the drug was soon discontinued for this reason. The voice changes were initially of weakness, followed after a few weeks by persistent huskiness and occasional loss of pitch control, 'squeaking' punctuating normal speech. The pitch of the voice when shouting was unpredictable, and weakness of the voice was exacerbated by prolonged talking. 16 months after drug withdrawal the changes persisted.

Efforts are being made to examine the value of danazol as a post-coital contraceptive. In a recent study (23[c]) only 3 out of 82 women treated with danazol became pregnant. The incidence of nausea (10%), vomiting (0%) and other side effects (4%) was low as compared with the agents used for this purpose so far.

Androgens, anabolics and sinus thrombosis

In a group of 27 patients with hypoplastic anemia treated with male hormone and 'protein-assimilating hormone' (i.e. anabolics) Shiozawa et al (24[C]) observed 3 cases of superior sagittal sinus thrombosis (SSST). The signs were seizures, hemiplegia, facial palsy, stupor and coma, the most important prodrome and consistent subjective complaint being headache. After discontinuation of the hormonal therapy the neurological signs and symptoms related to SSST gradually subsided. The authors concluded that administration of male hormone or 'protein-assimilating hormone' can be associated with development of SSST and if neurological symptoms or signs of SSST appear the administration of the hormones should be discontinued.

ESTROGENS

Exposure to diethylstilbestrol in utero *(SEDA-6, 347–51; SEDA-7, 390)*

Several reviews on the effect of prenatal diethylstilbestrol (DES) exposure have appeared during the past year (25[R], 26[R], 27[R], 28[R]); gradually, a more complete picture of the long-term effects is emerging.

It is estimated that up to six million persons were exposed to DES during its use for high-risk pregnancy between 1940 and 1971 (25[R]). The exposure in utero is as well documented during the last decade, associated with adverse effects on the reproductive tract in male and female progeny some of which become manifest at the time of puberty or even later. In male subjects epididymal cysts, microphallus, cryptorchidism and testicular hypoplasia have been observed, and in the female adenosis, clear cell adenocarcinoma and structural defects of the cervix, vagina, uterus and fallopian tube.

Recent case reports have suggested a possible relationship between in utero exposure to DES and ovarian cystadenofibroma (29[c]), prolactin-secreting pituitary adenoma (30[c]) and adenosquamous carcinoma (31[c]). The risk of development of clear cell cancer is estimated to be no more than 1.4 per 1,000 and could be as low as 1.4 per 10,000 exposed daughters (32[C]). Noncancerous changes appear in the vagina in about one-third and in the cervix in nearly every DES-exposed daughter (33[C], 34[C]). These conclusions are amply supported by recent reports (35[C]–37[C], 38[c]–40[c]).

Robboy et al (41[C]) have developed a remarkable model for the study of drug interaction with fetal development and tested it as regards human uterovaginal development in the presence and absence of diethylstilbestrol (DES).

Intact reproductive tracts from fragments of 29 human embryos and fetuses 5.0 to 17.7 weeks of age obtained after dilatation and curettage were grown for 4 weeks in vivo in athymic (nude) mice that were either untreated or implanted subcutaneously with a DES pellet. The control specimens continued their anticipated morphogenesis for equivalent in-utero ages; the normal processes observed included fusion of the paired embryonic müllerian ducts into a single uterovaginal canal, stratification of endometrial and tubal mesenchyma into inner (presumptive endometrial stroma) and outer (presumptive myometrium) layers; plication of tubal and endometrial mucosa; uterine gland formation; and stratification (transformation) of the simple columnar epithelium of the vagina and cervix into a stratified squamous plate. Specimens exposed in vivo to DES exhibited anomalies, many of which mimicked those observed clinically in young women exposed prenatally to DES. Glandular epithelium (adenosis) was found in the vagina. The upper genital tract was malformed; its growth was stunted, and the inner and outer stromal layers of the uterine corpus and fallopian tubes failed to segregate. The authors conclude that the in vivo model that they describe, with its built-in controls, provides a valid approach for examining the dynamics of morphogenesis and cytodifferentiation in developing human genital tracts under experimentally regulated conditions.

Concerning the screening of adolescents exposed to DES in utero nothing new can be added to the recommendations put forward in Annual 7 in 1983.

HORMONAL CONTRACEPTIVES*

Overall risks of contraceptive use *(SED-9, 669)*

On various occasions the point has been made that even where a contraceptive method involves certain risks to the users, these are negligible in comparison with the risks of pregnancy and childbirth. The argument is not accepted in all circles and it has not always been well documented. It is therefore interesting to cite an overview (Table 1) by Ory of the US Center for Disease Control of the mortality risks associated with various fertility control methods and with pregnancy and childbirth. The figures, which relate to the US population, incorporate both the latest obstetric statistics and current data on the risks of oral contraception (42[R]).

Oral contraceptives: congenital defects *(SEDA-4, 285; SEDA-5, 371; SEDA-6, 351)*

The general opinion to date is that oral contraceptives have at most a very slight effect on the fetus if taken in error in early pregnancy; it is quite possible that some slight derangement of endometrial function under hormonal influence could explain the non-specific patterns of abnormalities which have sometimes been attributed to these and other hormonal products.

McCredie et al (43[C]) have now conducted a retrospective case-control study on 155 live-born children with congenital limb reductions. 18 mothers (12%) were found to have taken oral contraceptives inadvertently during early pregnancy compared with only one mother in a control group. The relative risk (calculated by matched pair analysis) of a limb defect in the offspring of women who

*The progestagen 'mini-pill' is dealt with on p. 355.

Table 1. *Cumulative risk of death associated with fertility and fertility control methods (per 100,000 nonsterile women)*

Method	Age groups			Total 15–44
	15–34	35–39	40–44	
Condom/abortion	1	<1	<1	1
Condom	19	2	2	23
Pill/non-smoker	21	70	160	251
IUD	25	10	10	45
Abortion	26	9	6	41
Diaphragm/spermicide	28	11	14	53
Rhythm	36	14	18	68
Pill/smoker	132	257	588	977
No method	192	129	141	462

Source: Adapted from Ory (42[R]).

took oral contraceptives after conception was 23.9. 11 of the 18 mothers smoked, but the relative risk of occurrence of a limb defect when adjusted for smoking remained high (23.1). There was no evidence of a sex specific defect.

It is clear that this topic is not closed, but one must be extremely cautious in attaching conclusions to one study. The lower the dose of an oral contraceptive and the less complete cycle control is, the greater the risk that a woman will inadvertently continue to take the product early in pregnancy, the onset of which will not be readily recognized. It is however possible that the mothers of children having congenital defects may have a greater percentage of recall of possible factors deranging pregnancy than mothers of entirely normal children, and one must wonder whether in a control group such as that examined by McCredie the accidental use of the pill in early pregnancy really was limited to a single case.

Oral contraceptives: miscellaneous effects

Burns et al (44[c]) noted cold *urticaria* as an adverse effect to a low dose combination of norethindrone and mestranol in a 19-year-old woman. White non-pruritic swelling occurred on any part of the body exposed to temperatures lower than 10° centigrade. The effect disappeared when the oral contraceptive was withdrawn. Such an effect does not seem to have been described previously.

SEX HORMONES (GENERAL)

Sex steroids and cardiovascular complications: The state of knowledge *(SED-9, 659; SEDA-4, 280; SEDA-7, 386)*

During the past 20 years, a great deal of evidence has accumulated that current users of oral contraceptives have an increased risk of ischemic heart disease (45[R], 46[C], 47[C], 48[R], 49[C], 50[C], 51[C]). Cerebrovascular disease (52[C], 53[c], 54[c]), peripheral vascular disease (55[C], 64[c], 65[C]) and hypertension (66[c]–68[c]). However, much evidence indicates that the OC-induced risk for these diseases is very small for women under 35 years of age, whilst for those 35 to 45 years old the risk is about the same for users of OC's as it is for smokers. These conclusions have found support in a recent further report from The Royal College of General Practitioners Oral Contraception Study (45[R]). In addition this study found a 2- to 3-fold increased fatality rate in oral contraceptive users who smoke, an observation which has not been reported previously and requires confirmation. The risk of cerebrovascular disease was found to remain elevated in former users for at least 6 years after they had stopped oral contraceptives. The authors emphasize that this finding requires confirmation, since other published evidence is inconsistent (69[C]–72[C]). However, no increased risk of ischemic heart disease or peripheral vascular disease in former users could be detected.

The evidence is now very impressive that oral contraceptives raise the risk of thromboembolic disease, at least in women aged over 35 and more especially in smokers. Several explanations have been put forward in order to explain this association: abnormalities in the hemostasis system, changes in lipid and glucose metabolism and a direct vascular effect.

Effects on coagulation *The relationship between oral contraceptives and blood coagulation has recently been critically reviewed by Eberhard F. Mammen (73[R]), who looks particularly at the factors which have confused the issue.*

Three major problems exist. Firstly, the term hypercoagulability has been used to describe a hypothetical concept that postulates a prethrombotic state, identifiable by certain changes in the hemostasis system. Mammen emphasizes that at this time no laboratory test or combination of tests can clearly predict whether under certain circumstances a patient will develop a thromboembolic event or not. A second problem is that investigators have interpreted certain coagulation changes in vitro as being reflective of a thrombotic state in vivo without giving proof that the latter state ever existed. Furthermore, laboratory data obtained from patients with existing thrombotic events have been interpreted as having caused the thrombosis rather than being a reflection of the thrombosis. A third problem put forward by Mammen is that investigators have used epidemiologic data, retrospective and prospective, to claim cuase and effect without taking basic physiologic or pathologic principles into consideration. Epidemiologic data can at best demonstrate an association between two events but cannot be used to establish a causal relationship.

Effects on the vessel wall *As early as 1970, vascular wall lesions were described in 20 women who had taken oral contraceptives (74[C]). Later reports (75[C]–78[C]), however, showed that these lesions were not specific for users of oral contraceptives, and examination of the vessels is now considered to be of no predictive value in determining which individual might or might nor develop a thromboembolic episode during the use of oral contraceptives.*

The platelets and the interaction between platelets and the vessel wall have similarly been studied in women using oral contraception, but the findings have been contradictory and there is no clear proof that the platelet changes measured in vitro have a true relationship with the development of thromboembolism in vivo, especially venous thrombosis (79[C]).

The influence of oral contraceptives on clotting has been widely studied during recent years. According to Mammen, one of the major difficulties in interpreting the many data obtained in women who take oral contraceptives is that most investigators study a few selected parameters of either the clotting or the fibrinolytic system without necessarily taking the balance of the two systems into account. Even within the system there are factors that move the reaction forward, while there are others that inhibit this forward reaction. Therefore, a single abnormal finding does not necessarily mean that the entire system is out of balance. There are also few data to support the hypothesis that a certain abnormality in the clotting or fibrinolytic system in vitro has any relationship to either a 'prethrombotic' state or even to an ongoing thrombotic process in vivo.

Abnormalities detected in the blood of a patient with a massive thromboembolic event may be the result of the event and may not have necessarily led to the event. Moreover, the clotting and fibrinolytic test systems frequently utilized lack specificity, reliability and reproducibility. Many of the tests were designed to measure 'deficiency states' that lead to bleeding and not to measure intravascular clot formation (73[R]).

Fibrinolysis is initiated when plasminogen is converted to plasmin. Reports on changes in the fibrinolytic system of women taking oral contraceptive medications reveal conflicting data. While many investigations found no change in overall fibrinolytic activity (80[C]) several have reported increased fibrinolytic activity primarily based on increased plasma plasminogen activator activity and decreased antiplasmin activity (81[C]–87[C]). In contrast decreased levels of tissue activator of plasminogen have been reported in women who took contraceptives (88[C]–91[C]). These changes could be due to the thrombosis in reflecting an attempt by the organism to dissolve the clot.

Mammen (73[R]) draw attention to the presence of high-molecular-weight fibrinogen complexes, which are formed when thrombin converts the fibrinogen molecules to fibrin monomers; these complexes can be *determined in plasma by chromatography and quantified. A good correlation has been found between this procedure and the injection of ^{125}I-labelled fibrinogen, i.e. the levels of high-molecular-weight fibrinogen complexes were high in those patients in whom fibrin deposits were demonstrated by ^{125}I-fibrinogen tests (85[C]).*

During the past years several reports on the relationship between oral contraceptives and hemostasis have appeared (94[C]–100[C]). In one study on patients taking oral contraceptives 6.4% of the patients had elevated fibrinogen complexes prior to taking oral contraceptives, while the figure increased to approximately 27% when oral contraceptives were taken. These figures suggest a 4- to 5-fold greater risk of developing thrombosis in oral contraceptives users; these figures parallel to a certain extent the epidemiological observations (85[C], 92[C], 93[C]).

Effects on lipids *The action of sex steroid hormones on lipid metabolism has caused much concern, especially the inverse relationship between high-density-lipoprotein (HDL) and the subsequent development of atherosclerosis. As pointed out earlier in this chapter, recent reports seem to link the progestagens more closely to the changes in serum lipids, abnormal glucose tolerance and insulin secretion (101[C]–107[C]).*

Risks in elective surgery Although the increased risk of postoperative thromboembolism among oral contraceptive users has been known since the early 1970's it is not clear how much this knowledge has altered the preoperative management of women having elective operations. Accidents certainly continue to occur, and some may well be preventable.

A healthy 24-year-old white woman who did not smoke and had no history of thromboembolic disorders, had been using oral contraceptives for several years and continued their use until admitted to hospital for sterilization.

Tubal sterilization was performed under general anesthesia and an incidental appendectomy was performed. Exploration of the peritoneal cavity revealed no pathologic condition. The operation lasted 41 minutes. The patient tolerated the procedure well. The first 48 hours after operation the patient did well, except for some mild to moderate lower abdominal pain. Within 24 hours following operation, abdominal pain increased, and the following day she developed severe, acute abdominal pain and suffered cardiovascular collapse for which she required resuscitation. She was considered to be septic and dehydrated; treatment with intravenous fluids and antibiotics was initiated.

An echogram obtained on the 5th day after sterilization suggested the possibility of an abdominal mass on the right side; an exploratory laparotomy showed 2,000 ml of clear fluid in the peritoneal cavity. The cecum and ascending colon were necrotic with thrombosis of the colic and ileocolic veins. The pelvis and the appendectomy stump appeared normal. A right hemicolectomy and resection of the distal ileum were performed followed by a primary side-to-side ileocolostomy. Despite vigorous management, the patient's condition deteriorated after laparotomy and she died the next morning.

Significant findings at postmortem examination were thrombosis of both the ileocolic vein and the superior mesenteric vein and inflammation in the area of the colon adjacent to the anastomosis. The cause of death was determined to be endotoxic shock secondary to large bowel necrosis which resulted from thrombosis of the mesenteric veins (108[c]).

This case report leads us to recommend once more that other means of contraception should be used for several weeks before elective surgery (109[R]).

Sex steroids and liver disease *(SED-9, 665, 678; SEDA-4, 279; SEDA-5, 365; SEDA-7, 386)*

The association between oral contraceptives (in one case diethylstilbestrol and in one antiestrogen therapy was involved) and benign liver tumors has been supported by numerous new reports (110[c], 111[c], 112[C], 113[c], 114[c], 115[R], 116[c]–120[c], 121[R], 122[c], 123[R], 124[c]). A few malignant liver tumors have been reported in association with the use of oral contraceptives (125[c]–127[c]). Furthermore Helling et al (125[c]) advise an aggressive approach to ensure prompt diagnosis and surgical excision of liver tumors in young women who have taken oral contraceptives, since they can be malignant and even benign tumors can rupture causing fatal hemorrhage.

Goodman and Ishak (128[C]) have reviewed 128 cases of hepatocellular carcinoma (HCC) in order to investigate a possible association with oral contraceptives (OC). They found 48 cases under the age of 40 and 13 of these (27%) had used OC. However, 62% of HCC cases associated with OC and

58% of HCC cases in women under 40 not using OC were classified histologically as 'fibrolamellar' carcinoma. This subtype of HCC occurs predominantly in young people, both male and female. The authors conclude that the apparent increase in HCC in young women can be explained by the presence of cases of fibrolamellar carcinoma in this age group, and in their view the apparent association with oral contraceptives is probably coincidental.

Sex steroids and gall bladder disease

Previous reports have produced strong evidence of an increased incidence of gall bladder disease associated with the use of oral contraceptives (129[C]). The latest Royal College of General Practitioners Oral Contraceptive Study (130[C]) report provides data on 23,000 women using oral contraceptives. They conclude that no overall increased risk occurred in the long term and that the previously demonstrated short-term increase in risk is due to an acceleration of the onset of gall bladder disease in women already susceptible to it.

The acceleration may depend on the dose of estrogen in the combined oral contraceptive. The lithogenic effect of oral contraceptives has been confirmed by Kern et al (131[C]), who investigated bile-rich duodenal fluid in oral contraceptive users and non-users, all healthy non-obese women. They found a significant increase in biliary cholesterol saturation and in the lithogenic index of bile.

The effect of sex hormones on the central nervous system and on psychological function *(SED-9, 662–3)*

A number of studies suggest that a considerable group of women experience emotional side effects from sex steroids, but no consistent results have emerged. Some studies have implicated oral contraceptives in causing depression; the hormones implicated are thought to be estrogens by some, and progestagens by others; other well-conducted and carefully controlled studies have contradicted these findings and have found no adverse emotional effects with hormonal contraceptives (132[r]).

Chang et al (133[C]) report a series of sequential studies into the nature of mood changes reported by women taking the pill. Their results demonstrate the multidimensional nature of the reported emotional side effects of the pill. It seems doubtful whether the 'depression' as complained of by women taking the pill, is the same as depression in the psychiatric sense or can be meaningfully measured by the existing depression inventories.

Lobo and Gibbons (134[r]) have reviewed the role of progestagens on central nervous system function, pointing to studies in which progestagens administered to males induced characteristic changes in the electroencephalogram. Similar changes have been recorded after low doses of antidepressants such as diazepam. In animal studies a similar effect has been demonstrated. The neurological effect of progestagens appears to involve changes in the autonomic nervous system and mild central sedation.

There are only a few publications on the effect of progestagens on mood in postmenopausal women, but Lobo and Gibbons refer to preliminary data from their own ongoing studies in menopausal women which suggest a beneficial effect on mood and on the sense of well being and satisfaction.

Effect of sex steroids on lipid and lipoprotein metabolism

An increase in low-density-lipoprotein (LDL) is associated with an increase in coronary artery disease, while high-density-lipoprotein (HDL) seems to have some protective effect. Both progestagens and estrogens are known to alter plasmalipids and lipoprotein composition. Artificial estrogen (SEDA-7, 382) increased both HDL and LDL but the effect is dose-dependent. With natural estrogens (17β-estradiol) both LDL and VLDL decreases while HDL increases; these can be considered optimal changes.

Myocardial infarction seldom occurs in women prior to the menopause, but younger women who have had a bilateral oophorectomy show a higher incidence of myocardial infarction unless estrogen replacement therapy is begun soon after castration (135[C]).

Several recent clinical and epidemiological studies suggest that estrogens may exert a protective effect against cardiovascular disease (28[C], 136[C]–139[C]). In most of these studies estrogen alone has been used, but since the appearance of evidence pointing to the effectiveness of progestagens in protecting estrogen users from adenocarcinoma, estrogen-progestagen therapy after the menopause has become more popular. Progestagen (both norgestrel and norethindrone alone and in combination with estrogens) can alter plasma lipids and lipoprotein composition (140[C]), a rise in plasmatriglyceride levels and a decline in HDL being the most consistent findings. Most of the relevant studies have been conducted in women using oral contraceptives. Few data are available on lipid changes in postmenopausal women on estrogen-progestagen therapy, but the progestagen induced lipid changes could from a theoretical point of view negate the benefits of estrogens. Only the C-21 progestagens (medroxyprogesterone) and desogestrel seem not to have this unwanted effect on lipids (141[c]).

In a study from the Lipid Research Clinic (142[C]) the association of exogenous estrogen use and hysterectomy status with all-cause mortality was examined in 2,269 white women, aged 40 to 69. A total of 72 deaths occurred during this period. The relative risk of death in estrogen users as compared with non-users was 0.54 in gynecologically intact women, 0.34 in hysterectomized women and 0.12 in bilaterally oophorectomized women. The risk of death in estrogen users, irrespective of hysterectomy status, was 0.37 times that in non-users (3.4/1,000 vs 9.3/1,000). The significant negative association of estrogen use with mortality persisted after multivariate adjustment for confounding factors. Hysterectomy status alone was not a significant predictor of death. Some, but not all, of the lower risk mortality in estrogen users can be accounted for by increased levels of high-density lipoprotein cholesterol.

Sex hormones and cancer

Breast cancer *(SED-9, 682; SEDA-5, 365; SEDA-6, 339; SEDA-7, 382)* *Hormonal contraception* No major studies have demonstrated any relationship between breast cancer and hormonal contraception (SEDA-7, 383). In one study by Pikes et al (143[c]) it was found that oral contraceptive use before the first full-term pregnancy was associated with an elevated risk of breast cancer. In last year's review we suggested a possible explanation for the results in the Pikes study in terms of delay in the first pregnancy.

Pikes' group produced a further report in 1983 (144[C]), which gave rise to a great deal of discussion and some alarm.

> Using telephone interviews, the group compared the contraceptive histories of 314 Californian women with breast cancer diagnosed before the age of 37 with those of 314 neighborhood controls. Pike and his coworkers found that the women with cancer had used the pill for an average of 49.6 months, compared with 39.2 months among controls, and that they were more likely to have used the pill for long intervals before the age of 25.

Pikes' results, as pointed out by Drife (145[R]) are unique; they were not confirmed by the Oxford group's successive reports, and a major review of the entire field of breast cancer and oral contraceptives in 1983 found no overall association between the pill and breast cancer, apart from borderline trends among young users in two studies. The Oxford group is indeed currently of the opinion, in view of its own work (146[C]) that the pill may have some protective effect against breast cancer, a view which has been cautiously advanced earlier in the present series of volumes. Nevertheless the possibility can be excluded, as Drife points out, that young ladies in California are at greater risk than others, possibly by engaging in prolonged pill use very early in life. Another point is clearly that when the subjects interviewed by Pikes were asked to identify the brand of 'pill' they had used, most of those named were preparations with a high estrogen content. Such preparations if used for a number of years might indeed carry a degree of risk; since they are now obsolete it is unlikely that absolute certainty on this point will ever be attained.

In the meantime, two other studies of this topic must be noted.

> The Centers for Disease Control's Cancer and Steroid Hormone Investigation (147[C]) studied all women 20 to 54 years old with a first diagnosis of breast cancer as ascertained by eight cancer registries. Controls were selected at random from the general population of these eight areas. Analysis of the first 689 cases and 1,077 controls studied showed that women who had used oral contraceptives at some time in their lives had a relative risk of 0.9 compared with never-users (95% confidence interval, 0.8 to 1.2). Neither the duration of

oral contraceptive use nor the time elapsing since first use altered a user's risk of breast cancer; women whose first use was more than 15 years ago and who used oral contraceptives for 11 years or more had a relative risk of 0.8 (0.5 to 1.4). Oral contraceptive use did not increase the risk of breast cancer among women with benign breast disease or a family history of breast cancer. Oral contraceptive use before a woman's first pregnancy did not increase her risk of breast cancer significantly more than other methods of delaying the first pregnancy. This study provides no support for the hypothesis that oral contraceptive use increases a woman's risk of breast cancer.

A similar case control interview study (148[C]) conducted among participants in the Breast Cancer Detection Demonstration Project and involving 963 breast cancer cases and 858 controls, allowed evaluation of the risk of breast cancer associated with the use of oral contraceptives. Overall there was no association between use and risk of disease (RR = 1.1). In addition, there was no indication of increasing risk with years of use or years since initial use, despite slight excess risks observed among users of high-dose preparations. Premenopausal women who used the pill after the age of 40 showed an approximately 50% increase in risk, possibly as a result of artificial prolongation of a premenopausal rate of disease incidence. Non-significant excess risks associated with pill use were also seen among premenopausal women who reported a family history of breast cancer in a sister (RR = 3.6) or previous biopsies for benign breast disease (RR = 3.2). The latter excess was limited to women whose use of the pill preceded a first biopsy, suggesting that the types of lesions requiring biopsy among current long-term pill users may be those that predispose to breast cancer.

Cervical neoplasia and oral contraceptives *(SEDA-7, 385)* A new study by the Oxford Family Planning Association has examined the incidence of cervical neoplasia of all types in 6838 parous pill users (many of whom had been using relatively high-dose preparations) and comparing the results with a large group of IUD users. The women taking oral contraceptives had a 75% greater incidence of cervical neoplasia and the risk was related to the duration of oral contraceptive use (149[C]).

The authors of this study suggest that the 'pill' may have a direct effect upon the cervix but this is merely a supposition and one cannot exclude the possibility that other factors might explain the difference between the pill and IUD groups. Reviewing the evidence, Drife (145[R]) has pointed out that age at first intercourse and number of sexual partners which are known to be risk factors for cervical neoplasia, were not documented in this study, although the fact that the pill users in the Oxford study were somewhat younger at marriage and at first pregnancy than the comparison group suggests that there might have been differences. Drife also recalls the fact that the absolute risk, if present, is really very small: in the Oxford study the background risk of all types of cervical neoplasia (including dysplasia) was 1 in 1000 women years and this was doubled by use of the pill; preliminary data from the Royal College of General Practitioners' continuing study (150[c]) suggest that the excess risk of invasive cervical carcinoma in pill users is less than 1 in 14,000. All cancers in the Oxford study were detected at a curable stage.

Endometrial cancer, hormonal replacement therapy and contraceptives *(SED-9, 678; SEDA-5, 358; SEDA-6, 339; SEDA-7, 384)* The conclusion in SEDA-7 was that postmenopausal estrogen use may predispose to an increased incidence of endometrial cancer, but it appears that such use does not increase mortality from this condition. Use of combination oral contraceptives has been reported to decrease a woman's risk of developing endometrial cancer. A study from the Centers for Disease Control, Atlanta (151[C]) found that women who had used combination oral contraception some time in their lives had a relative risk of endometrial cancer of 0.5 compared with never-users. The protective effect occurred only in women who had used oral contraception for at least 12 months, and lasted for at least 10 years after cessation. It was estimated that approximately 2000 cases of endometrial cancer are averted each year by oral contraceptive use among women in the United States.

In view of the extent to which conclusions like this are often dependent upon American data, it is important to cite the results of a prospective cohort Swedish study, published late in 1983 by Persson. Starting in 1977, Persson sought to determine the risk of endometrial neoplasia in Swedish women as associated with estrogens and estrogen-progestagen combinations (152[C]).

A cohort comprising 22,233 women of ages from 35 years was obtained by registering and computerizing data from the prescription forms for estrogenic drugs received at the pharmacies in the Uppsala region during a three-year period. An efficient follow-up of the cohort was achieved by collecting incident cases of endometrial cancer from several sources and by identity number linkages. A histopathological review was undertaken to standardize diagnostic criteria for cases of endometrial cancer observed in the cohort and those occurring in the reference population and underlying the calculation of incidence rates.

A questionnaire study conducted in 735 cohort members permitted mapping of confounding factors, estimation of drug compliance and detailed characterization of estrogen and progestagen exposures. The results indicated that risk factors for endometrial cancer were not more prevalent in the cohort than in the background population. Furthermore, estrogen prescribing in this population during the period 1977–1980 was characterized by: low and decreasing rates of incidence and low rates of prevalent treatments; short treatment duration; predominant choice of estradiol valerate compounds; extensive usage of estrogen-progestagen combinations; preference for cyclic administration and low-strength tablets; and adherence to a few treatment indications.

The results of the cohort follow-up were based on an observation period of one to four completed years, corresponding to 89,306 person-years. In the analysis, the cohort was divided into subgroups according to duration of estrogen exposure and combinations with progestagens.

No significant increase in the risk of endometrial cancer was found in the cohort as a whole or in subgroups of it. Inclusion of premalignant endometrial lesions resulted in a significantly increased relative risk (RR = 1.6) in those exposed to estrogens alone for more than three years. When progestagens were added the relative risk was not elevated, indicating a possible protective effect. It was concluded that estrogen treatment in this cohort was associated with an increased risk of premalignant endometrial disease.

Other publications (153[C], 154[C], 155[r]) also seem to show that if progestagen is added to estrogen as a sequential therapy the risk of endometrial cancer can be decreased to less than that observed in untreated postmenopausal women. The explanation seems to be that estrogen and progestagen cause the atrophic endometrium to develop normal proliferative and secretory phases and nucleolar channel systems. The combination therapy is associated with increased glucoprotein production in the gland and stroma cells, while unopposed estrogen alone causes an irregular and unpredictable breakdown. Whitehead et al (156[C]) points out that, in the estrogen primed endometrium, progestagen opposes the mitotic stimulus, as can be shown by measuring the suppression of DNA synthesis and the antiproliferative effect. Progestagens are also responsible for changes in the pattern of intercellular protein production, which is mediated at least in part by the induction of various enzymes such as isocitric and estradiol-dehydrogenase. These enzymes predominantly convert the more potent intracellular estradiol into the less active estrone. The progestagen effect is not only dependent upon dose, but also upon time and it is now accepted that maximum protective effects are obtained if progestagen therapy is extended to 10 to 12 days each month.

With so much human data to hand, the debate on relevance of animal studies to this topic has somewhat receded into the background, but they continue to play a role, particularly as regards the dispute around medroxyprogesterone acetate (Depo-Provera). In 1983, an independent panel of pathology experts appointed by the US Food and Drug Administration's current board of enquiry into Depo-Provera reported that two controversial cancers found in a 10-year toxicity study in monkeys using 50 times the human dose were of endometrial, not endocervical, origin. This point has always been considered critical by the manufacturer since in monkeys the endometrium reacts to progestagens in a manner different to that of women, with the formation of plaques from which cancers can develop. In women, plaque formation does not occur. The same conclusion was voiced by a penal of pathologists convened by the World Health Organization (157[r]). In the light of these same findings the West German regulatory agency has similarly concluded that medroxyprogesterone acetate is not under suspicion as a cause of cancer in humans (158[r]).

REFERENCES

1. Edgren RA (1980) Progestagens, In: Givens I (Ed), *Clinical Uses of Sex Steroids.* Yearbook Publishers, Chicago.
2. *Drugs of Today* (1982) Desogestrel, *17,* 361.
3. Ruokonen A, Lund L, Nummi S et al (1982) Effects of two oral contraceptive combinations, 0.125 mg Desogestrel + 0.050 mg Ethinylestradiol and 0.125 mg Levonorgestrel + 0.05 mg Ethinylestradiol on the adrenal function of healthy female volunteers. *Eur. J. Obstet. Gynecol. Reprod. Biol., 13,* 259.
4. Weijers MJ (Ed) (1982) Development of an oral contraceptive containing a new pregestagen, desogestrel, and 30 pg ethinylestradiol. Report on clinical studies from Scandinavia. *Acta Obstet. Gynecol. Scand., Suppl. 1,* 11.
5. Graham S, Fraser IS (1982) The progestagen-only mini-pill. *Contraception, 26,* 4.
6. Detæuf M, Kuttenn F (1982) Hyperestrogénie sous contraception par micropilule progestative. *Contraception-fertilité-sexualité, 10,* 377.
7. Diaz S, Pavez M, Miranda P et al (1982) A five-year clinical trial of Levonorgestrel silastic implants (Norplant™). *Contraception, 25,* 5.
8. Swedish Health Authorities (1983) Depo-provera: Information from the Swedish Health Authorities. *Br. J. Fam. Plann., 8,* 129.
9. McGoldrick IA (1981) Depo-provera in perspective. *Papua New Guinea Med. J., 24,* 274.
10. Mateo JMR, Navarro AM, Calatoyud JMG (1982) Clinical experience with hormone contraceptives used by injectable route. *Toko-Gin. Pract., 41,* 63.
11. Dahlberg K (1982) Some effects of depo-medroxyprogesterone acetate: Observations in the nursing infant and in the long-term user. *Int. J. Gynaecol. Obstet., 20,* 43.
12. Coutinho EH, Souza JC, Barbusa IC, Silva VD (1982) Long-lasting ovulation inhibition with a new injectable progestagen. ORG-2154. *Contraception, 25,* 551.
13. Dukes MNG (1982) Parliaments, Prejudices and Pressure Groups. Paper presented to the W.H.O. Symposium on Clinical Pharmacological Evaluation in Drug Control, Schlangenbad. In press.
14. Søndergaard F, Ottesen B, Detlefsen GU et al (1983) Treatment with progesterone in threatened abortion, and low level of serum progesterone. A double blind randomized trial. *Steril. Fertil.,* in press.
15. Guilleminault C, Tilkian A, Dement W (1976) The sleep apnea syndrome. *Ann. Rev. Med., 27,* 465.
16. Sandblom RE, Matsumoto AM, Schoene RB et al (1983) Obstructive sleep apnea syndrome induced by testosterone administration. *N. Engl. J. Med., 9,* 508.
17. Skatrud J, Dempsey P, Kaiser D (1978) Ventilatory response to medroxyprogesterone in normal subjects. *J. Appl. Physiol., 44,* 939.
18. Reyniak JV, Lauersen NH (1982) Danazol – a versatile pharmacologic agent. *Fertil. Steril., 37,* 475.
19. Wentz AC (1982) Adverse effects of Danazol in pregnancy. *Ann. Intern. Med., 96,* 672.
20. Peress MR, Kreutner AK, Mathur RS, Williamson HO (1982) Female pseudohermaphroditism with somatic chromosomal anomaly in association with in utero exposure to Danazol. *Am. J. Obstet. Gynecol., 142,* 708.
21. Schwartz RP (1982) Ambiquores genitalia in a term female infant due to exposure to Danazol in utero. *Am. J. Dis. Child., 136,* 474.
22. Wardle PG, Whitehead MI, Mills RP (1983) Non-reversible and wide ranging voice changes after treatment with danazol. *Br. Med. J., 287,* 946.
23. Anon (1983) Danazol, a postcoital contraceptive? (News item from *J. Obstet. Gynaec., 3, S64*), *Scrip, 832,* 15.
24. Shio Zawa Z, Yamada H, Mabuchi C et al (1982) Superior sagittal sinus thrombosis associated with androgen therapy for hypoplastic anemia. *Ann. Neurol., 12,* 578.
25. Robboy SJ, Niller KL, Kaufman RH et al (1983) Prenatal diethylstilbestrol (DES) exposure. *Clin. Pediatr., 22,* 139.
26. Stillman RJ (1982) In utero exposure to diethylstilbestrol: Adverse effects on the reproductive tract and reproductive performance in male and female offspring. *Am. J. Obstet. Gynecol., 142,* 905.
27. Stolk JG, Vooijs GP, Aartsen EJ, Heintz AP (1983) Het teratogene effect van diethylstilbestrol in de zwangerschap in de omvang van het DES-probleem in Nederland. *Ned. Tijdschr. Geneeskd., 126,* 1350.
28. Holt LH, Herbst AL (1982) DES-related female genital changes. *Semin. Oncol., 9,* 341.
29. Schmidt G, Fowler WC (1982) Ovarian cystadenofibromas in three women with antinatal exposure to diethylstilbestrol. *Gynecol. Oncol., 14,* 175.
30. Cunningham JR, Gidwani GP, Gupta MS et al (1982) Prolactin-secreting pituitary adenoma: occurrence following prenatal exposure to diethylstilbestrol. *Cleveland Clin. Q., 49,* 249.
31. Vandrie DM, Puri S, Upton RT, Demeester LJ (1983) Adenosquamous carcinoma of the cervix in a woman exposed to diethylstilbestrol in utero. *Obstet. Gynecol., 61,* 845.
32. Herbst AL, Ulfelder H, Poskanzer DC (1971) Adenocarcinoma of the vagina: association of maternal stilbestrol therapy with tumor appearance in young women. *N. Engl. J. Med., 284,* 878.
33. Herbst AL, Cole P, Colton T et al (1977) Age-incidence and risk of diethylstilbestrol-related clear cell adenocarcinoma of the vagina and cervix. *Am. J. Obstet. Gynecol., 128,* 43.
34. O'Brian PC, Noller KL, Robboy SJ et al

(1979) Vaginal epithelial changes in young women enrolled in the national cooperative diethylstilbestrol-adenosis. (DESAD) project. *Obstet. Gynecol., 53,* 300.

35. Cabau A (1982) Malformations uterine chez les filler exposées en distilbene pendant leur vie embryonnaire. Consequence sur leur fécondité. *Contraception-fertilité-sexualité, 10,* 477.

36. Vericliano NP, Delke I, Rogers J, Tanger MI (1982) Reproductive performance of DES-exposed – female progeny. *Contraception-fertilité-sexualité, 10,* 315.

37. Buckley CH, Butler EB, Donnai P et al (1982) A fatal case of stilbestrol associated clear cell adenocarcinoma of the vagina. *J. Obstet. Gynaecol., 3,* 126.

38. Hudson CN, Crandon AJ, Baird PJ, Willcocks D (1983) Preservation of reproductive potential in diethylstilbestrol-related vaginal adenocarcinoma. *Am. J. Obstet. Gynecol., 145,* 375.

39. Caby J (1982) Anomalies hystérographiques chez de jeunes femmes exposées in utero au diéthylstilbestrol. *Gynecologie, 33,* 515.

40. Blythe JG, Michael H, Hodel KA (1983) Colposcopic and pathologic features in two cases of DES-related vaginal clear-cell adenocarcinoma. *J. Reprod. Med., 28,* 137.

41. Robboy SJ, Taguchi O, Cunka GR (1982) Normal development of the human female preproductive tract and alterations resulting from experimental exposure to diethylstilbestrol. *Pathol., 13,* 190.

42. Ory HW (1983) Mortality associated with fertility and fertility control: 1983. *Family Planning Perspective, 15,* 57.

43. McCredie J, Kricker A, Elliott J et al (1983) Congenital limb defects and the pill. *Lancet, 2,* 623.

44. Burns MP, Schoch DR, Grayzel AI (1983) Gold urticaria and an oral contraceptive. *Ann. Intern. Med., 98,* 1025.

45. Royal College of General Practitioners' Oral Contraception Study (1983) Incidence of arterial disease among oral contraceptive users. *J. R. Coll. Gen. Pract., 33,* 75.

46. Engel H-J, Engel E, Lichtlen PR (1983) Coronary atherosclerosis and myocardial infarction in young women – role of oral contraceptives. *Eur. Heart J., 4,* 1.

47. Salonen JT (1982) Oral contraceptives, smoking and risk of myocardial infarction in young women. *Acta Med. Scand., 212,* 141.

48. Meade T (1982) Effects of progestogens on the cardiovascular system. *Am. J. Obstet. Gynecol., 142,* 776.

49. Meade TW (1982) Recent developments on the association between oral contraceptives and cardiovascular disease. *Adv. Drug React. Ac. Pois. Rev., 1,* 243.

50. Kay CR (1982) Progestogens and arterial disease – evidence from the Royal College of General Practitioners' Study. *Am. J. Obstet. Gynecol., 142,* 762.

51. Mann JI (1982) Progestogens in cardiovascular disease: An introduction to the epidemiologic data. *Am. J. Obstet. Gynecol., 142,* 752.

52. Lidegaard Ø (1982) Tromboemboliske attakker i centralnervesystemet og p-piller. *Ugeskr. Laeg., 144,* 2769.

53. Mousa GY (1982) Migraine and oral contraceptives. *Am. J. Optom. Physiol. Optics., 59,* 821.

54. Blaul G (1983) Homonyme Hemianopsie als seltene Komplikation unter Antikonzeptivaeinnahme. *Fortschr. Ophthalmol., 79,* 453.

55. Lalonde G, Thécret G, Doloze P et al (1982) Inferior vena cava stenosis and Budal-Chian syndrome in a woman taking oral contraceptives. *Gastroenterology, 82,* 1452.

56. Cavin R, Boumghar M, Loosli H et al (1982) Les accidents digestifs aigues des contraceptifs oraux. *Chirurgie, 108,* 64.

57. Weinstein E, Silverman L (1982) Splenic artery thrombosis secondary to oral contraceptive medication: case report. *Mil. Med., 147,* 589.

58. Melodia G, Barbieri AG (1979) Infarto Intestinale De Trombosi venosa Mesenterica in corso di trattamento contraccettivo. *Chir. Ital., 31,* 1132.

59. Bouché RT, Medawar SJ, Dockery GL (1982) Oral contraceptives and deep venous thrombosis with pulmonary embolism. *J. Foot Surg., 21,* 297.

60. Goldman RS, Kettwich DL, Werdside JR et al (1983) Mild unilateral proteinuria and renal vein thrombosis associated with oral contraceptive usage. *Am. J. Kidney Dis., 2,* 471.

61. Barter JF, Addison A, Hidalgo H et al (1983) Inferior vena cava thrombosis with oral contraceptives documented by computer tomography. *Obstet. Gynecol., 61,* 595.

62. Givardin MS, Zarfani ES, Prigent A et al (1983) Unilobar small hepatic vein obstruction: possible role of progestogen given as oral contraceptive. *Gastroenterology, 84,* 630.

63. Strincker SJ, Sowers DK, Sowers JR et al (1981) "Effort thrombosis" of the subclavian vein associated with oral contraception. *Ann. Emerg. Med., 10,* 596.

64. Abet D, Pietri J (1982) Thrombosis veineuses patale et mésentérique supérieure, secondaires a un traitement contraceptif oral. *J. Mal. Vas., 7,* 59.

65. Berqvist A, Berqvist D, Hedner U (1982) Oral contraceptives and venous thromboembolism. *Br. J. Obstet. Gynecol., 89,* 381.

66. Lahtonen A, Perasalo J (1982) Relative Weight, Smoking and contraceptive pills: Interrelations to blood pressure in students. *Blood Pressure, 31,* 105.

67. Hodsman GP, Robertson JIS, Semple PF et al (1982) Malignant hypertension and oral contraceptives: four cases with two due to the 30 μg oestrogen pill. *Eur. Heart J., 3,* 255.

68. Wallace RB, Barrett-Connar E, Criqui M et al

(1982) Alteration in blood pressures associated with combined alcohol and oral contraceptive use – the lipid research clinics prevalence study. *J. Chron. Dis., 35,* 251.

69. Collaborative Group for the Study of Stroke in Young Women (1973) Oral contraception and increased risk of cerebral ischemia or thrombosis. *N. Engl. J. Med., 288,* 871.
70. Inman WHW (1979) Oral contraceptives and fatal subarachnoid haemorrhage. *Br. Med. J., 2,* 1468.
71. Petitti DB, Wingerd J, Pellegrin F et al (1979) Risk of vascular disease in women. *J. Am. Med. Assoc., 242,* 1150.
72. Thorogood M, Adam SA, Mann JI (1981) Fatal subarachnoid haemorrhage in young women: role of oral contraceptives. *Br. Med. J., 283,* 762.
73. Mammen EF (1982) Oral contraceptives and blood coagulation: A critical review. *Am. J. Obstet. Gynecol., 142,* 781.
74. Irey NS, Manion WC, Taylor HB (1970) Vascular lesions in women taking oral contraceptives. *Arch. Pathol., 89,* 1.
75. Irey NS, Norris HJ (1973) Intimal vascular lesions associated with female reproductive steroids. *Arch. Pathol., 96,* 227.
76. Irey NS, McAllister HA, Henry JM (1978) Oral contraceptives and stroke in young women: A clinicopathologic correlation. *Neurology, 28,* 1216.
77. Osterholzer HO, Grillo D, Kruger PS et al (1977) The effect of oral contraceptive steroids on branches of the uterine artery. *Obstet. Gynecol., 49,* 227.
78. Basdevant A, de Lignieres B, Mauvais-Jarvis P (1980) Effets des contraceptifs oraux sur le paroi des vaisseaux. *Nouv. Presse Méd., 16,* 519.
79. Hirsh J (1977) Hypercoagulability. *Semin. Hematol., 14,* 409.
80. Poller L (1978) Oral contraceptives, blood clotting and thrombosis. *Br. Med. Bull., 34,* 151.
81. Meade TW, Brozovic R, Horwarth COJ et al (1976) An epidemiological study of the haemostatic and other effects of oral contraceptives. *Br. J. Haematol., 34,* 353.
82. Ball AP, McKee PA (1977) Fibrin formation and dissolution in women receiving oral contraceptive drugs. *J. Lab. Clin. Med., 89,* 751.
83. Korsan-Bengtsen K, Larsson B (1978) Effect on blood coagulation and fibrinolysis in women using norethisterone or a combination of ethinylestradiol and quingestianol. *Gynecol. Obstet. Invest., 9,* 312.
84. Ghezzo F, Mele A, Pagoraro L (1980) Effects of oestroprogestogenic oral contraceptives on blood coagulation, fibrinolysis and platelet aggregation. *Haematologica, 65,* 737.
85. Alkjaersig N, Fletcher A, Burstein R (1975) Association between oral contraceptive use and thromboembolism: A new approach to its investigation based on plasma fibrinogen chromatography. *Am. J. Obstet. Gynecol., 122,* 199.
86. Ambrus JL, Mink IB, Courey NG et al (1976) Progestational agents and blood coagulation. VII. Thromboembolic and other complications of oral contraceptive therapy in relationship to pretreatment levels of blood coagulation factors: summary report of a ten-year study. *Am. J. Obstet. Gynecol., 125,* 1057.
87. Al-Khader AA, Aber GM (1980) Persistent abnormalities of fibrinolytic activity and platelet function in patients with reversible oestrogen-associated hypertension. *Br. J. Obstet. Gynecol., 87,* 672.
88. Astedt B (1971) Low fibrinolytic activity of veins during treatment with ethinyl estradiol. *Acta Obstet. Gynecol. Scand., 50,* 279.
89. Astedt B, Isacson S, Nilsson IM et al (1973) Thrombosis and oral contraceptives: Possible predisposition. *Br. Med. J., 4,* 631.
90. Drayer NA, Pizzo SV (1980) Blood coagulation and idiopathic thromboembolism among fertile women. *Contraception, 22,* 123.
91. Kjaeldgaard A, Larsson B (1983) Fibrinolytic activity in the walls of foot veins in women using combined contraceptive pills. *Gynecol. Obstet. Invest., 15,* 223.
92. Pilgeram LO, Ellison J, von dem Bussche G (1974) Oral contraceptives and increased formation of soluble fibrin. *Br. Med. J., 3,* 556.
93. Carvalho ACA, Vaillancourt RA, Cabral RB et al (1977) Coagulation abnormalities in women taking oral contraceptives. *J. Am. Med. Assoc., 237,* 875.
94. Wong V, Chan TK, Chan V et al (1982) The effects of oral contraceptives on coagulation and fibrinolytic parameters in the Chinese – A prospective study. *Thromb. Haemostasis, 48,* 263.
95. Jespersen J, Kluft C (1982) Decreased levels of histidine – rich glycoprotein (HRG) and increased levels of free plasminogen in women on oral contraceptive low in estrogen. *Thromb. Haemastasis, 48,* 283.
96. Meade TW (1982) Oral contraceptives, clotting factors, and thrombosis. *Am. J. Obstet. Gynecol., 142,* 758.
97. Hellstein P, Miyashita C, Köhler M et al (1982) Thrombin-induced platelet malon-dialdehyde (MDA) formation in normal suspects and in women taking oral contraceptives. *Thromb. Haemostasis, 48,* 325.
98. Jespersen J, Ingeberg S, Bach E (1983) Antithrombin III and platelets during the normal menstrual cycle and in women receiving oral contraceptives low in oestrogen. *Gynecol. Obstet. Invest., 15,* 153.
99. Hanington C, Jones RJ, Amess JAL (1982) Platelet aggregation in response to 5-HT in migraine patients taking oral contraceptives. *Lancet, 1,* 967.
100. Sabra A, Bonnar J (1983) Hemostatic system changes induced by 50 μg and 30 μg estrogen/progestogen oral contraceptives. *J. Reprod. Med., 28,* 85.

101. Wynn V, Niththyananthan R (1982) The effect of progestins in combined oral contraceptives on serum lipids with special reference to high-density lipoproteins. *Am. J. Obstet. Gynecol., 142,* 766.
102. Oster P, Arab C, Kohlmeier M et al (1982) Effects of estrogens and progestogens on lipid metabolism. *Am. J. Obstet. Gynecol., 142,* 773.
103. Basdevant A, Conard J, Guy-Grand B (1982) Influence de la dose d'Ethinyl-estradiol et de la nature du progestatif sur l'hyper triglyceridémie induite par les contraceptifs oraux. *J. Gynecol. Obstet. Biol. Reprod., 11,* 751.
104. Voors W, Srinivasan S, Hunter Mac D et al (1982) Smoking, oral contraceptives, and serum lipid and lipoprotein levels in youth. *Prev. Med., 11,* 1.
105. Knopp HR, Walden EC, Wahl PW, Hoover J (1982) Effects of oral contraceptives on lipoprotein triglyceride and cholesterol: Relationship to estrogen and progestin potency. *Am. J. Obstet. Gynecol., 142,* 725.
106. Rådberg T, Gustafson A, Skryten A, Karlsson K (1982) Metabolic studies in women with previrus gestational diabetes during contraceptive treatment: effects on serum lipids and high density lipoproteins. *Acta Endocrinol., 101,* 134.
107. Spellacy WN (1982) Carbohydrate metabolism during treatment with estrogen, progestogen and low-dose oral contraceptives. *Am. J. Obstet. Gynecol., 142,* 732.
108. Destefano F, Petersen HB, Ory HW, Layde PM (1982) Oral contraceptives and postoperative venous thrombosis. *Am. J. Obstet. Gynecol., 143,* 227.
109. Ratnoff OD, Kaufman R (1982) Arterial thrombosis in oral contraceptives users. *Intern. Med., 142,* 447.
110. Brooks JJ (1982) Hepatoma associated with diethylstilbestrol therapy for prostatic carcinoma. *J. Urology, 128,* 1044.
111. Gala KV, Griffiri TW (1983) Hepatomas in young women on oral contraceptives: report of two cases and review of the literature. *J. Surg. Oncol., 22,* 11.
112. Corboz A (1983) Hyperplasie focale nodulaire, adénome hépatocellulaire et contraceptifs hormonaux. *Schweiz. Rundschau Med., 72,* 177.
113. Vanderpool D, Lane RW, Winther JW (1982) Liver tumors and oral contraceptives. *South Med. J., 75,* 1118.
114. Malatjalian DA, Graham CH (1982) Liver adenoma with granulomas. *Arch. Pathol. Lab. Med., 106,* 244.
115. Hecht Y (1983) Stéroides sexuels et foie. *Contraception-fertilité-sexualité, 11,* 263.
116. Schonberg LA (1982) Peliosis hepatitis and oral contraceptives. *J. Reprod. Med., 27,* 753.
117. Verhamme M, Paulussen J, Fevery J (1983) Adenomen en focale nodulaire hyperplasie van de lever. Relatie met orale contraceptiva. *Tijdschr. Geneesk., 39,* 51.
118. Freund VE, Schröder H, Machnik G (1982) Ovulationshemmer und intraperitoneale Blutung durch Leberzelladenom. *Abl. Chirurgie, 107,* 1245.
119. Scully RE, Mark EJ, McNealy BU (1982) Weekly clinico pathological exercises. Case 40-1982. *N. Engl. J. Med., 307,* 934.
120. Voigt JJ, Pradére M, Cassigneul J et al (1982) Proliférations hépatiques et contraception orale. *Rev. Méd. Toulouse, 18,* 351.
121. Lie TS (1982) Lebererkrankungen durch hormonelle Kontrazeptiva. *Münch. Med. Wochenschr., 124,* 489.
122. Agha FP (1982) Clinical and roentgen features of hepatic cell adenomas associated with oral contraceptive use. *Clin. Roentgen., 7,* 63.
123. Christopherson WM (1982) Contraceptifs oraux et tumeurs hépatiques. Une mise au point. *Méd. Hyg., 40,* 2037.
124. Naud S, Gordon LI, Brestan E et al (1982) Benign hepatic cyst in a patient on antiestrogen therapy for metastatic breast cancer. *Cancer, 9,* 1882.
125. Helling TS, Wood WG (1982) Oral contraceptives and cancer of the liver. A review with two additional cases. *Am. J. Gastroenterol., 77,* 504.
126. Dudley AG, Sole P (1982) Hepatocellular carcinoma associated with oral contraceptive use and pregnancy. *Diagn. Gynecol. Obstet., 4,* 301.
127. Porter JB, Jick H, Ylvisaker JT (1981) Malignant liver tumor associated with oral contraceptive use. *Pharmacotherapy, 1,* 160.
128. Goodman ZD, Ishak KG (1982) Hepatocellular carcinoma in women: Probable lack of etiologic association with oral contraceptive steroids. *Hepatology, 2,* 440.
129. Evron S, Frankel M, Diamont Y (1982) Biliary disease in young women and its association with pregnancy on oral contraceptives. *Int. Surg., 67,* 448.
130. Royal College of General Practitioners' Oral Contraception Study (1982) Oral contraceptives and gallbladder disease. *Lancet, 2,* 957.
131. Kern F, Everson GT, DeMark B et al (1982) Biliary lipids, bile acids, and gallbladder function in the human female: Effects of contraceptive steroids. *J. Lab. Clin. Med., 99,* 798.
132. Synder K (1982) Psychische Nebenwirkungen oraler Kontrazeptiva (Vorläufige Ergebnisse). *Psychiatr. Neurol. Med. Psychol., 12,* 727.
133. Chang AMZ, Chick P, Milburn S (1982) Mood changes as reported by women taking the oral contraceptive pill. *Aust. NZ J. Obstet. Gynecol., 22,* 78.
134. Lobo RA, Gibbons WE (1982) The role of progestin therapy in breast disease and central nervous system function. *J. Reprod. Med., Suppl. 8,* 515.
135. Rosenburg BW, Armstrong B, Phil D (1976) Myocardial infarction and estrogen therapy. *N. Engl. J. Med., 294,* 1256.
136. Burch JC, Byrd Jr EF, Vaughn WK (1974)

The effects of long-term estrogen on hysterectomized women. *Am. J. Obstet. Gynecol., 118,* 778.

137. Gordon T, Kannel WB, Hjortland MC et al (1978) Menopause and coronary heart disease. *Ann. Intern. Med., 89,* 157.

138. Ross, RK, Paganini-Hill A, Mack TM et al (1981) Menopausal oestrogen therapy and protection from death from ischaemic heart disease. *Lancet, 1,* 858.

139. Hammond CB, Jelovsek RR, Lee K et al (1979) Effect of long-term estrogen replacement therapy. *Metabolic. Am. J. Obstet. Gynecol., 133,* 525.

140. Larsson-Cohn U, Wallentin L, Zador G (1979) Plasma lipids and high density lipoproteins during oral contraception with different combinations of ethinylestradiol and norgestreol. *Horm. Res., 11,* 437.

141. Samsio G (1982) Study on effect of 30 pg ethinylestradiol + 150 pg desogestrel on lipid and lipo-protein metabolism. *Acta Obstet. Gynecol. Scand. Suppl., 11,* 55.

142. Bush TL, Wowan L, Barret-Connor E et al (1983) Estrogen and all-cause mortality. *J. Am. Med. Assoc., 249,* 903.

143. Pikes MC, Henderson BE, Casagrande IT et al (1981) Oral contraceptive use and early abortion as a risk factor for breast cancer in young women. *Br. J. Cancer, 43,* 72.

144. Pikes MC, Henderson BE, Krailo MD et al (1983) Breast cancer in young women and use of oral contraceptives: possible modifying effects of formulation and age at use. *Lancet, 2,* 926.

145. Drife J (1983) Which Pill? *(Editorial). Brit. Med. J., 287,* 1397.

146. Vessey MP, McPherson K, Yeates D et al (1983) Oral contraceptive use and abortion before first term pregnancy in relation to breast cancer risk. *Br. J. Cancer, 45,* 327.

147. The Centers for Disease Control Cancer and Steroid Hormone Study (1983) Long-term oral contraceptive use and the risk of breast cancer. *J. Am. Med. Assoc., 249,* 1591.

148. Brinton LA, Hoover R, Szklo M et al (1982) Oral contraceptives and breast cancer. *Int. J. Epidemiol., 11,* 4.

149. Vessey MP, Lawless M, McPherson K et al (1983) Neoplasia of the cervix uteri and contraception: a possible adverse effect of the pill. *Lancet, 2,* 930.

150. Kay CR (1983) Oral contraceptives and cancer. *Lancet, 2,* 1018.

151. The Centers for Disease Control Cancer and Steroid Hormone Study (1983) Oral contraceptive use and the risk of endometrial cancer. *J. Am. Med. Assoc., 249,* 1600.

152. Persson I (1983) Climacteric treatment with estrogens and estrogen-progestogen combinations: The risk of endometrial neoplasia. *Acta Univ. Upsal., 471.*

153. Gambrelli RD (1982) Clinical use of progestins in the menopausal patients. Dosage and duration. *J. Reprod. Med., Suppl. 8,* 531.

154. Flowers Jr ChE, Wilborn H, Hyde M (1983) Mechanisms of uterine bleeding in postmenopausal patients receiving estrogen alone or with a progestin. *Obstet. Gynecol., 61,* 135.

155. Korenman SG (1982) Menopausal endocrinology and management. *Arch. Intern. Med., 142,* 1131.

156. Whitehead I, Townsend T, Pryse Davies J (1982) Effects of various types and dosages of progestagens on the postmenopausal endometrium. *J. Reprod. Med., Suppl. 8,* 539.

157. Anon (1983) Positive Depo-Provera Report. *Outlook,* September, 8.

158. Anon (1983) Regulation – Germany Restricts Injectable. *Outlook,* September, 7.

R. Bouillon

43 Thyroid and antithyroid drugs

THYROID HORMONES

The diagnosis of hypothyroidism and therefore the determination of indication for starting thyroid replacement therapy may be much more difficult than previously recognized. Indeed, many intercurrent illnesses, nutritional deficiencies or simply old age may profoundly alter thyroid function tests and falsely mimic hypothyroidism. A low free T4 concentration alone is, therefore, no longer a definite proof of hypothyroidism in such patients and requires further confirmation with TSH and/or rT3 measurements before replacement therapy is instituted (1[R], 2[R]). Obviously, if this precaution is not observed, a hyperthyroid state may be inadvertently induced by superfluous treatment.

Intoxication with thyroid hormones

Although some cases of fatal outcome after intoxication with oral thyroid hormones have been reported previously, most accidental or suicidal intoxications were only followed by minimal symptoms and favourable outcome (SEDA-5, 381). In some more severely affected patients plasmapheresis was found to be beneficial (SEDA-6, 363). It was therefore a surprise to encounter within 6 months in a single hospital 3 patients who died due to deliberate intake of excessive amounts of l-thyroxine (3[C]). The diagnosis is not always immediately recognized because the patients fail to admit to this drug abuse. An autopsy performed in 2 of these patients revealed focal myocarditis. The authors therefore raise the possibility that many cases of sudden cardiac death following unrecognized thyroxine intoxication may remain undiagnosed because of unfamiliarity with the disorder and an atypical presentation (3[C]).

Initiation of l-thyroxine therapy for juvenile hypothyroidism was associated with a syndrome of benign intracranial hypertension (pseudotumor cerebri) in two children. Two similar reports have appeared earlier. All symptoms started between 2 and 4½ months after the beginning of l-thyroxine therapy, and the initial complaints were usually increasing headaches. Bilateral papilledema was present without focal neurologic defects or other known reasons for intracranial hypertension. The neurologic symptoms disappeared after 1 to 10 months with or without supportive therapy (diuretics or corticosteroids) but with continued thyroid replacement therapy (38[CR]).

Triiodothyroacetic acid (Triac) is used in France to treat obesity (4[C]). An obese patient with a diffuse goiter, secondary hyperthyroidism (with low TSH levels) and signs of iodine saturation was found to have taken Triac for about 6 months (1 mg/day). After an interruption of 20 days all thyroid function tests became normal. Triac, therefore, seems to be able to induce a suppression of the hypothalamo-hypophysial TRF-TSH system, just as can prolonged thyroid replacement therapy (SEDA-4, 294; SEDA-6, 363).

ANTITHYROID DRUGS

An extensive review of the clinical pharmacology of antithyroid drugs has been published (5[R]). Both propylthiouracil (PTU) and the thioimidazoles (carbimazole and methimazole) have a high bio-availability (80–95%) and a relatively short half-life (1–2 h for PTU and 3–5 h for methimazole). Their effect is, however, more prolonged due to the active retention of these drugs in the thyroid gland for at least 24 h (6[C]). This might explain why once-a-day therapy is probably as effective as multiple daily doses; it is also likely to im-

Side Effects of Drugs Annual 8
M.N.G. Dukes, editor

ISBN 0 444 90339 9
$0.80 per article per page (transactional system)
$0.20 per article per page (licensing system)

prove patient compliance. No informative data on the metabolism of these drugs in children or in case of renal or hepatic insufficiency are available. The choice between the thiouracils and thioimidazoles cannot be based on strict pharmacological considerations, on the frequency of side effects or on differences in long-term effectiveness (5[R]).

Humoral and immune mechanisms

Several side-effects reported already in previous SEDA's continue to be described in case reports or short summaries. The more recent reports, however, provide better evidence for a humoral or immune mechanism of these side effects.

A transient methimazole-induced *bone marrow aplasia* (involving the erythroid and myeloid cells and shortly thereafter also the megakaryocytes) has been reported in a 31-year-old woman. In vitro lymphocyte studies with autologous sera obtained before and after recovery suggested a humoral, probably autoimmune mechanism for the transient bone marrow aplasia (7[C]).

Another case of *granulocytopenia, eosinophilia, skin reaction* and *hepatitis* due to PTU was observed in a 47-year-old black female with total recovery after withdrawal of therapy. In vitro lymphocyte transformation studies also revealed sensitization due to PTU during the acute phase of the disease which disappeared 5 months after recovery (8[C]).

Isolated transient *hepatitis* and *jaundice* was also found in association with PTU administration, and an immunologic mechanism was again documented by in vitro lymphocyte techniques (9[CR]). This in vitro test was positive for PTU but not for methimazole, confirming the general rule of non-cross-reacting drug sensitivity, although thiouracils and thioimidazoles produce virtually the same type of drug reaction and have a similar thioureum bond in their structure.

In a review of 15 reported cases of PTU-induced hepatic injury (9[CR]), all types of liver diseases have been described with a preponderance for hepatocellular injury due to PTU in contrast to a cholestatic hepatitis in case of methimazole-induced disease. Subsidence of jaundice and resolution of the abnormal liver function tests may require several months. Several cases (3 of the 15 reported) ended fatally, but these patients also had other drug-related symptoms (agranulocytosis or periarteritis). More recently a new case of fatal PTU-induced hepatitis was reported (10[CR]).

Dinsmore et al (37[c]) have described a case of postanesthetic jaundice attributable to carbimazole, an event which only seems to have been described on two previous occasions, namely by Prost et al in 1973 and by Lunzer et al in 1975 (37).

A woman of 24 who had been receiving carbimazole 40 mg dd for 3 months underwent a tubal ligation; anesthesia was with nitrous oxide; halothane was not used. Pruritus developed on the second post-operative day, followed by development of severe jaundice. Liver biopsy showed severe cholestasis. Carbimazole was stopped 24 days after the operation and recovery ensued. Some weeks later, rechallenge with carbimazole resulted in recurrence of jaundice.

The authors postulate that in this instance the anesthetic agents may have produced an alteration of the liver cell membranes, making them susceptible to carbimazole injury, possibly through an immunologic step.

Other types of allergic reactions described include a case of *'serum sickness'* during methimazole treatment. The 38-year-old woman developed a sore throat, pruritus, arthralgia, facial edema and fever 3 weeks after starting methimazole for Graves' disease. Her IgM concentration was elevated, but the in vitro lymphocyte reactions to methimazole were negative (11[C]). Diffuse *vasculitis* was also observed in 2 girls, one after PTU and another during methimazole treatment. In both cases purpuric skin rash, anemia, nephritis and especially pulmonary cavitation with hemoptysis were found. These pulmonary manifestations are, indeed, a very usual presentation of such vasculitis (12[C]). Recovery was complete in both cases after withdrawal of the drugs involved. Antithyroid drugs very rarely induce *neuritis* (SED-9, 697). A new case of polyradiculoneuritis during carbimazole treatment was observed. About 1 year later, after withdrawal of carbimazole and disappearance of the neuritis, the same 69-year-old patient developed a Sjögren syndrome (rheumatoid arthritis and drye eye syndrome). The causal relationship or more likely a genetic predisposition for an immune dysfunction is proposed (13[C]).

Antithyroid drugs during pregnancy

Antithyroid drugs for hyperthyroidism during pregnancy are usually preferred to surgery, and the discussion mainly concerns the dosage and duration of antithyroid drug therapy and its association with thyroid hormones. The fetal outcome of such drug-treated pregnancies is therefore important, and two such studies are fairly reassuring: the T4 and T3 concentration during the early days of life were normal in all 21 live infants, and only transient TSH abnormalities were found. Growth and psychomotor development at 6 months was normal. One child developed congenital Graves' disease (14[C]). Very similar results were obtained in the United Kingdom (15[CR]): again T4 was normal in 20 newborns, but serum T3 was slightly depressed and TSH significantly increased. One baby had a transient goiter and 1 developed neonatal thyrotoxicosis (15[CR]). An extensive literature review (1951-today) compares the fetal outcome after combined antithyroid and thyroid therapy versus antithyroid drugs alone. The combined therapy resulted in a lower frequency of fetal loss (9% *vs* 14%) and goiter (0.6% *vs* 4%) but with a higher rate of congenital malformations (5% *vs* 1%) and neonatal hypothyroidism (3% *vs* 1%). All these differences should, however, be regarded with some reservations, as many studies were performed before proper serum measurements for optimal dose adjustments were available. A randomized trial between the 2 therapy regimens is suggested by the authors, but on theoretical grounds a carefully controlled mono-therapy with antithyroid drugs would seem more logical and safer (SEDA-4, 294; SEDA-5, 381; SEDA-6, 364).

Other side effects

In a retrospective study of 102 patients with Graves' disease treated with antithyroid drugs between 1969 and 1979, 1 case of prolonged *agranulocytosis* and 1 of transient *granulocytopenia* was observed. Other minor side effects occurred in 9% of the PTU-treated patients and in 29% of carbimazole-treated subjects. The recurrence rate after withdrawal of therapy was high and increased from 45% to 57% from the first half to the second half of the observation period (16[C]). The authors therefore suggest that one should reserve antithyroid drugs for patients with a small goiter who are below 30 years of age.

Antithyroid drugs in children

Miceli et al (36[c]) have studied the kinetics of propylthiouracil in children with Graves' disease. Although their work was not directed towards side effects, their finding that the half-life of the drug appeared to be longer than that reported for adults does indicate what caution is likely to be needed in dosing the drug in children. Since the children studied ranged in age from 9 to 16 years the finding is clearly not one applicable only to the very youngest age groups.

IODINE PREPARATIONS

Iodine and iodine-containing drugs

Diagnostic radiographic procedures frequently involve the administration of iodine or iodine-containing contrast media which may alter thyroid function (17[c], 18[c]). For this reason some people recommend the use of antithyroid drugs in all patients with previous hyperthyroidism if they need an oral cholecystography (18[c]).

Povidone-iodine, a combination of polyvinylpyrrolidone (PVP) and iodine, is used in a local germicide, and the effect of a 14-day-period of vaginal douching with this drug has been studied. The serum and urinary iodine concentration increased, and the thyroid uptake of ^{123}I decreased, demonstrating the effective absorption of the topically applied iodine. The changes in serum T4 and TSH were minimal, and no cases of manifest hypothyroidism were observed (19[C]). This demonstrates its short-term safety in normal, non-pregnant subjects, but does not guarantee its long-term safety nor the absence of occasional side effects since the fetus, the newborn and some patients with thyroid diseases are especially sensitive to iodine. Isolated cases of Iod-Basedow due to povidone-iodine have again been reported (20[C]).

Amiodarone is increasingly being recognized as a very effective drug for long-term therapy of recurrent venticular tachyarrhythmias. The side effects of this drug are frequent but do not necessarily limit this therapy (21[CR]). Its high iodine content (a 200 mg tablet contains 75 mg of iodine) can, however, affect the thyroid function. In a series of 45 patients treated for a mean period of 1 year, 1 case of hyperthyroidism was observed (21[CR]). In another series of 100 patients treated for 6 weeks to 8 years *hyperthyroidism* was observed in 1 case and latent or overt *hypothyroidism* in another 6 patients (22[CR]). The true incidence may be somewhat higher, as in another study of 24 patients on amiodarone who were referred for extensive thyroid investigation 9 cases of hyperthyroidism and 4 cases of hypothyroidism were found (23[C]). The true incidence of thyroid disturbance due to amiodarone is therefore unclear, but it seems that patients needing this drug for severe cardiac arrhythmias should have at least a 2-yearly thyroid function test: tests indicating hypothyroidism are likely to represent true hypothyroidism. Simple evaluation of total or free T4 concentration is probably not diagnostic for hyperthyroidism due to the effect of amiodarone on the metabolic clearance of T4. Absence of TRF-induced TSH secretion and especially elevation of total and free T3 should be present before the diagnosis of amiodarone-induced hyperthyroidism is accepted (22[CR], 24[R]).

The pathogenic mechanism of iodine-induced hyperthyroidism is still unknown and is rendered even more obscure by a case report of an effective response to iodine treatment for iodine-induced thyrotoxicosis.

A 62-year-old female with typical iodine-induced hyperthyroidism (e.g. previous treatment with iodine for asthma, increased T4 and T3 concentration, low ^{131}I uptake and increased thyroidal ^{127}I content on fluorescent scan) was given Lugol's iodine (15 drops daily) with an immediate decrease in serum T3 and T4 (25[C]).

This case demonstrates that inhibitors of thyroid release (I) remain effective even in cases of iodine-induced hyperthyroidism.

Radioactive iodine

The incidence of hypothyroidism was studied in 4,473 patients treated with ^{131}I between 1951 and 1975. The mean age at therapy was 56 years and the mean ^{131}I dose was about 9 mc for diffuse goiters and 19 mc for nodular goiters. 6% developed hypothyroidism within 1 year of therapy whereas after 26 years 72% of the patients were hypothyroid. Previous treatment with antithyroid drugs did not affect the incidence of hypothyroidism, but a higher total dose or repeated administration of ^{131}I was associated with a higher incidence of hypothyroidism (26[CR]).

The frequency of hypothyroidism as a complication seems to have increased in more recent years (27[C]) even with the same general approach to treatment with ^{131}I. Very similar frequencies of ^{131}I-induced hypothyroidism were found in Hong-Kong Chinese (29[C]), in the Netherlands (28[C]) and in France (30[C]). A much higher incidence of hypothyroidism has, however, been observed in some other centers with a similarly increased incidence in later years (31[C]). In 454 patients treated at the Mayo Clinic between 1951 and 1978 the 1-year incidence of hypothyroidism was 40% during the earlier years and as much as 91% during more recent years. The mean dose of ^{131}I, however, increased during this observation period from 8.1 mc to 13.8 mc, mainly because of a higher estimated thyroid volume used for the calculation of the ^{131}I dose (31[C]).

A retrospective cohort study conducted at the Mayo clinic to evaluate the late effects of exposure to therapeutic doses of ^{131}I is especially interesting (32[CR], 33[CR]). A total of 1005 patients treated with a mean dose of 10.6 mc of ^{131}I at a mean age of 57 years between 1946 and 1964 were compared with 2141 patients (who were on average slightly younger: mean age 46 years), treated surgically for hyperthyroidism. The mean observation period was 15 and 21 years respectively. The incidence of hypothyroidism was higher in the ^{131}I treated group (54% *vs* 37%). No difference was found between the two groups as regards total cancer incidence (RR = 1), breast cancer (RR = 0.8) or leukemia (RR = 0.6). A slightly increased cancer risk was observed for organs that accumulate ^{131}I (salivary glands, digestive tract, kidney and bladder: RR = 1.8). Due to the small number of actual cancer deaths such observations on site-specific cancer are only suggestive and indicate the need for more extensive and prolonged observation (33[CR]). Nor was the number of cardiovascular, renal or cerebrovascular deaths altered by the ^{131}I treatment (32[CR]).

Newly reported side effects of ^{131}I treatment include a case of *diabetic ketoacidosis* associated with thyroid storm following repeated administration of ^{131}I for hyperthyroidism (34[c]). A case of *azoospermia* was documented after administration of a cumulative dose of 350 mCi ^{131}I for thyroid carcinoma. The testicular volume and androgen secretion remained normal. The reversibility of this azoospermia was not documented but estimated possible (35[c]).

REFERENCES

1. Wartofsky L, Burman KD (1982) Alterations in thyroid function in patients with systemic illness: the 'Euthyroid Sick Syndrome'. *Endocr. Rev., 3*, 164.
2. Burroughs V, Shenkman L (1982) Thyroid function in the elderly. *Am. J. Med. Sci., 283*, 8.
3. Bhasin S, Wallace W, Lawrence JB, Lesch M (1981) Sudden death associated with thyroid hormone abuse. *Am. J. Med., 71*, 887.
4. Heim J (1982) Hypothyroidie d'origine centrale réversible à l'arrêt d'un traitement par Triac. *Ann. Méd. Interne, 133*, 588.
5. Kampmann JP, Hansen JM (1981) Clinical Pharmacokinetics of antithyroid drugs. *Clin. Pharmacokin. 6*, 401.
6. Jansson R, Dahlberg PA, Johansson H, Lindström B (1983) Intrathyroidal concentrations of methimazole in patients with Graves' disease. *J. Clin. Endocr. Metab., 57*, 129.
7. Moreb J, Shemesh O, Shilo S et al (1983): Transient methimazole-induced bone marrow aplasia: in vitro evidence for a humoral mechanism of bone marrow suppression. *Acta Haematol. 69*, 127.
8. Pacini F, Sridama V, Refetoff S (1982) Multiple complications of propylthiouracil treatment: granulocytopenia, eosinophilia, skin reaction and hepatitis with lymphocyte sensitization. *J. Endocrinol. Invest., 5*, 403.
9. Parker WA (1982) Propylthiouracil-induced hepatotoxicity. *Clin. Pharm. 1*, 471.
10. Safani MM, Tatro DS, Rudd P (1982) Fatal propylthiouracil-induced hepatitis. *Arch. Intern. Med., 142*, 838.
11. Van Kuyk M, Van Laethem Y, Duchateau J, Bonnyns M (1983) Methimazole-induced serum sickness. *Acta Clin. Belg., 38*, 68.
12. Cassoria FG, Finegold DN, Parks JS et al (1983): Vasculitis, pulmonary cavitation and anemia during antithyroid drug therapy. *Am. J. Dis. Child., 137*, 118.
13. Mikol F, Simon F, Falcy M (1982) Syndrome de Gougerot-Sjögren et polyradiculonévrite au carbimazole. *Rev. Neurol. (Paris), 138*, 259;
14. Bricaire H, Viron B, Czernichow P, Luton JP (1983) Traitements par antithyroïdiens de synthèse au cours de la grossesse. *Presse Méd., 12*, 1057.
15. Ramsay I, Kaur S, Krassas G (1983) Thyrotoxicosis in pregnancy: results of treatment by antithyroid drugs combined with T4. *Clin. Endocrinol., 18*, 73.
16. Holm LE, Alinder I (1982) Relapses after thionamide therapy for Graves' disease. *Acta Med. Scand., 211*, 489.
17. Cavalieri RR (1982) 'Cold' thyroid-nodules seen with nonradioactive iodine. *N. Engl. J. Med., 307*, 1346.
18. Kleinmann RE, Braverman LE (1982) Feedback regulation of thyrotropin secretion by thyroid hormones. *N. Engl. J. Med., 306*, 1236.
19. Safrans M, Braverman LE (1982) Effect of chronic douching with polyvinylpyrrolidone-iodine on iodine absorption and thyroid function. *Obstet. Gynecol., 60*, 35.
20. Jacobson JM, Hankins GV, Murray JM et al (1981) Self-limited hyperthyroidism following intravaginal iodine administration. *Am. J. Obstet. Gynecol., 140*, 472.
21. Heger JJ, Prystowsky EN, Jackman WM et al (1981) Amiodarone. *N. Engl. J. Med., 305*, 539.
22. Jaggarao NSV, Sheldon J, Grundy EN, Vincent R (1982) The effects of amiodarone on thyroid function. *Postgrad. Med. J., 58*, 693.
23. Trip MC, Wiersinga WM, Düren DR et al (1983) Diagnostiek van hyper- en hypothyreoïdie bij patienten die amiodaron gebruiken. *Ned. Tijdschr. Geneeskd., 127*, 456.
24. Friocourt P, Coumel Ph (1983) Les effets indésirables de l'Amiodarone. *Ann. Méd. Interne, 134*, 55.
25. Boehm TM, McLain J, Burman KD et al (1980) Iodine treatment of iodine-induced thyrotoxicosis. *J. Endocrinol. Invest., 4*, 419.
26. Holm LE, Lundell G, Israelsson A, Dahlqvist I (1982) Incidence of hypothyroidism occurring long after Iodine-131 therapy for hyperthyroidism. *J. Nucl. Med., 23*, 103.
27. Holm LE (1982) Changing annual incidence of hypothyroidism after Iodine-131 therapy for hyperthyroidism, 1951–1975. *J. Nucl. Med., 23*, 108.
28. Kamphuis JJ (1980) Behandeling van hyperthyreoidie met ^{131}I: een retrospectief onderzoek. *Ned. Tijdschr. Geneeskd., 124*, 1045.
29. Best JD, Chan V, Khoo R et al (1981) Incidence of hypothyroidism after radioactive iodine therapy for thyrotoxicosis in Hong Kong Chinese. *Clin. Radiol., 32*, 57.
30. Rivière L, Muffragi J-M, Dartigue M et al (1982) Les différents types d'hypothyroidie après traitement par iode radioactif pour maladie de Basedow. *Rev. Fr. Endocrinol. Clin., 23*,

151.
31. Cunnien AJ, Hay ID, Gorman CA et al (1982) Radioiodine-induced hypothyroidism in Graves' disease: factors associated with the increasing incidence. *J. Nucl. Med., 23*, 978.
32. Hoffman DA, McConahey WM, Diamond EL, Kurland LT (1982) Mortality in women treated for hyperthyroidism. *Am. J. Epidemiol., 115*, 243.
33. Hoffman DA, Mc. Conahey WM, Fraumeni JF, Kurland LT (1982) Cancer incidence following treatment of hyperthyroidism. *Int. J. Epidemiol., 11*, 218.
34. Itoh M, Funauchi M, Fukuma N et al (1982) A case of hyperthyroidism complicated with diabetic ketoacidosis following ^{131}I therapy. *J. Jpn Diab. Soc., 25*, 1103.
35. Handelsman DJ, Conway AJ, Donnelly PE, Turtle JR (1980) Azoospermia after iodine-131 treatment for thyroid carcinoma. *Br. Med. J., 281*, 1527.
36. Miceli JN, McArthur B, Arora SK et al (1983) kinetics of propylthiouracil in children with Graves' disease. *Abstracts, World Conference on Clinical Pharmacology and Therapeutics, Washington*, No. 51.
37. Dinsmore WW, O'Hara MD, Callender ME (1983) Postanesthetic carbimazole jaundice. *N. Engl. J. Med.*, 438.
38. Van Dop C, Conte FA, Koch TK et al (1983) Pseudotumor cerebri associated with initiation of levothyroxine therapy for juvenile hypothyroidism. *N. Engl. J. Med., 308*, 1076.

H.M.J. Krans

44 Insulin, glucagon and oral hypoglycemic drugs

INSULIN

The UGDP study: a final report

A few years ago the final report of the University Group Diabetes Program (UGDP, see SEDA 4-301[R]) would have been considered to be of major interest (1). Since, however, the heat of the discussion over the UGDP study (SEDA 5-391) has been tempered, this report, which appeared in 1982, does not seem to have received much attention. In the eighth and final report insulin therapy is evaluated. This report also defends the entire study, explaining the choices made regarding assignment of patients to the various groups, the diagnostic criteria, and the means of dealing with neglectors. The protocol was based upon the insight into the treatment of diabetics and into the role of good control of blood glucose which prevailed at the end of the fifties when oral hypoglycemic agents had been available for no more than 5 years: the choices were made without the knowledge and insight of today.

The groups treated with a fixed dose of insulin (ISTD), with variable doses of insulin to maintain fasting and 1 hour glucose levels (IVAR), and with diet only (PLBO) were compared. Although the mean levels of glucose in the IVAR groups were closer to normal than in the other groups, no significant reduction of cardiovascular mortality or morbidity could be demonstrated. Only serum creatinine levels were significantly different ($P < 0.05$, not 0.001, for IVAR versus PLBO). Hypertension was seen more often in IVAR than in PLBO ($0.01 < P < 0.05$). There was some suggestive evidence that the overall mortality rate in the IVAR group was reduced as compared with the other groups. In the detailed life tables, however, the results of 13-year follow-up showed no difference for ISTD and IVAR. The variations in cardiovascular deaths were minimal. In this study no beneficial effect of strict control of blood glucose could be demonstrated, albeit that the method used differed widely from what nowadays is considered to be strict control.

Meticulous control and long-term effects of insulin

The trend towards rigorous maintenance of normoglycemia in the treatment of diabetes may induce chronic peripheral hyperinsulinism in patients. This renders the matter of the long- and short-term effect of hyperinsulinism relevant. The biochemical effects and clinical repercussions (including the Somogyi effect) of excessive insulin therapy have been reviewed (2[R]). In a comment (3) a warning is given, based both on theoretical considerations and on physiological and clinical intuitions, of the dangers which may arise when meticulous metabolic control is propagated. Dangers are hypoglycemia, hypoglycemic encephalopathy, accelerated retinopathy and absent secretion of catecholamines in neuropathy that may exclude a fail-safe warning system. Intensive training of the patient in self-care is essential. Meticulous control must be considered unsuitable for patients with a life expectancy under 5 years, cerebrovascular or coronary disease which makes hypoglycemic periods excessively dangerous, or patients with excessive insulin sensitivity because of renal failure, β-adrenergic blockade, autonomic neuropathy and hypophysectomy.

Side Effects of Drugs Annual 8
M.N.G. Dukes, editor

ISBN 0 444 90339 9
$0.80 per article per page (transactional system)
$0.20 per article per page (licensing system)

Stout (4) discusses the atherogenicity of insulin.

Hypoglycemia *(SED-9, 705; SEDA-4, 298; SEDA-5, 386; SEDA-6, 368; SEDA-7, 405)*

It is of interest to note that 113 of the 414 patients involved in both insulin groups in the UGDP study (1) had at least one prescription change for a suspected or observed episode of hypoglycemia (40% of the IVAR group, 15% of the ISTD group).

Hypoglycemia factitia was reported (5[C]) in a man without diabetes mellitus. Low C-peptide concentrations and high insulin concentrations were observed during hypoglycemic episodes.

Attempted suicide (6[C]) by a 24-year-old diabetic who lost his job was treated with excision of the injection site. This patient had injected 200 U protamine zinc insulin and 200 U of regular insulin after not having eaten for 12 hours except for consuming 3–4 liters of beer. He regretted his step and immediately went to the hospital. The injection site was macular and erythematous. Within half an hour a piece of skin and subcutaneous fat of 5 × 2 × 2 cm was excised. The blood insulin fell from 1240 U to 425 U within 14 hours when treated with 250 ml of 20% dextrose/hr after an initial injection of 20 ml of 50% dextrose. The patient remained conscious.

In 1978–79 18 cases of deliberate self-poisoning with insulin were reported in England, and 4 of the 204 severe hypoglycemic episodes in a casualty department were intentional overdoses. The situation may be less rare than is often thought.

Allergic reactions *(SED-9, 707; SEDA-4, 299; SEDA-5, 389; SEDA-6, 369; SEDA-7, 403)*

Insulin allergy was reported in a 19-month-old boy (7[C]), with newly diagnosed diabetes mellitus. 23 days after diagnosis treatment was with 1 unit of regular insulin and 3 units of NPH insulin daily. Small 'insect bite' lesions appeared which developed in 3 days into urticarial reactions. Angioedema appeared on the hands and face. The patient had positive skin reactions to single peak and monocomponent insulins. After desensitization he continued to have occasional local reactions for 1 month. The IgE/IgG ratio decreased only slightly after desensitization.

A case of persisting sclerosing granuloma after only 6 injections of insulin (depot Hoechst) has been reported (8[C]). The patient had forgotten to take his usual NPH and regular insulin with him during his holiday and he was prescribed this type of insulin. He had a positive skin test to 2 different batches of this type of insulin and to Surfen (see SEDA-7, p. 404). Red warm swellings (2 × 3–7 × 5 cm) were noticed at the injection site the day after the injection. A biopsy 4 months later revealed sclerosing granuloma. After 2 years the infiltrates could still be easily palpated.

4 different cases of serious allergic manifestations in patients treated with monocomponent insulin or other preparations of insulin have been reported (9[C]). A change-over to other more purified or human insulins was insufficient to alleviate complaints of itching, red plaques or urticarial eruptions. Desensitization was often not successful. These authors consider that, when the symptoms have not disappeared by the 10th day or have recurred, treatment with prednisone, beginning with 40 mg daily and reducing every week by 50%, may well lead to a permanent remission. However, no data on long-term success were presented. A fifth patient included in this report was a 'fresh' diabetic, with a glucose level of 680 mg/dl and an alkaline reserve of 5 mEq/l, who developed cardiac arrest after a second injection of subcutaneous insulin 4 hours after his first injection. The cause of the complication was not clear.

Local allergic reactions have been reported when using continuous subcutaneous infusion of insulin. Local hypertrophy (10[C]) was seen 6 months after a patient started continuous insulin infusion therapy in the abdominal wall. This did not affect the effectiveness of insulin. She had never developed local cutaneous reactions during the preceding 30 years of insulin injection in the thigh.

The question of localized skin reactions in patients using *insulin pumps* (i.e. mechanical devices for continuous insulin infusion) has been reviewed (11[R]). It was found that Squibb insulin induced more dermal hypersensitivity than other purified insulins, probably because of its higher proinsulin content. 35 patients treated with infusion pumps showed hypersensitivity reactions. Most reactions were induced by the adhesive tapes used to secure the needles and tubings to the skin. Pump-tubing may also induce an eczematoid reaction. The second most common reaction was infection. Cellulitis and abscess formation may require surgical and antibiotic treatment. Hard nodules may appear at the site of the insulin injection. These sometimes have a stone-hard consistency and may take months to subside. Changeover to other types of insulin may help.

The induction of antibodies by bovine insulin has been studied by Reeves and Kelly (12). A combination of soluble insulin and protamine zinc insulin was probably the most immunogenic insulin combination. The authors could not prove that antibodies induced by bovine insulin bound preferentially to regions of the insulin molecule where the sequence differed from that in human insulin. The antibodies may sequester a substantial part of the administered insulin.

In a study of the effects of a changeover to monocomponent insulin in the treatment of diabetes in Brazil (13) 30 patients with *lipoatrophy* recovered, but 2 patients developed lipohypertrophy.

A changeover to human insulin had no effect on a severe allergic reaction induced by purified beef insulin and later treated with monocomponent pork insulin. The lesions indeed tended to become worse (14[C]). The patient was hypersensitive to all types of insulin, including synthetic human and human DNA recombinant insulin. Desensitization with human insulin was successful.

A case of granulomatosis induced by *plastic syringes* has been presented (15[C]). A 14-year-old boy who had had diabetes for 7 years developed an acute vasculitis when he used a new type of insulin and plastic syringes. The syringes were used 3–10 times and stored in 94% alcohol. A change of insulin had no effect on the lesions. He gradually developed hyperpigmented and slightly scaling sclerotic plaques secondarily covered by hypertrichosis. After 9 years he shifted to glass syringes. His skin recovered its suppleness and normal appearance. The reduction in skin pliancy may be related to granulomatous infiltration in the subcutaneous septa. A pathogenically active agent may be released from the syringe or act as a Freund's adjuvant in a possible interaction with drugs. The alcohol used for syringe storage may have played a role.

NEW INSULINS *(SEDA-4, 299; SEDA-6, 368)*

The new insulins have recently been reviewed by Home and Alberti (16[R]). When intermittent insulin therapy is contemplated, the highly purified or human insulins are essential. The major advantages which they offer are in the authors' view a decrease in allergic reactions, decrease in antibody levels and sometimes a reduction in the amount of injected insulin required, albeit that the reduction of the dose is difficult to quantify. It may reflect over-insulinization with less pure insulins. In the 70 patients of the above mentioned study in Brazil (13) a transfer from nonpurified insulin to monocomponent insulin was accompanied by an average reduction in dose of 39%.

A double-blind crossover trial for transfer from bovine or pork insulin to biosynthetic insulin in 94 patients (17a, 17b) revealed that most patients had no trouble in making the change. 3 patients were withdrawn because of hypoglycemic episodes. Glucose profiles did not suggest a greater overall hypoglycemic potency of human insulin than of bovine or porcine insulin, but resorption was more rapid.

A report of a symposium on human insulin of recombinant DNA origin has appeared (18). Besides the above mentioned studies it contains various papers on antibodies and case reports on the treatment of insulin allergy.

Allergic reactions and the new human insulins

The new human insulins are taking a growing share of the market. Two types of human insulin are available, respectively by recombinant DNA techniques, or by chemical substitution of the COOH terminal aminoacid of the B-chain of porcine insulin, phenylalanine, with threonine.

Most reports in which human and porcine insulin are compared deal only with small numbers of patients or do not compare equivalent amounts of both types of insulin. For critical reviews of this subject see 16[R] and 19[R]. Small local areas of erythema, itching and induration are sometimes seen when insulin therapy is started, but this is in the majority of the cases a transient phenomenon. Major reactions like (generalized) urticaria or (anaphylactic) shock are extremely rare. They are most frequently seen when insulin therapy is reinstituted after an interruption, like the 'honeymoon period' in recently discovered diabetes, a period of treatment with oral hypoglycemic drugs, or when insulin has been used during pregnancy and stopped after delivery. The late local manifestations are sometimes related to increased IgE levels (20) or a high IgE/IgG ratio (21). The circulatory levels or IgG and IgM insulin antibodies are not related to sensitivity reactions. Some late local reactions may be IgG-mediated, cellular-mediated, or both. Recently a review on circulating insulin-binding antibodies has been published (22[R]). Insulin allergy is generally not related to insulin resistance (23[r]).

Other allergic reactions are lipoatrophy and lipohypertrophy developing on or near the injection sites. Most allergic reactions are seen with the older less pure insulins having a greater antigenicity. The allergic reactions may be induced by peptides or proteins from the isolating procedure, excipients added to change the duration of action of insulin like Zinc or Surfen or proinsulin. When highly purified insulins of animal origin were introduced, a general decrease of antibody titers was reported, but individual variations occurred and some antibody titers remained elevated. The allergic reactions have tended to diminish after a changeover to highly purified insulin, but occasionally no change in the reaction or even a deterioration has been reported (14). Desensitization or prednison treatment was sometimes necessary. Allergic reactions have been reported in patients only treated with monocomponent insulins (24).

Lipoatrophy can ameliorate when purified insulins are used. Lipohypertrophy is not influenced by highly purified insulins (25).

Data on allergic reactions in patients treated with human insulin are scarce. Persistence of severe allergic reactions after a changeover to human insulin has been reported (14[C]), and hypersensitivity to human insulins has been demonstrated in patients sensitized by earlier injections with insulin of animal origin. The number of patients treated exclusively with human insulin is small compared to the frequency of allergic reactions, but the above-mentioned report on human insulin prepared by recombinant DNA techniques (18) does touch on the topic.

In 7 patients treated with human insulin (26), insulin-specific IgG antibodies were seen in very low concentrations of no clinical significance. Insulin-specific IgE antibodies were increased after 2 months, but declined markedly to values slightly above normal within 4 months. In 101 patients exclusively treated with human insulin (27), 2 cases of lipohypertrophy were seen. Of 4 patients with immediate type I allergy (urticaria) (28), 3 had a (decreased) allergic reaction to human insulin. During 4 weeks of treatment no change in local reaction was observed. In 3 patients with delayed type allergy, no allergic reaction against human insulin prepared with recombinant DNA technique was shown, but 2 of them showed a delayed allergic reaction against semisynthetic human insulin. 2 patients with either asthma or allergic rhinitis who developed severe local reactions on beef or pork insulin had no trouble when they used NPH (recombinant DNA) human insulin (29). One of them developed local reactions on regular (recombinant DNA) human insulin.

A decrease in circulating insulin antibodies was seen in 2 patients treated with continuous subcutaneous insulin infusion when they were changed from highly purified insulin of animal origin to human insulin (30).

To summarize: The tendency to a decrease in allergic reaction and antibody levels, seen with highly purified insulins, is again encountered when human insulin is used. Some patients nevertheless continue to show allergic manifestations after a changeover to human insulin. Besides lipohypertrophy no other allergic reactions have yet been reported in patients who have been exclusively treated with human insulin, but the number of patients involved is still small.

Two cases of *insulin edema* (SEDA-4, 300; SEDA-7, 405; 31[c]) were reported following insulin treatment in patients with diabetic ketosis. Renal function was normal. Edema disappeared when the insulin dose was reduced. Elevated transaminases during insulin therapy (1 patient had chronic active hepatitis, and the other had no abnormalities on liver biopsy) returned to normal when glibenclamide was given after cessation of insulin therapy (32[c]).

A brief report from Kuwait relates to a 34-year-old pregnant diabetic woman receiving increasing doses of Actrapid and Monotard during her fourth pregnancy. The infant was born with an imperforate anus, and since all previous children had been normal, the question of a possible teratogenetic effect was raised. The Kuwait Adverse Drugs Reaction Monitoring Team no doubt correctly dismissed the incident as coincidental (44[c]).

ORAL HYPOGLYCEMIC DRUGS *(SED-9, 709; SEDA-4, 303; SEDA-5, 390; SEDA-6, 369; SEDA-7, 406)*

In the final report of the UGDP study referred to earlier in this Chapter (1), the intriguing question as to the effects of oral hypoglycemic drugs (tolbutamide and phenformin) on life expectancy is again discussed. Mortality figures following discontinuation of phenformin or tolbutamide therapy (protocol changes) until 1975 are presented. Before the discontinuation of oral therapy the number of deaths in the placebo group was unexpectedly low. The number of deaths in the placebo group had relatively increased during the period of follow-up of 5 years. In the new data, however, it was still impossible to detect any beneficial effect on life expectancy for patients treated with (a fixed dose of) tolbutamide or phenformin.

Sulfonylureas

Hypoglycemia induced by hypoglycemic agents may last for extended periods and tends to reccur. Diminished renal function may be a contributing factor.

A patient with chronic renal insufficiency (creatinine 475 μmol/l) treated for some years with tolbutamide was taken into hospital for a severe hypoglycemic episode lasting for 3 days (33[C]). Tolbutamide levels in the blood (maximal value 1110 μmol/l as compared with values in persons with normal kidney function of 74-288.6 μmol/l) remained elevated for at least 54 days after tolbutamide was stopped. Retarded carboxylation of tolbutamide in the liver and diminished excretion of inactive carboxytolbutamide contributed to the hypoglycemia.

In a recent Finnish case, purpura developed during glibenclamide therapy (34[C]). It disappeared after withdrawal of glibenclamide and reappeared when glibenclamide was reinstituted. IgA was found in the basement membrane but not in the dermal vessels.

Chlorpropamide (35[C]) induced a *nephrotic syndrome* and immune complex *glomerulonephritis* in an American patient with diabetes. He also developed *hepatitis* and *dermatitis* in association with the use of chlorpropamide. Renal biopsies were performed when the symptoms were manifest and again 6 months later, when all symptoms had disappeared. In both biopsies mild to moderate diabetic glomerulosclerosis was seen, but in the second biopsy the glomerular and interstitial inflammatory changes were completely resolved.

Transient diabetes insipidus was described in a child born of a diabetic mother treated with chlorpropamide in pregnancy (36[C]). After postnatal hypoglycemia the child became listless and dusky after 48 hours. On the fourth day of life serum sodium concentration was 162 mmol/l and urine osmolality was 91 mosm/l. The chlorpropamide in the mother may have increased either ADH release or the ADH-sensitivity of the kidney tubule in the unborn child, or both. The postnatal drug withdrawal may have induced a temporary ADH-deficiency.

The *chlorpropamide alcohol flushing test* (CPAF, see SEDA-7, 407) continues to intrigue physicians. Reduced macroangiopathy and peripheral neuropathy in CPAF-positive persons (37) was reported. Blood kinines do not play a role in mediating the flush (38).

Biguanides

Biguanides *inhibit intestinal absorption* of glucose and of many nutrients including other hexoses, aminoacids and vitamin B12. Of 46 diabetic patients treated with phenformin or metformin 30% had malabsorption of vitamin B12 (39). Half of these showed normal resorption after withdrawal of the drug. In the patients with permanent malabsorption coincident intrinsic factor deficiency could be demonstrated. Biguanides may induce a permanent depression of intrinsic factor secretion.

A case of *megaloblastic anemia* and *vita-*

min B12 deficiency, both of which disappeared after withdrawal of metformin and reappeared when the drug was reinstituted, has been published (40[C]).

Lactic acidotic coma (lactic acid 174 mg%, pH 6.7) is reported in a patient treated with 150 mg of phenformin (41[c]). She recovered with intensive treatment. Lactic acid levels are generally increased during phenformin treatment (42). The physiology and treatment of lactic acidosis is discussed in a recent review article (43[R]). It is still debatable whether glucose and insulin therapy is of value in biguanide-induced lactic acidosis. The role of sodium dichloroacetate (see SEDA-7, 410) remains unclear. It is certainly not suitable for long-term use.

REFERENCES

1. University Group Diabetes Program (1982) Effects of hypoglycemic agents on vascular complications in patients with adult-onset diabetes. VIII. Evaluation of insulin therapy: final report. *Diabetes, 19*, 1.
2. Wilson DE (1983) Excessive insulin therapy: biochemical effects and clinical repercussions. Current concepts of counterregulation in type I diabetes. *Ann. Intern. Med., 98*, 219.
3. Unger RH (1982) Meticulous control of diabetes: benefits, risks, and precautions. *Diabetes, 31*, 479.
4. Stout RW (1982) Is insulin atherogenic? *M. Sinai J. Med., 49*, 223.
5. Lüscher T, Kuhlmann U, Illig R et al (1982) Hypoglycaemia factitia: Klinik, Diagnostik und Verlauf bei einem Mann ohne Diabetes mellitus. *Schweiz. Med. Wochenschr., 112*, 832.
6. Campbell IW, Ratcliffe JG (1982) Suicidal insulin overdose managed by excision of insulin injection site. *Br. Med. J., 285*, 408.
7. Wishner KL, Fisher LK (1982) Insulin allergy in a 19-month-old boy with newly diagnosed diabetes mellitus. *Pediatrics, 70*, 137.
8. Elte JWF, Van der Schroeff JG, Van Leeuwen AWFM et al (1982) Sclerosing granuloma after short-term administration of depot-insulin Hoechst. *Klin. Wochenschr., 60*, 1461.
9. Darnaud J, Denard Y, Mouysset B (1982) Les manifestations graves de l'allergie a l'insuline. *Rev. Fr. Endocrinol. Clin., 23*, 434.
10. Mier A, Weerakoon J, Dandona P (1982) Bilateral abdominal lipohypertrophy after continuous subcutaneous infusion of insulin. *Br. Med. J.*, 1539.
11. Levandoski LA, White NH, Santiago JV (1982) Localized skin reactions to insulin: insulin lipodystrophies and skin reactions to pumped subcutaneous insulin therapy. *Diabetes Care, 5*, 6.
12. Reeves WG, Kelly U (1982) Insulin antibodies induced by bovine insulin therapy. *Clin. Exp. Immunol., 50*, 163.
13. Arduino F (1980) Experiência clínica com a insulina monocomponente. *Arq. Bras. Endocrinol. Metabol., 24*, 141.
14. Carveth-Johnson AO, Mylvaganam K, Child DF (1982) Generalized allergic reaction with synthetic human insulin. *Lancet, 2*, 1287.
15. Lapière CM, Pierard GE, Hermanns JF et al (1982) Unusual extensive granulomatosis after long-term use of plastic syringes for insulin injections. *Dermatologica, 165*, 580.
16. Home PD, Alberti KGMM (1982) The new insulins. Their characteristics and clinical indications. *Drugs, 24*, 401.

17a. Clark AJL, Knight G, Wiles PG et al (1982) Biosynthetic human insulin in the treatment of diabetes. A double-blind crossover trial in established diabetic patients. *Lancet, 2*, 354.

17b. Clark AJ, Wiles PG, Leiper JM et al (1982) A double-blind crossover trial comparing human insulin (recombinant DNA) with animal insulins in the treatment of previously insulin-treated diabetic patients. *Diabetes Care, 5 (Suppl. 2)*, 129.

18. Skyler JS (Ed) (1982) Symposium on human insulin of recombinant DNA origin. *Diabetes Care, 5 (Suppl. 2)*, 1.
19. Johansen K (1983) Human insulin – medical progress? *Metabolism, 32*, 528.
20. deShazo D, Boehm TM, Kumar D et al (1982) Dermal hypersensitivity reactions to insulin: correlations of three patterns to their histopathology. *J. Allergy Clin. Immunol., 69*, 229.
21. Kumar D (1981) Insulin allergy: differences in the binding of porcine, bovine, and human insulins with anti-insulin IgE. *Diabetes Care, 4*, 104.
22. Kurtz AB, Nabarro JDN (1980) Circulating insulin-binding antibodies. *Diabetologia, 19*, 329.
23. Grammer LC, Chen PY, Patterson R (1983) Evaluation and management of insulin allergy. *J. Allergy Clin. Immunol., 71*, 250.
24. Schernthaner G, Ludwig H, Jarisch R et al (1981) Immediate-type allergy against insulin itself: clinical and immunologic studies on a diabetic patient with insulin intolerance. *Diabetes Care, 4*, 196.
25. Sakamoto Y, Matsuba I, Itoh K et al (1981) Therapeutic effects of highly purified insulin on insulin allergy and insulin lipodystrophy induced by conventional insulin treatment. *Jikeikai Med. J., 28*, 41.
26. Velcovsky HG, Federlin KF (1982) Insulin-specific IgG and IgE antibody response in type I diabetic subjects exclusively treated with human insulin (recombinant DNA). *Diabetes Care, 5*

(Suppl. 2), 126.

27. Galloway JA, Peck Jr FB, Fineberg SE et al (1982) The U.S. 'new patient' and 'transfer' studies. *Diabetes Care, 5 (Suppl. 2)*, 135.
28. Schlüter KJ, Kerp L (1982) Receptor binding studies and clinical effects of human insulin (recombinant DNA): studies in patients with newly diagnosed type I diabetes, type II diabetes, insulin resistance (type A and type B), insulin antibodies, insulin allergy, and 'brittle' diabetes. *Diabetes Care, 5 (Suppl. 2)*, 152.
29. De Leeuw I, Delvigne C, Bekaert J (1982) Insulin allergy treated with human insulin (recombinant DNA). *Diabetes Care, 5 (Suppl. 2)*, 168.
30. Spijker AJ, Poortman J, Thijssen JHH et al (1982) Decrease of circulating insulin antibodies in two patients treated with continuous subcutaneous infusion of human insulin (recombinant DNA). *Diabetes Care, 5 (Suppl. 2)*, 171.
31. Matsuura M, Kawara A, Doi K et al (1983) Two cases of insulin edema. *J. Jpn Diab. Soc., 26*, 79.
32. Hiramatsu K, Arimori S (1982) Increased serum GOT and GPT during treatment with insulin in two diabetic patients. *J. Jpn Diab. Soc., 25*, 1221.
33. Bureš J, Fixa B, Kaut V et al (1982) Severe hypoglycemia after Dirastan (tolbutamide) in a diabetic patient with chronic renal insufficiency. *Vnitř. Lék., 28*, 678.
34. Väätäinen N, Fräki JE, Hyvönen M et al (1983) Purpura with a linear epidermo-dermal deposition of IgA. *Acta Derm. Venereol., 63*, 169.
35. Appel GB, D'Agati V, Bergman M et al (1983) Nephrotic syndrome and immune complex glomerulonephritis associated with chlorpropamide therapy. *Am. J. Med., 74*, 337.
36. Uhrig JD, Hurley RM (1983) Chlorpropamide in pregnancy and transient neonatal diabetes insipidus. *Can. Med. Assoc. J., 128*, 368.
37. Jerntorp P, Almér LO (1981) Chlorpropamide-alcohol flushing in relation to macroangiopathy and peripheral neuropathy in non-insulin dependent diabetes. *Acta Med. Scand. Suppl., 656*, 33.
38. Jerntorp P, Hulthén UL, Almér LO (1981) Chlorpropamide-alcohol flushing and blood kinins. *Acta Med. Scand. Suppl., 656*, 37.
39. Adams JF, Clark JS, Ireland JT et al (1983) Malabsorption of vitamin B_{12} and intrinsic factor secretion during biguanide therapy. *Diabetologia, 24*, 16.
40. Mourits-Andersen T, Ditzel J (1983) Megaloblastic anaemia caused by malabsorption of vitamin B_{12} during long-term metformin therapy. *Ugeskr. Laeg., 145*, 25.
41. Fumelli P, Giansanti R, Romagnoli F et al (1981) Acidosi lattica: Un episodio di patologia iatrogena nel vecchio. *Rass. Geriatr., 17*, 137.
42. Sitprija S, Vajanamarhutue C, Bunnag S (1982) Blood lactate and pyruvate levels in diabetic patient treated with sulphonylureas with and without biguanides. *J. Med. Assoc. Thailand, 65*, 63.
43. Cohen RD, Woods HF (1983) Lactic acidosis revisited. *Diabetes, 32*, 181.
44. Insulin (1983) *Kuwait Univ. Drug Adverse Reactions Series, 2*, 21.

R. Bouillon and F.A. van Assche

45 Miscellaneous hormones and prostaglandins

MISCELLANEOUS HORMONES

Calcitonin *(SED-9, 719)* and elcatonin

The favourable effects of calcitonin on the evolution of pagetic bone are well documented (SEDA-5, 397; SEDA-6, 374; SEDA-7, 413). The long-term effect of calcitonin on nonpagetic bone was studied in a longitudinal prospective study (3 years; 12 patients) using the monoenergetic photon absorptiometric method as a measurement for bone mineral content (1[CR]). The control group showed a progressive decrease in bone mineral content which could be entirely prevented by synthetic salmon calcitonin (50 MRC units s.c. per day for 3 years). Calcitonin thus seems to provide protection against age-dependent bone loss. No clear side effects were noted (1[CR]). A derivative of salmon calcitonin, elcatonin, a 31-amino-acid calcitonin in which the L-cysteine at the first and seventh position is replaced by α-aminosuberic acid, can be used as a long-acting calcitonin for the treatment of Paget's disease. Preliminary experience in man reveals a general pattern of side effects similar to that of the other calcitonins (2[R]).

Vasopressin and analogs

Intravenous or intraarterial administration of vasopressin is effective for the control of gastroesophageal bleeding of patients with or without liver cirrhosis. Due to its vasoconstrictive effects, gangrene of the perfused organs or even at distant sites remains a constant threat.

Side Effects of Drugs Annual 8
M.N.G. Dukes, editor

ISBN 0 444 90339 9
$0.80 per article per page (transactional system)
$0.20 per article per page (licensing system)

A case of upper extremity gangrene was observed in a 71-year-old man with massive upper gastrointestinal bleeding and liver cirrhosis. 2 hours after disconnecting the vasopressin infusion, complete resolution of the ischemic changes in the upper extremities and in one arm was observed, but dry gangrene continued in several fingers of the other arm necessitating limited elective amputations 2 weeks later (3[C]).

In another patient with a vasopressin infusion, gangrene was observed in various cutaneous regions subject to pressure and around the infusion sites (4[c]). The authors also suggest that *continuous* infusion might predispose to such complications since no report of *local* ischemia has been published after bolus administration of the drug. Hyponatremia is also very frequent but rarely severe (5[c]).

A more complete review on the use of vasopressin in the management of bleeding esophageal varices stresses that this therapy is effective in controlling upper gastrointestinal bleeding, but should mainly be viewed as a means of buying time to organize surgical correction of the primary lesions. The cardiovascular complications (hypertension, decreased cardiac output, arrhythmias) can largely be prevented by careful control of the pulse rate, bradycardia being the alarming symptom (6[R]). Abdominal pain and nausea sometimes occur, but infarction of small bowel segments, myocardium or other organs is certainly the most dangerous complication. Simultaneous isoproterenol infusion might be helpful in reducing its cardiovascular toxicity (6[R]).

One analog of vasopressin, TGLVP or n-triglycyl-8-lysine vasopressin might offer better effectiveness with less in the way of side effects than vasopressin itself (6[R]). Another analog, DDAVP or Minirin, has only minimal pressor effects but more antidiuretic effects and is the drug of choice for treating diabetes insipidus. Allergic reactions are rare (7[c]); hyponatremia remains a possibility but is mainly related to abuse of this (expensive) drug (8[c]). Vasopressin and DDAVP have definite blood clotting effects: they induce fibrinolysis via the release of plasminogen activator (6[R]). Because they also induce the release of autologous F VIII:VWF from tissue storage sites into plasma and since DDAVP has less marked cardiovascular side effects than vasopressin, this drug has been successfully used in Van Willebrand's disease (SEDA-2, 354) and is now also reported to correct temporarily the increased bleeding time due to uremia (9[CR]). DDAVP can therefore be used for temporary correction of bleeding time in uremic patients. The side effects of this medication were minor, comprising only transient facial flushing, headache or dizziness. No significant changes in blood pressure or cardiac rhythm were observed.

Growth hormone

Experience with human growth hormone (HGH) for growth-retarded children is now sufficiently great to be summarized in detail (10[R], 11[R]). Moreover, the pending explosion of HGH supplies due to recombinant DNA technology will greatly enlarge its possible fields of application. The growth hormone should be of human origin and is to be injected several times a week, preferably intramuscularly. There is a dose-dependent growth rate increase, but the slope of this ratio is shallow, so that doubling the dose doubles the cost but does not double the response.

The side effects are unimportant: there is variable (but usually minimal) *local pain and discomfort* and scattered reports of local *lipoatrophy*. A few cases of *slipped capital femoral epiphyses* have also been reported, but their causal relation with HGH therapy is unclear. HGH does *not accelerate existing tumor growth* (e.g. intracranial tumors).

Several authors have described the development of *hypothyroidism* during HGH therapy. The incidence has however, varied from less than 1% to 100% in the several studies summarized in 2 recent reviews (10[R], 11[R]) without any clear explanation for such variable findings. If hypothyroidism develops it need not necessarily to be due to the HGH therapy itself, but could simply be a reflection of the natural history of the primary pituitary disorder, unmasked by HGH treatment. Whatever its cause, such hypothyroidism needs to be treated immediately as it otherwise seriously impairs the growth-promoting effect of the therapy (10[R]).

Antibody development during HGH treatment is quite frequent, its incidence varying from 31 to 60% of all patients according to a literature review (10[R]), but these antibodies do not usually lead to clinical resistance to therapy (seen only in 0 to 5% of all patients). The antibody response depends on the extraction procedure used for HGH isolation (acetone-dried pituitaries induce more antibodies), and patients with severe congenital isolated HGH deficiency are more likely to produce neutralizing antibodies (10[R], 11[R]). Resistance due to antibodies may be overcome by either increasing doses or switching to more purified preparations (10[R]).

Growth hormone releasing hormone

Pancreatic tumors associated with clinical acromegaly contain a 44-aminoacid peptide (or somewhat shorter chain break-down products) capable of stimulating growth hormone release from cultured pituitary glands even when present in femtomolar concentrations (12[C]). Immunochemical staining demonstrates its presence in the hypothalamic area (13[R]). The clinical activity of this hormone, which has now been synthesized, was proven in several experiments (14[C]): intravenous bolus injection (100 μg) induced GH release in all normal subjects, no GH release in hypopituitarism, and a variable response in acromegaly. No side effects were noted; this is a major advantage over existing GH testing procedures such as insulin-induced hypoglycemia (14[C], 15[C]).

Gonadotropin-releasing hormones (LH-RF or GnRH) and their analogs

Although GnRH initially stimulates the secretion of the gonadotropins, the long-term use of agonists or even superagonists without the typical endogenous pulsatile pattern produces a downward regulation of the hypothalamic-hypophysial gonadal system, possibly even with direct inhibitory effects on the gonads. It was there-

fore logical to explore the possible benefits of prolonged GnRH therapy as an alternative to orchidectomy or stilboestrol treatment in prostatic cancer. Two British studies (16[C], 17[C]) with a synthetic GnRH agonist demonstrate a favorable effect in patients with advanced or metastatic prostatic cancer: clinical regression of the tumor and pain relief were observed in 8 of 10 and 9 of 12 patients respectively. The hormonal pattern obtained with GnRH administration (either subcutaneously or intranasally) is very similar to that obtained after castration. Loss of libido and a considerable reduction in sexual activity were therefore regularly observed (16[C], 17[C]); mild facial flushing reminiscent of menopausal flushing was sometimes observed (17[C]). It is therefore tempting to assume, as is done in a recent review (18[R]), that use of GnRH analogs in continuous high-dose therapy will acquire a therapeutic dimension in the palliative treatment of prostatic cancer, since it has potentially the same therapeutic effect as other procedures without the side effects which the latter involve (orchidectomy, estrogens or antiandrogens). A study, published in abstract, on a large number of patients with prostatic cancer claims objective and subjective positive results in 74% and 90%. Beside the side effects mentioned in the British studies above (16[C], 17[C]), a possible flare-up of the disease activity during the first weeks of injection (i.e. during the period of positive stimulatory effect of GnRH) was observed in 4 out of 18 patients (19[c]).

Another application of the downwards regulation of the gonadotropin function by prolonged nonpulsatile administration of GnRH is found in a reversible inhibition of testicular steroidogenesis and spermatogenesis (20[C]). 8 normal men were treated daily with a subcutaneous injection of a potent GnRH against for 6 to 10 weeks. Plasma testosterone fell substantially in all. Impotence developed in 5 men with resolution in each case within 2 weeks after stopping treatment. Sperm count and mobility fell to a nadir during the 7th-18th week after therapy with thereafter a return to pretreatment levels. Hot flushes were noted by 4 patients. It is therefore clear that such therapy could result in a reversible inhibition of spermatogenesis and provide an approach to male contraception, but the associated loss of libido and impotence makes it unacceptable in its present form (20[C]). Similar data were obtained in monkeys (21[c]). The possible use of GnRH as a female contraceptive was further evaluated (22[c], 23[c]). Hot 'menopausal' flushes were observed even in the absence of pulsatile LH pulses (22[c]).

The normal physiologic effect of GnRH can, of course, also find therapeutic applications beside its diagnostic potential (18[R]). Pulsatile administration of GnRH is able to restore normal ovarian function in women with hypothalamic amenorrhea (SEDA-6, 377). A similar approach with episodic GnRH administration (25 ng/kg every 2 hours s.c. for up to 43 weeks) by a portable pump was used for the induction of puberty in 6 men with idiopathic hypogonadotropic hypogonadism (24[C]). Serum gonadotropin levels rose to normal adult levels within 1 week and reached supraphysiologic levels after 2 weeks. Serum testosterone levels became normal after 1 month. The testicular size increased and spermatogenesis was achieved in 3 patients after 43 weeks of therapy. Androgen-induced skin changes (e.g. acne and seborrhea) were frequent but expected. Transient mild breast discomfort occurred in all patients and a mild but persistent gynecomastia in 3 out of 6 patients was observed (24[C]).

The effect of intranasal, synthetic GnRH on undescended testes was reported in 2 studies (25[C], 26[c]). In a double blind study (50 patients), a complete descent of the testes was observed in 40% with incomplete results in another 20% of the testes. The best results were observed in young patients (under 6 years of age) and with the higher doses of GnRH. No significant hormonal changes were observed during the 4 week treatment period (25[c]). Side effects were minor and included the mentioning of more active and/or aggressive behavior, furunculosis, impetigo and local nasal irritation. A similar study compared the effect of GnRH and a potent analog on the testicular descent of 67 boys. The natural hormone gave a positive result in about 30% after 7 days of treatment. The long-acting analog resulted in a similar percentage of results when given as a 25 µg dose every other day for a total of 8 doses (26[c]). No serious side effects were observed either during or after treatment.

Gonadotropins

A recent review by Rily on the use and side effects of gonadotropins mainly discusses the indications for the several gonadotropins now available and their pharmacokinetics. The major side effect is ovarian hyperstimulation resulting in mild to gross ovarian enlargement, accompanied by nausea, vomiting, abdominal pain and ascites. Ovarian cysts may also rupture, and oliguria and fluid retention can occur. Multiple pregnancy can be the result of treating female infertility with gonadotropins. Allergic reactions have also been reported (27[R]). The use of gonadotropins for the treatment of testicular maldescent has also been reviewed (28[R]). Even if some success has been achieved with these drugs as far as testicular descent is concerned, the prognosis as to fertility remains generally bad. Treatment during early life may have a better long-term prognosis, but no data are yet available to substantiate this hypothesis (28[R]). Large doses (>5.000 IU of HCG) may be followed by local edema and painful swelling of the testis and even cause histological lesions (28[R]). Antibodies against HLH have been found in some children treated with HGH, bovine TSH and posterior pituitary extract for hypopituitarism (29[c]). These antibodies certainly interfered with the serum assay of the gonadotropins. Of three such children, none had shown spontaneous puberty, although the causal relation with their circulating antibodies is difficult to prove. To reduce the risk of generating neutralizing antibodies, pituitary hormones of the highest purity should be used whenever possible (29[c]).

Oxytocin

Oxytocin use was not associated with an increased morbidity or mortality in 641 patients or their newborns as compared with an equal number of deliveries without oxytocin administration. Oxytocin was therefore considered safe and effective provided strict critera and protocols for its use are maintained (30[C]). Rupture and necrosis of the pregnant uterus after injudicious use of oxytocin as well as water intoxication have, however, been reported (31[C], 32[C]), suggesting that treatment is not always as judicious as it might be.

PROSTAGLANDINS

Use in cardiovascular diseases

Prostaglandins can be used during early life to keep the ductus arteriosus open until palliative or corrective surgery for congenital heart defects can be performed (SEDA-6, 378). Two recent reviews are devoted to this subject (33[R], 34[R]). Prostaglandin E_1 (alprostadil, Prostin) has been most widely used and is of proven efficacy. The side effects include *peripheral dilatation, hypotension* and, most importantly, *apnea. Hyperpyrexia* and *jitteriness* have also been observed as has been discussed previously (SEDA-6, 378). The incidence of these side effects may be as much as 20%, but they are usually reversible and the benefit of the therapy certainly outweighs its risks (34[R]). Careful monitoring is needed and ventilatory assistance must be at hand because of the risk of drug-induced bradycardia or apnea. Pyrexia or hypotension can usually be corrected by reduction of the dose. Flushing usually subsides after repositioning of the intraarterial catheter (33[R]).

The use of drugs which interfere with prostaglandin E synthesis may also increase the frequency of patency of the ductus arteriosus. Furosemide used in the treatment of respiratory distress resulted in open ductus arteriosus in 18 out of 39 infants in contrast to only 8 out of 33 patients treated with chlorothiazide (which does not stimulate the PGE_1 synthesis) (35[C]).

Prostacyclin (PGI_2) was used in 5 patients with myocardial infarction to reduce the size of the infarct. Moderate *hypotension* and *tachycardia* was frequently observed. All 5 patients returned with a *status anginosus* within 5 to 25 days after first admission. The authors therefore suggest that after acute PGI_2 treatment other drugs improving the tromboxane-prostacyclin ratio should be started (36a[C]). Other applications for prostacyclin are discussed in another recent review (36b[R]). Its antiplatelet activity could be exploited during extracorporal circulation and peripheral, cerebral or coronary arterial diseases. Prevention of kidney transplant rejection is also a possible indication.

The side effects of prostacyclin infusion have been described as few and minimal (36b[R]).

A better study of the side effects of PGI_2 reports facial flushing, headache, tachycardia and decreased diastolic blood pressure in almost all subjects (37[CR]). Erythema over the infusion site was also frequently encountered. Other complaints included restlessness, abdominal discomfort, nausea and drowsiness. Vagal reflexes (sudden bradycardia, pallor and sweating) and chest pain were noted occasionally. The authors also discuss the potential relation between the observed side effects and the dosage and infusion techniques employed, and advise heart rate monitoring in all patients. This article should be required reading for those who want to explore further the potential application of this drug (37[CR]).

Use in gastroenterology

A multicenter double-blind study, conducted on 173 patients with active duodenal ulcer, revealed that 100 μg of arbaprostil (15(R)-15-methyl-PGE_2) given 4 times daily for 28 days increased the incidence of peptic ulcer healing to approximately the same degree as reported in most studies using cimetidine. At 28 days 67% of the arbaprostil-treated patients were healed compared to 39% in the placebo group. The side effects consisted primarily in loose stools and diarrhea (34%). The favourable effect of this drug was ascribed to its ability to decrease gastric acid production (38a[C]).

Use in urology and nephrology

The intravesical application of PGE_2 resulted in a marked improvement of the detrusor function in 21 patients with bladder motor disturbances. Transient painful urgency of micturition was experienced by half of the patients, but no systemic side effects were observed (38b[C]).

Continuous PGE_1 infusion into a patient with rapidly progressive glomerulonephritis improved the kidney function without changing the urinary protein loss. The effect was ascribed to the drug's vasodilatory action (39[c]).

Use in obstetrics *(SEDA-7, 416)*

There have been no substantial changes in the therapeutic use of prostaglandins and oxytocin in obstetrics over the last year. For the induction of labor the prostaglandins of the third generation (40[C]) seem to offer a safe procedure, provided there is close supervision of the mother and the fetus (41[C], 42[C]). Neonatal jaundice was not increased after induction of labor with prostaglandins (43[C]). 2 cases of severe *bradycardia* and *bronchospasm* have been reported after intramyometrial injection of PGF_2 for uterine atony (50[c]).

The most frequent indication for prostaglandin administration still remains termination of pregnancy. Prostaglandin E_2 derivates are mostly used (sulprostone and 9-deoxo-16,16-dimethyl-9-methylene prostaglandin E_2) (40[C], 44[CR], 49[C]). Sulprostone was recorded as having too low a success rate and on the other hand nausea and vomiting were substantial problems. The success rate of 9-deoxo-16,16-dimethyl-9-methylene prostaglandin E_2 was no higher than that with previously used prostaglandins.

Wislicki (45[C]) reported adverse reactions such as nausea and vomiting in half of the patients who underwent prostaglandin-induced abortion. For the extra amniotic administration of prostaglandins $F_{2\alpha}$ a tylose gel is recommended (46[C]).

In 16 women out of 17 undergoing prostaglandin induced abortions, no change in the *intraocular pressure* occurred; in the other patient there was a transient moderate pressure elevation (47[c]).

For the induction of labour after intrauterine fetal death, sulprostone was less effective than $PGF_{2\alpha}$ or 15-methyl-$PGF_{2\alpha}$. Gastrointestinal side effects, however, were lower with sulprostone (48[C]).

REFERENCES

1. Toh SH, Claunch BC, Brown PH (1983) Effect of calcitonin treatment on the natural course of bone demineralization in Paget's disease. *J. Clin. Endocr. Metab.*, *56*, 405.
2. Anon (1983) Elcatonin. *Drugs future, 8*, 105.
3. Colombani P (1982) Upper extremity gangrene secondary to superior mesenteric artery infusion of vasopressin. *Digest. Dis. Sciences*, *27*, 367.
4. Wormser GP, Kornblee LV, Gottfried EB (1982) Cutaneous necrosis following peripheral intravenous vasopressin therapy. *Cutis, 29*, 249.

5. Brivet F, Naveau S, Delfraissy J-F et al (1983) Complications de la vasopressine dans le traitement des hémorragies digestives graves du sujet non cirrhotique. *Gastroenterol. Clin. Biol.*, *7*, 323.
6. Schweitzer EJ, Kerr JC, Swan KG (1982) Clinical use of vasopressin in the management of bleeding esophageal varices. *Am. Surg.*, *48*, 558.
7. Anon (1982) Ueberempfindlichkeit auf Vasopressin-Analogon? *Münch. Med. Wochenschr.*, *124*, 13.
8. Stone E, Zinman B (1980) Hyponatremia from 1-deamino-8-d-arginine (dDAVP) abuse. *Ann. Intern. Med.*, *92*, 711.
9. Mannucci PM, Remuzzi G, Pusineri F et al (1983) Deamino-8-d-arginine vasopressin shortens the bleeding time in uremia. *N. Engl. J. Med.*, *308*, 8.
10. Frasier SD (1983) Human pituitary growth hormone (hGH) therapy in growth hormone deficiency. *Endocr. Rev.*, *4*, 155.
11. Preece MA (1982) Diagnosis and treatment of children with growth hormone deficiency. *Clin. Endocrinol. Metab.*, *11*, 1.
12. Rivier J, Spiess J, Thorner M, Vale W (1983) Characterisation of a growth hormone releasing factor from a human pancreatic islet tumour. *Nature*, *300*, 276.
13. Lewitt PA, Chase TN (1983) Discovery of a new peptide with growth hormone releasing activity. *Trends Neurosci.*, *55*, 1.
14. Wood SM, Ch'ng JLC, Adams EF et al (1983) Abnormalities of growth hormone release in response to human pancreatic growth hormone releasing factor (GRF (1–44)) in acromegaly and hypopituitarism. *Br. Med. J.*, *286*, 1687.
15. Thorner MO, Rivier J, Spiess J et al (1983) Human pancreatic growth hormone releasing factor selectively stimulates growth hormone secretion in man. *Lancet*, *1*, 24.
16. Allen JM, O'Shea JP, Mashiter K et al (1983) Advanced carcinoma of the prostate: treatment with a gonadotrophin releasing hormone agonist. *Br. Med. J.*, *286*, 1607.
17. Waxman JH, Wass JAH, Hendry WF et al (1983) Treatment with gonadotrophin releasing hormone analogue in advanced prostatic cancer. *Br. Med. J.*, *286*, 1309.
18. Jacobi GH, Wenderoth UK (1982) Gonadotropin-releasing hormone analogues for prostatic cancer: untoward side effects of high-dose regimens acquire a therapeutical dimension. *Eur. Urol*, *8*, 129.
19. Glode LM (1982) Leuprolide therapy of advanced prostatic cancer. *Proc. Am. Soc. Clin. Oncol.*, Abstract C-426.
20. Linde R, Doelle GC, Alexander N et al (1981) Reversible inhibition of testicular steroidogenesis and spermatogenesis by a potent gonadotropin-releasing hormone agonist in normal men. *N. Engl. J. Med.*, *305*, 663.
21. Akhtar FB, Marshall GR, Wickings EJ, Nieschlag E (1983) Reversible induction of azoospermia in rhesus monkeys by constant infusion of a gonadotropin-releasing hormone agonist using osmotic minipumps. *J. Clin. Endocrinol. Metab.*, *56*, 534.
22. DeFazio J, Meldrum DR, Laufer L et al (1983) Induction of hot flashes in premenopausal women treated with a long-acting GnRH agonist. *J. Clin. Endocrinol. Metab.*, *56*, 445.
23. Werlin LB, Hodgen GD (1983) Gonadotropin-releasing hormone agonist suppresses ovulation, menses, and endometriosis in monkeys: an individualized, intermittent regimen. *J. Clin. Endocrinol. Metab.*, *56*, 844.
24. Hoffman AR, Crowley WF (1982) Induction of puberty in men by long-term pulsatile administration of low-dose gonadotropin-releasing hormone. *N. Engl. J. Med.*, *307*, 1237.
25. Cacciari E, Fréjaville E, Becca A (1982) Treatment of cryptorchidism by intranasal synthetic LH-RH and its analogue D-Ser $(TBU)^6$-LHRH-EA^{10}. *Eur. J. Pediatr.*, *139*, 280.
26. Hagberg S, Westphal O (1982) Treatment of undescended testes with intranasal application of synthetic LH-RH. *Eur. J. Pediat.* *139*, 285.
27. Riley AJ (1982) Clinical pharmacology of drugs used in sexual medicine: II. Gonadotropins and antigonadotropins. *Br. J. Sexual Med.*, *9*, 31.
28. Bierich JR (1982) Undescended testes: treatment with gonadotropin. *Eur. J. Pediatr.*, *139*, 275.
29. Burstein S, Kaplan SL, Grumbach MM (1983) The induction of antibodies to human luteinizing hormone by contaminated clinical pituitary hormone preparations. *J. Clin. Endocrinol. Metab.*, *56*, 192.
30. Belsky DH (1982) Statistical observations on the elective induction of labor with oxytocin. *J. AOA*, *81*, 524/55.
31. Biswas BP (1982) Rupture and necrosis of pregnant uterus after injudicious use of oxytocin. *Calcutta Med. J.*, *79*, 136.
32. Feeney JG (1982) Water intoxication and oxytocin. *Br. Med. J.*, *285*, 243.
33. Roehl SL, Townsend RJ (1982) New drug evaluations: Alprostadil. *Drug Intell. Clin. Pharm.*, *16*, 823.
34. Heymann MA, Clyman RI (1982) Evaluation of Alprostadil (Prostaglandin E_1) in the management of congenital heart disease in infancy. *Pharmacotherapy*, *2*, 148.
35. Green TP, Thompson TR, Johnson DA, Lock JE (1983) Furosemide promotes patent ductus arteriosus in premature infants with the respiratory-distress syndrome. *N. Engl. J. Med.*, *308*, 843.
36a. Levy M (1983) Prostacyclin infusion in patients with acute myocardial infarction (preliminary report). *N. Engl. J. Med.*, *308*, 1032.
36b. Moncada S (1983) Progress in cerebrovascular disease. Biology and therapeutic potential of prostacyclin. *Stroke*, *14*, 157.

37. Picles H, Grady JO (1982) Side effects occurring during administration of epoprostenol (prostacyclin, PGI_2), in man. *Br. J. Clin. Pharmacol.*, *14*, 177.

38a. Vantrappen G, Janssens J, Popiela T et al (1982) Effect of 15(R)-15-Methyl Prostaglandin E_2 (Arbaprostil) on the healing of duodenal ulcer. *Gastroenterology*, *83*, 357.

38b. Koller A, Nürnberger N, Plüger H (1983) Prostaglandin E_2 – eine Bereicherung in der Therapie der Blasenentleerungsstörungen? *Z. Urol. Nephrol.*, *75*, 145.

39. Niwa T, Maeda K, Asada H et al (1983) Beneficial effects of prostaglandin E_1 in rapidly progressive glomerulonephritis. *N. Engl. J. Med.*, *308*, 969.

40. Godicke HD (1982) Ergebnisse der Klinischen Prüfung des neuen Prostaglandin E_2-Derivatis Nalador^R (Sulproston). *Ther. Gegenw.*, *121*, 312.

41. Lorrain J, Beaumont L, Desaulniers G, Chemaly R (1982) Etude comparative des prostaglandines synthétiques et naturelles pour l'induction du travail. *Union Méd. Canada*, *111*, 563.

42. Merveille JJ, Godefoid L, Pestiau J (1982) Déclenchement électif du travail par PGE_2 orale. *J. Gynecol. Obstet. Biol. Reprod.*, *11*, 877.

43. Lange PK, Sestergaard G, Secher J, Skovgaard I (1982) Neonatal jaundice after labour induced or stimulated by prostaglandin E_2 or oxytocin. *Lancet*, *1*, 992.

44. Brenner PF, Marrs RP, Roy S, Mishell DR (1982) Termination of early gestation with 9-deoxo-16,16-dimethyl-9-methylene prostaglandin E_2. *Contraception*, *26*, 261.

45. Wislicki L (1982) Systemic adverse reactions to prostaglandin F_2 (PGF_2, dinoprostone, Prostin F_{2a}, Prostalmon F). *Biol. Res. Pregnancy*, *3*, 158.

46. Smith DH, Dalrymple JC (1983) A comparison of intraamniotic prostaglandin and estraamniotic prostaglandin gel for midtrimester termination of pregnancy. *Aust. N.Z. J. Obstet. Gynaecol.*, *23*, 32.

47. Ober M, Scharrer A (1982) Entwicklung des Augeninnendruckes bei prostaglandininduziertem Schwangerschaftsabbruch. *Klin. Monatsbl. Augenheilk.*, *180*, 230.

48. Keirse MJNC, Lobatto R (1983) Synthetische prostaglandine-analoga voor het inleiden van de baring bij intra-uteriene vruchtdood. *TGO*, 1561.

49. Fylling P (1982) Experience with 16-phenoxy-ω-tetranor-PGE_2-methylsulfonamide (Sulprostone) for termination of second trimester pregnancy. *Contraception*, *4*, 279.

50. Pottecher T, Freys G, Schon E and Jeanmougin J (1982) Effets indésirables de l'injection intra-myométriale de prostaglandines. *J. Méd. Strasbourg*, *13*, 448.

O.R. Ødegaard

46 Drugs affecting lipid metabolism

CLOFIBRATE *(SED-9, 728; SEDA-4, 316; SEDA-5, 401; SEDA-6, 384; SEDA-7, 421)*

The clofibrate controversy, which started after the WHO cooperative study 1978/79, still continues. In this study, it was found that administration of clofibrate resulted in a lowering of serum cholesterol by about 9%. The incidence of ischemic heart disease and myocardial infarction was reduced by about 20–25% as compared to the placebo groups. The incidence of lethal heart infarction was not influenced. In the clofibrate group, the total mortality was increased due to diseases of the liver and gallbladder, intestinal disturbances and carcinoma.

The study has been criticised: some authors have found that, when correcting for age and differences between the centers involved, the mortality rate in the clofibrate group was not increased. Recently it has been claimed that the only documented serious side effect of clofibrate is the increased incidence of gallstone formation. The well-known side effects diarrhea, increased liver transaminases, myositis, and allergic disease, are mostly transient and reversible. As a result of this criticism, an expert committee in the GDR has recommended the use of clofibrinic acid in hyperlipoproteinemia types IIb, III, IV and V, if the serum triglyceride concentration does not respond adequately to diet. If serum cholesterol is increased in hyperlipoproteinemia types IIa and IIb, the committee has recommended combining clofibrinic acid with nicotine acid or cholestyramine (1[R]).

Side Effects of Drugs Annual 8
M.N.G. Dukes, editor

ISBN 0 444 90339 9
$0.80 per article per page (transactional system)
$0.20 per article per page (licensing system)

Concerning the long-term effect of clofibrate, a case report from Japan was recently published which unfortunately raises more questions than it answers.

A 76-year-old woman with hypercholesterolemia had been taking clofibrate for 7 years. She died of cerebral infarction. At autopsy, preneoplastic and other adenomatous hepatocellular lesions were observed in a noncirrhotic liver. The patient had also taken other drugs but no information on these was provided (2[c]).

At present, it still seems that the use of clofibrate should be limited to patients with elevated lipids who have failed to respond adequately to diet and who are at high risk of coronary artery disease because of other risk factors. It should be borne in mind that the importance of increased serum lipid concentration as a risk factor diminishes with advancing age.

Bezafibrate *(SED-9, 733; SEDA-7, 421)*

Prager et al have reported on the use of this clofibrate congener in hyperlipidemic, non-insulin-dependent diabetics. 600 mg bezafibrate daily, divided into 3 doses, was given to 16 patients for 8 weeks. A significant decrease in plasma triglycerides, cholesterol, VLDL triglycerides and VLDL cholesterol was found. A significant increase of HDL cholesterol was observed, while LDL cholesterol remained unchanged, as did LCAT activity, blood glucose and serum insulin concentrations. Side effects were not reported. The authors conclude that long-term studies are needed to clarify the possible therapeutic benefits of bezafibrate (3[c]).

In another study, 10 patients with familial hypercholesterolemia were given placebo for 4 weeks, following bezafibrate 600 mg daily, divided in 3 doses for 12 weeks. After a placebo period of 6 weeks, clofibrate 2 g daily was given for 12 weeks. The effect of bezafibrate was analogous to that of clofibrate. During bezafibrate treatment, transitory pollakisuria occurred in 1 patient. In about half of the patients, a slight increase in liver size was observed both with bezafibrate and clofibrate. The enlargement regressed in all patients following the placebo administration (4[C]).

The effect of bezafibrate 600 mg daily divided over 3 doses has been compared with that of etofibrate retard, 500 mg daily, in 41 patients with hyperlipoproteinemia (IIa, IIb and IV). The treatment period was 12 weeks twice for each medication. The insufficient efficacy of etofibrate was considered to be due to an inadequate dose. In 4 patients etofibrate caused flushing, and the treatment had to be stopped in 2 of these. In the bezafibrate period, well-known transient complaints occurred in 3 patients (headache, nausea, abdominal pain). The treatment could be continued in all patients. In this study, bezafibrate significantly reduced the fasting glucose values (5[c]).

It would seem that headache can occur as a troublesome isolated side effect to bezafibrate, as evidenced by a report from Kuwait (17[c]):

> Bezafibrate was given to 4 patients, 2 men aged 30 and 40, and 2 women aged 32 and 35 for the treatment of hyperlipidemia. The dose was 200 mg t.d.s. The 4 patients started suffering immediately from severe headache after receiving the first tablet. The headache was generalized with no associated vomiting or other gastrointestinal symptoms. 2 patients received paracetamol to relieve the headache.

Ciprofibrate *(2-(p-(2,2-dichlorocyclopropyl) phenoxy)-2-p-methylpropionic acid)*

A daily dose of 50–200 mg of this compound was given to 50 patients with hyperlipoproteinemia for 6 months. In 5 patients the drug was stopped because of insufficient effects on serum lipoprotein concentrations. 45 patients continued with 200 mg for an additional 6 months. No patient complained of subjective side effects at any of the doses taken. The erythrocyte sedimentation rate and alkaline phosphatase decreased significantly. Serum transaminases, lactate dehydrogenase and creatinine concentrations increased. Similar changes have been observed with related drugs, e.g. bezafibrate (6[C]).

The long-term effects of ciprofibrate are at present unknown.

Clinofibrate *(cyclohexylidenebis(4,1-phenyleneoxy)bis(2-butyl-2-carboxylic acid))*

The effect of this compound in a dosage of 600 mg daily divided in 3 doses has been investigated in Japan in some 1300 patients. The effect on serum cholesterol and triglycerides was similar to that of clofibrate. Weakness, malaise, headache and skin eruptions occasionally occurred. Alopecia led to the discontinuation of the drug in some cases. Diaphoresis, increase in dandruff, angular stomatitis, abdominal pain, feeling of enlarged abdomen, anorexia, nausea, vomiting, diarrhea and constipation occasionally occurred (7[r]).

Fenofibrate *(SED-9, 733; SEDA-5, 405; SEDA-6, 384; SEDA-7, 421)*

A long-term study of the effect of fenofibrate 200–400 mg/day in 435 patients with hyperlipoproteinemia has recently been published (8[c]). At the time of its compilation, 83 of the patients had been taking fenofibrate for 5 years, 17 for 7 years. Dyspepsia occurred in 3.7% of the patients, myalgia in 1.8%, alopecia in 0.7%, impotence in 5%. 10 patients died during the study; 81 patients left the study for different reasons. The value of the study is limited, as no placebo group was included.

Gemfibrozil *(SED-9, 733; SEDA-6, 384; SEDA-7, 422)*

Gemfibrozil was given to 349 patients with hyperlipidemia for 13 months. Triglycerides and VLDL cholesterol decreased by 43–48% during the double-blind, placebo-controlled 18-week period of treatment and HDL cholesterol increased by 19–25%, all changes being significant as compared with the placebo group (9[C]). Abdominal pain occurred in 3.7% of the patients, diarrhea in 2%, nausea in 0.8%, epigastric pain in 0.8% and dizziness in 0.8%. In 3.4% of the patients the drug had to be withdrawn because of adverse reactions.

In diabetic patients treated with gemfibrozil, it has been found that plasma glucose levels were slightly elevated and that the requirement for insulin and oral hypoglycemic agents increased (10[c]).

Probucol *(SEDA-3, 359–360)*

Reports on the use of probucol in man have appeared since 1969. Although the lipid lowering effect in short-term studies is well documented, its use has been limited. In 1980, the nonprofit publication Medical Letter on Drugs and Therapeutics advised against its use for lack of knowledge of long-term effects (11r). Probucol is slowly released from fat stores, and it has been found that the drug is still present in plasma 6 months after discontinuing administration. A matter of concern is that, in addition to mean plasma cholesterol and LDL cholesterol level reductions, the major apolipoprotein of the HDL, apoprotein A-1 and HDL cholesterol are reduced as well. Accordingly, the ratio of major atherogenic to antiatherogenic lipoprotein cholesterols is increased on probucol as compared with placebo (12C 13C).

Recently, McCaughan (14C) reported the results of a long-term study. 118 patients with at least 3 serum cholesterol values above 250 mg/dl were randomized in a double-blind trial, in a ratio of 3 on drug (88) to 1 on placebo (30). The probucol dose was 500 mg twice daily. At the end of 1 year, 2 patients in the treatment group and 3 in the placebo group died, and 8 dropped out or moved. After 6 months of probucol treatment, a significant reduction of serum cholesterol of 17.2% was found in the probucol group. A long-term open trial was continued during the next 8 years. It was found that probucol continued to lower mean serum cholesterol values throughout the trial period. During the first year, loose stools or diarrhea occurred in 19.3% of the patients. Flatulence, constipation, dizziness, vertigo, a changed odor of the skin, itching, pruritus and impotence were reported. No patients were withdrawn from the study due to the side effects.

In all, 11 patients died during the 9-year period. The causes of death were: coronary heart disease (8), an automobile accident (1), pneumonia (1), and cerebrovascular accident (1). No cancer deaths occurred. As no placebo group existed, the morbidity and mortality was compared with the data obtained in the coronary Drug Project and the WHO studies, which strongly limits the value of the investigation.

In a recent review, Tedeschi et al (15R) have summarized clinical studies of 1133 patients more than 300 of whom were treated with probucol for as long as 5 years. The only conclusion which can be drawn from these investigations, is that no unexpected overall excess of morbidity or mortality was found. As long as long-term placebo controlled studies are lacking, it will be impossible to pronounce final judgement on the efficacy and risks of long-term probucol treatment.

Acarbose (α-glucoside hydrolase inhibitor) *(SEDA-7, 410)*

α-Glucoside hydrolase inhibitor is of microbial origin, and inhibits α-amylase and disaccharidase in the intestinal lumen. The compound therefore has a retarding effect on glucose and fat absorption, and has been recommended for use in the treatment of diabetes. In a recent study, 300 mg/day was administered to 9 healthy volunteers for 3 weeks. Plasma triglyceride and VLDL cholesterol levels decreased significantly. Total plasma cholesterol, LDL-cholesterol and HDL-cholesterol levels remained unchanged. Nothing was reported as to side effects (16). It is still too early to decide whether this substance has a future either in antidiabetic therapy (see Chapter 44) or in hyperlipidemic states.

REFERENCES

1. Reuter W (1982) Zur aktuellen Stand der Therapie mit Clofibrat bzw. Clofibrinsäure (Regadrin(R)). *Z. Ärztl. Fortbild., 76*, 437.
2. Mori H, Tanaka T, Sugie S et al (1982) Adenoma with multiple hyperplastic nodules in noncirrhotic liver possibly related to long-term administration of a hypolipidemic drug. *Acta Pathol. Jpn, 32*, 671.
3. Prager R, Schernthaner G, Kostner GM et al (1982) Effect of bezafibrate on plasma lipids, lipoproteins, apolipoproteins AI, AII and B and LCAT activity in hyperlipidemic non-insulin dependent diabetics. *Atherosclerosis, 43*, 321.
4. Martini S, Valerio G, Fellin R et al (1982) Bezafibrate and clofibrate effects on plasma lipids, lipoproteins and apoproteins compared in familial hypercholesterolamia. *Curr. Ther. Res., 31*, 354.

5. Luley C, Schwartzkopff W, Holler HD (1982) Bezafibrat and Etofibrat retard. Vergleichsuntersuchung zur Wirksamkeit auf die Lipide des Blutes bei Hyperlipoproteinämie. *Therapiewoche, 32,* 6469.
6. Olsson AG, Orö L (1982) Dose-response study of the effect of ciprofibrate on serum lipoprotein concentrations in hyperlipoproteinaemia. *Atherosclerosis, 42*, 229.
7. Anonymus (1982) Clinofibrate. *Drugs Today, 18*, 5, 221.
8. Bakir R, Chanu B, Goy-Loeper J et al (1983) Langzeitstudie über lipidsenkende Wirkung und Verträglichkeit von Fenofibrat. *Therapiewoche, 33*, 1935.
9. Lewis JE (1982) Long-term use of gemfibrozil (Lopid[R]) in the treatment of dyslipidemia. *Angiology, 33*, 603.
10. Konttinen A, Kuisma I, Ralli R (1979) The effect of gemfibrozil on serum lipids in diabetic patients. *Am. Clin. Res., 11,* 240.
11. Anon (1980) Lipid lowering drugs. *Med. Letter Drugs Therapeutics, 22*, 16, 66.
12. Mellies MJ, Gartside DS, Glatfelder L et al (1980) Effects of probucol on plasma cholesterol, high and low density lipoprotein cholesterol, and apolipoproteins A1 and A2 in adults with primary familial hypercholesterolemia. *Metabolism, 29,* 956.
13. Hunninghake DB, Bell C, Olson L (1980) Effects of probucol on plasma lipids and lipoproteins in type IIB hyperlipoproteinemia. *Atherosclerosis, 37*, 469.
14. McCaughan D (1982) Nine years of treatment with Probucol. *Artery, 10*, 56.
15. Tedeschi RE, Martz BL, Taylor BJ et al (1982) Safety and effectiveness of probucol as a cholesterol lowering agent. *Artery, 10,* 22.
16. Homma Y, Irie N, Yano Y et al (1982) Changes in plasma lipoprotein levels during medication with a glucoside-hydrolase inhibitor (Acarbose). *Tokai J. Exp. Clin. Med.*, 7, 393.
17. Anon (1982) Report in Drug Adverse Reaction's Series, Kuwait University, Nr 1, October.

K. Wierzba, B. Wańkowicz, A. Piekarczyk
and A. Danysz

47 Cytostatics and immunosuppressive drugs

CARDIOTOXICITY *(SEDA-4, 322; SEDA-5, 407; SEDA-6, 386; SEDA-7, 425)*

The cardiotoxic effects of cytostatics should be borne in mind whenever a patient develops a cardiac disorder during and/or following chemotherapy. It is, however, not always easy to distinguish them from (1) preexisting heart disease, (2) involvement of the heart or pericardium by the tumor, (3) nonbacterial thrombotic endocarditis, (4) infectious complications of therapy affecting the heart, and (5) complications of radiotherapy. These other factors can moreover accentuate the cardiotoxic effects of some cytostatics.

Early toxicity

Adriamycin The incidence of electrocardiographic abnormalities associated with administration of ADR ranges from 0 to 41% of patients receiving the drug (1[R]). The acute electrocardiographic changes occurring with ADR are generally nonspecific. Von Hoff et al (1[R]) have pointed out that

1. most commonly noted abnormalities have included nonspecific ST-T wave changes, sinus tachycardia, premature ventricular and arterial contractions, and low voltage of the QRS complex;
2. ECG changes have been noted both during and after intravenous administration;
3. the ECG changes appear to be unrelated to total dose of ADR administered;
4. an increased incidence of ECG changes is seen in patients with an abnormal baseline electrocardiogram;
5. the ECG changes usually revert to baseline values within periods ranging from a few days to 2 months;
6. the development of transient ECG changes is usually not an indication to discontinue ADR therapy.

Ganz et al (2[C]) have recently described a patient who had developed angina pectoris with ischemic changes on the ECG shortly after receiving ADR with mitomycin C (40 and 14 mg i.v. respectively). The patient experienced a severe and crushing retrosternal chest pain with shortness of breath. An ECG taken approximately 7 hours after drug administration showed persistent but improving T wave inversion.

4′-epi-Doxorubicin 4′-epi-Doxorubicin is a new isomer of ADR with a different steric configuration at position 4 of the sugar moiety. Ferrazzi et al (3[c]) administered 4′-epi-doxorubicin to 65 patients with advanced solid tumors (75 mg/m^2 i.v., once every 21 days). The pattern of acute toxicity was similar to that of ADR. Transient ECG abnormalities consisting of flattening of the T wave were found in about 25% of patients. The ratio of pre-ejection period to the left ventricular ejection time (PEP/LVET) increased within 1 hour after drug administration and returned to near basal values after 24 hours.

Amsacrine (m-AMSA) m-AMSA is an investigational agent that has activity in the treatment of acute leukemia. The dose-limiting toxicity is myelosuppression, but recently serious cardiac arrhythmias and congestive heart failures were noted in some patients receiving the drug; a few patients died.

Weiss et al (4[C]) observed ECG changes in 3 patients receiving infusion of m-AMSA, in the form of prolongation of QT interval. The prolongation of the QT interval was noted about 30 min after starting the infu-

Side Effects of Drugs Annual 8
M.N.G. Dukes, editor

ISBN 0 444 90339 9
$0.80 per article per page (transactional system)
$0.20 per article per page (licensing system)

sion of 160 mg/m^2 of m-AMSA. 2 of the 3 patients had received prior ADR treatment, the total dose being 455 and 340 mg/m^2. Since QT interval prolongation due to m-AMSA may evoke a potentially fatal arrhythmia in hypokalemic patients, it has been suggested that serum potassium should be measured before m-AMSA is administered.

Miller and Rajder (5[c]) have observed acute ECG changes (transient and not related to electrolyte abnormalities) in patients treated with m-AMSA. The ECG, taken 1 hour after m-AMSA infusion, revealed ST-segment alterations and T wave inversion; 24 hours later the ECG reverted to the normal pretreatment pattern. The transient nature of ECG changes may represent a local irritant-like effect on the myocardium.

5-Fluorouracil (5-FU) The cause of 5-FU cardiotoxicity is unknown. The most reasonable hypothesis seems to be that of coronary artery spasm induced by 5-FU or by a vasoactive metabolite, since there is an interval, usually of some hours, between the administration of 5-FU and the appearance of cardiotoxic effects. Labianca et al (6[Cr]) define the clinical characteristics of 5-FU-induced cardiotoxic manifestations as follows:

1. appearance (usually within a few hours after 5-FU administration) of angina and/or myocardial infarction;
2. onset of cardiomyopathy usually after the 4th to 5th administration of the drug;
3. ECG abnormalities (in most cases);
4. changes in cardiac enzymes (in some cases);
5. good response to cardioactive drugs.

A retrospective analysis performed by Labianca et al (6[Cr]) has shown that the incidence of 5-FU-induced cardiotoxicity was not related to the age of patients or to the prior chemotherapy, but was significantly increased (4.5% versus 1.1%) in patients with a positive history of cardiac disease.

2 new cases of 5-FU-induced cardiotoxicity have been reported by Antonelli et al (7[C]) and Vorobiof (8[C]).

Mitoxantrone In contrast to the anthracyclines, preclinical studies with mitoxantrone have not demonstrated cardiotoxicity. Wynert et al (10[C]) have observed only minor, clinically insignificant ECG changes (nonspecific ST-T wave changes) in 5 of 25 patients treated with the drug. 2 of the patients had previously received ADR.

Vindesine Although vindesine has not been reported to induce cardiac ischemia before, Yancey and Talpaz (11[C]) have now described 3 patients on this drug who developed acute chest pain and ECG changes suggestive of acute myocardial ischemia. The ECGs revealed inverted T waves in 1 patient and ST-segment elevation in the 2 others. The cardiac enzyme levels were within normal limits. All 3 patients had an acute episode of chest pain and shortness of breath. The symptoms resolved within 24 hours, and the ECG returned to normal limits within 10 days. An acute coronary spasm can cause angina and was probably the cause of the acute cardiac ischemia in these patients; a release of vasoconstricting substances induced by vindesine may underlie this complication.

Late cardiotoxicity

Adriamycin Late cardiotoxicity is a well-recognized complication of ADR administration. The single most important determinant for the development of congestive heart failure is the total cumulative dose of ADR, and the incidence of cardiomyopathy was presented in Table 1 of SEDA-7, 427. Other factors affecting the degree of risk are age, prior cardiac or liver disease, high dose mediastinal irradiation, route and schedule of administration, and other drugs administered: synergistic cardiotoxicity was reported with cyclophosphamide, vincristine, bleomycin, mitomycin C, mithramycin, dactinomycin, DTIC, beta-blocking agents, halothane (narcosis), and tricyclic antidepressants.

Isner et al (12[Cr]) have designed studies to determine the extent of morphological cardiotoxicity at autopsy in patients treated with anthracyclines (ADR and daunorubicin), and the degree to which the results of morphological examination of autopsy hearts correlate with clinical evidence of cardiac dysfunction. It was found that of 64 patients, 20 (31%) had clinical evidence of cardiotoxicity, and histological signs of cardiotoxicity were observed in 13 of these 20 patients at autopsy. Of the 64 patients, 44 (69%) had shown no clinical signs of cardiotoxicity; histological signs of cardiotoxicity were nevertheless observed in 23 of these 44 patients. This investigation suggests that prediction of ADR cardiotoxicity, even on the basis of histological changes, is uncertain because the correlation between morphological and functional changes is incomplete. Histological signs of toxicity unassociated with clinical toxicity have been frequently observed in patients studied by endomyocardial biopsy, and, if extensive, have been interpreted as a contraindication to continued administration of ADR. On the other hand, the finding of morphological toxicity in asympomatic patients may suggest that such subclinical morphological alterations can be the basis for the development of latent cardiac dysfunction. More complex monitoring is therefore required in patients on ADR chemotherapy.

Richter et al (13[C]), who examined 150 patients treated with ADR to determine the risk of cardiomyopathy using noninvasive techniques, concluded that echocardiography was the most specific noninvasive technique for detecting cardiomyopathy in such patients; the systolic time interval method was less specific but highly sensitive. They considered that the administration of cardiotoxic agents should be stopped when these values were abnormal, even in the absence of symptoms. Richter et al lost no patients from cardiomyopathic complications after adopting this policy.

Daunorubicin Daunorubicin-induced cardiotoxicity is a well-documented phenomenon, but there is very little information available as regards its incidence and risk factors for its development. Von Hoff and Layard (14[Cr]), who analyzed the records of 5613 patients who had received daunorubicin, found that only 110 (1.96%) developed cardiotoxicity. 65 cases showed drug-induced congestive heart failure (1.16%). Daunorubicin-induced cardiomyopathy appeared to be dose-related; in the population that received up to 550 mg/m^2 of daunorubicin, there was only a 4% incidence of congestive heart failure, but at a total dose of 1050 mg/m^2 there was a 14% incidence. The time between the last dose of daunorubicin and the development of congestive heart failure ranged from 14 to 280 days. It was found that the incidence of congestive heart failure was much higher in children than in adults.

Aclacinomycin A Aclacinomycin A is a new antitumor agent of the anthracycline group. In animals it seems to have less cardiac toxicity than ADR, while in humans data currently available indicate that aclacinomycin has only infrequently produced alopecia and cardiac toxicity, even at cumulative doses up to 1350 mg.

Wolley et al (15[C]) have administered aclacinomycin to 22 patients with advanced cancers, monitoring the effects on cardiac function prospectively. One patient developed atrial fibrillation following 3 doses of 15 mg/m^2. This converted spontaneously to normal sinus rhythm, but he was digitalized and subsequently received 2 more drug courses without problems. A patient with advanced breast cancer developed changes in cardiac function. She had previously received 380 mg/m^2 ADR, but no chest irradiation. On day 43 after receiving 100 mg/m^2 of aclacinomycin, she developed congestive heart failure. Repeat scan showed that the ejection fraction had fallen from 49 to 21%.

Anthracyclines in children Favrot et al (16[Cr]) have evaluated 481 children treated with daunorubicin. 13 developed cardiac changes, consisting in 1 case of acute and transient failure of the ventricular extrasystole type, in another of cardiac failure superimposed on preexistent cardiomyopathy, and in the other 11 cases of typical cardiomyopathy. The younger the child, the greater the risk of cardiomyopathy.

Cardiac irradiation, even partial, during ADR administration has resulted in fatal cardiomyopathy. Pinkel et al (17[c]) have reported on 2 children with left-sided Wilms' tumor who died of ADR cardiomyopathy after receiving tumor bed irradiation and doses of ADR normally considered to be within cardiac tolerance. The two 5-year-old girls had received total ADR doses of 450 and 410 mg/m^2, as well as postnephrectomy irradiation that included the lower portion of the heart (2950 and 2100 rads). The combination of ADR and left Wilms' tumor bed irradiation is now used frequently, so that one may expect further reports of cardiomyopathy in children. Some recent cases of cardiomyopathy in children with Wilms' tumor are presented in Table 1. The dose of 350 mg/m^2 should be consid-

Table 1. *Fatal and severe cardiomyopathies in children with Wilms' tumors following ADR and radiotherapy (17Cr)*

Patient	Total ADR dose (mg/m^2)	Radiotherapy
1	450	Prior cardiac irradiation
2	500	Prior cardiac irradiation
3	350	1260 rads to the entire heart
4	400	1250 rads to the entire heart
5	450	Total 2950 rads irradiation of lower portion of heart
6	410	Total 2100 rads irradiation of lower portion of heart
7	330	Thoracic irradiation

ered as a threshold dose for ADR for children who are going to receive irradiation to the left lower heart when the left tumor bed is treated.

Children appear to be relatively more sensitive to the cardiotoxic effects of daunorubicin. Von Hoff and Layard (14Cr) found the incidence of congestive heart failure at total doses greater than 300 mg/m^2 to be significantly higher in children than in adults. At 550 mg/m^2 the risk is 6% for children and 1.3% for adults, while at 1100 mg/m^2 the risk is 16% for children and 6% for adults. This unexpected finding remains unexplained, but it has also been encountered by other investigators with both daunorubicin and ADR.

Mitoxantrone Mitoxantrone (DHAD) was developed in the hope of providing a quinone-containing antitumor agent devoid of cardiotoxicity by replacing the amino sugar with an amino alkyl side chain.

Schell et al (18c) administered mitoxantrone to 31 high-risk patients with refractory breast cancer. Congestive heart failure was observed in 4 of 31 patients, which was surprising and in excess of what one would normally expect in a similar population of patients. Whether congestive heart failure was directly related to the drug cannot be determined from these patients, since this population carried multiple risk factors for cardiovascular decompensation, including pretreatment with ADR (300–450 mg/m^2), precordial radiation therapy, and generally poor performance status. However, this would not alter the observation that this drug is apparently potentially cardiotoxic, either directly or possibly synergistically with ADR.

Congestive heart failure was also observed in 2 children receiving mitoxantrone (total doses 128 and 90 mg/m^2) who had previously been treated with ADR and CDDP (19c).

Prevention of cardiomyopathy The prevention of anthracycline cardiomyopathy has been the object of numerous studies. The free radical scavengers are still a very popular area for investigation because of the hope that the antineoplastic activity will not be impeded while cardiac toxicity will be diminished. Vitamin E has been investigated in some animal systems because it is a lipid soluble antioxidant which can prevent destructive peroxidation of lipids and stabilize biological membranes. Vitamin E deficiency, moreover, produces lesions in both skeletal and cardiac muscle similar to the tissue damage due to ADR.

Legha et al (20C) studied this question in man. Vitamin E was given orally in a dose of 2 g/m^2 daily, starting 7 days prior to ADR therapy. The response rate was similar to that achieved with this chemotherapeutic regimen without vitamin E. No obvious side effects were observed that could be related to vitamin E therapy. 3 of 21 evaluable patients developed congestive heart failure at ADR dose levels of 470, 550 and 820 mg/m^2. The cardiac biopsy findings showed pathological changes in approximately half of the patients at ADR dose levels in the range of 450 to 660 mg/m^2. These results are similar to the author's current experiences with conventional use of ADR. Vitamin E therapy may at best have allowed administration of an additional 100 mg/m^2 of ADR.

Another free radical scavenger, N-acetylcysteine (NAC) is also currently undergoing clinical trials. Dresdale et al (21C) have conducted a randomized prospective trial in 19 patients with ADR-induced cardiomyopathy to determine the efficacy of NAC in reversing the drug's cardiotoxic effects. 11 received oral NAC (5.5 g/m^2 daily for 30 days) and 8 patients served as controls. NAC was not effective in reversing the cardiomyopathy, though this does not exclude the possibility that it might protect against ADR cardiomyopathy when administered prior to, or during, chemotherapy.

Villani et al (22[C]) tried an alternative means of prophylaxis, treating 21 patients with 60–75 mg/m^2 of ADR every 3 to 4 weeks and intermittently with β-methyldigoxin. During treatment, the dose-related changes in left ventricular function (PEP/LVET) in digitalized patients did not differ significantly from basal values even at the highest doses. After completing the ADR treatment and stopping digitalis administration, however, systolic time intervals significantly increased: mean values were not significantly different from those in patients who had received ADR alone. 2 patients developed congestive heart failure. It therefore seems possible to conclude that digitalis, at least when administered intermittently, is not able to prevent ADR-induced cardiomyopathy, but temporarily masks the cardiotoxic effect of the drug by stimulating the heart's functional reserve capacity.

It has recently been shown that L-carnitine, an endogenous amino acid, may protect cardiac cells from the toxic effects of the anthracyclines. Carnitine is known to be essential for the transport of fatty acid groups from the cytoplasm to the mitochondria where it stimulates beta-oxidation. It therefore promotes energy production (especially in those tissues where lipids are the main energy source), and counters the pathological accumulation of free fatty acids in blood and cells, which causes serious toxic effects.

Neri et al (23[C]) have performed a preliminary clinical study on the cardioprotective value of carnitine (3 g daily, 2 days before and 2 days after ADR administration). Carnitine treatment appears to reduce the risk of acute anthracycline cardiotoxicity significantly without introducing new risks. This will obviously require confirmation.

NEUROTOXICITY *(SEDA-6, 392; SEDA-7, 428)*

Many drugs in the expanding arsenal of cytotoxic chemotherapeutic agents are occasionally neurotoxic and a few are regularly neurotoxic. Several agents were reviewed in SEDA-6 (p. 392); in the interest of compactness some recent reports are outlined in Table 2.

Vincristine overdose Vincristine toxicity is mainly related to total dose as well as to the time course over which the drug is taken. The usual course of toxicity related to vincristine as a single agent consists of fever, nausea and vomiting occurring within 24 hours and persisting for 1 week. Peripheral neuropathy, with loss of deep tendon reflexes, development of paresthesias, and muscle weakness (developing over the course of weeks), is often fully established within 4 to 6 weeks and in time partially or completely reversible if it is recognized early and no further drug is given.

Life-threatening toxicity of vincristine has been described (24[c]) in a patient who had received 5 doses of vincristine (1 mg/m^2, total dose 9.5 mg), given in error on consecutive days instead of at much greater intervals. The patient developed weakness, respiratory collapse, fever, and peripheral neuropathy, but recovered within 2 weeks.

When 25 mg of vincristine was administered in error to another patient (25[C]), it caused more dangerous toxic effects, comprising the syndrome of inappropriate secretion of antidiuretic hormone (days 6–10), hepatotoxicity (days 3–10), alopecia, cerebral dysfunction (anxiety, depression, and hallucinations lasting for several weeks), and neurotoxicity. The latter was severe, with paresthesias (days 2–80) and generalized pain in muscles, jaws and abdomen, paralytic ileus (days 5–16), muscular weakness and loss of tendon reflexes (days 4–80), and bladder atony (days 7–16). 6 months after the vincristine overdose, neurological examination still showed a slight paresis of both feet and atrophy of the muscles of both hands.

Manelis et al (26[c]) have reported on a case of fatal toxicity following accidental intrathecal injection of vincristine (0.9 mg)

Table 2. *Neurotoxicity of cytostatic drugs: recent reports*

Drug	Complication	Ref.
m-AMSA	Grand mal seizures in hypokalemic patients; it is recommended to keep a minimum serum potassium value of 3.5 mEq/l	27[c]
Ara-C	Cerebellar dysfunction (marked changes in the Purkinje cell population) in patient treated intravenously with high-dose Ara-C (3000 mg/m² every 12 hours for 3 days)	28[c]
CDDP	Peripheral neuropathy (paresthesia, pain, sensory atoxia)	29[c], 30[Cr]
	Epileptic seizures in 10% of treated patients; hyponatremia and pretreatment impairment of renal function considered possible contributory factors	31[c]
5-FU with allopurinol	Neurotoxicity dose-limiting; consisting of intermittent blurring of vision, decreased sense of balance and dizziness	32[c]
Mechlorethamine	Acute effects: confusion, disorientation, headache, hallucination, lethargy, tremor; delayed effects: personality change, confusion, seizures, dementia	33[c]
Methotrexate	White and grey matter necrosis, following intrathecal administration of 54 times standard dose (650 mg versus 12 mg)	34[c]
Methyl-GAG	Peripheral paresthesias, malaise, vertigo, confusion and tinnitus	35[c]
Misconodazole	Axonal neuropathy with loss of large fibers and secondary demyelination	36[Cr]
	Misonidazole-induced peripheral neuropathy lessened by concomitant administration of dexamethasone (2 mg orally, 3 times a day)	37[Cr]
PALA	Seizures and encephalopathy as cumulative effect over several doses, particularly affecting patients with previously existing brain lesions	38[Cr]
Prednimustine	Grand mal and myoclonic seizures in 10 of 99 evaluable children, associated in 4 patients with intracranial hemorrhage	39[c]
Vincristine	Laryngeal nerve paresis (hoarseness) resolving after drug withdrawal	40[Cr]
	Bilateral peroneal nerve palsies, resulting in paralysis of extensor muscles of foot and ankle (children)	41[c]
Vindesine	Peripheral neuropathy, dose-related	42[c]

to a 5-year-old child. The first sign was severe headache followed by bladder paresis, loss of deep tendon reflexes, progressive sensory loss, and alteration in the state of consciousness. Subsequently respiratory difficulties developed and resulted in respiratory paralysis.

Intrathecally administered vincristine has been fatal in all recorded cases; no treatment is known and no antidote has been found. The removal of cerebrospinal fluid did not diminish the progressive course of the toxic effect.

PULMONARY TOXICITY

Pulmonary disease produced by chemotherapeutic agents is a very significant problem for clinicians for 2 reasons: it is often fatal and it simulates other diseases such as pneumonia or the pulmonary manifestations of leukemia or lymphoma (43[R]). Increased awareness that anticancer drugs may cause pulmonary toxicity has led to more frequent diagnoses and descriptions of this phenomenon. Pulmonary toxicity is usually characterized by dyspnea, cough, abnormal pulmonary auscultation, and chest X-ray changes in a febrile patient. Early detection of such toxicity prior to the onset of X-ray changes may have a significant impact on morbidity and mortality.

Cytotoxic drugs implicated in pulmonary toxicity are shown in Table 3.

Bleomycin Bleomycin is clearly the chemotherapeutic agent most frequently associated with pulmonary toxicity. The effect is dose- and age-related. The incidence of bleomycin-induced lung disease, ranging from nonspecific pneumonitis to pulmonary fibrosis, varies from 2 to 10%. With high doses of bleomycin (more than 450 mg) the mortality rate will be significant (3–5%).

Wilson et al (44[c]) have described a patient who developed histologically proven pulmonary fibrosis following the administration of as little as 30 units of bleomycin.

Open lung biopsy revealed focal interstitial pneumonitis and fibrosis with scattered aggregates of lymphoid and plasma cells. After treatment with prednisone, the patient recovered.

Many factors, including impaired renal failure, can increase the risk. Perry et al (45[c]) observed moderate interstitial pulmonary fibrosis in a patient who had developed deficient renal function due to cisplatin treatment. Reduced renal function can significantly prolong bleomycin elimination since it is primarily excreted in the urine.

The risk of bleomycin-induced lung complications may also be greater in patients receiving bleomycin as a component of combination chemotherapy regimens. Bauer et al (46[C]) in this respect compared 2 therapeutic protocols, i.e. M-BACOD (methotrexate, bleomycin, adriamycin, cyclophosphamide, oncovin, and dexamethasone; median total dose 36 units of bleomycin) and VBP (vinblastine, bleomycin and cisplatin; total bleomycin dose 360 units). An acute pulmonary reaction developed in 18% of patients undergoing M-BACOD treatment, substantially more than one would expect among patients receiving bleomycin alone in comparable total doses. This suggests that interactions with other cytostatics may potentiate its toxicity. The incidence of symptomatic pulmonary complications in patients treated with the VBP regimen was much lower (6.5%), but residual fibrosis on chest X-ray was common among patients surviving for at least 6 months after VBP therapy.

Peplomycin This new bleomycin analog is claimed to have reduced pulmonary toxicity; clinical investigations have been performed primarily in Japan. Clinical trials with the drug were initiated in Europe by Sørensen et al (47[C]). They treated 18 patients with peplomycin twice weekly at different dose levels (from 5 to 15 mg/m^2). 6 patients received 5 mg/m^2 of peplomycin to a cumulative total dose which ranged from 120 to 280 mg; none of these patients developed any signs of pulmonary toxicity. At the dose level of 10 mg/m^2 (cumulative dose 112 to 315 mg), carbon monoxide diffusion capacity and forced vital capacity showed a progressive fall with increasing doses of peplomycin; in 2 of 8 patients dyspnea, nonproductive cough, and diffuse infiltrative changes on the chest X-rays developed. Peplomycin given in a dose of 15 mg/m^2 (total doses ranging from 190 to 350 mg) caused respiratory dysfunction in all treated patients. 2 patients died from severe pulmonary insufficiency despite discontinuation of treatment and initiation of treatment with prednisone. Histological examination of the lungs revealed severe pulmonary fibrosis but no evidence of tumor. As compared with the pulmonary toxicity of bleomycin given in the same way (i.v. twice weekly) and in the same doses (10–15 mg), the pulmonary toxicity of peplomycin actually appeared to be more pronounced.

In a phase II trial also performed by Sørensen et al with peplomycin in 21 treated patients (48[c]), only 1 developed clinical symptoms and a decrease in the lung function test. The 21 patients were here treated using a reduced dose schedule of 5 mg/m^2 given twice weekly intravenously.

Azathioprine Azathioprine-associated pulmonary toxicity appears to be a rare occurrence. Krowka et al (49[c]) have presented a patient who developed a reversible alveolitis after azathioprine treatment. The pulmotoxic effect was characterized by fever, a normal chest radiograph, but a diffusely abnormal gallium scan of both lungs. Pulmonary dysfunction in this patient, who had no respiratory symptoms, was documented by abnormally low single-breath diffusing capacities and restrictive lung vol-

Table 3. *Cytotoxic drugs inducing lung damage*

Drug	Incidence	Dose-relationship	Risk factor
ANTIBIOTICS			
Bleomycin	2–10% severe; 1% fatal	Dose-schedule related (above 500 mg); duration therapy 15 days – 3 months	Age (above 70 years) Radiotherapy (prior or concomitant) Drugs: Bleomycin (previous exposure Cyclophosphamide (concurren High oxygen concentration (during anesthesia)
Peplomycin	12 cases	Dose-related; total dose 195–250 mg	Not known
Mitomycin C	5–12%	At low total doses (50–350 mg); duration of therapy 8 weeks	Previous exposure cyclophosphamide High oxygen concentration Concurrent 5-FU or DTIC administration
Neocarzinostatin	2 cases	Duration of therapy 1 month	–
ALKYLATING AGENTS			
Busulfan	2–11%	Total dose 500–5700 mg; duration of therapy 1–13 years	Radiotherapy to chest may enhance development of interstitial pneumonitis
Cyclophosphamide	Rare reports (16 cases)	More common after total dose of 10 g; duration of therapy 9–120 months	Not known
Chlorambucil	Rare reports (9 cases)	Total dose above 2 g; duration of therapy days up to 2 years	Not known
Melphalan	Rare reports (5 cases)	Total dose 180–360 mg	Age (above 70 years)
NITROSOUREAS			
BCNU	1–30%	1200–1500 mg/m²	Preexisting lung disease Thoracic irradiation Concurrent cyclophosphamide administration
CCNU	Rare reports	Total dose 600–1040 mg; duration of therapy 3 and 26 months	Not known
methyl-CCNU	1 case	Total dose of 4100 mg	Not known
Chlorozotocin	5 cases	240–670 mg/m²	Not known
ANTIMETABOLITES			
Azathioprine	Rare reports (2 cases)	Not determined	Not known
Ara-C	Rare reports (3 cases)	High doses (3000 mg/m² twice daily for 6 days)	Not known
6-Mercaptopurine	Rare reports (3 cases)	Not determined	Not known
Methotrexate	8.5%	High doses; dose-related	Not known

Table 3 (continued)

Drug	Incidence	Dose-relationship	Risk factor
OTHERS			
2′-Deoxycoformycin	First report (1 case)	Not determined	Not known
Procarbazine	5 cases	Not determined (acute onset within some days of first dose)	Not known
VM-26	1 case	Not determined	Not known
Vinblastine	3 cases	Not determined	Mitomycin C

umes. These abnormalities reversed when azathioprine therapy was stopped.

2′-Deoxycoformycin Kahn et al (50[c]) have reported the occurrence of respiratory failure, presenting with sudden onset of severe hypoxia, tachypnea, and rapid evolution of diffuse alveolar infiltrates and pleural effusions, in a pediatric patient who had received deoxycoformycin (0.25 mg/kg for 5 days). He experienced increasing respiratory distress. On physical examination breath sounds were markedly decreased over both lungs. Chest radiographs revealed large bilateral confluent alveolar infiltrates.

NEPHROTOXICITY AND OTHER URINARY COMPLICATIONS *(SEDA-4, 325; SEDA-5, 410; SEDA-6, 393; SEDA-7, 431)*

A number of commonly used antineoplastic agents are associated with renal toxicity. Renal failure may, however, also develop in patients receiving cancer chemotherapy because of the rapid release of intracellular ions and metabolites following destruction of a large mass of tumor cells. Cytotoxic drugs implicated in renal toxicity are shown in Table 4, derived from Weiss and Poster (51[R]).

cis-Dichlorodiammine platinum (CDDP) CDDP is predominantly excreted via the kidney with recovery of up to 90% of the administered dose. Like other heavy metals, platinum is nephrotoxic, but the presence of platinum is not the only factor in renal toxicity; the configuration of the compound is also important. Of this platinum compound, only the cis isomer is nephrotoxic (51[R]). The molecular basis of CDDP renal toxicity is still unknown. CDDP can reduce sulfhydryl groups in kidneys, and this reduction may mediate the renal injury. The initial clinical manifestation of CDDP renal toxicity is a rise in the BUN and/or serum creatinine; creatinine clearance is usually decreased. Proteinuria is not seen, because glomerular injury is not part of the nephrotoxic process. Recently, measurement of the urinary excretion of β_2-microglobulin has been used as a specific and sensitive indicator of proximal tubular dysfunction, even when the serum creatinine has been normal.

Buamah et al (52[C]) have monitored subtle changes in renal function in patients receiving CDDP (100 mg/m^2 at 3-weekly intervals). The mean serum creatinine and creatinine clearance did not change significantly during treatment, provided there

Table 4. *Cancer chemotherapeutic agents and their risk of nephrotoxicity (51[R])*

High risk of immediate nephrotoxicity:
CDDP
MTX (high-dose)
Mithramycin (high-dose)
Streptozotocin
High risk of nephrotoxicity from long-term use:
CCNU
Mitomycin C
Methyl-CCNU
Low to moderate risk of nephrotoxicity:
5-Azacytidine
6-Thioguanine (high-dose i.v.)
MTX (low-dose)
Azotemia without risk of nephrotoxicity:
Dacarbazine
L-Asparaginase
Very low risk of nephrotoxicity:
BCNU
Cyclophosphamide
Daunorubicin
ADR

was adequate hydration and diuresis. There was, however, an overall decline in the excretion of β_2-microglobulin during treatment, with a mean value of 148 μg/mmol creatinine before treatment and 86 μg/mmol creatinine before the 5th course of CDDP. β_2-Microglobulin excretion has earlier been thought to rise after CDDP (SEDA-7, p. 432), but it was then assessed mainly before and shortly after CDDP administration. The excretion of β_2-microglobulin increased in most patients within 5 days of treatment and then fell.

Another indicator of renal tubular dysfunction, hypomagnesemia, has recently been reported with CDDP.

Gonzalez and Villasanta (53[C]) have reported severe magnesium wastage resulting in severe symptomatic hypocalcemia and hypokalemia in patients being treated with CDDP. 6 weeks after the 7th course of CDDP (50 mg/m^2 every 4 weeks), the patient showed severe hypomagnesemia (0.5 mg/dl), hypocalcemia (6.5 mg/dl), hypophosphatemia (6.8 mg/dl), and hypokalemia (3.2 mEq/l).

Studies by Schilsky et al (54[c]) have clearly demonstrated that in many patients hypomagnesemia and renal magnesium wasting are problems that may persist for years following completion of CDDP therapy. 22 of their patients (76%) became hypomagnesemic (serum magnesium lower than 1.4 mEq/l) during chemotherapy, and 11 of these remained persistently hypomagnesemic for a median of 1.3 years following discontinuation of CDDP. In the remaining patients, serum magnesium levels returned to normal 0.2 to 2.1 years after completion of chemotherapy. Symptoms attributable to hypomagnesemia were rarely reported, although muscle cramps, twitching, or mild tremor were noted by the most severely affected patients.

Usually, the incidence of hypomagnesemia is dose-related. Bitran et al (55[C]) have found, however, that even the first dose of CDDP (30–50 mg/m^2) can cause tubular dysfunction with increased urinary losses of calcium, magnesium and amino acids.

Schilsky et al (54[C]) have stated that symptomatic (hypomagnesemic) patients should initially be treated with parenteral $MgSO_4$. These individuals may then require a dietary Mg supplement in an attempt to prevent recurrence of symptoms. The dose of oral Mg prescribed should be determined on the extent of urinary losses and after consideration of the fact that the average daily diet contains approximately 25 mEq of Mg, of which only 30 to 50% is absorbed. It is rarely necessary to raise the serum Mg level to normal, since symptoms are uncommon at serum levels below 1 mEq/L.

Macaulay et al (56[C]) have investigated the prophylactic addition of 3 g $MgSO_4$ to a high-dose CDDP regimen. Hypomagnesemia was rapidly corrected by $MgSO_4$, and the incidence of clinical manifestations significantly decreased.

The most sensitive laboratory test in detecting nephrotoxicity is the measurement of the activity of renal parenchymal enzymes in the urine (enzymuria). Giannattasio et al (57[C]) have assayed the activity of alanine aminopeptidase, γ-glutamyl transpeptidase and alkaline phosphatase as specific markers for the brush border region of proximal tubule in patients on CDDP chemotherapy. There was no alteration in the serum creatinine and BUN, but there was a high urinary excretion rate of brush border membrane enzymes. Maximum excretion of enzymes occurred on the 1st-2nd day and returned to the pretreatment value on the 4th day.

Protection against CDDP-induced nephrotoxicity Heavy metals in general, and CDDP in particular, can injure the kidney in various ways. It is therefore not surprising that many concepts in prevention have been developed and sometimes tested in the clinical situations. Several manoeuvres to keep nephrotoxicity within acceptable limits are presented in Table 5.

Adriamycin Intravesical ADR administration is used in the management of superficial bladder tumors. Yu et al (58[c]) treated 35 patients with intravesical ADR; 12 of them had microscopic hematuria before and after treatment; 4 patients showed evidence of tubulo-proteinuria (excretion of α_1-microglobulin, β_2-microglobulin or N-acetyl-glucosamidase); and 4 had detectable fibrinogen degradation products. The fibrinogen degradation levels were always increased in patients with microscopic hematuria. 27 patients demonstrated an increased excretion of carcinoembryonic antigen. It is well established that urinary carcinoembryonic antigen originates from

Table 5. *Factors diminishing CDDP-induced nephrotoxicity*

Factor	Rationale	Ref.
1. Hydration and/or furosemide- or mannitol-induced diuresis	Swelling of tissues possibly inhibited by hyperosmotic agent, mannitol and suppression of renin-angiotensin system by hydration with saline	51[R]
2. Probenecid	May inhibit peritubular uptake of heavy metals	51[R]
3. SH-groups containing compounds - cysteamine - WR 2721 - Na-thiosulfate	Application for nephrotoxicity prevention based on theory that Pt tubular toxicity is mediated through Pt binding to SH-groups on tubular transport enzymes. They may act as effective Pt chelator	67[C] 68[Cr]
4. CDDP circadian timing	Renal toxicity of CDDP markedly dependent upon circadian stage of drug administration	69[r]

the lower urinary tract and is not filtered from the plasma by the glomeruli.

Cyclosporin A Keown et al (59[c]) have examined the adverse effects of cyclosporin on the kidney in relation to serum concentrations of the drug in 15 patients. Acute nephrotoxicity, defined by a transient rise in serum creatinine in the absence of clinical or immunologic evidence of graft rejection, was observed in 8 patients. None of these episodes occurred with serum cyclosporin levels of less than 200 ng/ml; 1 occurred with levels between 200 and 400 ng/ml, and 7 with levels exceeding 400 ng/ml.

Cyclophosphamide Vesical irritability and hemorrhage have been recognized as common side effects of cyclophosphamide administration. Moreover, the increasing use of high doses of cyclophosphamide has been accompanied by many instances of massive hemorrhage. The occurrence of hemorrhagic cystitis is thought to be a toxic effect of cyclophosphamide metabolites (acrolein) directly on the bladder mucosa.

Droller et al (60[C]) have used a new regimen of hydration, diuresis and bladder drainage to diminish the concentration of cyclophosphamide or its metabolites and the time of their contact with the bladder mucosa. Their patients received 50 mg/kg cyclophosphamide (for 4 days) and 4–5 l of parenteral fluids every 24 hours, beginning 24 hours prior to infusion of cyclophosphamide, to maintain urine output at 150–200 ml/hour. Patients were asked to void every hour, even at night. If there was any evidence of residual urine, a catheter was inserted. Of 97 patients who had been treated with high-dose cyclophosphamide prior to the diuresis regimen, 8 developed massive hemorrhages, which were directly fatal in 6 cases. After institution of this new regimen, massive, clot-producing cystitis developed in only 1 of 198 treated patients.

Ifosfamide Ifosfamide, like cyclophosphamide, is an alkylating agent that must be metabolized in order to become an active cytotoxic agent. One of the metabolites is again acrolein, which is considered to be the principle bladder irritant.

Morgan et al (61[C]) have confirmed earlier findings that the oral use of N-acetylcysteine is promising in providing protection against ifosfamide-induced bladder toxicity with no compromise of the therapeutic response.

Earlier clinical study in Germany showed that mesnum (2-mercaptoethane sulfonate) significantly lowers the frequency of microhematuria during therapy with ifosfamide. Recently, similar effects were observed by Falkson et al (62[C]). It is evident that with mesnum urotoxicity is very much decreased, but that there is little, if any, protective effect against the hemopoietic toxicity. The uroprotective effect of mesnum has also been confirmed by Araujo and Tessler (63[C]) in 45 patients treated with ifosfamide (2250 mg/m^2 plus mesnum 840 mg/m^2).

Streptozotocin Nephrotoxicity of streptozotocin, in the form of transient proteinuria, azotemia, abnormalities of tubular function, and acute renal failure, is dose-limiting.

Hall-Craggs et al (64[C]) have reported on a patient who received streptozotocin for 4 months (total dose 38.2 g) and developed acute renal failure. At autopsy the kidneys showed acute tubular necrosis. Although these changes predominantly involved the proximal tubules, the cortical ducts were also affected. Cellular debris and polymorphonuclear leukocytes were found in the collecting duct lumens. No interstitial inflammation was present but some interstitial fibrosis was seen.

Methyl-CCNU The nephrotoxicity of methyl-CCNU has previously been reported; the effect is dose-related. A virtually 100% incidence of severe renal damage has been demonstrated in children receiving a cumulative dose of 1500 mg/m^2 of methyl-CCNU or CCNU. Recently, Micetich et al (65[C]) have observed abnormalities of renal function in 7 of 45 patients treated with methyl-CCNU; all these 7 patients had received more than 1400 mg/m^2. No clinical signs of renal insufficiency were detected at lower doses. The renal damage comprised globerulo-interstitial changes.

Methotrexate (MTX) Nephrotoxicity is one of the potentially serious problems encountered in the use of MTX. Pathological reports have noted renal tubular damage, probably due to intratubular precipitation of MTX. The incidence of renal toxicity has been markedly reduced with the use of adequate hydration and alkalization.

Freeman-Narrod et al (66[C]) have shown elevated urinary concentrations of lysozyme in patients treated with high-dose MTX. The lysozyme is a low molecular weight protein found in the highest concentrations in the kidneys; generally, lysozyme will not appear in the urine except in cases of renal tubular damage. Lysozyme was measured in 88 patients and detected in 10% of instances after an MTX dose, levels ranging from 2 to 120 μg/ml. There was no relationship to age, dose or to rises in serum creatinine, but there was a correlation with the administration of aminoglycoside antibiotics. Most of these elevations occurred early and lasted for 24 to 48 hours. The rises occurring after 5 days were persistent and were associated with prolonged exposure to MTX. Increased lysozyme excretion, which is due to renal tubular damage, did not parallel increased serum creatinine concentrations, which are indicative of glomerular filtration.

HEPATOTOXICITY *(SEDA-4, 326; SEDA-5, 411; SEDA-6, 393; SEDA-7, 433)*

Amsacrine (m-AMSA) The sometimes fatal hepatic toxicity now known to be associated with m-AMSA was predicted by the preclinical toxicology studies, but was not noted in the phase I trials.

Recently, a case of fatal hepatic toxicity has been reported in a patient who had been given m-AMSA (120 mg/m^2 for 5 consecutive days) (70[c]). On day 17 her liver function tests first became abnormal, with a bilirubin 2.3 mg/100 ml and an alkaline phosphatase 286 U/l. Over the next 10 days, liver dysfunction progressed to liver failure, which was fatal. The patient's bilirubin increased to 16.5 mg/100 ml; alkaline phosphatase increased to 460 units/l. Finally, she developed hepatic encephalopathy and coma. A diffuse and severe hepatocellular injury was found at autopsy.

Another case of fatal hepatotoxity after m-AMSA administration has been described by Dupont et al (71[c]). A 10-year-old girl developed liver failure and died in hepatic coma 2 weeks after the first m-AMSA cycle was completed. The serum transaminases were repeatedly normal, but the total bilirubin rose to 21 mg/100 ml prior to death. The patient had a positive hepatitis B antigen titer but no history of overt hepatitis.

Life-threatening hepatotoxicity has been reported by Lawrence (72[c]) in 23 cycles of m-AMSA therapy (120 mg/m^2 every 3 weeks). 4 patients had bilirubin elevations above 10 mg/100 ml and alkaline phosphatases greater than twice normal. One of these patients developed progressive hepatic failure; percutaneous liver biopsy revealed severe centrilobular necrosis and fatty degeneration. 3 months after receiving his first course of m-AMSA the patient relapsed and died.

m-AMSA is an important new antileukemic agent. However, the occurrence of fatal toxicity in the patients reported here should alert physicians to the fact that liver function abnormalities arising during the course of m-AMSA chemotherapy may be due to this drug, and m-AMSA should be used with caution in patients with known hepatic dysfunction.

Dacarbazine (DTIC) DTIC has been considered a relatively safe drug, but hepatotoxicity of the drug has previously been reported. Recently, Doering et al (73[c]) have described an additional case of a patient with the Budd-Ghiari syndrome following DTIC administration. The disease was manifested by severe liver disease with acute thrombosis of intrahepatic veins and parenchymal cell necrosis (veno-occlusive disease). The pathological findings and the appearance of the clinical symptoms only during the second injection suggested an allergic reaction of the liver.

Estramustine phosphate Estramustine phosphate is a compound incorporating an alkylating agent and a steroid hormone. Dawes (74[c]) gave the drug (560 mg/day orally) to 16 patients with advanced breast cancer. When 2 patients with biochemical evidence of liver disease started estramustine therapy, their livers became painful and tender. One patient became jaundiced. The jaundice and pain regressed when estramustine was discontinued. The second patient died of advanced breast cancer while taking estramustine, without any improvement in the hepatic symptoms.

5-Fluorouracil and 5-fluorodeoxyuridine (5-FU and 5-FUdR) Intra-arterial administration of 5-FU (5–10 mg/kg/day) followed by 5-FUdR (0.2 mg/kg/day) permits higher drug exposure than intravenous administration. Barone et al (75[C]) have studied the effect of intra-arterial 5-FU/5-FUdR administration with whole liver irradiation in patients with metastatic colon carcinoma to the liver. They found a close inverse relationship between hepatotoxic effects and survival time. In those patients whose liver function tests (bilirubin and alkaline phosphatase) were less than twice normal, the median survival was 770 days; it decreased to 178 days in those patients with liver tests values greater than two times normal.

Mitomycin C Toxic reactions to conventional doses of mitomycin C include alopecia, nausea, vomiting, diarrhea, stomatitis and dysfunction of the renal, cardiac and pulmonary systems. The dose-limiting toxicity is bone marrow suppression, which is typically delayed in onset and may be cumulative.

Intensive therapy with increasing doses of mitomycin C and autologous bone marrow transplantation was employed in 29 patients with refractory malignancies (76[C]). 6 of 29 patients developed the clinical syndrome of hepatic veno-occlusive disease characterized by progressive abnormalities in liver function, abdominal pain, and ascites some 15–70 days after starting mitomycin C therapy. The patients in whom veno-occlusive disease occurred had all previously received cyclophosphamide, ADR or 5-FU, but it was difficult to pinpoint these as clear risk factors.

Rubidazone and 5-azacitidine 29 patients with advanced acute nonlymphocytic leukemia were treated with intensive chemotherapy consisting of 5-azacitidine and rubidazone (77[c]). 15 patients developed hepatic function abnormalities usually manifested by an elevation of the serum alkaline phosphatase and the SGOT to twice normal. 5 patients became jaundiced and hepatic failure was thought to have played a role in the death of 1 patient.

6-Thioguanine (6-TG) 6-Thioguanine, an antimetabolite of purine, elevated hepatic enzymes (alkaline phosphatase and aspartate aminotransferase) in 3 of 29 patients treated for polycythemia rubra vera (78[c]). One patient developed cholestatic jaundice which resolved when therapy with 6-TG was stopped.

A case of reversible veno-occlusive disease of the liver caused by 6-TG has been reported by Krivoy et al (79[c]).

Vincristine Radiation hepatitis is well known, and the incidence of the disease increases with higher doses of irradiation. Usually, radiation hepatitis appears when the whole liver is irradiated with more than 2500–3000 rads in adults; children are more sensitive. Increased sensitivity of the liver has been described whether there is concomitant or early subsequent chemotherapy with ADR, actinomycin D and 5-FU.

Recently, Hansen et al (80[c]) have reported a case of total hepatotoxicity caused by vincristine-induced increased radiosensitivity.

A 30-year-old woman was treated with vincristine (1.6 mg weekly) for 4 weeks. 4 weeks after the last dose of vincristine, irradiation was initiated (2250 rads during 49 days) to a large abdominal field, including the liver. During the course of radiation therapy, reinduction treatment was given with prednisone, 65 mg daily for 1 week every month, and vincristine, 0.8 mg, 2 weeks before terminating the irradiation. 1 week after radiotherapy termination the patient experienced severe jaundice with a strong rise in transaminase and a very low prothrombin value. At the same time, a high fever and gradually increasing ascites developed. Hepatic coma developed terminating in death 4 weeks after the first signs of liver disease. The liver lesions corresponded to the lesions which might be observed after high irradiation doses.

OTOTOXICITY *(SEDA-6, 393; SEDA-7, 434)*

Cisplatin (cis-dichlorodiammine platinum, CDDP) The most important adverse effects of CDDP are nephrotoxicity (see above) and ototoxicity; the latter is both cochlear and vestibular. The hearing loss generally increases in severity with age, dose, and frequency of treatment. Young children and individuals with preexisting hearing loss impairments are also highly susceptible to CDDP ototoxicity. It has been suggested that the audiometric abnormalities are correlated with the mode of administration of CDDP, the highest incidence being associated with bolus injection.

Vermorken et al (81[C]) studied hearing acuity in 48 patients prior to and following CDDP administration as (1) a single low dose of 25–50 mg/m², (2) a single high dose of 70–120 mg/m², and (3) a daily dose of 20 mg/m² for 5 days. The doses were variously given by rapid infusion (4–15 min), 2-, 3-, or 24-hour infusion. Clinical hearing loss occurred in 12.5% of patients. The incidence of audiographic changes (65% overall, 81% bilaterally) increased with increasing cumulative dose independent of the treatment schedule. The median cumulative doses at which audiographic changes occurred in a single high dose and a low daily dose for 5 days were 110 and 400 mg/m² respectively. The incidence was correlated with the daily dose, and changes were more severe after a single high dose. Rapid infusion of a single high dose was more ototoxic than a 24-hour infusion of the same dose.

The most prominent ototoxic effects of CDDP are observed at 8000 Hz. It is very important to determine the changes in hearing threshold, following CDDP therapy, within a frequency range which includes 2000 Hz, because accurate perception of speech is dependent upon acoustic information contained within that range. Most studies have not reported significant ototoxicity at 2000 Hz. Fleming et al (82[c]) have, however, observed significant changes in hearing threshold at both 2000 and 8000 Hz in patients treated with CDDP as a combination therapy. The prechemotherapy hearing threshold at 2000 Hz was initially 21.9 decibels and it increased to 28.57 decibels following drug treatment.

McHaney et al (83[c]) have investigated ototoxic effects in children following CDDP therapy. The first significant threshold shift (more than 10 decibels from the baseline) was observed at 8000 Hz in 5 of 10 patients who received a cumulative dose of 270 mg/m^2; above 450 mg/m^2 all patients experienced hearing losses at 8000 Hz. At 6000 and 4000 Hz, the percentage of affected patients increased more slowly with increasing cumulative dosage. A threshold shift at 2000 Hz was observed in all patients treated with CDDP in a cumulative dosage higher than 1080 mg/m^2.

Regardless of CDDP dosage or test frequency, younger children showed greater hearing loss (hearing loss inversely related to age). There was no recovery of hearing loss in any child during a period of 15 months following cessation of therapy. Hearing abnormalities can delay speech and language development in very young children, creating learning difficulties.

OCULAR TOXICITY *(SEDA-5, 413; SEDA-6, 314; SEDA-7, 434)*

Ocular toxicity with cytostatics is generally uncommon, but can cause all gradations of ocular and visual complaints, including blindness. Cytotoxic and immunosuppressive drugs implicated in ocular toxicity are shown in Table 6, derived from SEDA-7, p. 434, but here expanded with data from Frauenfelder et al (84[R]).

5-Trifluoromethyldeoxyuridine (trifluridine) Trifluridine is used for the treatment of herpes simplex keratitis and is known to induce hypersensitivity and toxic reactions affecting the eyes.

Recently, Maudgal et al (85[c]) have reported the development of corneal epithelial

Table 6. *Cytotoxic and immunosuppressive drugs exerting ocular toxicity*

Drug	Eye toxicity	Incidence cases reported
Adriamycin	Lacrimation	25%
2-Anhydro-β-D-arabinofuranosyl-5-fluorocytosine	Eye pain, conjunctivitis (in 6% dose-limiting reaction)	41%
Ara-C	Conjunctivitis, photophobia	17 cases
Busulfan	Posterior subcapsular cataract	7 cases
Corticosteroids	Posterior subcapsular cataract	21–36%
Cis-platinum	Optic neuritis	2 cases
Cyclophosphamide	Blurred vision	5 cases
Dibromomannitol	Posterior subcapsular cataract	5 cases
5-Fluorouracil	Excessive lacrimation or conjunctivitis	23 cases
	Cicatricial ectropion	4 cases
	Oculomotor disturbances	
Methotrexate	Ocular irritation	25%
	Conjunctivitis	7 cases
Methyl-GAG	Bilateral ocular keratopathy	1 case
Mitotane	Blurred vision, lens opacities, retinal hemorrhage	rare
Nitrosoureas	Optic neuritis	9 cases
	Intraretinal hemorrhage	3 cases
Tamoxifen	Retinopathy	4 cases
Vinca alkaloids	Diplopia, ptosis	23 cases
	Optic neuropathy	3 cases

dysplasia in 3 patients treated topically with trifluridine for 1 to 6 months. The corneal epithelial dysplasia in these old patients was characterized by severe cellular atypism, pleomorphism, loss of polarity and a few mitotic figures. After scraping and cessation of therapy, the edema and opaque cells disappeared in 3 to 4 months.

BCNU The ocular toxicity of the nitrosoureas is not extensively documented. However, Shingleton et al (86^{Cr}) have now reported on 9 patients with ocular complications after BCNU therapy. Evidence of delayed bilateral ocular toxicity developed in 2 of 50 patients treated with high dose intravenous BCNU (800 mg/m^2). 7 of 10 patients, treated with intra-arterial carotid doses of BCNU to a cumulative level of at least 450 mg/m^2, developed evidence of delayed ocular toxicity ipsilateral to the side of the infusion. The symptoms began 2 to 14 weeks following infusion. BCNU ocular toxicity appeared to be secondary to segmental introretinal vasculitis and obstruction. This produced nerve fiber-layer infarcts and retinal hemorrhages.

CARCINOGENECITY *(SEDA-6; 394; SEDA-7, 435)*

Most cytotoxic agents are known to be mutagens, as are the forms of radiation used in radiatherapeutic procedures. Cytotoxic treatment can therefore lead to the development of cell variants, which have either an enhanced or diminished malignant phenotype. The indication from a number of studies that treatment does not alter the life-span of cancer patients is compatible with this view, for if bulk reduction of a life-threatening cancer does not prolong life, it could be that the growth rate and malignancy status of the tumor have been changed by the treatment (87^{r}).

Schmähl et al (88^{R}) of DKFZ (Heidelberg) have reviewed 303 case reports of patients who had developed second tumors following chemotherapy. It was found that the second tumors were reported most frequently after chemotherapy of Hodgkin's disease. The incidence of cytotoxic drug-induced second malignancy in patients with various primary diseases is presented in Table 7. Cyclophosphamide and other alkylating agents were the drugs most often implicated in second malignancy induction.

Table 7. *Incidence of cytotoxic drug-induced second malignancies as correlated with primary disease, derived from Schmähl et al (88[R])*

Primary disease	Incidence	
	N	%
Hodgkin's disease	51	32
Multiple myeloma	43	27
Ovarian carcinoma	26	16
Breast cancer	19	12
Chronic lymphoid leukemia	11	7
Bronchial carcinoma	9	6
Total	159	100

The median doses and the latent periods required to induce second malignancy are presented in Table 8.

Coltman and Dixon (89[Cr]) have described 32 second malignancies (21 acute leukemias and 11 solid tumors) among 659 patients with all stages of Hodgkin's disease. The actuarial risk of developing leukemia at 7 years was 6.2% for chemotherapy alone, 6.4% for combined modality, and 7.7% for salvage chemotherapy. The actuarial risk of solid tumor development was lower. There was an increased incidence of second malignancy with respect to age. The actuarial risk of acute leukemia among those who began treatment of their Hodgkin's disease at more than 40 years of age is 20.7 ± 6.2% at 7 years. Among patients with solid tumors the age factor was also evident.

A very high risk of leukemia was observed in women receiving chemotherapy for ovarian cancer who had survived for more than 2 years.

Recently, Einhorn et al (90[Cr]) have studied the late side effects of chemotherapy in 51 women who had received at least 300 mg of melphalan for ovarian cancer and had survived for at least 3 years. Within some years of the start of chemotherapy, an irreversible hematological disturbance was noted in 6 of 51 patients. In 5 cases the changes were characterized by hypercellularity of the bone marrow, including all the blood cell precursors, with concurrent pancytopenia in the peripheral blood. These changes were followed by a picture of acute myeloid or erythroblastic leukemia. The risk of leukemia in women who survived for 3 or more years after melphalan treatment was estimated to be 950 times greater than the leukemia risk in the total female population.

Table 8. *Median dose of cytotoxic drugs administered and latent periods of second malignancy, derived from Schmähl et al (88[R])*

Cytotoxic drug	Median total dose (mg)	Median latent period (months)
Cyclophosphamide	74,000	54
Chlorambucil	2,505	60
Nitrogen mustard	42	44
Busulfan	643	62
Thio-TEPA	150	50
Azathioprine	108,000	48
Melphalan	1,550	48

Greene et al (91[Cr]) have evaluated the occurrence of acute nonlymphocytic leukemia (ANL) among 1399 women with ovarian cancer. Of these, 998 had been treated with alkylating agents, and among these patients 12 cases of ANL were observed. No ANL developed in patients treated only with surgery or radiation or both. This study showed that there was an excess risk of ANL in patients with ovarian cancer who had been treated with alkylating agents and that melphalan and chlorambucil were 2 specific agents associated with this risk. 9 of the 10 cases treated with melphalan received more than 700 mg, whereas the chlorambucil-related cases received more than 2000 mg.

Second malignant neoplasms were also reported in children. However, the information on the incidence is limited because of the rarity of pediatric cancer.

Miké et al (92[Cr]) have estimated the incidence of second malignancies in 14,610 children. There were 113 cases of second malignancy. The average age at diagnosis was 7 years (0–14) for the first malignant disease, and 17 years (2–35) for the second. The mean interval between the 2 diagnoses was 10 years (0–27). The estimated rate of second malignant disease 5 to 15 years after the first disease was 188/100,000 a year. The corresponding age-adjusted rate for all races was 19/100,000 a year, i.e. there is approximately a tenfold increase in the risk of second cancer during a 5–15 follow-up period.

Recently, Elliott et al (93[c]) have reported on 2 patients who developed bladder carcinoma following cyclophosphamide therapy for systemic lupus erythematosus. The patients had taken cyclophosphamide 50–100 mg daily for 6 and 7 years respectively.

OCCUPATIONAL HEALTH HAZARDS OF HANDLING CYTOTOXIC AGENTS *(SEDA-7, 438)*

The first known report on the possible occupational hazard of handling cytostatics was published by Falck and related to nurses. Concern about the potential occupational exposure of pharmacy personnel to cytotoxic agents was the subject of studies by Anderson et al (94[Cr]).

8-day continuous urine collections in 24-hour sample lots were obtained from persons who prepared intravenous admixture solutions containing chemotherapeutic agents (12–90 admixtures per working day). These persons worked in the normally used horizontal-flow hoods. Urine samples were also collected from persons who worked in the pharmacy but did not mix or handle anticancer drugs. Mutagenicity was observed in the urine of all personnel during periods when they prepared admixtures in horizontal laminar-flow hoods, both when using no protection and while wearing gloves or masks. When admixtures were prepared in the vertical-flow biological safety hoods by personnel wearing gloves, no urine mutagenicity was detected. The control group showed no urine mutagenicity.

The relevance of drug exposure to these personnel is not known. Effects may be subclinical or remain latent for many years following exposure.

Gallelli (95[r]) has commented on Anderson's article and stressed the need for personnel handling antineoplastic drugs to take extensive precautions to prevent exposure.

GONADAL TOXICITY *(SEDA-4, 326; SEDA-5, 412; SEDA-6; 395; SEDA-7, 438)*

Cytotoxic drugs implicated in gonadal toxicity are presented in Table 9.

Male gonads

Amsacrine (m-AMSA) Da Cunha et al (97[C]) treated a male melanoma patient with m-AMSA (40 mg/m^2/day for 3 days every 3 weeks) and tested gonadal function. Semen analysis of specimens collected before, during, and after 9 courses of m-AMSA revealed an increase in abnormally shaped sperm at the end of treatment as well as a steady decline of sperm concentration and motility followed by a rapid recovery. 13 weeks after cessation of therapy, the patient's sperm count returned to its pretreatment level. The rapid recovery of normal spermatogenesis observed during the interruption of chemotherapy indicates that m-AMSA has only a temporary, reversible effect on differentiating germinal cells with no toxicity to the stem cells.

MVPP (nitrogen mustard, vinblastine, prednisolone, procarbazine) Waxman et al (98[C]) have reported the results of a long-term study of gonadal function in 46 men in prolonged remission of advanced Hodgkin's disease after cyclical MVPP combination chemotherapy. In this study, 36 (88%) of the 41 men became azoospermic or severely

Table 9. *Cytotoxic drugs known to induce gonadal dysfunction (100[R])*

Males	Females
Radiation	Radiation
Busulfan	Busulfan
Chlorambucil (2.4–79 mg/kg)	Chlorambucil (150 mg)
Cyclophosphamide (1–52 g)	Cyclophosphamide (12–63 g)
Nitrogen mustard (400 mg)	Nitrogen mustard
Vinblastine	Vinblastine
Adriamycin (625 mg/m^2)	
Corticosteroids (500 mg)	
Ara-C	
Methotrexate	
Probarbazine (7–101 g)	
Vincristine	

oligospermic. A small proportion of men who had been under 30 years of age at the start of treatment (20%) showed partial recovery, although this was delayed by up to 10 years. None of the men developed impaired testosterone secretion or impotence.

MOPP (nitrogen mustard, vincristine, prednisolone, procarbazine) Whitehead et al (99[Cr]) have studied survivors of childhood Hodgkin's disease who had received MOPP treatment. 12 of 15 males showed normal progression of pubertal development after completing their treatment. 9 out of 10 late pubertal or adult subjects had small testes, but only 1 developed gynecomastia. Each of the 6 males who provided semen analysis was azoospermic after an interval of 2.4 to 8 years following completion of treatment.

Female gonads

Ovarian susceptibility to injury by cytotoxic agents is clearly correlated with age at the time of treatment. The ovaries of prepubertal girls are fairly resistant to the toxic effects of chemotherapeutic agents. In adult women, cytotoxic therapies have variable effects on fertility and gonadal function (100[R]). From their late twenties onwards, women exposed to cytotoxic drugs have an increased risk of sustaining complete ovarian failure. The clinical picture includes amenorrhea, postmenopausal levels of gonadotropins and estradiol as well as associated climacteric symptoms. The occurrence and intensivity of these symptoms vary according to the age at which the menopause occurs. They are worse in young women, but they may be troublesome even in some women in their late forties. 85% of women over the age of 25 develop complete irreversible ovarian failure after 6 cycles of MOPP or MVPP therapy.

Dnistrian et al (101[Cr]) investigated the effect of CMF (cyclophosphamide, MTX, 5-FU) adjuvant therapy on endocrine function in both pre- and postmenopausal breast cancer patients. CMF therapy resulted in suppression of ovarian function in some premenopausal patients, but pituitary and adrenal function were unaffected. There was an inverse relationship between age and the duration of treatment required to induce ovarian suppression. Although amenorrhea was achieved within 2 to 4 months in patients aged 40 or older, younger women required large cumulative doses to induce ovarian dysfunction.

Waxman et al (98[C]) have reported on 28 women who had received MVPP therapy for advanced Hodgkin's disease. 22 of the 28 women with regular menses before chemotherapy became amenorrheic. There was no late return of menstruation if periods had failed to return within 3 months after the completion of treatment. 5 of the 6 patients whose menses remained normal had been aged under 30 at the time of treatment, and 2 of these subsequently had normal pregnancies and delivered normal children.

Cases of pregnancy following MOPP chemotherapy have been reported by Andrieu et al (102[C]). They retrospectively studied 62 women who had been given 3 to 6 cycles of MOPP chemotherapy. After treatment, 30 pregnancies were recorded in 22 of the 50 women who were still menstruating.

NAUSEA AND VOMITING

Nausea and vomiting induced by cancer chemotherapeutic agents is a common and often dose-limiting problem for cancer patients. It can lead to anorexia and malnutrition (107[R]). Cytotoxic drugs implicated in the induction of nausea and vomiting are shown in Table 10, derived from Borison and McCarthy (108[R]).

Pharmacological management of chemotherapy-induced nausea and vomiting

The site of action of emetic cytotoxic drugs has been little studied. Mechlorethamine seems to stimulate the chemoreceptor trigger zone and to have a cortical and peripheral action. The effects of CDDP have been variously attributed to stimulation at peripheral sites and through the chemoreceptor trigger zone. Cytotoxic drugs may inhibit the synthesis in the chemoreceptor trigger zone of those enzymes which are responsible for the breakdown of enkephalin (109[r]). The subsequent accumulation of enkephalin would then stimulate receptors in the chemoreceptor trigger zone with the release of dopamine, which acts as an intermediary.

Whatever may be the mode of action of these drugs, the immediate problem is to

Table 10. *Cytotoxic drugs inducing nausea and vomiting (108[R])*

Drug	Time in hours onset	duration	Remarks
Incidence >90%			
CDDP	1–6	24–48	Vomiting generally severe
Dacarbazine	1–3	1–12	Vomiting often dose-limiting
Mechlorethamine	0.5–2	8–24	
Streptozotocin	1–4	12–24	Vomiting can be dose-limiting
Incidence 60–90%			
BCNU	2–4	4–24	Delayed anorexia
CCNU	2–6	4–6	Severe
Cyclophosphamide	4–12	4–10	Dose-related
Actinomycin D	2–6	12–24	Vomiting can be dose-limiting
Mithramycin	4–6	12–24	
Mitotane	Delayed	Persistent	Dose-limiting
Methyl-CCNU	4–6	6–8	Delayed anorexia
Procarbazine	24–27	Variable	Dose-related
Incidence 30–60%			
Adriamycin	4–6	6	Severe
Azacytidine	1–4	3–4	Dose-related
L-Asparaginase	1–3	–	
Daunomycin	2–6	24	Severe
5-Fluorouracil	3–6	–	Dose-limiting
Hexamethylmelamine	3–6	–	Dose-limiting
Mitomycin C	1–4	48–72	
Incidence 10–30%			
Ara-C	6–12	3–5	Dose-related
Bleomycin	3–6	–	Emetic tolerance develops
Estrogens	24–48	Extended	Emetic tolerance develops
Etoposide	3–8	–	Severe with oral route
Hydroxyurea	6–12	–	Dose-related
Ifosfamide	1–2	Extended	
Melphalan	6–12	–	

reduce vomiting. The widely used dopamine antagonists are believed to block receptors at the chemoreceptor trigger zone. The phenothiazines have been effective in several trials (113[C]), the most useful probably being prochlorperazine and thiethylperazine. The clinical effectiveness of phenothiazines and related drugs for managing chemotherapy-induced nausea and vomiting has been presented in a review article by Wampler (110[R]).

Metoclopramide, another dopamine antagonist, appears to be more effective in preventing vomiting due to CDDP than placebo or prochlorperazine (111[C], 112[C]).

Anticipatory nausea and vomiting (ANV)

So-called anticipatory nausea and vomiting is characterized by nausea and vomiting prior to, and in anticipation of, cytotoxic drug administration (105[c], 106[c]).

Morrow and Morrell (103[Cr]) observed ANV in 120 of 500 cancer patients (24%). A similar incidence of ANV was found in women receiving cyclophosphamide, methotrexate and 5-fluorouracil (CMF) adjuvant chemotherapy for breast cancer (104[C]). Among the 52 patients, ANV occurred in 17 (33%), while postchemotherapy nausea and vomiting was experienced by 46 (88%). There was a significant relationship between both higher doses of CMF and severe postchemotherapy nausea and vomiting on the one hand and the development of ANV on the other. Since no patient developed ANV without first developing postchemotherapy nausea and vomiting, it seems likely that the relationship between the higher dose of CMF and ANV is mediated through the severe postchemotherapy nausea and vomiting caused by that regimen.

Since ANV has a large psychological component and may represent a learned or conditioned phenomenon, systematic desensitization and relaxation techniques might be helpful for some patients.

DERMATOLOGICAL TOXICITY

Skin changes in patients receiving cytotoxic drugs may have a variety of causes. Direct toxic effects of the agent on skin and cutaneous appendages cause the most frequent and clinically distinctive reactions.

Alopecia

The most common cutaneous effect of chemotherapy is diffuse hair loss, due to a toxic effect of the drug on the rapidly dividing cells of the hair bulb. Adriamycin and cyclophosphamide are particularly toxic to hair bulbs, both as a single agents or in combination with other drugs. Other agents that commonly produce alopecia when given in sufficient doses include MTX, 5-FU, vincristine, daunomycin, bleomycin and hydroxyurea.

The appearance of horizontal hyperpigmentated bands on the hair is an unusual and a unique effect of cytostatics. Wheeland et al (114[c]) recently reported a patient who had developed such symptoms following high-dose MTX chemotherapy.

Stomatitis

The normal oral mucosa is maintained by rapidly dividing cells, and is consequently very susceptible to the effects of cytostatic drugs, notably MTX, Ara-C, cyclophosphamide, ADR, daunorubicin, and 5-FU (115[C]). Infection can occur, and mucositis may impair the patient's nutritional intake because of the discomfort of eating (116[Cr]).

Phlebitis

Adriamycin Extravasation of cytotoxic drugs can cause a full thickness loss of skin above the affected area. In areas having little subcutaneous fat, such as the dorsum of the hand and around the joints, severe damage to nerves, tendons and muscle can also occur. Local necrosis is most commonly seen with ADR. Extravasation of ADR into the skin or subcutaneous tissue can lead to a painful slowly enlarging subcutaneous lesion which, if not diagnosed and treated promptly, will develop over a period of weeks or months into a chronic, severe, frequently painful ulceration. The reaction progresses through the usual 4 stages that have been described for burns. This chemical necrosis associated with the administration of ADR is a significant problem with a reported incidence of 0.5% to 2%.

Cohen et al (117[c]) have reported 3 patients who suffered extravasation leading to deep tissue necrosis requiring skin grafts. The necrotic areas of skin containing ADR were localized directly under a UV lamp or after fluorescein administration (i.v. 10 mg/kg). It is possible to identify non-necrotic tissue in this way since fluorescein will only enter viable perfused cells. The residual necrotic tissue which does not fluoresce should be removed.

Amsacrine (m-AMSA) Mild phlebitis was reported by Micetich et al (118[C]) in 22 patients treated with m-AMSA (30–40 mg/m^2 for 3 days). Initially, the daily dose of drug was administered in a total volume of 1000 ml over 24 hours. Under these conditions, the phlebitis was severe, causing significant discomfort after about 6 hours and usually necessitating a change in the i.v. site. Administering each day's dose of drug in total volume of 2000 ml with 2 mEq of sodium bicarbonate solution significantly lessened the phlebitis.

The incidence of m-AMSA-induced phlebitis also decreased when m-AMSA infusion was followed by a heparin (1000 units) injection (119[c]).

Mitomycin C Mitomycin C extravasation produces a chronic painful ulceration similar to that caused by ADR (120[c]).

INFECTIONS

Cohen et al (121[Cr]) studied the infective complications in a group of 75 patients with immunologically-mediated disease who required high dose immunosuppression. The mean infection rate was 3.7 infections per patient, or 0.74 infections per patient during 1 week of immunosuppression. Bacteria were the commonest infecting organism (76%); serious viral and fungal infections were less frequent (11%) but an important cause of death. There was no single factor predisposing to infections, but renal impairment and increasing doses of prednisolone played a role.

Dreizen et al (122[C]) have reported a 33% incidence of oral (often fungal) infections in patients with acute leukemia while receiving remission-induction therapy. Infection is the proximate cause of death in 75% of patients with acute leukemia.

The frequency of chemotherapy-associated oral infections in adult patients with solid tumors was much lower (123[C]). The total number of documented oral infections in a series of 1000 patients was 97 (9.7%), with rates of 8.4, 11.7, and 18.3% for carcinoma, sarcoma and lymphoma patients respectively. Most of the infections were caused by fungi (69%).

The experience with oral infections in acute leukemia and solid tumor patients strongly suggests that the more aggressive the chemotherapy, the greater the tendency to stomatologic infections.

Herpes zoster

Herpes zoster is seen most commonly in children and adults with hematologic malignancies, particularly Hodgkin's disease (4–25%).

Feld et al (124[C]) encountered herpes zoster only in 4 of 250 (1.6%) patients with small cell lung carcinoma who had been treated with 6 courses of cyclophosphamide, ADR and vincristine. 3 patients had localized lesions and one had disseminated lesions. Infection developed in the patients from 2 to 7 months following initiation of chemotherapy.

Cunningham et al (125[Cr]) noted that 82 of 263 patients with Hodgkin's disease experienced herpes zoster infections during or after chemotherapy with MOPP regimen and/or total nodal irradiation. These were localized cutaneously in 71 patients and disseminated in 11 patients. 63 (77%) patients developed herpes zoster either during or within the first year after treatment. The 6-year actuarial risk of developing herpes zoster was 14% for patients treated with MOPP alone, and 18% when total nodal irradiation was used. The risk increased to 57% in patients treated with MOPP combined with total nodal irradiation. Many other infections occurring in the immune compromised host and the measures to cure them are presented in the review by Hughes et al (126[R]).

TOXIC EFFECTS OF SOME NEW AND INVESTIGATIONAL SUBSTANCES

Table 11 provides a summary of side effects which have been reported of a number of less-known or experimental agents during the period under review. Some of these drugs have been listed in earlier volumes but are included once again because additional information has become available.

MISCELLANEOUS REPORTS

Table 12 provides a brief review of some miscellaneous reports of interest which relate to topics not selected for detailed discussion in this Annual.

Table 11. *Toxic effects of some new or investigational cytostatics*

Drug	Remarks	Severe or abnormal side effects (dose)	Other side effects
Acronine (127[C])	Alkaloid prepared from the bark of Achronychia baueri	Nausea Vomiting (dose-related; more than 300 mg/m^2)	Hepatotoxicity Ataxia (400 mg/m^2 daily for 93 weeks)
ACNU (128[Cr])	1-(4-Amino-2-methylpyrimidine-5-yl)-methyl-3-(2-chloroethyl)-3-nitrosourea. Possesses antitumor activity against various animal and human solid and cerebral tumors	Myelotoxicity (10–150 mg)	Nausea Vomiting Anorexia Malaise Hepatotoxicity (3.5–12 mg/kg/day)

Table 11. *(continued)*

Drug	Remarks	Severe or abnormal side effects (dose)	Other side effects
Acyclovir (129[C])	9-(2-Hydroxyethoxymethyl) guanine. Active against herpes simplex virus in vitro and in animal models; i.v. acyclovir may be effective for treatment of established herpes simplex virus infection in immunosuppressed patients	Phlebitis (250 mg/m² every 8 hours for 7 days)	Rash
ADR-DNA complex (130)	Formed by directly mixing herring sperm DNA with ADR. Taken up selectively only into cells with capacity for endocytosis; excluded from cardiac muscle cells (with low pinocytotic activity); taken up by neoplastic cells (increased pinocytotic activity)	Fever Chills (dependent on infusion rate) Nausea Vomiting	Myelotoxicity Cardiotoxicity (patients with predisposing factors)
L-Alanosine (NSC-15 353) (131[C])	Antibiotic derived from Streptomyces alanosinicus. Presumed mechanism of action: as antipurine by interfering with aspartate-nucleotide interactions, not (as initially suggested) as glutamine antagonist	Musitis (dose limiting) Myelotoxicity (increased in patients with extensive prior radio- and/or chemotherapy)	Hypotension
Ametantrone acetate (NSC-287 513) (132[r])	One of series of compounds related to anthracycline antibiotics. Antitumor activity in animals similar to that of adriamycin; developed in attempt to reduce adriamycin's cardiotoxicity	Myelotoxicity (dose-related and -limiting)	Alopecia Blue skin Discoloration
Aziridinyl-benzoquinone (AZQ) (NSC-182 986) (133[c], 134[c], 135[c], 136[c], 137[c], 138[c], 139[c], 140[c])	1,4-Cyclohexadiene-1,4-dicarbamic acid, 2,5-bis(1-aziridinyl)-3,6-dioxodiethyl ester. Of interest for 2 major reasons: (1) significant activity against number of transplantable murine tumors; (2) possesses chemical structure in which properties of lipid solubility, low ionization and water solubility are optimized; important in penetration into CNS	Myelotoxicity (dose-related)	Anorexia Nausea Vomiting Fever of unknown origin Alopecia Constipation
Bisantren (141[c], 142[c])	9,10-Anthracene-dicarboxyaldehyde(bis(4,5-dihydro-1H-imidazole-2-yl) hydrazone) dihydrochloride. Anthracene hydrazone analog developed in effort to identify compound with antitumor activity devoid of cardiotoxicity. Seems to be DNA-reactive agent	Myelotoxicity (dose-related, 120–180 mg/m²) Phlebitis	General malaise (accompanied by flu-like illness) Hypotension

Table 11. *(continued)*

Drug	Remarks	Severe or abnormal side effects (dose)	Other side effects
Bruceantin (NSC-165 563) (143[c])	Plant product isolated from stem bark of Brucea antidysenterica. Specific inhibitor of peptide band formation; has little effect on RNA synthesis	Hypotension	Fever Nausea Vomiting (related to abnormal liver function)
Carminomycin (NSC-180 024) (144[c])	Anthracycline antitumor antibiotic; structurally a demethyldaunorubicin derivative. Claimed to be less cardiotoxic than adriamycin	Myelotoxicity (dose-limiting, 15–25 mg/m^2) Phlebitis	Abnormalities in ECG Local toxicity (erythema, pain) Alopecia, nausea, vomiting
Cis-diammine-1,1-cyclobutane dicarboxylate platinum II (145[c])	Selected on account of reduced nephrotoxicity in rats coupled with increased antitumor selectivity in several test systems; claimed to be less emetic than cisplatin	Myelotoxicity (dose-related 100–500 mg/m^2) Nephrotoxicity (dose-related, 320–520 mg/m^2; below 320 mg/m^2 no nephrotoxic effects) Nausea, vomiting (over 120 mg/m^2)	Peripheral neuropathy (after cumulative doses of 1.6–1.8 g/m^2)
DACC P(II) (146[c])	Analog of CDDP; 4′-carboxyphthalato(1,2-diaminocyclohexane) platinum(II); second generation platinum compound. Demonstrated in vitro activity in L 1210 cell lines resistant to CDDP; less nephrotoxic	Myelotoxicity (dose-limiting thrombocytopenia 360–800 mg/m^2) Nephrotoxicity (over 360 mg/m^2) Nausea, vomiting	Peripheral neuropathy Allergic reactions
4-Demethoxydaunorubicin (NSC-256 439) (147[c])	New daunorubicin analog; lacks methoxygroup at C-4 position in the aglycone. Claimed to have better therapeutic index, particularly as regards cardiotoxicity	Myelotoxicity (15 mg/m^2)	Nausea Vomiting
Dichloromethotrexate (NSC-29 630) (148[c])	Halogenoted derivative of methotrexate	Myelotoxicity Infections	Fever Conjunctivitis
5-Deoxy-5-fluorouridine (DFUR) (149[c])	New fluoropyridine derivative with 5-FU molecule attached to pseudopentose (5′-deoxy- instead of 2′-deoxypentose). Possesses higher therapeutic index in animals; substrate for intracellular nucleoside phosphorylase	Myelotoxicity (dose-related 1000–4000 mg/m^2/day)	Stomatitis ECG changes Tremor Ataxia Somnolence
HCFU (150[c])	1-Hexylcarbamoyl-5-fluorouracil; antimetabolite interfering with pyrimidine synthesis	Psychoneurotoxicity (heat sensations, frequent urinations)	Nausea Vomiting Fatigue Fever

Table 11. *(continued)*

Drug	Remarks	Severe or abnormal side effects (dose)	Other side effects
Indicine-N-oxide (NSC-132 319) (151[C])	Water-soluble pyrrolizidine alkaloid isolated from Heliotropium indicum. These alkaloids produced antimitotic and mutagenic activity, and chromosomal breakage indicating possible antitumor activity; their hepatotoxic effect dampened enthusiasm for clinical trials	Myelotoxicity (dose-related 3.3–5 g/m^2) Hepatotoxicity	Nausea Vomiting
Malonato-platinum (152[Cr])	Malonato(1,2-diamminecyclohexane)platinum; analog of CDDP. Shows no cross-resistance with CDDP	Nausea Vomiting	Myelotoxicity
Mitoxantrone (DHAD) (NSC-301 739) (153[C])	1,4-Dihydroxy-5,8-bis-2,2-hydroxyethylaminoethylamino-9,10-anthracenedione dihydrochloride. New anthraquinone derivative designed to have good antitumor activity without cardiotoxicity; main structural difference from ADR: absence of aminosugar moiety	Myelotoxicity (predisposing factors: prior chemo-, radiotherapy, advanced age, extensive liver metastasis)	Mild hair loss Dry mouth Nausea Vomiting
1-Octadecyl-2-methylglycero-3-phosphocholine (154[C])	Synthetic alkyl-lysophospholipid, inhibiting growth and metastasis of different tumors in mice. Mechanism of antitumor activity may involve derangement of phospholipid metabolism, selective for tumor cells; in contrast to normal tissue, neoplastic cells lack alkyl cleavage enzymes	Nephrotoxicity (20 mg/kg daily) Hepatotoxicity	Nausea Vomiting
PCNU (NSC-95 466) (155[r], 156[C], 157[C])	1-(2-Chloroethyl)-3-(2,6-dioxo-3-piperidyl)-1-nitrosourea. Shows antitumor activity against variety of intracerebrally implanted tumors; has greater in vitro alkylating activity and lower carbamylating activity than other nitrosoureas	Myelotoxicity (cumulative, dose-related)	Nausea Vomiting Fever of unknown origin Photosensitivity
Pipobroman (158[C])	N,N'-bis(bromopropionyl) piperazine; piperazine derivative with antitumor properties; neutral amide derivative of nitrogen mustard. Mechanism of action of alkylating type		Myelotoxicity (moderate)
Pumitepa (159[r])	2-Dimethylamino-6-diethyleniminophosphamido-7-methylpurine; water-soluble 6-mercaptopurine derivative characterized by relatively low toxicity		Headache Burning sensation Allergy

Table 11. *(continued)*

Drug	Remarks	Severe or abnormal side effect (dose)	Other side effects
RFCNU (160[C], 161[C])	(Chloro-2-ethyl)-1-(ribofuranosylisopropylidene-2′,3-paranitrobenzoate-5′)-3-nitrosourea. Derivative of nitrosourea; produces excellent antitumor activity in several murine tumors	Myelotoxicity (prior treatment related)	Nausea Vomiting
RPCNU (161[C])	(Chloro-2-ethyl)-1-ribopyranosyl triacetate-2′,3′,4′-(3-nitrosourea); derivative of nitrosourea	Myelotoxicity	Nausea Vomiting
SOAz (162[C])	Pentaziridinocyclodiphosphathiazene; inorganic cyclic derivative of unknown mechanism of action	Myelotoxicity (dose-related)	Nausea Vomiting Fever
Spirogermanium (NSC-192 965) (163[r], 164[C])	Derivative of azaspirane with the substitution of 1 carbon atom with germanium. Inhibits protein and nucleic acid synthesis	Neurotoxicity (dose-limiting 32–160 mg/m²)	Myelotoxicity Nausea Vomiting
WR-2721 (165[C])	Organic thiophosphate. In animal model provides selective protection of normal tissues against toxicity of radiation and alkylating-agent chemotherapy; may provide normal tissue protection when administered prior to cyclophosphamide or nitrogen mustard	Not observed	
Yoshi 864 (NSC-102 627) (166[C], 167[C])	1-Propanol-3,3′-iminodimethanesulfonate (ester) hydrochloride. Busulfan analog active against experimental tumors.	Myelotoxicity	Neurotoxicity Nausea Vomiting

Table 12. *Miscellaneous reports 1982–1983*

Drug	Nature of report	Ref.
1. Hydroxy-9-methyl-2-ellipticinium	Inhibition of salivary secretion, causing other complications (tongue mycosis, anorexia and asthenia)	168[C]
2. 5-FU	Severe stomatitis followed by nasal cartilage necrosis (high-dose, 2.8 g/m²/day)	169[c]
3. CDDP	Mallory-Weise syndrome requiring surgical intervention because of digestive tract bleeding	170[C]
4. Vinblastine	Inappropriate ADH secretion following administration of 30 mg instead of 10 mg vinblastine	171[c]

Table 12. *(continued)*

Drug	Nature of report	Ref.
5. L-Asparaginase	Pancreatitis and pseudocyst of pancreas	172[C]
6. Cyclosporin A	Fluid retention and hypertension associated with convulsions in children	173[C]
7. Ara-C	Severe gastrointestinal tract toxicity (severe diarrhea, abdominal distension absence of bowel sounds)	174[C]
8. Thiotepa	Symptoms of intestinal obstruction (abundant intestinal adhesions found at autopsy) following intraperitoneal drug administration	175[C]

REFERENCES

1. Von Hoff BD, Rozencweig M, Piccart M (1982) The cardiotoxicity of anticancer agents. *Sem. Oncol., 9,* 23.
2. Ganz PA, Gold BS, Tandron I (1983) Angina pectoris after doxorubicin and mitomycin therapy. *Cancer Treat. Rep., 67,* 98.
3. Ferrazzi E, Nicoletto O, Vinante O et al (1982) Phase II study 4'epi-doxorubicin. *Tumori, 68,* 431.
4. Weiss RB, Moquin D, Adams J et al (1983) Electrocardiogram abnormalities induced by amsacrine. *Cancer Chemother. Pharmacol., 10,* 133.
5. Miller CF, Rajder N (1982) Acute ECG changes associated with AMSA treatment. *Cancer Treat. Rep., 66,* 1678.
6. Labianca R, Beretta C, Clerici M et al (1982) Cardiac toxicity of 5-fluorouracil: a study on 1083 patients. *Tumori, 68,* 505.
7. Antonelli D, Beker B, Barzilay J (1981) Precoce cardiotossicita da 5-fluorouracile. *J. Ital. Cardiol., 11,* 1758.
8. Vorobiof DA (1982) Cardiotoxicity of 5-fluoro-uracil. *S. Afr. Med. J., 61,* 634.
9. Gasser AB, Tieche M, Brunner KW (1982) Neurologic and cardiac toxicity following iv. application of methotrexate. *Cancer Treat. Rep., 66,* 1561.
10. Wynert WR, Harvey HA, Lipton A et al (1982) Phase I study of a 5-day schedule of mitoxantrone (dihydroxyanthracenadione). *Cancer Treat. Rep., 66,* 1303.
11. Yancey RS, Talpaz M (1982) Vindesine-associated angina and ECG changes. *Cancer Treat. Rep., 66,* 587.
12. Isner JM, Ferrans VJ, Cohen SR et al (1983) Clinical and morphologic cardiac findings after anthracycline chemotherapy. *Am. J. Cardiol., 51,* 1167.
13. Richter v-Arnauld HP, Kleeberg UR, Hassel C. et al (1982) Überwachung der Myokardfunktion während der Therapie mit kardiotoxischen Zytostatika. *Onkologie, 5,* 168.
14. von Hoft DD, Layard M (1981) Risk factors for development of daunorubicin cardiotoxicity. *Cancer Treat. Rep., 65 (Suppl. 4),* 19.
15. Woolley PV, Ayoob MJ, Levenson SM, Smith FP (1982) A phase I clinical trial of aclacinomycin A administered on a five-consecutive-day schedule. *J. Clin. Pharmacol., 22,* 359.
16. Favrot MC, Pouyan G, Souillet G et al (1981) Cardiotoxicité des anthracyclines. *Pédiatrie, 36,* 437.
17. Pinkel D, Camitta B, Kun L et al (1982) Doxombicin cardiomyopathy in children with left-sided Wilms' tumor. *Med. Pediatr. Oncol., 10,* 483.
18. Schell FC, Yap H-Y, Blumenschein G et al (1982) Potential cardiotoxicity with mitoxantrone. *Cancer Treat. Rep., 66,* 1641.
19. Pratt CB, Crom DB, Wallenberg J et al (1983) Fatal congestive heart failure following mitoxantrone treatment in two children previously treated with doxombicin and cisplatin. *Cancer Treat. Rep., 67,* 85.
20. Legha GS, Wang Y-M, Mackay B et al (1982) Clinical and pharmacologic investigation of the effects of α-tocopherol on adriamycin cardiotoxicity. *Ann. NY Acad. Sci., 393,* 411.
21. Dresdale AR, Barr LH, Bonow RC et al (1982) Prospective randomized study of the role of N-acetyl cysteine in reversing doxorubicin-induced cardiomyopathy. *Am. J. Clin. Oncol., 5,* 657.
22. Villani F, Comazzi R, Di Fronzo G et al (1982) Evaluation of doxombicin cardiotoxicity in patients treated intermittently with betamethyldigoxin. *Tumori, 68,* 349.
23. Neri B, Comparini T, Miliani A, Torcia M (1983) Protective effects of L-carnitine (carnitene) on acute adriamycin and daunomycin cardiotoxicity in cancer patients. *Clin. Trials J., 20,* 98.

24. Jochimsen PR (1982) Subacute vincristine toxicity following five consecutive daily doses. *Am. J. Clin. Oncol.*, *5*, 437.
25. Thomas LL, Braat PC, Somers R, Goudsmit R (1982) Massive vincristine overdose: failure of leucovorin to reduce toxicity. *Cancer Treat. Rep.*, *66*, 1967.
26. Manelis J, Freundlich E, Ezekiel E, Doron J (1982) Accidental intrathecal vincristine administration. *J. Neurol.*, *228*, 209.
27. Mittelman A, Arlin ZA (1983) AMSA-induced seizures in patients with hypokalemia. *Cancer Treat. Rep.*, *67*, 102.
28. Salinsky MC, Levine RL, Aubuchon JP, Schutta HS (1983) Acute cerebral dysfunction with high-dose Ara-C therapy. *Cancer*, *51*, 426.
29. Gastaut JL, Pellissier JF, Jean Ph et al (1982) Neuropathie périphérique au cisplatine. *Nouv. Presse Méd.*, *11*, 1113.
30. Wright DE, Drouin P (1982) Cisplatin-induced myasthenic syndrome. *Clin. Pharm.*, *1*, 76.
31. Mead GM, Arnold AM, Green JA et al (1982) Epileptic seizures associated with cisplatin administration. *Cancer Treat. Rep.*, *66*, 1719.
32. Campbell TN, Howell SB, Pfeife C, House BA (1982) High-dose allopurinol modulation of 5-FU toxicity: phase I trial of an outpatient dose schedule. *Cancer Treat. Rep.*, *66*, 1723.
33. Sullivan KM, Storb R, Shulman HM et al (1982) Immediate and delayed neurotoxicity after mechlorethamine preparation for bone marrow transplantation. *Am. Intern. Med.*, *97*, 182.
34. Ettinger LJ (1982) Pharmacokinetics and biochemical effects of a fatal intrathecal methotrexate overdose. *Cancer*, *50*, 444.
35. Killen JY, Mitchel EP, Hoth DF et al (1982) Phase II studies of methyl glyoxal bis-guanylhydrazone (NSC 32946) in carcinoma of the colon and lung. *Cancer*, *50*, 1258.
36. Melgaard B, Hausen HS, Kamieniecka Z et al (1982) Misonidasole neuropathy: a clinical electrophysiological and histological study. *Ann. Neurol.*, *12*, 10.
37. Urtasun RC, Tanasichuk H, Fulton D et al (1982) High dose misonidasole with dexamethasone rescue: a possible approach to circumvent neurotoxicity. *Int. J. Radiat. Oncol. Biol. Phys.*, *8*, 365.
38. Wiley RG, Gralla RJ, Casper ES, Kemedy N (1982) Neurotoxicity of the pyrimidine synthesis inhibitor N-phosphonoacetyl-L-aspartate. *Ann. Neurol.*, *12*, 175.
39. Gaymon PS, Baum ES, Krivit W, Hammond D (1982) Phase II trial of prednimustine in children with recurrent cancer: a children's cancer study group report. *Cancer Treat. Rep.*, *66*, 1583.
40. Delaney P (1982) Vincristine-induced laryngeal nerve paralysis. *Neurology*, *32*, 1285.
41. Ryan JR, Emami A (1983) Vincristine neurotoxicity with residual equinocarus deformity in children with acute leukemia. *Cancer*, *51*, 423.
42. Fuks JZ, Egorin HJ, Aisner J et al (1983) Therapeutic efficacy and pharmacocinetics of vindesine and vindesine-cisplatin in previously treated patient with non-small cell lung carcinoma. *Cancer Chemother. Pharmacol.*, *10*, 104.
43. Rosenow EC (1980) Chemotherapeutic drug-induced pulmonary disease. *Sem. Respir. Med.*, *2*, 89.
44. Wilson KS, Worth A, Richards AG, Ford HS (1982) Low-dose bleomycin lung. *Med. Pediatr. Oncol.*, *10*, 283.
45. Perry DJ, Weiss RB, Taylor HG (1982) Enhanced bleomycin toxicity during acute renal failure. *Cancer Treat. Rep.*, *66*, 592.
46. Bauer KA, Skarin AT, Balikian JP (1983) Pulmonary complications associated with combination chemotherapy programs containing bleomycin. *Am. J. Med.*, *74*, 557.
47. Sørensen PG, Rørth M, Hansen HH (1983) Phase I evaluation of peplomycin with special reference to pulmonary toxicity. *Eur. J. Cancer Oncol.*, *19*, 319.
48. Sørensen PG, Rørth M, Hansen HH et al (1983) A phase II trial of peplomycin in squamous cell carcinoma of the lung. *Eur. J. Cancer Oncol.*, *19*, 25.
49. Krowka MJ, Breuer RJ, Kehoe TJ (1983) Azathioprine-associated pulmonary dysfunction. *Chest*, *4*, 696.
50. Kahn RC, Carlon GC, Miller L et al (1982) Acute respiratory failure due to 2'deoxyformycin. *Intensive Care Med.*, *8*, 101.
51. Weiss RB, Poster DS (1982) The renal toxicity of cancer chemotherapeutic agents. *Cancer Treat. Rev.*, *9*, 37.
52. Buamah PK, Howell A, Whitby H et al (1982) Assessment of renal function during high-dose cis-platinum therapy in patients with ovarian carcinoma. *Cancer Chemother. Pharmacol.*, *8*, 281.
53. Gonzalez C, Villasanta U (1982) Life-threatening hypocalcemia associated with cisplatin chemotherapy. *Obstet. Gynecol.*, *59*, 732.
54. Schilsky RL, Barlock A, Ozois RF (1982) Persistent hypomagnesemia following cisplatin chemotherapy for testicular cancer. *Cancer Treat. Rep.*, *66*, 1767.
55. Bitran JD, Desser RK, Billings AA et al (1982) Acute nephrotoxicity following cis-dichlorodiammine-platinum. *Cancer*, *49*, 1784.
56. Macaulay VM, Begent RHJ, Phillips ME, Newlands ES (1982) Prophylaxis against hypomagnesemia induced by cis-platinum combination therapy. *Cancer Chemother. Pharmacol.*, *9*, 179.
57. Giannattasio M, Antonelli M, Montanaro AA et al (1982) Enzymuria as a marker of renal damage caused by cis-dichlorodiammine-platinum II (CDDP) administered to patients with ovarian carcinoma. *Chemioterapia*, *1*, 437.

58. Yu H, Glashan R, Robinson MRG et al (1982) Changes in the urine protein following intravesical doxorubicin. *J. Urol.*, *128*, 272.
59. Keown PA, Stiller CR, Laupacis AL et al (1982) The effects and side effects of cyclosporine: relationship to drug pharmacokinetics. *Transplant. Proc.*, *14*, 659.
60. Droller MJ, Saral R, Santos G (1982) Prevention of cyclophosphamide-induced hemorrhagic cysticis. *Urology*, *20*, 256.
61. Morgan LR, Donley PJ, Harrison EF, Hunter HL (1982) The control of ifosfamide-induced hematuria with N-acetylcysteine in patients with advanced carcinoma of the lung. *Sem. Oncol.*, *9 (Suppl. 1)*, 71.
62. Falkson G, Van Dyk JJ, Stapelberg R, Falkson HC (1982) Mesnum as a protector against kidney and bladder toxicity with high-dose ifosfamide treatment. *Cancer Chemother. Pharmacol.*, *9*, 81.
63. Araujo CE, Tessler J (1983) Treatment of ifosfamide-induced urothelial toxicity by oral administration of sodium 2-mercaptoethane sulphonate (MESNA) to patients with inoperable lung cancer. *Eur. J. Cancer Clin. Oncol.*, *19*, 195.
64. Hall-Craggs M, Brenner DE, Vigorito RD, Sutherland JC (1982) Acute renal failure and renal tubular squamous metaplasia following treatment with streptozotocin. *Hum. Pathol.*, *13*, 597.
65. Micetich KC, Jensen-Akula M, Mandarol JC, Fischer RS (1981) Nephrotoxicity of semustine (methyl-CCNU) in patients with malignant melanoma receiving adjuvant chemotherapy. *Am. J. Med.*, *71*, 967.
66. Freeman-Narrod M, Kim JS, Onanissian H et al (1982) The effect of high-dose methotrexate on renal tubules as indicated by urinary lysozyme concentration. *Cancer*, *50*, 2775.
67. Howell SB, Pfeifle CE, Wung WE, Olshen RA (1983) Intraperitoneal cis-diamminedichloroplatinum with systemic thiosulfate protection. *Cancer Res.*, *43*, 1426.
68. Shrieve DC, Harris JW (1982) Protection against cis-dichlorodiamine Pt(II) cytotoxicity in vitro by cysteamine. *Int. J. Radiat. Oncol. Biol. Phys.*, *8*, 585.
69. Levi FA, Hrushesky WJM, Halberg F et al (1982) Lethal nephrotoxicity of cis-diamminedichloroplatinum ameliorated by optimal circadian timing and hydration. *Eur. J. Cancer Clin. Oncol.*, *18*, 471.
70. Appelbaum FR, Shulman HM (1982) Fatal hepatotoxicity associated with AMSA therapy. *Cancer Treat. Rep.*, *66*, 1863.
71. Dupont JC, Garay GE, Seaglione C, Pavlovsky S (1982) Trial of AMSA in acute leukemia. *Cancer Treat. Rep.*, *66*, 1596.
72. Lawrence HJ, Ries CA, Reynolds RD et al (1982) AMSA – A promising new agent in refractory acute leukemia. *Cancer Treat. Rep.*, *66*, 1475.
73. Doering Ch, Piekartz H, Orfanos CE, Altenahr E (1982) DTIC bei malignem Melanom – seltene, schwere Komplikation: Budd-Chiari Syndrom. *Z. Hautkr.*, *57*, 971.
74. Dawes PIDK (1982) A pilot study of estracyt in advanced breast cancer. *Cancer Treat. Rep.*, *66*, 581.
75. Barone RM, Byfield JE, Goldfarb PB et al (1982) Intra-arterial chemotherapy using an implantable infusion pump and liver irradiation for the treatment of hepatic metastases. *Cancer*, *50*, 850.
76. Lazarus HM, Gottfried MR, Herzig RH et al (1982) Veno-occlusive disease of the liver after high-dose mitomycin C therapy and autologous bone marrow transplantation. *Cancer*, *49*, 1789.
77. Peterson BA, Bloomfield CD, Gottlieb AJ et al (1982) 5-Azacitidine and zorubicin for patients with previously treated acute nonlymphocytic leukemia: a cancer and leukemia group B pilot study. *Cancer Treat. Rep.*, *66*, 563.
78. Milligan DW, Thein SL, Roberts BE (1982) Secondary treatment of polycythemia rubra vera with 6-thioguanine. *Cancer*, *50*, 836.
79. Krivoy N, Raz R, Carter A, Alroy G (1982) Reversible hepatic veno-occlusive disease and 6-thioguanine. *Ann. Intern. Med.*, *96*, 788.
80. Hansen MM, Ranek L, Walbom S, Nissen NJ (1982) Fatal hepatitis following irradiation and vincristine. *Acta Med. Scand.*, *212*, 171.
81. Vermorken JB, Kapteijn TS, Hart AAM, Pinedo HM (1983) Ototoxicity of cis-diamminedichloroplatinum (II): influence of dose, schedule and mode of administration. *Eur. J. Cancer Clin. Oncol.*, *19*, 53.
82. Fleming SM, Peters GM, Weaver AW et al (1983) Ototoxicity associated with cis-platinum in three chemotherapy multi-drug regimens. *Cancer*, *51*, 610.
83. McHaney VA, Thibadoux G, Hayes FA, Green AA (1983) Hearing loss in children receiving cisplatin chemotherapy. *J. Pediatr.*, *102*, 314.
84. Fraunfelder FT, Meyer SM (1983) Ocular toxicity of antineoplastic agents. *Ophthalmology*, *90*, 1.
85. Maudgal PC, van Damme B, Missotten L (1983) Corneal epithelial dysplasia after trifluridine use. *Grafe's Arch. Clin. Exp. Ophthalmol.*, *220*, 6.
86. Shingleton BJ, Bienfang DC, Albert DM et al (1982). Ocular toxicity associated with high-dose carmustine. *Arch. Ophthalmol.*, *100*, 1766.
87. Kerbel RS, Davies AJS (1982) Facilitation of tumor progression by cancer therapy. *Lancet*, *2*, 977.
88. Schmähl D, Habs M, Lorenz M, Wagner J (1982) Occurrence of second tumors in man after anticancer drug treatment. *Cancer Treat. Rev.*, *9*, 167.
89. Coltman CA, Dixon DO (1982) Second malignancies complicating Hodgkin's disease: a

southwest oncology group 10-year followup. *Cancer Treat. Rep., 66*, 1023.

90. Einhorn N, Eklund G, Franzen S et al (1982) Late side effects of chemotherapy in ovarian carcinoma. *Cancer, 49*, 2234.
91. Greene MH, Boice JD, Greer BE et al (1982) Acute nonlymphocytic leukemia after therapy with alkylating agents for ovarian cancer. *N. Engl. J. Med., 307*, 1416.
92. Miké V (1982) Incidence of second malignant neoplasms in children: Results of an international study. *Lancet, 2*, 1326.
93. Elliott RW, Essenhigh DM, Morley AR (1982) Cyclophosphamide treatment of systemic lupus erythematosus: risk of bladder cancer exceeds benefit. *Br. Med. J., 284*, 1160.
94. Anderson RW, Puckett WH, Dana WJ et al (1982) Risk of handling injectable antineoplastic agents. *Am. J. Hosp. Pharm., 39*, 1881.
95. Gallelli JF (1982) Evaluating the potential hazard of handling antineoplastic drugs. *Am. J. Hosp. Pharm., 39*, 1877.
97. Da Cunha MF, Meistrich ML, Haq MM et al (1982) Temporary effects of AMSA (4'-(acridin-9-ylamino)methanesulfon-m-anisidide) chemotherapy on spermatogenesis. *Cancer, 49*, 2495.
98. Waxman JHX, Terry YA, Wrigley PFM et al (1982) Gonadal function in Hodgkin's disease: long-term follow-up of chemotherapy. *Br. Med. J., 285*, 1612.
99. Whitehead E, Shalet SM, Jones PHM et al (1982) Gonadal function after combination chemotherapy for Hodgkin's disease in childhood. *Arch. Dis. Childh., 47*, 287.
100. Chapman RM (1983) Gonadal injury resulting from chemotherapy. *Am. J. Ind. Med., 4*, 149.
101. Dnistrian AM, Schwartz MK, Fracchia AA et al (1983) Endocrine consequences of CMF adjuvant therapy in premenopausal and postmenopausal breast cancer patients. *Cancer, 51*, 803.
102. Andrieu JM, Ochoa-Molina ME (1982) Grossesses et progèniture aprés chimiothérapie MOPP. *Nouv. Presse Méd., 11*, 3623.
103. Morrow GR, Morrel Ch (1982) Behavioral treatment for the anticipatory nausea and vomiting induced by cancer chemotherapy. *N. Engl. J. Med., 307*, 1476.
104. Wilcox PM, Fetting JH, Nettesham KM, Abeloff MD (1982) Anticipatory vomiting in women receiving cyclophosphamide, methotrexate, and 5-FU (CMF) adjuvant chemotherapy for breast carcinoma. *Cancer Treat. Rep., 66*, 1601.
105. Morrow GR (1982) Prevalence and correlates of anticipatory-nausea and vomiting in chemotherapy patients. *J. Nat. Cancer Inst., 68*, 585.
106. Weddington WW (1982) Psychogenic nausea and vomiting associated with termination of cancer chemotherapy. *Psychother. Psychosom., 37*, 129.
107. Laszlo J (1983) Nausea and vomiting as major complications of cancer chemotherapy. *Drugs, 25, Suppl. 1*, 1.
108. Borison HL, McCarthy LE (1983) Neuropharmacology of chemotherapy-induced emesis. *Drugs, 25, Suppl. 1*, 8.
109. Trounce JR (1983) Antiemetics and cytotoxic drugs. *Br. Med. J., 286*, 327.
110. Wampler G (1983) The pharmacology and clinical effectiveness of phenotiazines and related drugs for managing chemotherapy-induced emesis. *Drugs, 25, Suppl. 1*, 35.
111. Strum SB, McDermed JE, Opfell RW, Riech LP (1982) Intravenous metoclopramide. *J. Am. Med. Assoc., 247*, 2683.
112. Cox R, Newman CE, Leyland MJ (1982) Metoclopramide in the reduction of nausea and vomiting associated with combined chemotherapy. *Cancer Chemother. Pharmacol., 8*, 133.
113. Colbert N, Izrael V, Lotz JP et al (1983) Action anti-émétique de l'ACTH chez les malades traités par cisplatine. *Presse Méd., 12*, 1077.
114. Wheeland RG, Burgdorf WHC, Humphrey GB (1983) The flag sign of chemotherapy. *Cancer, 51*, 1356.
115. Carl W (1983) Oral complications in cancer patients. *AFP, 27*, 161.
116. Peterson DE, Sonis ST (1982) Oral complications of cancer chemotherapy: present status and future studies. *Cancer Treat. Rep., 66*, 1251.
117. Cohen FJ, Manganaro J, Bezozo RC (1983) Identification of involved tissue during surgical treatment of doxorubicin-induced extravasation necrosis. *J. Hand Surg., 8*, 43.
118. Micetich KC, Zwelling LA, Gormley P, Young RC (1982) Phase I-II study of m-AMSA administered as a continuous infusion. *Cancer Treat. Rep., 66*, 1813.
119. Case DC (1982) Prevention of amsacrine-induced phlebitis with heparin. *Clin. Pharm., 1*, 490.
120. Argenta LC, Manders EK (1983) Mitomycin C extravasation injures. *Cancer, 51*, 1080.
121. Cohen J, Pinching AJ, Rees AJ, Peters DK (1982) Infection and immunosuppression. *Q. J. Med. (New Series), 51*, 1.
122. Dreizen S, McCredie KB, Keating MJ, Bodey GP (1982) Oral infections associated with chemotherapy in adults with acute leukemia. *Postgrad. Med., 71*, 133.
123. Dreizen S, Bodey GP, Valdivieso M (1983) Chemotherapy-associated oral infections in adults with solid tumors. *Oral Surg., Oral Med., Oral Pathol., 55*, 113.
124. Feld R, Evans WK, De Boer G (1982) Herpes zoster in patients with carcinoma of the lung. *Am. J. Med., 73*, 795.
125. Cunningham J, Mauch P, Rosenthal DS, Canellos GP (1982) Long-term complications of MOPP chemotherapy in patients with Hodgkin's disease. *Cancer Treat. Rep., 66*, 1015.
126. Hughes WT, Tufenkeji H, Bartley DL (1983) The immune compromised host. *Pediatr.*

Clin. North Am., *30*, 103.
127. Scarffe JH, Beaumont AR, Crowther D (1983) Phase I-II evaluation of acronine in patients with multiple myeloma. *Cancer Treat. Rep.*, *67*, 93.
128. Kimura K (1982) Early clinical trials of new antitumor drugs. *Jpn Pharmacol. Ther.*, *10*, 3787.
129. Meyers JD, Wade JC, Mitchel CD et al (1983) Multicenter collaborative trial of intravenous acyclovir for treatment of mucocutaneous herpes simplex virus infection in the immunocompromised host. *Am. J. Med.*, *229*, Acyclovir Symposium.
130. Hall SW, Benjamin RS, Burgess MA et al (1982) Doxorubicin-DNA complex: a phase I clinical trial. *Cancer Treat. Rep.*, *66*, 2033.
131. Goldsmith MA, Ohnuma T, Spigelman M et al (1983) Phase I study of L-alanoside (NSC 15353). *Cancer*, *51*, 378.
132. Hillier K (1982) Ametantrone acetate. *Drugs Future*, *7*, 303.
133. Bedikian AY, Strochlein JR, Karlin DA et al (1982) Phase II clinical evaluation of AZQ in colorectal cancer. *Am. J. Oncol.*, *5*, 535.
134. Creagan ET, Schutt AJ, Ahmann DL, Green SJ (1982) Phase II study of aziridinylbenzoquinone (AZQ) in disseminated malignant melanoma. *Cancer Treat. Rep.*, *66*, 2089.
135. Yap BS, Bedikian AY, Burgess MA, Bodey GP (1982) AZQ therapy in patients with disseminated malignant melanoma. *Am. J. Clin. Oncol.*, *5*, 623.
136. Forastiere AA, Crain SM, Callahan K et al (1982) Phase II trial of aziridinylbenzoquinone (AZQ) in head and neck cancer. *Cancer Treat. Rep.*, *66*, 2097.
137. Rubin J, van Hazel GA, Schutt AJ et al (1982) A phase II study of aziridinylbenzoquinone (AZQ) in advanced large bowel carcinoma. *Am. J. Clin. Oncol.*, *5*, 539.
138. Yap HY, Bedikian AY, Schell FC et al (1982) Phase II clinical evaluation of AZQ in metastatic breast cancer. *Am. J. Clin. Oncol.*, *6*, 31.
139. Griffin JP, Newman RA, McCornack JJ, Krakoff IH (1982) Clinical and clinical pharmacologic studies of aziridinylbenzoquinone. *Cancer Treat. Rep.*, *66*, 1321.
140. Van Echo DA, Schulman P, Budman DR et al (1982) A phase I trial of aziridinylbenzoquinone (NSC 182986) in patients with previously treated acute leukemia. *Am. J. Clin. Oncol.*, *5*, 405.
141. Yap B-S, Yap H-Y, Blumenshein GR et al (1982) Phase I clinical evaluation of 9,10-anthracenedicarboxyaldehyde (bis(4,5-dihydro-1H-imidazol-2-yl)hydrazone) dihydrochloride (Bisantrene). *Cancer Treat. Rep.*, *66*, 1517.
142. Perry MC, Forastiere AA, Richards F et al (1982) Phase II trial of bisantrene in advanced colorectal cancer: a cancer and leukemia group B study. *Cancer Treat. Rep.*, *66*, 1997.
143. Fong KLL, Ho DHW, Benjamin RS et al (1982) Clinical pharmacology of bruceantin by radioimmunoassay. *Cancer Chemother. Pharmacol.*, *9*, 169.
144. Comis RL, Issell BF, Pittman K et al (1982) A phase I and clinical pharmacology study of intravenously administered carminomycin in cancer patients in the United States. *Cancer Res.*, *42*, 2944.
145. Calvert AH, Harland SJ, Newell DR et al (1982). Early clinical studies with cis-diammine-1,1,-cyclobutane dicárboxylate platinum II. *Cancer Chemother. Pharmacol.*, *9*, 140.
146. Kelsen DP, Scher H, Alcock N et al (1982) Phase I clinical trial and pharmacokinetics of 4′-carboxyphthalato(1,2-diaminocyclohexane) platinum II. *Cancer Res.*, *42*, 4831.
147. Kaplan S, Martini A, Varini M et al (1982) Phase I trial of 4-demethoxydaunorubicin with single i.v. doses. *Eur. J. Cancer Clin. Oncol.*, *18*, 1303.
148. Tester WJ, Donehower RC, Eddy JL et al (1982) Evaluation of weekly escalating doses of dichloromethotrexate in patients with hepatocellular carcinoma and other solid tumors. *Cancer Chemother. Pharmacol.*, *8*, 305.
149. Abele R, Alberto P, Seematter RJ et al (1982) Phase I clinical study with 5′-deoxy-5-fluorouridine, a new fluoropirimidine derivative. *Cancer Treat. Rep.*, *66*, 1307.
150. Robinson CP (1982) Carmofur. *Drugs Today*, *18*, 424.
151. Ohnuma T, Sridhar KS, Ratner LH, Holland JF (1982) Phase I study of indicine N-oxide in patients with advanced cancer. *Cancer Treat. Rep.*, *66*, 1509.
152. Ribaud P, Gouvela J, Bonnay M, Mathe G (1981) Clinical pharmacology and pharmacokinetics of cis-platinum and analogs. *Cancer Treat. Rep.*, *65*, *Suppl. 3*, 97.
153. Stuart-Harris RG, Smith IE (1982) Mitoxantrone: a phase II study in the treatment of patients with advanced breast carcinoma and other solid tumors. *Cancer Chemother. Pharmacol.*, *8*, 179.
154. Berdel WE, Schlehe H, Fink V et al (1982) Early tumor and leukemia response to alkyllysophospholipids in a plase I study. *Cancer*, *50*, 2011.
155. Poster DS, Penta JS, Bruno S (1982) A new nitrosourea in clinical oncology. *Am. J. Clin. Oncol.*, *5*, 9.
156. Bedikian AY, Strochlein JR, Karlin DA et al (1983) Phase II evaluation of 1-(2-chloroethyl)-3-(2,6-dioxo-3-piperidyl)-1-nitrosourea (PCNU, NSC 95466) in patients with metastatic colorectal cancer. *Am. J. Clin. Oncol.*, *6*, 49.
157. Kavanagh JJ, Yap HY, Blumenschein GR et al (1982) Phase II trial of PCNU in refractory advanced breast cancer. *Am. J. Clin. Oncol.*, *5*, 249.
158. Najman A, Stachowiak J, Parlier Y et al (1982): Pipobroman therapy of polycythemia

vera. *Blood, 59*, 890.

159. Socolova AS (1983) Pumitepa. *Drugs Future, 8*, 132.

160. Mathe G, Schein P, MacDonald JS et al (1982) Study of nitrosourea glycosyl analogs – V. An oriented phase II trial of RFCNU. *Eur. J. Cancer Clin. Oncol., 18*, 127.

161. Mathé G, Schein PS, De Vassal F et al (1982) Etude phase II des trois nouvelles nitrosourées: une américaine: la chlorozotocine, et deux francaises: le RFCNU et le RPCNU. *Sem. Hôp. Paris, 58*, 1867.

162. Nasca S, Jezekova D, Coninx P et al (1982) Phase I study of SOAz. *Cancer Treat. Rep., 66*, 2039.

163. Slavik M, Saires JH (1981) Spirogermanium: a new metallic anticancer drug without bone marrow toxicity. *Cancer, 11*, 25.

164. Budman BR, Ginsberg S, Perry M et al (1982) Phase II trial of spirogermanium in breast adenocarcinoma: a cancer and leukemia group B study. *Cancer Treat. Rep., 66*, 1667.

165. Glick JH, Glover DJ, Weiler C et al (1982): Phase I clinical trials of WR-2721 with alkylating agent chemotherapy. *Int. J. Oncol. Biol. Phys., 8*, 575.

166. Altman SJ, Stephens RL, Bonnet JD (1982) Yoshi 864 plus medroxyprogesterone acetate in adenocarcinoma of the kidney: a southwest oncology group study. *Cancer Treat. Rep., 66*, 1781.

167. Slavik M, Muss H, Blessing JA, Delgado G (1982) Phase II clinical study of Yoshi 864 in epithelial ovarian carcinoma: a gynecologic oncology group study. *Cancer Treat. Rep., 66*, 1775.

168. Juret P, Heron JF, Couette JE et al (1982) Hydroxy-9-methyl-2-ellipticinium for osseous metastases from breast cancer: a 5-year experience. *Cancer Treat. Rep., 66*, 1909.

169. Ashford RFU, Mughal T, Goold MA et al (1982): Nasal cartilage necrosis following high-dose 5-FU: a case report. *Cancer Treat. Rep., 66*, 1884.

170. Lubicz S, Shafir M, Diamond S et al (1982) Mallory-Weiss syndrome secondary to cisplatinum chemotherapy: an unusual complication. *J. Surg. Oncol., 20*, 247.

171. Stahel RA, Oelz O (1982) Syndrome of inappropriate ADH secretion secondary to vinblastine. *Cancer Chemother. Pharmacol., 8*, 253.

172. Bertolone SJ, Fuenfer MM, Groff DB, Patel CC (1982) Delayed pancreatic pseudocyst formation. *Cancer, 50*, 2964.

173. Joss DV, Barrett AJ, Kendra JR et al (1982) Hypertension and convulsions in children receiving cyclosporin A. *Lancet, 1*, 906.

174. Slevin ML, Rohatiner AZS, Dhaliwal HS et al (1982) A comparison of two schedules of cytosine arabinose used in combination with adriamycin and 6-thioguanine in the treatment of acute myelogenous leukemia. *Med. Pediatr. Oncol., Suppl., 1*, 185.

175. Appelqvist P, Silvo J, Salmela L, Kostiainen S (1982) On the treatment and prognosis of malignant ascites: is the survival time determined when the abdominal paracentesis is needed? *J. Surg. Oncol., 20*, 238.

G. Ansell

48 Radiological contrast media and radiopharmaceuticals

ALIMENTARY TRACT

Barium sulfate *(SED-9, 750; SEDA-6, 404; SEDA-7, 450)*

12 cases of *perforation of the colon* by barium enema with 4 deaths are reported in three recent publications (1[CR]–3[CR]). The incidence of perforation was approximately 1 in 6,000 examinations. In 4 cases, perforation occurred following double-contrast procedures; 2 of these resulted in pneumoperitoneum and 2 showed retroperitoneal emphysema. In a majority of these cases perforation occurred through apparently normal bowel. In 1 patient a tear of the rectum was thought to be due to expulsion of an inflated balloon catheter. In another patient, perforation occurred during the evacuation of the enema. The present author is also aware of three recent unpublished cases of retroperitoneal emphysema which occurred during double-contrast examinations in patients with ulcerative colitis.

Eklof et al (4[CR]) reported 4 cases of *barium peritonitis* in neonates and one in an older child. Recovery occurred but in one neonate there were severe circulatory disturbances and convulsions during treatment and there was residual slight mental impairment and spastic diplega.

Occasional cases of *barium appendicitis* have been reported in the past following prolonged retention of barium in the appendix. In a further case report, acute appendicitis occurred 2 months after a barium enema. At operation there was a necrotic perforated appendix with a barium faecolith in its base (5[CR]).

Side Effects of Drugs Annual 8
M.N.G. Dukes, editor

ISBN 0 444 90339 9
$0.80 per article per page (transactional system)
$0.20 per article per page (licensing system)

Water-soluble contrast media *(SED-9, 751)*

Accidental inhalation of hypertonic iodinated contrast media may cause *pulmonary edema.* Two further examples have been reported following use of these media. In one patient with an esophageal fistula, there was a severe respiratory distress syndrome with pulmonary edema and superimposed infection, requiring prolonged positive pressure ventilation, and there was residual pulmonary impairment (6[CR]). In the other case, a patient with esophageal perforation, leakage into the mediastinum and pleura caused severe shock requiring intensive treatment (7[CR]). Where there is a risk of inhalation of contrast medium, low osmolar media are preferable. Intratracheal injection of large volumes of Gastrografin in animals causes acute respiratory distress and pulmonary edema. With metrizamide, these changes may also occur but they are considerably less severe. Clearance of metrizamide from the lungs tends to be somewhat slower that with Gastrografin (8[R]). Metrizamide may also cause a chemical inflammatory response in the alveoli (9[R]).

The literature on complications of gastrointestinal radiology and endoscopy has recently been comprehensively reviewed in German (10[R]).

CHOLEGRAPHY

Elevation of serum lactate dehydrogenase-5 was noted in 2 patients 12-24 hr following infusion of 40 ml of Cholegrafin (iodipamide) for intravenous cholangiography, suggesting hepatocellular toxicity. There were no overt clinical signs of adverse reaction (11[CR]).

Certain *risk factors* may be determined by sexual function. An increased incidence of adverse reactions to intravenous cholangiography with ioglycamide was noted in fertile women during the last third of the menstrual cycle. This was attributed to high levels of circulating progesterone. In men, the incidence of adverse reactions was lower in those over the age of 70 and it was suggested that this was due to lowered testosterone levels. However, the risk of severe reactions in older patients should not be ignored (12[CR]).

EXCRETION UROGRAPHY

Idiosyncratic reactions

In a consecutive series of 300,000 urograms performed at the Mayo Clinic between 1964 and 1982 (13[CR]) there were 4 *deaths*, all in patients over the age of 50. It seems probable that the relatively low mortality rate in this series (1 in 75,000) may in part have been due to the efficiency of resuscitation. In addition, the dose of contrast medium used in the majority of cases was also smaller than that currently used in many centres.

Routine electrocardiographic monitoring during intravenous urography has shown that significant *ECG abnormalities* may occur (SEDA-6, 405). These appear to be more common in older patients and in those with pre-existing ECG changes (14[CR]). Iodamide appeared to produce a lower incidence of ECG changes than diatrizoate (15[CR]) but variations in the dose of iodine administered in this investigation makes assessment difficult. Preliminary results suggest that non-ionic media such as iopamidol and iohexol are likely to cause fewer ECG changes (16).

Subclinical *bronchospasm* can be demonstrated following the bolus injection of ionic urographic contrast media (SEDA-7, 452). The incidence of subclinical bronchospasm is much reduced with iopamidol and iohexol and it has been suggested that these media should be used when urography is required in patients with asthma or chronic obstructive airways disease (17[CR]). However, non-ionic media may still give rise to allergic phenomena such as urticaria (18[CR]) and possibly anaphylactic collapse (50[CR]).

Animal studies can throw some light on *risk factors* and on the *treatment* of generalized reactions. Injection of methylglucamine diatrizoate into dehydrated dogs may produce a syndrome with many of the features that occur in severe contrast media reactions in patients. In 4 out of 12 dogs, there was prolonged hypotension and 1 dog died. In this dog there was severe vomiting, slowing of the heart rate, heart block and S-T depression. Plasma histamine was also markedly elevated. While this may have aggravated the toxic effect, it did not appear to be the primary mechanism, since plasma histamine was not elevated in the other hypotensive dogs, one of which was severely shocked (19). The degree of dehydration in these dogs was considerably more severe than would be expected in the clinical situation. This study nevertheless indicates that dehydration could be an adverse factor in patients undergoing urography; it also emphasizes the importance of blood volume expansion in the treatment of contrast medium-induced shock reactions. It is suggested that dopamine should also be used for the treatment of hypotension in these cases.

Some authorities advocate the use of intravenous adrenaline in the treatment of contrast media reactions. In a recent case report, angina and severe myocardial ischemia with S-T depression lasting 5 hr, occurred following the intravenous injection of 0.3 mg of adrenaline to treat a suspected anaphylactic reaction to penicillin in a 23-year-old woman. An intravenous infusion of nitroglycerine was required to relieve the pain and the ECG then reverted to normal (20[CR]). This report emphasizes the potential hazard of *intravenous* adrenaline; this route should be confined to 'cardiac arrest' emergencies.

Intravenous steroids are routinely used in the treatment of contrast media reactions. Intravenous hydrocortisone succinate or phosphate may rarely cause severe anaphylactic reactions (SEDA-5, 354). Bronchospasm has also been noted in aspirin-sensitive asthmatics following intravenous hydrocortisone sodium succinate. Dexamethasone appeared to be preferable for these patients. Sudden deaths have also been reported after *pulse therapy* with very large doses of corticosteroids (SEDA-7, 379).

Effects on renal function *(SED-9, 755; SEDA-4, 334; SEDA-5, 420; SEDA-6, 406; SEDA-7, 452)*

The effects of contrast media on renal function continue to be of interest. In a prospective series of 378 patients undergoing non-renal angiography, the most important single *risk factor* was azotemia. Whereas non-azotemic patients had a 2% incidence of acute renal failure, patients with chronic azotemia had a 33% incidence. The most useful screening test was serum creatinine determination 24-48 hours after the angiogram (21[CR]). In another prospective series of 2216 consecutive medical and surgical admissions, contrast medium administration caused renal failure in 16 cases and one patient died. The incidence of renal insufficiency following major angiographic studies was 3.2%. Following transluminal renal angioplasty it was 30% (22[CR]).

Earlier reports suggested that contrast media examinations in renal allografts might precipitate *acute tubular necrosis or rejection*. In a series of 211 patients receiving renal transplants, the incidence of renal allograft dysfunction did not appear to differ significantly between those who received contrast medium and those who did not. However, the risk was related to the level of serum creatinine at the time of the contrast medium exposure. The yield of significant findings from routine contrast medium examinations was small. With the advent of non-invasive technics such as ultrasound and nuclear studies, it is therefore suggested that excretion urography or renal arteriography should be limited to patients where there are specifically suspected lesions such as ureteric leaks or arterial stenosis (23[CR]).

Renal arteriography with ionic contrast media such as metrizoate and diatrizoate produces transient *proteinuria* which may be massive. The low-osmolar non-ionic medium metrizamide also produced similar proteinuria. A similar investigation using one of the newer low osmolar media ioxaglate showed that this produced only negligible proteinuria after renal arteriography (24[CR]). Ioxaglate is a dimer. The two new non-ionic media iohexol and iopamidol also cause negligible proteinuria in renal angiography (25). The fact that metrizamide caused proteinuria indicates that this was due to a chemotoxic factor rather than to osmolality and this may have been the reason for renal failure which occurred after excretion urography with metrizamide (SEDA-3, 378). In azotemic patients the contrast medium-induced proteinuria may be of greater significance and it may be a factor in causing renal failure. If this is the case, the risk of renal failure following contrast media examinations in high risk cases may be expected to be reduced with ioxaglate, iohexol and iopamidol (25).

The risk of renal failure following intravenous urography in *multiple myeloma* has been the subject of dispute. In 26 cases of myeloma, where urography was performed with methylglucamine iothalamate, there was no significant deterioration of renal function. Review of the literature however indicates that there may be a moderately increased risk of renal failure in such cases. It is concluded that if there is a definite indication for urography, this may be performed. It is recommended that compression and dehydration should be avoided and that the urine should be made alkaline (26[CR]). It may be that ioxaglate, iohexol or iopamidol may be preferable in such cases.

Crystalluria may occur in some patients if the urine is cooled to room temperature after excretion urography with diatrizoate. This is more marked in acid urine. Examination by polarized light microscopy, scanning electron microscopy and energy dispersive X-ray analysis confirms that these were crystals of diatrizoate. Diatrizoate crystalluria may be confused with the other types of crystalluria in routine microscopy of the urine. It is uncertain whether diatrizoate crystalluria plays any part in contrast medium-induced renal failure (27[CR]).

ANGIOGRAPHY

Renal arteriography

Severe reactions occurred in 2 azotemic diabetic patients with evidence of immunopathy, following renal arteriography and biopsy. Both patients developed transient hypertension, hyperglycemia and hyperpotassemia, resistant to treatment. One patient had a sudden cardiac arrest; he was resuscitated but remained unconscious until his death 3 months later. The other patient developed oliguria, requiring a renal transplant. Both patients had been dehydrated and this may have been an aggravating factor (28[CR]).

Coronary arteriography

A transitory *fall in free ionic calcium* occurs following the intravascular administration of Renografin (SEDA-7, 452). The fall in ionic calcium is greater with Renografin-76 than with Hypaque-76. Both of these contrast media contain diatrizoate, but Renografin contains the chelating agent disodium edetate and sodium citrate which both bind calcium, whereas Hypaque contains calcium sodium edetate (29[cR]). However, the diatrizoate ion itself also binds calcium and this is more marked with sodium diatrizoate than with methylglucamine diatrizoate. Iopamidol does not bind calcium (30). Hypocalcemia due to contrast media may be responsible for some of the myocardial abnormalities which occur during coronary arteriography. Diastolic cardiac arrest occurred during coronary arteriography in a patient with Prinzmetal angina receiving verapamil. The patient was resuscitated by external cardiac massage but the heart failed to show electrical activity. After 110 min, extracorporeal circulation was commenced and 10 min later, electrical activity returned and the patient recovered. In this case, there may have been a synergic effect between the calcium antagonist action of verapamil and hypocalcemia caused by the contrast medium (31[Cr]).

In coronary arteriography, the non-ionic contrast media iohexol and metrizamide produced fewer alterations than ionic contrast media in coronary sinus blood chemistry and myocardial contractile state. The adverse effect of ionic contrast media on regional myocardial contraction is accentuated in the presence of coronary artery stenosis, possibly due to longer exposure of the myocardium to contrast medium as a result of the decreased flow rate (32[R]).

Coronary arteriography with Renografin produces an ECG change with transient prolongation of the Q-T interval. In a patient with an improperly positioned sensing ventricular demand pacemaker electrode, the coincidence of this Q-T prolongation and a premature pacemaker capture beat resulted in ventricular fibrillation (33[CR]).

Cerebral arteriography

In the syndrome of *transient global amnesia,* there is a single short episode when a patient is unable to assimilate new information even though he or she is otherwise alert. Seven cases of this syndrome were found in a review of a series of patients undergoing either carotid or vertebral arteriography. Symptoms cleared within 6 to 24 hours but there was no recall of events occurring during the period of amnesia (34[Cr]).

COMPUTERIZED TOMOGRAPHY

Possible non-random *clustering of adverse reactions* was found in a consecutive series of 6453 patients receiving contrast media injections for computer tomography. The overall incidence of adverse reactions was 3.3%. If a patient had a reaction, the relative risk of the next patient having a reaction was calculated to be 1.3 times greater than would be expected on a random basis. The reason for such clustering is uncertain. In some cases it might be due to the batch of contrast medium (35[cr]). However, the attitude of the doctor injecting the medium and evaluating the reaction may also be relevant (SEDA-6, 405).

In patients with cerebral metastases, injection of contrast medium for computed tomography may cause *seizures* (SEDA-6, 407). The effect of prophylactic diazepam (5 mg i.v., immediately before the contrast injection) was assessed in 284 consecutive patients with known or suspected brain metastases undergoing contrast CT. In the non-diazepam group, the incidence of seizures was 15% (14 out of 92 patients with brain metastases) whereas in the diazepam group the incidence was only 3% (3 out of 96 patients). In 6 patients, seizures commenced after less than 20 g of iodine had been given. No seizures occurred in 96 patients without metastases (36[CR]).

Narcotic premedication used in children to minimize motion during brain CT may cause *CNS depression, vomiting* or *voiding problems.* In 4 infants who were less than 3 months old there was life-threatening cardiorespiratory depression or arrest (37[CR]).

Effects on the blood

Hypertonic contrast media make the erythrocyte wall more rigid so that the red cells are unable to negotiate capillaries thereby producing *capillary blockage* (SEDA-4, 335). These changes in the red cells also increase the microviscosity of the contrast medium blood mixture. The greatest increase in microviscosity occurs with diatrizoate. Despite its lower osmolality, metrizamide also causes a marked increase of microviscosity, apparently due to an action of metrizamide on the red cell membrane, causing crenation of the cells. Ioxaglate has only a minor influence on the red cell membrane and causes a much lower increase in the microviscosity (38[R]). Iohexol and iopamidol also cause only minor changes in the red cell membrane and shape (39).

Large doses of contrast media may cause an anticoagulant effect (SED-8, 1038). In vitro experiments with normal plasma showed that contrast medium potentiates the anticoagulant action of heparin. This effect is more marked with plasma from patients with liver disease or coagulation diseases. Clotting time measured in a patient shortly after administration of contrast media may show abnormally elevated levels and may cause problems in monitoring anticoagulant therapy (40[r]).

Particulate contamination of contrast media

Contrast media used for arteriography contain a variety of microscopic particles which can be demonstrated by scanning electron microscopy and energy dispersive X-ray analysis. When glass ampoules are opened they contain a larger number of particles than rubber capped vials due to the vacuum effect on glass particles during the opening of the ampoule (41). Renal arteriography in rabbits using the centrifuged deposit from contrast media ampoules causes arterial obstruction and infarction, and the incidence of these lesions was decreased with filtered contrast medium (SEDA-5, 422). Angiographic catheters and guide-wires also contain a very large number of particles derived from the manufacturing process and the release of these particles is increased some 6-fold after the insertion of the guide-wire into the catheter (42). The various aspects of these problems have been reviewed in detail (43). Vials should be opened by removing the cap and not by puncture of the membrane, since the needle usually pushes large rubber particles into the solution. Ideally, contrast media should be filtered before injection but this will often not be practicable.

In the case of glass ampoules, if the ampoule is allowed to stand for 30–60 sec after opening, most of the larger particles will have sedimented to the bottom of the ampoule. These can then be avoided by leaving the lower 2–3 mm of contrast medium in the ampoule (44). With catheters, the guide-wire should be moved in and out of the dry catheter several times, followed by high-pressure flushing of the catheter. The guide-wire itself should then be rinsed in a large amount of sterile water. Furthermore, bending of the catheter should be avoided when it is moved over the guide-wire. The friction of the hard metal against the soft plastic increases considerably when bent and long plastic shavings (up to 3.8 cm) can be scraped from the wall of the catheter and released into the artery (43).

VENOGRAPHY *(SEDA-1, 356; SEDA-4, 335; SEDA-5, 421)*

The effects of meglumine iothalamate 280 (Conray), and the low-osmolar medium sodium and meglumine ioxaglate 320 (Hexabrix) were compared in a double-blind, within-patient study. Bilateral venography was performed in 100 patients and alternate contrast media were used in each leg. The incidence of *pain* in the foot and leg at the time of the examination was significantly lower after ioxaglate (35%) than after iothalamate (50%). A postal questionnaire on delayed effects was returned by 55 patients. There was also a significant difference in the incidence of *delayed pain* in the foot or leg (ioxaglate 24%, iothalamate 49%) and *swelling* of the foot or leg (ioxaglate 15%, iothalamate 38%) (45[CR]).

Gangrene of the toes occurred 3 days after venography with meglumine iothalamate 282 as a result of extravasation of contrast medium. An additional factor may have been arterial damage by submalleolar compression during the examination (46[Cr]).

MYELOGRAPHY

Iophendylate

In a series of 68 cervical myelograms using iophendylate, some contrast medium entered the cisterna magna in 35 patients and immediately gave rise to *headache*. In 22 patients, when contrast medium reached the sella there was severe headache. 12 patients complained of headache for 6 months or longer after myelography and in these cases there were residues of iophendylate in the hypophyseal region (47[cr]).

Starch glove-powder (Biosorb), injected into the subarachnoid space of rabbits, causes *arachnoiditis*. The combination of iophendylate and glove-powder was synergistic. It is important to avoid contamination of the spinal needle with glove-powder during myelography (48).

Water-soluble media

A variety of side effects have been reported in the previous annuals (SEDA-4, 335; SEDA-5, 422; SEDA-6, 407; SEDA-7, 453). Additional side effects described in a recent analysis include *muscle pains* in various parts of the body, *auditory symptoms* of a high frequency tone or bell-ringing, and *visual disturbances* of various types. One hypermetropic patient was able to read a newspaper without glasses for several hours whereas usually without glasses he could only read the larger headlines. In one patient a generalized *allergic rash* lasted for 2 weeks (49[CR]).

In another study an *anaphylactic reaction* occurred 2 hours after cervical myelography. There was dyspnea and acute hypotension. The patient responded to treatment but developed a blotchy rash (50[cR]).

Transient *motor aphasia* occurred in 2 patients. In one of these, measurements of regional blood flow showed areas of relative hypoperfusion in the right frontal region and left Sylvian region. The hypoperfusion might have been a predisposing factor (51[CR]).

3 cases of bilateral *sixth nerve palsy* occurred, 1–3 weeks after water-soluble myelography. The condition was benign and symptoms cleared over a period of 5 months. The main cause was probably post-puncture leakage of CSF but an additional toxic effect of the contrast medium could not be excluded. The authors in this paper refer to the use of iophendylate but the context suggests that metrizamide was probably used (52[Cr]). In another paper 2 similar cases of sixth nerve palsy were reported after metrizamide myelography (53[CR]).

In an analysis of metrizamide myelography in *children and adolescents* to determine the *incidence of complications* minor adverse reactions occurred in 58% of cases, moderate reactions in 17%, marked reactions in 8% and severe reactions in 1.6% of cases. The incidence of moderate, marked and severe reactions was related to dose and to the intracranial extension of the medium. Dose should therefore be calculated in relation to a child's age (and hence according to the size of the CNS); it should therefore not be based on the physical size or weight of the child (54[CR]). In a series of 605 pediatric myelograms with metrizamide the lumbar puncture needle penetrated a lesion below the conus in 10 cases but only 1 patient developed a paraplegia due to puncture of the lesion and injection of contrast medium. The risk of myelography by lumbar puncture is therefore minimal (55[CR]).

It has been suggested earlier that neurotropic drugs increase the risk of *epilepsy* in metrizamide myelography. The use of levomepromazine (20–50 mg/day) in combination with paracetamol to control severe pain in the lumbago sciatica syndrome did not increase the incidence of EEG abnormalities after metrizamide myelography and it is concluded that it is not necessary to discontinue such treatment before myelography is performed (56[CR]).

When iophendylate is used for myelography, the presence of blood in the CSF is commonly believed to increase the risk of *arachnoiditis*. An experimental study in monkeys indicates however that a mixture of blood and metrizamide does not increase the risk of arachnoiditis, and a bloody CSF is therefore not a contraindication to metrizamide myelography (57).

8 cases of streptococcal *meningitis* occurred after myelography with metrizamide or iophendylate. In 6 patients, the Gram stain of the CSF was positive and helped to differentiate the condition from a chemical meningitis. In 2 patients, the Gram stain was negative leading to an initial diagnosis of chemical meningitis which was at first treated by steroids. In 1 patient there was a temporary improvement followed by a relapse. The other patient showed no improvement. Both patients subsequently had positive cultures in the CSF and responded to chemotherapy (59[CR]).

Iopamidol is now tending to replace metrizamide for myelography. Several papers report a lower incidence of side effects following iopamidol, particularly in relation

Table 1. *Summary of reports received on adverse reactions from radiopharmaceuticals (70)*

Radiopharmaceutical		1980			1981			1982 (1st half)		
		Number of reports	Types of reaction	Number of patients requiring treatment	Number of reports	Types of reaction	Number of patients requiring treatment	Number of reports	Types of reaction	Number of patients requiring treatment
^{99m}Tc	colloid SbS	1	a		1	a	1	2	a	
	RhS	1	a	1	–			–		
	S-colloid	1	a		–			–		
	Albumin	1	a		–			–		
	Microspheres	1	a	1	1	b		1	b	
	Millimicrospheres	2	b	1	–			–		
	DTPA	–			1	a	1	–		
	MDP	4	a	1	3	a,b		2	b	
	Plasmin	–			–			1	a	1
^{51}Cr	Chromate RBC, ^{125}I HSA	1	d		–			–		
	EDTA	–			1	c		1	a	
^{67}Ga	Citrate	1	c		1	d	1	1	a	
^{123}I	NaI	–			1	d		–		
	Hippuran	1	c	1	–			–		
$^{125/131}$I	Hippuran	1	a	1	1	a	1	–		
^{131}I	Cholesterol	9	a	9	1	a	1	–		
	NaI	–			–			1	d	
^{198}Au	Colloid	1	a		–			–		
^{131}I	HSA-cisternography	–			1	d	1	1	b	
^{111}In	DTPA-cisternography	–			1	d		–		
^{169}Yb	Ca-DTPA-cisternography	–			3	d	3	–		
Total		25		15	16		9	10		1

Types of reaction: a: Allergic; b: Vasovagal; c: Local effects; d: Other effects.

to the psychosyndrome characteristic of metrizamide (60[CR]–62[CR]). Computed tomography of the brain following iopamidol myelography shows penetration of the contrast medium into the cortex, similar to that occurring with metrizamide. The lower incidence of side effects with iopamidol therefore suggests that the psychosyndrome was due to a chemical effect on the brain cells by metrizamide. However, if used in excess, iopamidol is potentially also neurotoxic (63[CR]). In patients with a narrow lumbar sac contrast density in the spine decreases more rapidly and is accompanied by a more rapid intracranial accumulation of contrast medium suggesting a more active transport of CSF in this group of patients (64[CR]).

THOROTRAST *(SED-9, 767)*

Delayed neurotoxicity occurred 20 years after thorotrast myelography in 5 patients. All the patients developed a cauda equina syndrome. Unenhanced CT studies showed dense opacification of the subarachnoid space by the thorotrast, maximal in the basal cisterns and this was associated with obstructive hydrocephalus. One patient had dense opacification in the sella and hypothalamus with panhypopituitarism (65[CR]).

HYSTEROSALPINGOGRAPHY

The side effects of Dimer-X (iocarmate), Hexabrix (ioxaglate), Vasurix Polyvidone (acetrizoate) and Endografine (iodipamide) were compared in 142 patients undergoing hysterosalpingography. Endografine caused considerably more *pain,* particularly in patients under the age of 30. In this paper Endografine is incorrectly stated to consist of diatrizoate. Endografine is iodipamide. Dimer-X tended to cause more *nausea.* In this series, no increase of pain was noted in patients with hydrosalpinx (66[CR]). In another series of 220 hysterosalpingograms using Isopaque Amin 200, contrast medium in bilaterally closed tubes caused longer lasting pain (67). In both series delayed onset of pain was a problem in a number of patients.

HEPATIC OIL EMBOLISM

Hepatic oil embolism after lymphography is a rare complication. It does not give rise to clinical symptoms but usually indicates a severe degree of malignant node obstruction, causing a lympho-venous fistula. Thrombosis of the inferior vena cava may be an adjuvant factor. Hepatic oil embolism has also been seen in filariasis, tuberculosis and retroperitoneal fibrosis (68[CR]).

EFFECTS ON THRYOID FUNCTION

Varying effects on thyroid function tests have been reported after administration of iodine containing contrast media, more particularly after cholecystographic media. In one series of cases there was an increase in serum T3, after 6 weeks and in another case there was frank thyrotoxicosis (SEDA-6, 408). Other authors have reported that the main action of the oral cholecystographic media (iopanoate and ipodate) is to block the de-iodination of thyroxine (T4) to tri-iodothyronine (T3) in the central nervous system, pituitary gland and in the peripheral tissues such as the liver and kidney. This causes a decrease in serum T3 levels and an increase in serum concentrations of T4, free T4 and TSH. There is also an increase in the inactive metabolite reverse T3 (rT3). The anti-arrhythmic agent amiodarone has a similar action (69[CR]).

RADIOPHARMACEUTICALS

The European Nuclear Medicine Society has recently instituted a reporting system for adverse reactions to radiopharmaceuticals (Table 1). The group 'other effects' included *vomiting, headache, pain* in the thyroid region after administration of radioactive iodine, one *pyrogen* reaction and a fatal case of *cardiac arrest* 1 hour after the injection of gallium citrate. The cause of the cardiac arrest could not be found but it did not appear to be related to the radiopharmaceutical (70[CR]).

A severe *anaphylactic reaction* occurred 7 min after injection of orthoiodohippurate for renography in a patient who had previously had a severe reaction following intravenous urography with Conray 400. It was estimated that the dose of radiopharmaceutical contained approximately 11 μg of iodine (71[CR]). A delayed anaphylactoid reaction with respiratory embarassment, hypotension and an urticarial rash occurred 1 hour after injection of 99 Technetium diethylenetriaminepentaacetic acid (99mTc DTPA) for a brain scan (72[CR]). Experience with under-reporting of reactions in contrast media surveys, suggests that the incidence of reactions after radiopharmaceuticals is likely to be higher than the few reported cases might suggest.

REFERENCES

1. Peterson N, Rohrman CA, Lennard ES (1982) Diagnosis and treatment of retroperitoneal perforations complicating the double-contrast barium-enema examination. *Radiology, 144,* 249.
2. Han SY, Tishler JM (1982) Perforation of the colon above the peritoneal reflection during the barium-enema examination. *Radiology, 144,* 253.
3. Nelson RL, Abcarian H, Prasad ML (1982) Iatrogenic perforation of the colon and rectum. *Dis. Col. Rect., 25,* 305.
4. Eklöf O, Hald J, Thomasson B (1983) Barium peritonitis. Experience of five pediatric cases. *Pediatr. Radiol., 13,* 5.
5. Sisley JF, Wagner CW (1982) Barium appendicitis. *South. Med. J., 75,* 498.
6. Blanloe Y, Colomb P, Vairon A et al (1983) Syndrome des détresse respiratoire aiguë après inhalation accidentelle de produit de contraste hydrosoluble. *Sem. Hôp. Paris, 59,* 762.
7. Radberg C, Tibbling L (1982) Väly ratt kontrast vid röntgen av misstänkt esofagusperforation. *Läkartidningen, 79,* 4305.
8. Rust RJ, Cohen MD, Ulbricht TM (1982) Clinical, radiographic and pathologic effects of amipaque on rabbit lung. Comparison with barium and gastrografin. *Acta Radiol. Diagn., 23,* 553.
9. Alford BA, Dee P, Feldman P (1983) The effects of metrizamide on the lung. *Pediatr. Radiol., 13,* 1.
10. Von Vogel H, Oesterrich F-U (1983) Art und Häufigkeit von Komplikationen bei Röntgenuntersuchungen des oberen Gastrointestinaltraktes. *Röntgenpraxis, 36,* 104.
11. Hutton LC, Tuckerman JF, Henderson AR (1982) Elevation of serum lactate dehydrogenase-5 following methylglucamine iodipamide (Cholografin/Biligrafin) infusion for intravenous cholangiography. *Clin. Chim. Acta, 122,* 279.
12. Wirell S (1982) Adverse reactions to intravenous cholegraphy with ioglycamide. Correlation with the level of circulating sex hormones. *Acta Radiol. Diagn., 23,* 405.
13. Hartman GW, Hattery RR, Witten DM, Williamson B (1982) Mortality during excretory urography: Mayo Clinic experience. *Am. J. Roentgenol., 139,* 919.
14. Lawton G, Phillips T, Davies R (1982) Alteration in heart rate and rhythm at urography with sodium diatrizoate. *Acta Radiol. Diagn., 23,* 107.
15. Pfister RC, Hutter AM, Newhouse JH et al (1983) Contrast-medium-induced electrocardiographic abnormalities: comparison of bolus and infusion of methylglucamine iodamide and methylglucamine/sodium diatrizoate. *Am. J. Roentgenol., 140,* 149.
16. Dawson P (1983) Unpublished data.
17. Dawson P, Pitfield J, Britton J (1983) Contrast media and bronchospasm: a study with iopamidol. *Clin. Radiol., 34,* 227.
18. Hagen B (1982) Iopamidol, a new non-ionic x-ray contrast medium. Results of angiographic investigations of more than 300 patients with special regard to pain sensations. *Radiologe, 22,* 581.
19. Katzberg RW, Morris TW, Schulman G et al (1983) Reactions to intravenous contrast media. Part 1: Severe and fatal cardiovascular reactions in a canine dehydration model. *Radiology, 147,* 327.
20. Horak A, Raine R, Opie LH, Lloyd EA (1983) Severe myocardial ischaemia induced by intravenous adrenaline. *Br. Med. J., 286,* 519.
21. D'Elia JA, Gleason RE, Alday M et al (1982) Nephrotoxicity from angiographic contrast media. A prospective study. *Am. J. Med., 72,* 719.
22. Hou SH, Bushinsky DA, Wish JB et al (1983) Hospital-acquired renal insufficiency: a prospective study. *Am. J. Med., 74,* 243.
23. Peters C, Delmonico FL, Cosimi AB et al (1983) Risk versus benefits of contrast medium exposure in renal allograft recipients. *Surg. Gynec. Obstet., 176,* 467.
24. Nillson PE, Holtäs SL, Tejler LT (1982) Subjective responses and albuminuria induced by ioxaglate during renal angiography in man. *Radiology, 144,* 509.
25. Holtäs SL (1983) Personal communication.
26. Gassman W, Haferlach T, Schmitz N et al (1983) Zur Problematik der intravenösen Urographie bei Patienten mit Plasmozytom. *Schweiz Med. Wschr., 113,* 301.
27. Ramsay AW, Spector M, Rodgers AL et al (1982) Crystalluria following excretory urography. *Br. J. Urol., 54,* 341.
28. Hietala S-O, Lindqvist B, Lithner F, Wirell M (1982) Fatal reaction following renal angiography and biopsy in diabetic patients with azotaemia. *Acta Med. Scand., 212,* 179.
29. Mallette LE, Gomez LS (1983) Systemic hypocalcaemia after clinical injections of radiographic contrast media: amelioration by omission of calcium chelating agents. *Radiology, 147,* 677.
30. Morris S, Sahler LG, Fischer HW (1982) Calcium binding by radiopaque media. *Invest. Radiol., 17,* 501.
31. Gressier M, Beaune J, Amouroux C et al

(1980) Arrêt cardiaque prolongé en diastole au cours d'une coronarographie chez un patient atteint d'un angor de Prinzmétal traité par le Vérapamil. Réversibilité sous circulation extra-corporelle. *Nouv. Presse Méd., 9,* 1521.
32. Gerber KH, Higgins CB, Yuh Y-S et al (1982) Regional hemodynamic and metabolic effects of ionic and non-ionic contrast media in normal and ischaemic states. *Circulation, 65,* 1307.
33. Lehman MH, Case RB (1983) Reduced human ventricular fibrillation threshold associated with contrast-induced Q-T prolongation. *J. Electrocardiol., 16,* 105.
34. Cochran JW, Morrell F, Huckman MS, Cochran EJ (1982) Transient global amnesia after cerebral angiography. Report of seven cases. *Arch. Neurol., 39,* 593.
35. Winter J (1982) Non-random clustering of adverse reactions to iodinated radiographic contrast media used for computed tomography. *J. Comput. Tomogr., 6,* 109.
36. Pagani JJ, Hayman LA, Bigelow RH et al (1983) Diazepam prophylaxis of contrast media-induced seizures during computed tomography of patients with brain metastases. *Am. J. Neuroradiol., 4,* 67.
37. Mitchell AA, Louik C, Lacoutoure P et al (1982) Risks to children from computed tomographic scan premedication. *J. Am. Med. Assoc., 247,* 2385.
38. Staubli M, Braunschweig J, Tillman U (1982) Changes in the rheologic properties of blood as induced by sodium/meglumine ioxaglate compared with sodium/meglumine diatrizoate and metrizamide. *Acta Radiol. Diagn., 23,* 71.
39. Aspelin P (1983) Personal communication.
40. Parvez R, Moncada R, Messmore HL, Fareed J (1982) Ionic and non-ionic contrast media interaction with anti-coagulant drugs. *Acta Radiol. Diagn., 23,* 401.
41. Winding O (1980) Intrinsic particles in angiographic contrast media. *Radiology, 134,* 317.
42. Winding O (1981) Particle release from angiographic utensils. *Europ. J. Radiol., 1,* 114.
43. Hegedos V, Winding O, Grønvall J, Faarup P (1982) Manufacturing-derived impurities in angiography. In: Baert AL, Boijsen E, Fuchs WA, Heuck FHW (Eds), *Frontiers in European Radiology, Vol. 1,* p. 109. Springer, Berlin.
44. Winding O (1983) Personal communication.
45. Lea Thomas M, Walters HL, Briggs GM (1982) A double-blind comparative study of the tolerance of sodium and meglumine ioxaglate (Hexabrix) with meglumine iothalamate (Conray) in ascending phlebography of the leg. *Australas. Radiol., 26,* 288.
46. Von Kinnunen J, Reinikainen M, Laasonen EM (1982) Hautnekrose nach aszendierender Beinphlebographie. *Fortschr. Röngenstr., 136,* 104.
47. Avrahami E, Cohn DF (1982) Zur Problem der postmyelographischen Kopfschmerzen. *Schweiz. Arch. Neurol. Neurochir. Psych., 130,* 157.
48. Williams AG, Seigel RS, Kornfield M, Whorton JA (1982) Experimental production of arachnoiditis with glove powder contamination during myelography. *Am. J. Neuroradiol., 3,* 121.
49. Hauge O, Falkenberg H (1982) Neuropsychologic reactions and other side effects after metrizamide myelography. *Am. J. Neuroradiol., 3,* 229.
50. Gelmers HJ (1979) Adverse side effects of metrizamide in myelography. *Neuroradiology, 18,* 119.
51. Masdeu JC, Glista GG, Rubino FA et al (1983) Transient motor aphasia following metrizamide. *Am. J. Neuroradiol., 4,* 200.
52. Miller EA, Savino PJ, Schatz NJ (1982) Bilateral sixth-nerve palsy. A rare complication of water-soluble contrast myelography. *Arch. Ophthalmol., 100,* 603.
53. Heredero EB, Gutierrez JA, Estaban F et al (1982) Neuropatia del sexto par craneal por metrizamida. A proposito de dos observaciones. *Arch. Neurobiol., 45,* 291.
54. Petterson H, Fitz CR, Harwood-Nash DCF et al (1982) Adverse reactions to myelography with metrizamide in infants, children and adolescents. I. General and CNS effects. *Acta Radiol. Diagn., 23,* 323.
55. Petterson H, Fitz CR, Harwood-Nash DCF et al (1982) Adverse reactions to myelography with metrizamide in infants, children and adolescents. II. Local injury caused by lumbar puncture and injection of contrast medium. *Acta Radiol. Diagn., 23,* 331.
56. Stadnes B, Oftedal SI, Weber H (1982) Effect of levomepromazine on EEG and clinical side effects after lumbar myelography with metrizamide. *Acta Radiol. Diagn., 23,* 111.
57. Haughton VM, Ho K-G (1982) Effect of blood on arachnoiditis from aqueous myelographic contrast media. *Am. J. Roentgenol., 139,* 569.
58. Auer RN, Fox AJ, Kaufman CE (1982) The histologic effect of intraventricular injection of metrizamide. *Arch. Neurol., 39,* 60.
59. Schlesinger JJ, Salit IE, McCormack G (1982) Streptococcal meningitis after myelography. *Arch. Neurol., 39,* 576.
60. Bassi P, Cecchini A, Dettori P, Signorini E (1982) Myelography with iopamidol, a non-ionic water-soluble contrast medium: incidence of complications. *Neuroradiology, 24,* 85.
61. McAllister VL, Hall K (1983) A randomised blind trial of iopamidol (Niopam) and metrizamide (Amipaque) in lumbar myelography. *Neuroradiology, 24,* 217.
62. Drayer BP, Warner MA, Sudilovsky A et al 982) Iopamidol vs metrizamide: a double blind study for cervical myelography. *Neuroradiology, 24,* 77.
63. Drayer BP, Vassalo C, Sudilovsky A et al (1983) A double-blind trial of iopamidol versus

metrizamide for lumbosacral myelography. *J. Neurosurg., 58,* 531.
64. Stoeter P, Bergleiter R, Schneider I, Kubina FG (1982) Nebenwirkungen und Kontrastmittelresorption von Iopamidol und Iocarmat bei der lumbalen Myelographie. *CT-Sonographie, 2,* 179.
65. Hanson M, Weinstein M, Duchesneau P (1982) Delayed thorotrast neurotoxicity: a clinical radiologic study. *Neurology (NY), 32,* 148.
66. Schutte HE (1982) Comparative study: Endografine (diatrizoate), Vasurix Polyvidone (acetrizoate), Dimer-X (iocarmate) and Hexabrix (ioxaglate) in hysterosalpingopelvigraphy. *Diagnostic Imaging, 51,* 277.
67. Zimmer J (1983) Isopaque Amin (200) (meglumin metrizoas) a contrast medium for use in hysterosalpingopelvigraphy. Registration of late reactions. *Tidskr. Nor. Laegeforen, 103,* 534.
68. Bruneton JN, Le Treut A, Abbes M et al (1982) Hepatic oil embolization following lymphangiography. A report of 12 cases. *Lymphology, 15,* 70.
69. Borst GC, Eil C, Burman KD (1983) Euthyroid hyperthyroxinaemia. *Ann. Intern. Med., 98,* 366.
70. Joint Committee on Radiopharmaceuticals of the European Nuclear Medicine Society and the Society of Nuclear Medicine – Europe (1982) The system for 'Reporting of adverse reactions and drug defects' (1980–1982) – First report. *Nucl. Med., 21,* 274.
71. Stφckel M, Ennow K, Kristensen K, Rφdbro P (1983) Anaphylactic reactions to orthoiodohippurate. *Eur. J. Nucl. Med., 8,* 89.
72. Hurman DC, Critchley M, Shanahan CV (1982) Adverse reaction to a radionuclide brainscanning agent. *Nucl. Med. Commun., 3,* 373.

B.C.P. Polak

49 Drugs used in ocular treatment

Ophthalmic drugs topically applied have significant absorption, which may result in widespread adverse side effects. As previously in this series, ophthalmic drugs will for the sake of convenience, if somewhat arbitrarily, be classified into two main groups: diagnostic and therapeutic agents.

DIAGNOSTIC OPHTHALMIC DRUGS

CYCLOPLEGICS AND MYDRIATICS

Anticholinergic agents

Atropine *(SED-9, 772; SEDA-5, 295; SEDA-6, 412; SEDA-7, 355)* The effect of atropine on the central nervous system is due to its anticholinergic central action affecting stimulation of the medulla and higher cerebral centers. In toxic dosages this accounts for irritability, hallucinations, tachypnea and the probable thermoregulatory center dysfunction in homeostatic body temperature control. Children are especially sensitive.

31 children aged from 1 to 14 years who had been given atropine eye drops to measure refraction presented with the following side effects: increased temperature (9/31), dry red skin (8/31), reddened eye (3/31) and periorbital dermatitis (2/31) after single (22/31) or repeated (9/31) administration of atropine. In the epicutaneous test with atropine 1% (readings after 24, 48 and 72 hours) not a single child showed an allergic or toxic reaction. The rarity of allergy after administration of atropine eye drops is emphasized by the fact that periorbital dermatitis was observed in only 2 cases (1^R).

Recently atropine toxicity has been reported in identical twins.

Both infants were 5-month-old white males, born after a full-term, uncomplicated pregnancy. Because of developmental delay and parental concern about their vision they were referred to an ophthalmologist. Approximately 30 minutes after instillation of one drop of 0.5% atropine sulfate solution into each eye the day prior to examination, both children developed irritability and fever prompting the parents to bring them to the emergency room. Both infants showed a fine maculopapular rash, warm dry skin, distended abdomen with decreased bowel sounds and dilated unreactive pupils. There was a temperature of 39°C and 41°C respectively, a pulse rate of 200 and 180, a respiratory rate of 80 and a blood pressure of 106/30 and 94/44 respectively. After treatment with 0.5 mg of physostigmine intravenously the children became more alert; flushing and abdominal distension decreased, as well as pulse rate and temperature. Funduscopic examination revealed moderate optic nerve hypoplasia in one eye and marked optic nerve hypoplasia in the other eye of both children, with bilateral pale optic discs (2^C).

Optic nerve hypoplasia or atrophy and atropine toxicity or hypersensitivity have not been reported as occurring together before, and the association here may be purely coincidental. Careful instruction to parents about dosage schedules should be routinely provided, so that improper usage is minimized. Parents should also be informed about the toxic effects and be alerted to the signs and symptoms to watch for when using atropine eye drops.

THERAPEUTIC OPHTHALMIC DRUGS

Cholinergic agents

Acetylcholine *(SED-9, 776)* Hypotension and mild bradycardia have been reported as systemic reactions following ophthalmologic use of acetylcholine. Recently a 83-year-old man, scheduled for cataract extraction under local anesthesia, developed bradycardia, hypotension, flushing, sweating and breathing difficulty after instillation of acetyl-

Side Effects of Drugs Annual 8
M.N.G. Dukes, editor

ISBN 0 444 90339 9
$0.80 per article per page (transactional system)
$0.20 per article per page (licensing system)

choline chloride solution into the anterior chamber following the removal of the lens (3[C]).

Antiglaucomatous drugs. Sympathomimetic agents

Dipivefrine (dipivalylepinephrine; DPE; Propine) *(SED-9, 780; SEDA-5, 429)* Potential advantages of this epinephrine pro-drug include increased duration of action, increased bioavailability, increased potency, increased stability and a decreased incidence of side effects. The effect on pupil size is minor and insignificant, no objective sight-threatening effects are observed, and central visual acuity and visual fields are not affected after application of 0.1% solution of dipivalylepinephrine into the eye. However, minor sporadic and transient burning or stinging sensations may be observed (4[C]).

In aphakic glaucomatous eyes undergoing topical epinephrine therapy, cystoid macular edema may occur, which is completely reversed by discontinuing therapy. A similar untoward reaction was seen in a glaucomatous phakic eye after treatment with dipivefrine hydrochloride (Propine) (5[C]).

Beta-blockers

Beta-blockers have a brief local anesthetic effect when applied to the cornea in drop form. With the electronic optical esthesiometer accurate, reproducible sensibility measurements are now possible. In a randomized study the local anesthetic side effects of the beta-blockers metipranolol and timolol were found to be comparable and dosage-dependent (6[r]).

Timolol (Timoptol; Timoptic) *(SED-9, 779; SEDA-5, 425; SEDA-7, 458)* Systemic adverse effects of timolol ophthalmic solution include bradycardia, palpitations, hypotension, syncope, cardiac failure, sudden death, bronchospasm (asthma attacks), gastrointestinal distress (nausea and diarrhea), impotence, disorientation, anxiety, loss of memory, sedation, depression and fatigue. Ocular adverse reactions may be observed as burning sensations and dryness of eyes.

The incidence of side effects in two prospective studies was about 20%, and some 40% of these had to discontinue timolol treatment. Most side effects are usually experienced after administration of the 0.5% solution.

Bilateral glaucoma simplex was diagnosed in a 70-year-old male patient, who had been suffering from moderate asthma since adolescence. Topical treatment with timolol in ophthalmic solution of 0.25% twice a day was initiated. During the following year the patient noticed that his dyspnea became consistently worse for 1–2 hours following application of the eyedrops. He was advised to discontinue timolol therapy, and his asthma subsequently ameliorated. In a provocation test, carried out 2 months later with the patient's informed consent, forced expiratory volume in the first second was reduced by 56% and bradycardia was induced after application of 2 drops of timolol (7[c]).

The timolol 0.25% solution has so far been considered less prone to result in systemic beta-blockage. Even this concentration may, however, cause severe bronchoconstriction and bradycardia in patients with chronic airflow obstruction, and it represents a potential risk to patients suffering from cardiac failure or chronic obstructive pulmonary disease.

The results of a 12-month blind randomized trial comparing the intraocular pressure lowering effect of timolol 0.25% with timolol 0.5% revealed little difference in effectiveness (8[c]). Timolol 0.25% should be the initial treatment of choice, and if this proves ineffective (either early or late), then alternative or additional therapy should be considered in preference to the common clinical practice of changing the concentration of timolol to 0.5%. However, one has to be aware of the existence and importance of long-term drift (or loss of control with continuous long-term topical timolol).

An additional ocular side effect of timolol is a marked (e.g. 40%) reduction in the magnitude of the light-insensitive component of the standing potential of the eye. This corresponds to the "dark trough" of the electro-oculogram (EOG) and might be attributed to the effect of timolol on the ciliary epithelium which contributes, as does the retinal pigment epithelium, to the standing potential. The other component of the EOG, the light rise, remains unaffected. The result would be a significant increase in the value of the EOG ratio (or Arden index) (9[R]).

Antibiotics *(SEDA-5, 428)*

Chloramphenicol Marrow aplasia from ophthalmic chloramphenicol has been reported.

A 73-year-old woman died of aplastic anemia less than 2 months after undergoing cataract extraction and beginning topical therapy with chloramphenicol. The first signs of pancytopenia began within 1 month, and the pattern of aplastic anemia was associated with an idiosyncratic response to chloramphenicol (10[R]). Chloramphenicol is the agent most frequently associated with drug-induced aplastic anemia, but physicians faced with blood dyscrasias may fail to ask patients if they have ever received this agent topically in an ocular medication, and especially because significant hematopoietic reactions may occur many months after the drug is discontinued, the patient may not even remember having undergone topical ophthalmic treatment. The hematologic risk associated with topically administered ocular chloramphenicol may therefore in fact be higher than the 4 earlier reported cases seem to indicate (SEDA-5, 428). Recently 2 patients were seen in The Netherlands with marrow aplasia associated with ocular chloramphenicol therapy: one patient died because of thrombocytopenia, the other recovered from marrow aplasia (unpublished data).

Antivirals

Ara-A (adenine arabinoside, vidarabine) and acycloguanosine (aciclovir, Zovirax) *(SEDA-7, 459)* In a double-blind clinical trial of 3% aciclovir and 3% adenine arabinoside in 93 patients with herpetic corneal ulceration, patients treated with aciclovir healed more rapidly than those treated with Ara-A. 1 patient on aciclovir experienced an *allergic response*, which could also have been caused by the atropine drops being administered concurrently; 1 patient on Ara-A complained of *gritty feeling* of the eye after application of the ointment (11[c]).

A combination of 3% aciclovir and 0.01% betamethasone eye drops was found to be effective in the management of disciform keratitis in a double-blind at-random treatment of 40 patients. The combination therapy showed a faster rate of healing, while other clinical parameters also improved more favourably. 3 patients showed mild transient *punctate keratopathy* (12[c]).

Newly developed therapeutic ophthalmic agents

Silicone oil The use of silicone oil injection in the treatment of retinal detachment with massive periretinal proliferation has been found to induce macular attachment in a high percentage of treated patients when followed up over more than 5 years. There is no difference in the success rate between phakic and aphakic eyes. The filling of the vitreous cavity with silicone oil may, however, cause *changes in refraction* (13[R]). Complications attributed to intraocular silicone oil include *cataract, keratopathy* and *glaucoma*. Of 103 phakic eyes, 73% developed lens opacities after 1 to 3 years. 87% after 3 to 5 years, and 90% after 5 years or longer. Few of these cataracts were sufficiently dense to require surgery, and those that did were managed with intra- or extracapsular lens extraction without difficulty. Keratopathy developed in 9 eyes, and in 2 of these penetrating keratoplasty was undertaken successfully. In 16 eyes persistently raised intraocular pressure (greater than 25 mm Hg) occurred; although silicone oil was found to be present in the chamber angle on gonioscopy in 33% of the cases, in only 6 eyes raised IOP was associated with oil in the anterior chamber (14[r]).

REFERENCES

1. Gallasch G, Schütz R, Götz ML, Kraus-Mackiw E (1982) Atropinebewirkungen: pharmakologische, allergische, pseudoallergische oder toxische Reaktionen? *Klin. Monatsbl. Augenheilkd., 181*, 96.
2. Sanitato JJ, Burke MJ (1983) Atropine toxicity in identical twins. *Ann. Ophthalmol., 15*, 380.
3. Gombos GM (1982) Systemic reactions following intraocular acetylcholine instillation. *Ann. Ophthalmol., 15*, 529.
4. Fajardo RV, Noche RR (1982) Ocular reactions of Filippino eyes to topical dipivalyl epinephrine. *Philipp. J. Ophthalmol., 14*, 8.
5. Mehelas TJ, Kollarits CR, Martin WG (1982) Cystoid macular edema presumably induced by dipivefrin hydrochloride (Propine). *Am. J. Ophthalmol., 94*, 682.
6. Draeger J, Schneider B, Winter R (1983) Die

lokalanästhetische Wirkung von Metipranolol im Vergleich zu Timolol. *Klin. Monatsbl. Augenheilkd.*, *182*, 210.

7. Ostergaard Laursen S, Bjerrum P (1982) Timolol eyedrop-induced severe bronchospasm. *Acta Med. Scand.*, *211*, 505.
8. Mills KB (1983) Blind randomised non-crossover long-term trial comparing topical timolol 0.25% with timolol 0.5% in the treatment of simple chronic glaucoma. *Br. J. Ophthalmol.*, *67*, 216.
9. Levine L (1982) Clinical implications of reported timolol-induced side effects. *Am. J. Optom. Physiol. Opt.*, *59*, 523.
10. Fraunfelder FT and Bagby GC (1982) Fatal aplastic anemia following topical administration of ophthalmic chloramphenicol. *Am. J. Ophthal.*, *93*, 356.
11. Young BJ, Patterson A, Ravenscroft T (1982) A randomised double-blind clinical trial of acyclovir (Zovirax) and adenine-arabinoside in herpes simplex corneal ulceration. *Br. J. Ophthalmol.*, *66*, 361.
12. Collum LMT, Logan P, Ravenscroft T (1983) Acyclovir (Zovirax) in herpetic disciform keratitis. *Br. J. Ophthalmol.*, *67*, 115.
13. Launay F, Laroche G, Limon S (1982) Modifications de la réfraction après injections intraoculaires de silicone liquide. *J. Fr. Ophtalmol.*, *5*, 417.
14. Leaver PK, Lean JS (1982) Results and complications of silicone oil injection in the treatment of massive periretinal proliferation. *Int. Ophthalmol.*, *5*, 86.

Henk Buurma and Arnold G. Vulto

50

Drugs used in nonorthodox medicine

Because of the still increasing use of nonorthodox approaches in the hope of curing illness and relieving suffering in many developed countries, interest from the side of 'official' medical sciences in these principles is rising. With respect to herbal remedies, an enormous research effort continues to isolate new and useful therapeutic substances from traditionally used plant material (1^r, 2^r). Classically this was the field of pharmacognosy, but with the emergence of a more integrated approach together with representatives of other sciences (e.g. anthropologists), a new discipline defined as ethnopharmacology has come into existence (3). Along with the search for potential alternative means of therapy, the body of knowledge available on the side effects of such treatments also increases. Several recent reviews (4^R, 5^R) deal with the possible side effects of 'natural' treatments, giving some counterweight to the often over-optimistic description of these treatments in publications directed to the lay public, an over-optimism which is reflected in the expectations regarding efficacy as well as safety. Fortunately, general practitioner trainees have shown considerable interest (more than 85% of respondents) in training in one or more alternative methods, with particularly high scores for acupuncture, hypnosis, homeopathy and osteopathy (6). It must be added, however, that such interest was much less among junior hospital doctors and less still among senior physicians. It is striking that, for example, in a country such as Great Britain the number of lay practitioners was about 27,800 (in 1981), of whom some 10,000 were organized in professional associations. This contrasts with the number of 29,800 general practitioners (in 1982), of whom only about 2000 have been trained to some degree in hypnosis, acupuncture, homeopathy or other 'alternative' means of treatment.

As pointed out in earlier volumes in this series we still have no reliable data as to the extent of use of nonorthodox remedies in developed countries or the use of traditional treatments in developing countries. A survey carried out in the Netherlands (8) showed that about a quarter of a representative sample had sought medical advice from nonorthodox healers in the past 3 years. Higher education, rural living area and relative low age (under 34 years) were determinants for a higher incidence of contacts with nonorthodox practitioners. In an English study it was found that 33% of patients with rheumatoid arthritis and 39% of those with backache admitted to having consulted an alternative practitioner (7).

In a 'Letter from ... Africa' in the British Medical Journal (9), Anne Savage reports that of 100 severely ill children admitted to a hospital in Transkei, 50% had received some treatment prior to coming to the clinic. 33 children had received enemas, predominantly of herbal origin, and 22 children had received some kind of oral herbal treatment. It turned out to be almost impossible to determine the nature of the components. Professor D'Arcy reports from Zimbabwe (10) the use of *nhowa muti* (orifice medicines) in babies and infants. The status of the anterior fontanel of an infant is used as an index of the health of a child. Any deviation from what is regarded as normal is taken as comprising a need for *nhowa* medicines. The paste for application to the fontanel invariably has cow dung as the vehicle, to which can be added powdered aspirin, aloe (*Aloe capensis*) or *rapoko* (a deep brown cereal

Side Effects of Drugs Annual 8
M.N.G. Dukes, editor

ISBN 0 444 90339 9
$0.80 per article per page (transactional system)
$0.20 per article per page (licensing system)

frequently infested with ergot), sugar, starch etc. The extent of this use of fontanel medicines is such that 80–90% of African infants admitted to hospitals around Harare (the capital of Zimbabwe), for any indication, show evidence of nhowa applications. The possible side effects are numerous. The scalp of the infant in the fontanel region is highly permeable and allows the entry of drugs (e.g. salicylates), toxins (e.g. tetanus), toxic substances (e.g. ergot alkaloids, anthraquinones from aloe), and infection (bacterial and fungal) into the systemic circulation. Faith in these treatments is such that efforts to stop the use of dung-mixtures are likely to fail.

From these examples it will be clear that if a patient presents symptoms that are difficult to explain by physiological or pathological mechanisms, one must bear in mind the very likelihood of his or her having taken 'alternative' or 'traditional' medicines of unknown composition and therefore unpredictable therapeutic outcome, either positive or negative.

In this chapter we will discuss in detail one group of alkaloids of highly toxic potential, as well as present 2 examples of folk remedies that may cause confusion in diagnosis.

Toxicity of plants containing pyrrolizidine alkaloids *(SEDA-6, 418; SEDA-7, 463, 467)*

Over the last 15 years a tremendous growth of interest in pyrrolizidine alkaloids (PA) could be noticed (for reviews see 11, 12, 17). This increased interest is due to the recognition that many of these substances may be the cause of illness and death, not only in livestock, but also in man. Plants containing PA are of worldwide distribution, and in many countries some species have been traditionally used as food or medicine for man and animals (13). Many, though not all, of the PA are hepatotoxic. The structural features necessary for hepatotoxic action are: a double bond at C(1)C(2) of the pyrrolizidine moiety and esterification of at least 1 of its hydroxyl groups (R′ and/or R″) (see 11, 12) (Fig. 1).

At this moment more than 350 plant species belonging to 10 botanical families (mostly to the Boraginaceae, Compositae and Leguminosae) are known to contain

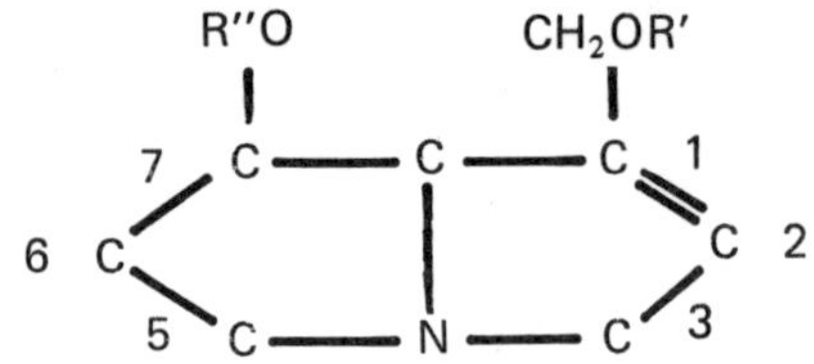

Fig. 1. Elemental structure of pyrrolizidine alkaloids.

PA, and this figure increases every year. In several parts of the world, but more especially in developing countries, PA poisoning poses a serious problem to public health. The two major sources of human exposure are accidental contamination of foodstuffs and the deliberate use of PA containing plants in herbal preparations. There are several reports of outbreaks of hepatic veno-occlusive disease that indicate the extent of this cultural problem in many areas of Africa, Asia and South- and Central America. In the latter, particularly on Jamaica, veno-occlusive disease in children has taken on almost epidemic proportions. In that country, for example, an undefinable 'bush tea' is prepared of which Crotalaria species are the major source. The high incidence of chronic liver disease in Sri-Lanka and Africa is also thought by some to be caused by the extensive consumption of PA-containing plants or foods (13). However, in many developed countries all kinds of preparations containing PA are highly valued by proponents of 'natural' treatments and are marketed as a consequence. In particular Comfrey (Symphytum officinale) and Senecio longilobus are widely used both in internal and external preparations.

An outbreak of veno-occlusive disease in Northwest Afghanistan during 1974–1975 has been correlated with the consumption of bread made from unwinnowed wheat, contaminated with seeds of Heliotropium popovii H. Riedl, subsp. gillianum H. Riedl (see below). A general problem in recognizing such intoxications is that the victims have rarely been exposed to only one possibly causative factor. Often, they have been exposed to parasitic infestations and the effects of malnutrition as well as to the toxic effects of herbal preparations. Moreover, the toxicological profile of a whole plant or a preparation may differ quite substantially from that of an isolated, purified active principle. Therefore it can be misleading to extrapolate findings from laboratory experiments involving the administration to animals of large doses of purified compounds.

Roitman (14) points out that human toxicological data are scarce as compared with experimental data from animal studies. The most reliable report emanated from an incident in which a large number of people (>7200) were examined after consuming an estimated 2 mg/day of PA from Heliotropium-contaminated wheat flour over a 2-year time span. After this period, 23% of the subjects had severe liver impairment. It was concluded that the regular use of Comfrey root tea, containing 3–13 times the amount of alkaloid taken in the above episode, would have serious consequences for human health and that its use should therefore be discouraged. Roitman estimated the total alkaloid content in both the roots and the leaves of Comfrey and also determined how much alkaloid is consumed by drinking a cup of Comfrey root tea after having prepared an infusion according to directions on the package of a locally purchased product (in the USA). The amount of alkaloid could be from 8.5 mg up to as much as 26 mg per cup. With respect to the use of Comfrey leaves it was suggested that consumption should similarly be avoided because of the carcinogenicity demonstrated in rats fed a diet containing Symphytum officinale. Although only few of the known PA have as yet been tested for possible carcinogenic action in long-term experiments, there are reports of tumors in rats having been fed with (mixtures of) PA. For these reasons, some over-the-counter drugs containing S. officinale have been withdrawn from the market by their manufacturers. The German health authorities are preparing a general warning against the use of pyrrolizidine-containing preparations (15). As yet a direct correlation between the use of PA and the occurrence of liver cancer has not been confirmed. A further cause for concern is that in experimental animals exposure to low levels of the alkaloids resulted in the appearance of lung, rather than liver, lesions. These lesions progressed to pulmonary arterial hypertension and right-ventricular hypertrophy. It has indeed been observed that in several human cases of pyrrolizidine poisoning lung disease was a concomitant complication.

In a well documented paper Huxtable (16[C]) has presented the case histories of 2 instances of poisoning in children in the state of Arizona (USA).

One case involved a 6-month-old Mexican-American girl, admitted to hospital with a diagnosis of typical hepatitis. It was found that the child had been given a herbal tea, known as Gardolobo Yerba, over a 2-week period prior to admission. The remainder of this herb was identified as Senecio longilobus, which is probably identical with Senecio douglasii. After analysis of the sample it was found that the alkaloid fraction (which was 0.3%) was largely ridelliine and the N-oxide fraction (ca. 1%) was largely retrorsine N-oxide, together with the N-oxides of seneciphylline and senecionine. Based on the mother's recipe a tea was prepared in which the alkaloid contents were analyzed. The investigators estimated that the child had received between 70 (minimum) and 147 (at a maximum) mg of alkaloid over a 2-week period. A complicating factor in evaluating these figures is that chronic exposure is likely to be more toxic than an acute intake. Some indication of relative toxicity however can be obtained from the LD50 in rats over a 72-hour period, following a single i.p. injection: senecionine 85 mg/kg, seneciphylline 77 mg/kg and retrorsine 35 mg/kg. The minimum estimated ingested dose of 70 mg of a retrorsine-rich mixture is therefore clearly in the toxic range (especially if one considers the age of the child). The child developed cirrhosis but survived.

A second case involved a 2-month-old Mexican-American boy with a diagnosis of Reye's syndrome on hospital admission, who died after 5 days. Two weeks prior to admission he had been given Gardolobo. This had been sold in popcorn packets as a sore throat remedy by a pharmacy. The authors obtained the material, which was consequently identified as Senecio longilobus; they demonstrated the presence of pyrrolizidine alkaloids in a slightly higher concentration than in the first case (0.5% free alkaloids). They estimated the likely ingested amount to be about 66 mg, albeit over a shorter period and by a lighter infant.

The estimations of Huxtable et al are in agreement with the approximations of Roitman.

Huxtable et al have also encountered in Arizona a number of cases of suspected pyrrolizidine poisoning, 4 of which they have described briefly. No definite confirmation was possible because no herbal samples were available, nor was it possible to assay for the alkaloids in body fluids or tissue samples. Ingested alkaloids are predominantly excreted within 24 hours, yet symptomatology may not appear for days, weeks, or even months. They point out that diagnosis of pyrrolizidine poisoning rests largely on (1) liver symptoms indicative of this type of poisoning (especially veno-occlusive disease), (2) analysis for the presence of PA in samples of herbs or foods taken by the patient, and (3) pathognomonic changes in liver architecture (histology of biopsy or autopsy material).

Regarding long-term effects of PA consumption it is of interest to observe, as these authors do, that mortality rates from cirrhosis in Arizona are consistently higher than the national average (ranging from 3 to 41% over the years). It is postulated that exposure to PA is at least a contributory factor to this.

HERBAL REMEDIES

Acute renal failure *(SEDA-7, 468)*

Miura et al (18^C) have reported in great detail on a case of acute *interstitial nephritis* in a 30-year-old patient after taking a herb medicine during the course of a nephrotic syndrome, for which he also received a daily maintenance dose of 15 mg prednisolone orally. The case was confirmed histologically. The constituents of the herbal preparation ingested by the patient were: *Fungus Hoelen* (pachyman, pachymic acid, ergosterol, eburicoic acid, tumulosic acid), *Fungus umbellatus* (α-hydroxytetracosanoic acid), *Alismae rhizoma* (alisol A and B, β-sitosterol, choline), *Atractyloides rhizoma* (atractylone, β-eudesmol, hinesol) and *Cinnamoni cortex* (cinnamic aldehyde, cinnamic alcohol acetate). The components between parentheses are, according to the authors, possibly causative agents for the nephritis. However, one must take into consideration the fact that the onset of the acute interstitial nephritis coincided with the relapse of a preexistent nephrotic syndrome.

Liquorice *(SED-9, 619; SEDA-6, 420)*

The regular consumption of large amounts (more than ca 20 g/day) of liquorice is likely to cause iatrogenic disease. This is due to one of the 'active' ingredients, glycyrrhizinic acid. The exact concentration depends on the extraction process. The intake of about 0.5 g daily for a month of this ingredient may cause pseudo(hyper) *aldosteronism*, with the expansion of the extracellular fluid volume, *hypertension, hypokalemia* and a depressed renin-angiotensin-aldosterone system. Another effect is a rise in the concentration of progesterone and other steroids in the blood (competition for liver metabolism). This may result in amenorrhea, hyperprolactinemia and subsequent infertility in females.

Cereda et al have reported the case of a patient who was admitted to hospital because of progressive fatigue and uncontrolled hypertension (200/110 mm Hg) (19). Urinary aldosterone was below 1 μg per 24 hr and peripheral renin activity undetectable. Worthy of note was also a decreased serum potassium of 1.6 mEq/l. The authors related these findings with a daily consumption of at least 0.3 g glycyrrhizinic acid in a French alcohol-free pastis (Blancard) which he took to curb his drinking habits. One month after discharge his serum potassium was 4.1 mEq/l and, on 50 mg atenolol daily, the blood pressure was 140/80 mm Hg.

Extract of *Glycyrrhiza glabra* is widely used as flavoring in foods and candy, and medically as a supposed mild expectorant and as a vehicle for masking the unpleasant taste of some pharmaceutical compounds. In Japan and other oriental countries nearly 70% of Chinese medicines on sale contain liquorice, and these are used commonly without any restrictions. Kamei and Arakawa (20^C) have described in great detail the case of a 50-year-old man who had been using *Jintan* granules (a mouth refresher) in large doses, corresponding to 150–220 mg glycyrrhizinic acid per day, for more than 10 years. Hypertension (220/120 mm Hg) and hypokalemia (2.5 mEq/l) were correctable by spironolactone. Following cessation of Jintan ingestion, the blood pressure and the serum potassium level were normalized within 40 days (120/80 mm Hg and 4.3 mEq/l). In Japan glycyrrhizinic acid and its derivatives are widely used for their supposed efficacy in various diseases such as allergic dermatitis and chronic hepatitis (!). For this reason, the incidence of pseudoaldosteronism has tended to increase in recent years.

Another case of severe hypokalemia followed by coma after the inadvertent ingestion of 1 kg of liquorice was reported by Hupperets et al (21^C).

A 25-year-old woman was treated for relapsed acute myelogenous leukemia. After a 7-day period of diarrhea, a slight improvement in the clinical condition was noted. A day after the ingestion of 1 kg liquorice she became unconscious. Neurological examination revealed decerebrate rigidity followed by flaccid paresis, symmetrical absence of tendon reflexes, and indifferent plantar responses without signs of intracranial hypertension. Severe hypokalemia (1.2 mEq/l) was found. Several predisposing factors, including starvation and diarrhea, may have contributed to the development of the severe hypokalemia; diarrhea is a common complication of chemotherapy for malignant disease. In this case, the authors suggest that the mineralocorticoid action of glycyrrhizinic acid on the renal tubular sodium-potassium exchange site may have contributed considerably to the seriousness of the complications. Intravenous suppletion of potassium chloride (170 mmol/ 24 hr) led to an uneventful recovery. As little as 8 hours after the start of the infusion the patient regained consciousness.

NON-HERBAL PREPARATIONS

Lead poisoning and traditional practices

In SEDA-6 (p. 420) we reviewed a wide range of traditional medicines and cosmetics containing heavy metals. Lead-containing products are encountered particularly on the Indian subcontinent and within the Asian community in the United Kingdom. Fernando et al (22[C]) have presented data obtained in Kuwait indicating the extensive use of lead, in many cases the major component of the traditional medical preparation and eye cosmetic known as *Al Kohl.* Al Kohl is not only used by women, but it is also applied by mothers to their children's eyes and as a pack on the raw umbilical stump in an erroneous belief in its beneficial adstringent action. In addition to Al Kohl another traditional practice, known as *Bokkoor,* is described in this paper. In this practice, the patient is exposed to fumes from heated lead or lead sulfide. 4 cases of children with clinical manifestations associated with lead poisoning are presented. In the light of these case histories it is suggested that infants under the age of 6 months are especially sensitive to lead, with a rapid onset of symptoms after exposure. Together with the practices mentioned, another possible source of lead is breast milk of mothers who are regular users of an injurious type of Al Kohl. The observations of these authors suggest that a high maternal lead level may be associated with preterm labor. The abortifacient nature of lead is well known. In addition the lasting mental impairment that may result from lead intoxication represents a very real risk. Of 13 samples of Al Kohl which were analyzed, 8 contained more than 80% lead. Only 3 products contained no lead at all or less than 5%. It is concluded by the authors that the use of such preparations poses a grave hazard to the health of a major section of the population, especially in the Moslem world.

Acute bicarbonate intoxication from a folk remedy

Brown et al (23) have described the case of a 4-month-old cyanotic girl, who was in moderate respiratory distress (apnea) on admission to hospital. No satisfactory explanation could at first be found to account for the symptoms. On closer questioning the grandmother of the baby admitted that she had given the child a home remedy for the symptoms of a cold. She had added approximately one tablespoon of baking soda to an 8-oz (ca. 250 g) feed. This dose of bicarbonate is approximately equivalent to a dose of 30 mEq/kg and resulted in *hypernatremia*, an acute metabolic *alkalosis*, and *apnea*. The clinical impression of acute volume depletion was most likely due to acute intraintestinal sequestration of fluids and osmotic diuresis. Both symptoms were easily corrected by saline infusion and volume expansion. According to the authors, combinations of baking soda with turpentine, castor oil, lemon and sugar are still popular in folk remedies in Arkansas, USA.

Precocious sexual development

There has been correspondence over the striking increase in the incidence of precocious sexual development in children from the early age of 6 months up to 8 years in Puerto Rico over the period 1978–1981. Schoental (24) suggests that several environmental estrogenic agents may have contributed to this phenomenon. Environmental estrogenic agents can include, besides the residues from anabolic agents in meat, milk, eggs and their products, 'naturally' occurring phyto-estrogens such as coumestrol (present, for instance, in alfalfa and soya beans) and zearalenone and its derivatives, the secondary metabolites of Fusarium spp., the common soil microfungi sporadically present in maize (corn) and in livestock fodder. The weather is of great influence on the growth of moulds and their production of zearalenone. The evidence is insofar only hypothetical.

Makwa and tetanus

Tetanus is still a serious problem in many developing countries. Yagil and Heyman (25) of the Hadassah University Hospital in Jerusalem point to a possibly underestimated cause of tetanus in the Middle East. They describe the admission to hospital of 4 adult Arab villagers with tetanus. Because they had earlier been suffering from low back pain, the village 'folk-doctors' had treated them with *Makwa*; this is a widely used therapeutic practice in the Middle East and elsewhere. Makwa involves the cauterization of the skin at nonsterilized predesignated sites with a red-hot iron, and the dressing of the resulting third-degree burn with mud and herbs. The mud dressing creates an ideal situation for infection with anaerobic organisms such as *Clostridium tetani.* Indeed, the necrotic wounds at the sites of Makwa proved to be the foci of the tetanus infection. It would seem advisable to discourage the practice of Makwa.

Skin disorders and folk medicine

Factitial dermatitis in children should alert the physician to the possibility of child abuse. A discrepancy between history and physical findings are common features of such an entity with skin abnormalities. Sometimes, however, other reasons, related to traditional medical practices, play a role.

An 11-year-old Vietnamese boy was brought to hospital for treatment of cough, sore throat and fever. On examination, non-blanching, erythematous patches were found along the intercostal spaces of the thorax and along the paraspinal muscles of the back (26). These symptoms were thought to be unrelated to the prime reason for taking the boy to hospital. However, the father told that when his son became ill, he had attempted to cure him with *Cao Gio* ('scratch the wind'), a Vietnamese folk medicine practice of treating illnesses by massaging the skin with a medicated substance such as mentholated ointment or oil. The skin is then rubbed with an object like a coin, comb or spoon until purpura occurs. This procedure rids the body of 'bad winds' which are the cause of the patient's symptoms. This practice is in itself not harmful, and the lesions usually resolve spontaneously without sequelae in about 7 to 10 days.

Another reason for confusion in diagnosis can be the practice of cupping (27). *Dry cupping* is a technique of bruising the skin painlessly. It is performed by placing a glass over the skin and creating a partial vacuum in the glass, e.g. by exhausting the available oxygen with some spirit burning in the glass. Occasionally, the skin is scarified before cupping (*wet cupping*), and the resulting blood loss can be impressive.

The technique of cupping antedates Hippocrates' symptomatic view of asthma as an illness characterized by panting, but the practice still persists. In Russia, cupping is today performed in a cultural rather than a medical context. Dearlove et al have described 2 cases of Russian girls (6 and 14 years old) suffering from asthma and presenting with a bruised skin (27). One of the mothers thought that cupping 'drew the congestion out of her chest and made the blood flow faster'. As stated already, the appearance of bruises or other skin abnormalities can lead to the suspicion of child abuse.

REFERENCES

1. Xu B (1981) Pharmacology of some natural products of China. *Trends Pharmacol. Sci., 2*, 271.
2. Baerheim Svendsen A, Scheffer JJC (1982) Natural products in therapy, prospects, goals and means in modern research. *Pharm. Weekbl. (Sci. Edit.), 4*, 93.
3. Holmstedt B, Bruhn JG (1982) Is there a place for ethnopharmacology in our time? *Trends Pharmacol. Sci., 3*, 181.
4. Humphreys J (1982) Plants that bring health – or death. *New Scientist, 93*, 513.
5. Röder E (1982) Nebenwirkungen von Heilpflanzen. *Dtsch. Apothek.-Ztg., 122*, 2081.

6. Reilly DT (1983) Young doctors' views on alternative medicine. *Br. Med. J., 287*, 337.
7. Higham C, Ashcroft C, Jayson MW (1983) Non-prescribed treatments in rheumatic diseases. *Practitioner, 227*, 1201.
8. Lagendijk (1983) *Public Opinion Poll on Alternative Treatments, January 1983, Apeldoorn, The Netherlands.*
9. Savage A (1982) Do-it-yourself medicine. *Br. Med. J., 285*, 560.
10. D'Arcy PF (1983) Traditional medicines can be toxic. *Pharm. Int., 4*, 29.
11. Robins DJ (1982) The pyrrolizidine alkaloids. *Prog. Chem. Org. Nat. Prod., 41*, 115.
12. Schoental R (1982) Health hazards of pyrrolizidine alkaloids: a short review. *Toxicol. Letters, 10*, 323.
13. Arseculeratne SN, Gunatilaka AAL, Panabokke RG (1981) Studies on medicinal plants of Sri Lanka: occurrence of pyrrolizidine alkaloids and hepatotoxic properties in some traditional medicinal herbs. *J. Ethnopharmacol., 4*, 159.
14. Roitman JN (1981) Comfrey and liver damage. *Lancet, 1*, 944.
15. Anon (1982) Bundesgesundheitsamt plant Massnahmen gegen Naturstoffe. *Arzneitelegramm*, 16.
16. Huxtable RJ (1980) Herbal teas and toxins: novel aspects of pyrrolizidine poisoning in the United States. *Perspect. Biol. Med., 24*, 1.
17. Steigl P, Wiedenfeld H, Röder E (1982) Lebertoxische Pyrrolizidinalkaloïde in Symphytum Präparaten. *Dtsch. Apothek. Ztg., 122*, 851.
18. Miura H, Nakayama M, Sato T (1982) A case of acute interstitial nephritis induced by herb medicines. *Jpn. J. Med., 21*, 192.
19. Cereda JM, Trono D, Schifferli J (1983) Liquorice intoxication caused by alcohol-free pastis. *Lancet, 1*, 1442.
20. Kamei H, Arakawa K (1982) A case of pseudoaldosteronism due to addiction of Jintan, a mouth refresher popular among Japanese. *Jpn. Heart J., 23*, 651.
21. Hupperets P, De Pauw BE, Holdrinet RSG et al (1983) Reversible coma due to hypokalaemia in a patient treated for acute leukaemia. *Neth. J. Med., 26*, 21.
22. Fernando NP, Healy MA, Aslam M et al (1981) Lead poisoning and traditional practices: the consequences for world health. A study in Kuwait. *Public Health London, 95*, 250.
23. Brown AL, Whaley S, Arnold WC (1981) Acute bicarbonate intoxication from a folk remedy. *Am. J. Dis. Child., 135*, 965.
24. Schoental R (1983) Precocious sexual development in Puerto Rico and oestrogenic mycotoxins (Zearalenone). *Lancet, 1*, 537.
25. Yagil Y, Heyman S (1982) Makwa (nonsterile skin cauterisation) as a cause of tetanus. *Lancet, 1*, 1027.
26. Silfen E, Wyre CDR HW (1981) Factitial dermatitis – Cao Gio. *Cutis, 28*, 399.
27. Dearlove J, Verguei AP, Birkin N et al (1981) An anachronistic treatment for asthma. *Br. Med. J., 283*, 1684.

Z. Fastner

51 Miscellaneous drugs

SURGICAL MATERIALS

Acrylic bone cement *(SEDA-5, 436; SEDA-6, 426)*

An isolated case was reported in which on two occasions a patient receiving treatment with acrylic bone cement developed transient second-degree atrioventricular block ([1c]). The patient, a 29-year-old woman, had been operated on twice with an interval of 1 month, receiving acetabular prostheses bilaterally. In both operations, 5 min after acrylate application, a 2:1 AV block appeared, but resolved spontaneously after 30 and 10 sec respectively.

No similar observation was ever made previously. Although in this case no further cardiodynamic consequences were seen, due to transient nature of the dysrhythmia, such an incident in the presence of cardiac disease, would probably cause more worry.

Suture material *(SEDA-6, 426)*

New surgical materials, such as polyester yarn, are becoming increasingly popular in surgery due to their tensile strength and good tissue tolerance. However, certain warnings seem to be warranted as several cases have been reported in which these sutures acted as stone matrix material, leading in 2 patients to the formation of biliary stones several years after biliary tract surgery ([2c]). An analogous urethral complication occurred in a patient 4 years after a uretherolithotomy, in which a nonabsorbable polyester suture was used ([3c]).

In view of the widespread use of these materials, such isolated observations do not seem to have any great significance, but they should be borne in mind as new suture materials come into use.

Side Effects of Drugs Annual 8
M.N.G. Dukes, editor

ISBN 0 444 90339 9
$0.80 per article per page (transactional system)
$0.20 per article per page (licensing system)

HEMODIALYSIS ACCIDENTS

Fluoride contamination of water supply

Following fluoride leakage into a public water supply, fluoride levels in the water rose to 30 ppm, persisting for 7 days until the concentration fell to the normal level of 1.6 ppm. Two days after the leakage 8 patients at a local hemodialysis center developed gastrointestinal symptoms. One patient was found dead at home and another developed chest pain with dyspnea after 2.5 hours of dialysis. Dialysis was discontinued, and the symptoms receded. 14 hours later, his dyspnea reappeared at home and during transport to hospital he had cardiopulmonary arrest. Resuscitation was successful, but the blood analysis showed highly elevated potassium, 10.5 mEq/l. With cation exchange and peritoneal dialysis his serum electrolytes were normalized.

The mechanism of hypokalemia is not known, but a high fluoride level may have toxic effects on cellular membranes, allowing the escape of intracellular potassium into the blood ([4C]).

During normal dialysis, about 36 mg of fluoride is absorbed. In the case described here, the fluoride load was almost 20 times this and far in excess of what can be cleared by the kidney.

Faulty procedures

In 4 hemodialysis patients described by Popli et al ([5C]), 5 reactions occurred. In all cases the condition was life-threatening and 1 patient died. All patients were using Cuprophan capillary dialysers and it is notable that all these accidents happened in a self-care dialysis unit.

It seems that Cuprophan capillary dialysers are prone to produce this type of reaction more frequently than are Cuprophan plate or coil dialysers. The exact etiology of these reactions remains unclear, but it seems that improper care and inadequate rinsing of dialysers prior to use are the main source of problems rather than any identifiable individual substance.

INORGANIC COMPOUNDS

Potassium *(SEDA-4, 354; SEDA-5, 439; SEDA-6, 180)*

As potassium deficit remains a worldwide obsession, potassium supplementation continues to be, if not a life-saving medical treatment, at least a flourishing trade (6[R]). When slow-release potassium formulations based on the wax-matrix principle failed to prevent gastrointestinal lesions, microencapsulated formulations of potassium chloride were developed.

A comparison of these two formulations in healthy volunteers with gastroscopy, revealed a significant fall in gastrointestinal lesions, when the microencapsulated preparation was used, but lesions were not absent (7[C], 8[C]). As these studies were performed with a limited number of patients (12 per group) the fact that lesions were encountered at all with the microencapsulated form must be taken seriously. Even if one assumes that the new formulation produces lesions at a rate 6–10 times less than the old, the total number of lesions occurring when the product is widely used will still be very great, even if they are not all clinically manifest.

ORGANIC COMPOUNDS

Dimethylsulfoxide *(SEDA-4, 351; SEDA-5, 440; SEDA-6, 429; SEDA-7, 159)*

A new presentation of dimethylsulfoxide (RIMSO 100) has introduced a new problem since, when it is diluted with water, a strong exothermic reaction results. This can lead to thermal injury on intracystic instillation unless one waits until the mixture cools off (9[c]).

Diphosphonates *(SEDA-5, 440)*

In patients with Paget's disease treated with dichloromethane diphosphonate (Cl_2-MDP), serum parathyroid hormone levels were found to be increased during treatment; they returned to normal within 6 months of treatment withdrawal. As an increase of PTH does not automatically indicate parathyroid hyperfunction, a study was undertaken to establish whether in treated patients secondary hyperparathyroidism also appears. Six Pagetic patients were treated with Cl_2MDP during 3 months. Alkaline phosphatase and hydroxyproline decreased. The PTH secretory reserve was assessed by EDTA infusion; after 3 months of treatment, an EDTA infusion raised immunoreactive PTH to a higher level than before the treatment. It was concluded that the PTH secretory reserve is increased during Cl_2MDP treatment. The hyperparathyroidism is partly reversible. The cause of these changes is not clear. Whether these findings may be of clinical significance is not known, but they certainly contribute to our knowledge of bone turnover (10[C]).

More important is another clinical observation in diphosphonate-treated patients with hypercalcemia due to malignancy. Bounameaux et al (11[C]) described 3 such patients, suffering from malignancies associated with hypercalcemia in whom following treatment with intravenous diphosphonates, renal failure occurred, with a fatal outcome in 2 cases. The 3rd patient died 2 months later of gastrointestinal bleeding. As the clinical conditions here involved (2 patients with metastatic breast carcinoma, and 1 patient with myeloma) can themselves produce kidney failure, diphosphonates must be considered merely as triggering the lethal chain of events.

Disulfiram *(SEDA-4, 351; SEDA-5, 440; SEDA-6, 430)*

Interaction disulfiram-marijuana A curious recent case suggests that disulfiram and marijuana can interact, producing a hypomaniac reaction (12[c]).

A 28-year-old patient was admitted to be treated for his addiction (alcohol, amphetamines, cocaine and marijuana). He was treated with 250 mg of disulfiram but after the second dose became hyperactive and euphoric. Disulfiram was reduced to 125 mg, but the symptoms persisted and disulfiram was stopped. It was established that he had smoked several marijuana cigarettes during his disulfiram days, but he denied previously having experienced this feeling during marijuana use. 48 hours after disulfiram withdrawal, his behaviour normalized despite continued use of marijuana.

9 months later he was readmitted because of his alcohol abuse, and was given 250 mg disulfiram daily, initially with no ill effects. After a period of uneventful treatment he again became irritable and uncooperative; he admitted to smoking one marijuana cigarette; his behavior normalized within a day.

Neuropathy It has been suggested earlier that reduction of Antabuse dosage may reduce the incidence of side effects. In a recent report, a patient was described who developed *peripheral neuropathy* after 1 year of treatment with 250 mg Antabuse a day. The dosage was then reduced to 125 mg daily, accompanied by intensive vitamin treatment and the symptoms of neuropathy subsided within 1 month. It is difficult to know whether the improvement was due to the reduction of dosage or to the vitamin treatment (13[c]).

Arthritis Two patients have been described who displayed arthritic pain in various joints after 6–8 weeks of disulfiram use. Tests for rheumatism were negative, and even ESR was within normal limits in one patient and only slightly elevated in the other. Once disulfiram was stopped, the symptoms abated. Several months later, the patients were rechallenged with disulfiram and the symptoms reappeared within a week or two. One of these patients displayed also the symptoms of carpal tunnel syndrome (14[C]).

Isaxozine *(SEDA-7, 477)*

Isaxozine used to treat neuropathies, has produced *acute hepatitis* in 4 patients, presented in two different reports. No clinical details are available for 3 of these patients, except that icterus appeared 16, 30 and 83 days respectively after the start of treatment. In 2 cases treatment was continued with resulting hepatic insufficiency and fatal outcome. One patient recovered. In one case reported in detail, jaundice appeared after 2 months of treatment with 750 mg isaxozine daily. All hepatic functions had grossly deteriorated and hepatic biopsy revealed hepatocellular necrosis. Isaxozin was withdrawn immediately after the onset of icterus, and within 6 weeks the clinical and laboratory picture had cleared (15[c]).

It therefore seems that during isaxozine treatment regular laboratory tests for liver functions are mandatory, and that treatment should be withdrawn immediately if liver functions show abnormalities.

Ketanserin *(SEDA-7, 477)*

Ketanserin is a 5-hydroxytryptamine receptor blocker which has vasodilator properties. It has variously been proposed for use in the treatment of hypertension and Raynaud's disease. Experience is still limited but to date the drug appears to be well tolerated. In a group of 9 patients, treated with 10 mg i.v. daily, only transient *sedation* and *dizziness* was observed in 4 patients (16[c]).

Tiopronin (α-mercaptopropionylglycine) *(SEDA-5, 440)*

Three cases of *liver injury* were described in adult patients treated orally with tiopronin. Biochemical disturbances persisted up to nine months after the onset of jaundice (17[c]).

SWEETENERS

Aspartam

Aspartam has been widely regarded as a break-through in the field of sweeteners. It is a dipeptide, consisting of the amino acids aspartic acid and phenylalanine, which disintegrates in the gastrointestinal tract. Aspartam is some 200 times sweeter than sugar. Due to its composition it is not calorie-free, but in the small amounts used, the calorific effect will be negligible.

The compound was extensively tested for safety and no ill effects have been found to date, even in patients with phenylketonuria (18).

However in August 1983 the UK Department of Health did point out in a public statement that consumption of the sweetener either in soft drinks or in the form of sweetening tablets could in principle result in an undesirable intake of phenylalanine by phenylketonuric patients, and in such individuals some caution would seem indicated (21[r]). However, another public statement by Britain's Chief Medical Officer a month later indicated that there was 'no suggestion' that aspartam might harm mere carriers of phenylketonuria or be harmful to the unborn infant of a mother who was a phenylketonuria carrier if taken in pregnancy (22[R]).

Palatinit

The sugar substitute palatinit appears to be well tolerated provided the total daily dose does not exceed 50 g divided over several portions. When this quantity is taken in one dose, diarrhea resulted in 11 of 24 patients tested (19[C]).

MISCELLANEOUS PRODUCTS

Vicks Vaporub

Lipoid pneumonia is well known as a complication in patients using mineral oil laxatives, or inhaling oil dispersed in air.

A case was recently described in which lipoid pneumonia appeared as the consequence of 5 years use of Vicks Vaporub (an ointment containing various aromatic oils) in and around the nostrils. Histologic study revealed fibrosis and infiltration with lipoid laden macrophages, lymphocytes and neutrophils. When the offending agent was withdrawn, total clinical clearance ensued, with no other medication than diuretics, within 8 weeks (20[C]).

Benign as it seems to be, this complication cannot be disregarded, as many people use over-the-counter preparations of similar composition, and only the fever betrayed the fact that the lung was affected. It can reasonably be postulated that the number of lipoid lung infiltrations is much greater than reported, in view of the many 'sniffers' of oil and fat-based common cold preparations. As superimposed infection can add to the hazard, unlimited and prolonged use of these preparations must be warned against. There is no reason to think that they will be harmful with occasional use.

EXCIPIENTS

Polyvinylpyrrolidone (PVP)

In July 1983, the West German Federal Health authorities issued an edict forbidding the sale of medicaments for injection containing PVP as excipient. In fact, the excipient appears to have been replaced before that time as a result of an earlier decree, at least insofar as registered drugs were concerned. As is well known from earlier literature, PVP can cumulate in the body and give rise to foreign body granulomata (23[R]).

Listing of inactive ingredients

A common problem for the student of adverse reactions and interactions is to distinguish between those effects due to an active component and those elicited by an excipient. In many countries, these excipients are still, regrettably, not specified on the label of a medicament. Pointing to this problem, Brown (24[R]) has published a list, issued by the US FDA in 1982, of several hundred inactive ingredients approved for use in prescription drug products in the United States. The list at least illustrated the extent of the potential problems, since it is clear that the published literature at least does not provide adequate evidence of the safety of many of these agents, though such evidence may be available to manufacturers or regulatory authorities.

REFERENCES

1. Brown DL, Parmley CL (1982) Second-degree atrioventricular block after methyl methacrylate. *Anesthesiol., 56,* 391.
2. Dell'Orto V, Genoni E, Biccazzi G, Bonzi F (1982) Una causa ancora poco valutata di litiasi coledocica: i calcoli su materiale di sutura non riassorbibile. *Minerva Chir., 37,* 1243.
3. Androulakakis P, Deliveliotis A (1982) Ureteric stone formed upon polyester suture: case report. *Int. Surg., 61,* 83.
4. McIvor M, Baltazar RF, Beltran J et al (1983) Hyperkalemia and cardiac arrest from fluoride exposure during hemodialysis. *Am. J. Cardiol., 51,* 901.
5. Popli S, Todd S, Daugirdas JT et al (1982) Severe reactions to Cuprophan capillary dialysers. *Artif. Organs, 6,* 312.
6. Harrington JT, Isner JM, Kassirer JP (1982) Our national obsession with potassium. *J. Am. Med. Assoc., 73,* 155.
7. McMahon FG, Ryan JR, Akdamar K, Ertan A (1982) Upper gastrointestinal lesions after potassium chloride supplements: a controlled clinical trial. *Lancet, 2,* 1059.
8. Barkin JB, Harary AM, Shamblen CE, Lasseter KC (1983) Potassium chloride and gastrointestinal injury. *Ann. Intern. Med., 98,* 261.
9. Albert NE (1982) Exothermal reaction with

RIMSO 100. *Urology, 20,* 662.

10. Harris ST, Neer RM, Segre GV et al (1982) Secondary hyperparathyroidism associated with dichlormethane diphosphonate treatment of Paget's disease. *J. Clin. Endocrinol. Metab., 55,* 1100.
11. Bounameaux HM, Schifferli J, Montani J-P et al (1983) Renal failure associated with intravenous diphosphonates. *Lancet, 1,* 471.
12. Lacoursiere RB, Swatek R (1983) Adverse interaction between disulfiram and marijuana: a case report. *Am. J. Psychiat., 140,* 243.
13. Worner TM (1982) Peripheral neuropathy after disulfiram administration: reversibility despite continued therapy. *Drug Alcohol Dependence, 10,* 199.
14. Howard JF (1982) Arthritis and carpal tunnel syndrome associated with disulfiram (Antabuse) therapy. *Arthr. Rheum., 25,* 1494.
15. Papazian A, Galian A, Capron J-P et al (1983) Hépatite cytolitique aiguë réversible due à l'isaxozine. *Presse Méd., 12,* 770.
16. Strande E, Roald OK, Krohg K (1982) Treatment of Raynaud's phenomenon with the 5-HT_2-receptor antagonist ketanserin. *Br. Med. J., 285,* 1069.
17. Kusakabe A, Yoshioka K, Okayama M et al (1982) Three cases of Tiopronin-induced liver injury. *Acta Hepatol. Jap., 23,* 432.
18. Manufacturers' data.
19. Petzoldt R, Lauer P, Spengler M, Schöffling K (1982) Palatinit bei Typ-II-Diabetikern. *Dtsch. Med. Wochenschr., 107,* 1910.
20. Subramanian S, Kherdekar SS, Babu PGV, Christianson CS (1982) Lipoid pneumonia with Criptococcus neoformans colonisation. *Thorax, 37,* 319.
21. Anon (1983) Aspartame and phenylketonuria. *Lancet, 2,* 411.
22. Yellowlees H (1983) Aspartame. *Br. Med. J., 287.*
23. Bundesgesundheitsamt (1983) Änderung PVP-haltiger Arzneimittel. *BGA Pressedienst, 8.*
24. Brown JL (1983) Incomplete labeling of pharmaceuticals: A list of 'inactive' ingredients (Letter to the editor). *N. Engl. J. Med., 309,* 439.

National centers for adverse reaction monitoring

Introductory note: International drug monitoring

For nearly a decade the World Health Organization has fostered international collaboration in monitoring suspected adverse drug reactions. The system is based upon the interchange of information between national drug monitoring centers in 22 countries. Collectively these centers provide each month some 2000 reports of individual reactions suspected of being drug-induced and which, for the most part, have been notified spontaneously by practising physicians. The cumulative data base that has been constructed from these reports now comprises over 130,000 records of individual reactions suspected of being drug-induced.

In addition to collating and commenting on the reports received, the international coordinating center administered by WHO has contributed to the development of a uniform recording system among the participating countries. In particular, it has assumed responsibility for developing a standardized adverse reaction terminology and comprehensive index of marketed drugs, both of which have a utility beyond their importance to the monitoring system.

The national centers contributing to the scheme, and which are listed below, vary in size and complexity. In addition to their basic function of collecting, analyzing, evaluating and commenting upon the individual reports submitted to them, some of the larger centers have sponsored or developed other related activities, including intensive monitoring within selected hospital centers, systematized collection of data on the use and effects of drugs in a defined population, and of drugs newly released for routine use.

Australia
Telephone: 89 85 38
Telegrams: HEALTH, CANBERRA
Telex No: AA 62149

The Secretary
Australian Drug Evaluation Committee
P.O. Box 100
WODEN, A.C.T. 2606
Australia

Belgium
Telephone: (02) 564.10.47

Monsieur l'Inspecteur général
Inspection de la Pharmacie
Ministère de la Santé publique et de la Famille
Cité administrative de l'Etat
Quartier Vésale
20, rue Montagne de l'Oratoire
1010 BRUSSELS
Belgium

Bulgaria
Telephone: 44 65 66
Telex No.: 22430

Institute for State Control of Drugs
Bul. 'Vl. Zaimov' 26
1040 SOFIA
Bulgaria

Canada
Telephone: 613-9929160
Telex No.: 0533679
with mention:
for Chief, Poison Control and Adverse Reaction Programs Division

Chief, Poison Control and Adverse Reaction Reporting Programs Division
Bureau of Epidemiology, Laboratory Centre for Disease Control
Health Protection Branch
Department of National Health and Welfare
Tunney's Pasture
OTTAWA, Ontario K1A 1B8
Canada

Czechoslovakia
Telephone: 72 27 51
73 39 51
Telex No.: 1HE C I 2362
with mention:
for Committee on Adverse Drug Reactions

The Secretary
Committee on Adverse Drug Reactions
State Institute for Drug Control
Srobarova 48
100 41 PRAGUE 10
Czechoslovakia

Denmark
Telephone: (01) 94 37 73
Telex No.: 34333 ipharm dk
with mention:
for SFL

Danish National Health Service
Board on Adverse Reactions to Drugs
Frederikssundsvej 378
DK-2700 BRØNSHØJ
Denmark

Finland
Telephone: 71 85 11
Telex No.: 12 17 74

Chief Medical Officer Pharmacology
The National Board of Health
Siltasaarenkatu 18A
SF-00530 HELSINKI 53
Finland

France
Telephone: (01) 5675544

Monsieur le Chef du Service central de la Pharmacie et du Médicament
Ministère de la Santé et de la Sécurité Sociale
1 Place Fontenoy
F-75007 PARIS
France

Federal Republic of Germany
Telephone: (0221) 4004-1
Telex No.: 8882161/8882308/8882428

Arzneimittelkommission der Deutschen Ärzteschaft
Hädenkampstrasse 5
5000 COLOGNE 41
Federal Republic of Germany

Indonesia

Vice-Chairman
National Centre for Monitoring of Adverse Reactions to Drugs
c/o Directorate General of Food and Drug Control
Ministry of Health
J. Percetakan Negara 23
JAKARTA
Indonesia

Ireland
Telephone: 68 10 98 or 68 14 11 or 78 28 86
Telex No.: 4894
with mention:
for the Medical Director, National Drugs Advisory Board

The Medical Director
National Drugs Advisory Board
57C Harcourt Street
DUBLIN 2
Ireland

Israel Telephone: 428632	Department of Clinical Pharmacology Ministry of Health 38, Keren Hayessor str. JERUSALEM Israel
Italy Telephone: 071-42 28 9	Istituto di Medicina Sperimentale University of Ancona Via Grotte di Posatora 1-60100 ANCONA Italy
Japan Telephone: 03-503-2066 Telex No.: 2225132 QUA JPN with mention: for ANZENKA	Head, Pharmaceuticals and Chemicals Safety Division Pharmaceutical Affairs Bureau Ministry of Health and Welfare 2-2, 1-Chome, Kasumigaseki Chiyoda-ku TOKYO 100 Japan
The Netherlands Telephone: 070-27 99 86/20 96 20 Telex No.: 32362 vm nl	Head, Bureau of Adverse Drug Reactions Ministry of Public Health and Environmental Hygiene Koopmanstraat 1 2288 BC RIJSWIJK The Netherlands
New Zealand Telephone: 40-069 Telex No.: NZ 5706	The Medical Assessor Committee on Adverse Drug Reactions P.O. Box 913 DUNEDIN New Zealand
Norway Telephone: (02) 257550	Secretary Norwegian Adverse Drug Reaction Committee Statens Legemiddelkontroll Sven Oftedals Vei 6 OSLO 9 Norway
Poland Telephone: 410652	Head, Department of Organization of Drugs Investigations Chelmska 30/34 00-725 WARSAW Poland
Romania Telephone: 17 22 70 Telex No.: 11595 O.C.F.R. with mention: pour le Directeur, Institut de l'Etat/Contrôle du Médicament	Monsieur le Directeur Institut de l'Etat pour le Contrôle du Médicament et Recherches Pharmaceutiques 48, rue Av. Sănătescu BUCAREST, Sectorul I. Romania
Sweden Telephone: (018) 100360	The Medical Officer in Charge Adverse Drug Reaction Section Pharmacotherapeutic Division Department of Drugs National Board of Health and Welfare Box 607 S-75125 UPPSALA Sweden

United Kingdom of Great Britain and Northern Ireland
Telephone: 01 7202188

Principal Medical Officer
Committee on Safety of Medicines
Market Towers
1 Nine-Elms Lane
LONDON SW8 5NQ
United Kingdom of Great Britain and Northern Ireland

United States of America
Telephone: 301-443-4580
Telex No.: 898488

Special Assistant to the Associate Director for Biometrics, Epidemiology (HFD-200)
Bureau of Drugs
Food and Drug Administration
ROCKVILLE, MD 20852
U.S.A.

Yugoslavia
Telephone: 519-933

Centar za Lijekove
Zajednica zdravstvenih organizacija SR Hrvatske
Savska cesta 41/VII
41000 ZAGREB
Yugoslavia

Index of drugs

Page numbers in **bold** type indicate where a given drug is discussed in detail.

Index of side effects